AF477341

CARDIOVASCULAR PATHOLOGY DECENNIAL

1966–1975

SERIES EDITOR

SHELDON C. SOMMERS, M.D.

Director of Laboratories, Lenox Hill Hospital, New York, New York;
Clinical Professor of Pathology, Columbia University College of
Physicians and Surgeons, New York, New York; Clinical Professor
of Pathology, University of Southern California School of Medicine,
Los Angeles, California

CARDIOVASCULAR PATHOLOGY

DECENNIAL

1966–1975

APPLETON-CENTURY-CROFTS/New York
A Publishing Division of Prentice-Hall, Inc.

CONTRIBUTORS

Ralph Alley, M.D.

Professor of Surgery, Albany Medical Center Hospital, Albany, New York

Alfred Angrist, M.D.

Chairman Emeritus and Professor of Pathology, Albert Einstein College of Medicine of Yeshiva University, Bronx, New York

Saroja Bharati, M.D.

Pathologist and Research Associate, Congenital Heart Disease Research and Training Center, Hektoen Institute, Chicago, Illinois

Joseph Davis, M.D.

Professor of Pathology, University of Miami School of Medicine, Miami, Florida

Garabed A. Fattal, M.D.

Director of Laboratories, Binghamton General Hospital, Binghamton, New York

Gerald Fine, M.D.

Associate Pathologist, Henry Ford Hospital, Detroit, Michigan

Maurice Lev, M.D.

Director, Congenital Heart Disease and Training Center, Hektoen Institute, Chicago, Illinois

Samuel Levy, M.D.

Fellow in Cardiology, University of Miami School of Medicine, Miami, Florida

Jacqueline A. Mauro, M.D., F.A.C.P.

Department of Pathology, Albany Medical Center Hospital, Albany, New York

Vincent J. McGovern, M.D.

Director, Fairfax Institute of Pathology, Royal Prince Alfred Hospital, Sydney, N.S.W., Australia

Azorides R. Morales, M.D.

Professor and Chairman, Department of Pathology, University of Miami School of Medicine, Miami, Florida

John J. Moran, M.D.

Chairman, Division of Laboratory Medicine, Geisinger Medical Center, Danville, Pennsylvania

Komei Nakao, M.D.

Assistant Professor of Pathology, Albert Einstein College of Medicine of Yeshiva University, New York, New York

Masamichi Oka, M.D.

Assistant Professor of Pathology, Cornell University Medical College, North Shore University Hospital, Manhasset, New York

Cassius M. Plair, M.D.

Chief, Department of Anatomical Pathology, New York Veterans' Administration Hospital, New York, New York

Leopold Reiner, M.D.

Director, Department of Pathology, The Bronx–Lebanon Hospital Center, New York, New York

Shirley Siew, M.D.

Associate Professor of Pathology, The University of Pittsburgh School of Medicine, Pittsburgh, Pennsylvania

Arthur A. Stein, M.D.

Professor of Pathology, Albany Medical College and Albany Medical Center Hospital, Albany, New York

Lloyd Thibodeau

Electron Microscopy Senior Technician, New York State Department of Health, Albany, New York

Dragoslava Vesselinovitch, M.D.

Research Associate (Associate Professor), Department of Pathology, The Pritzker School of Medicine of the University of Chicago, Chicago, Illinois

Bernard M. Wagner, M.D.

Clinical Professor of Pathology, Columbia College of Physicians and Surgeons, New York, New York

Sigmund L. Wilens, M.D. (deceased)

Chief, Laboratory Service, Veterans' Administration Hospital, New York, New York

Robert W. Wissler, M.D.

Professor of Pathology, The University of Chicago School of Medicine, Chicago, Illinois

John P. Wyatt, M.D.

Director, Tobacco and Health Research Institute, The University of Kentucky School of Medicine, Lexington, Kentucky

PREFACE

This year's *Pathology Annual 1975* is the tenth volume of the series begun in 1966. *Pathology Annuals* now have an established readership among practitioners of pathology. Since several volumes are out of print and the original plates have been preserved by the publisher, it was decided to collect the articles by organ systems and to republish them in seven decennial volumes. Not every article in the ten *Pathology Annuals* is included.

All authors were invited to prepare addenda updating their contributions to late 1974. About two-thirds were able to do so. One completely new essay was provided by Drs. Dixon and Cochrane for the *Kidney Pathology Decennial 1966–1975,* and Drs. Pierce and Abell rewrote their paper in the *Genital and Mammary Pathology Decennial 1966–1975.* The *Endocrine Pathology Decennial 1966–1975* differs from the others in that articles were included from the *Pathobiology Annuals* edited by Dr. Harry L. Ioachim and from other sources to provide a more complete coverage.

It is hoped that the *Pathology Decennial* volumes may appeal to clinical specialists as well as to pathologists. Better communication between clinician and pathologist in part involves a mutual familiarity with the special literature that each may read.

I would like to express my appreciation to the personnel at Appleton-Century-Crofts: David Stires, Doreen Berne, Berta Steiner Rosenberg, Laura Bird, and Joann Lindner, who have assisted me in the preparation and production of these volumes.

The seven volumes are as follows: *Kidney Pathology Decennial 1966–1975; Pulmonary Pathology Decennial 1966–1975; Gastrointestinal and Hepatic Pathology Decennial 1966–1975; Genital and Mammary Pathology Decennial 1966–1975; Hematologic and Lymphoid Pathology Decennial 1966–1975; Cardiovascular Pathology Decennial 1966–1975;* and *Endocrine Pathology Decennial 1966–1975.*

Sheldon C. Sommers

CONTENTS

CARDIOVASCULAR PATHOLOGY DECENNIAL
1966–1975

TRANSPOSITION OF THE ARTERIAL TRUNKS IN LEVOCARDIA *

MAURICE LEV AND
SAROJA BHARATI

The term transposition of the arterial trunks has included many concepts. The older literature concerning these concepts was reviewed by Lev and Saphir,[1] and Harris and Farber.[2] More recent contributions to the overall concept of transposition have been made by Lev and Saphir,[3] Taussig,[4] Shaner,[5] Doerr,[6] Goerttler,[7] Cardell,[8] De la Crux et al,[9] Witham,[10] Edwards,[11] Neufeld et al,[12] Grant,[13] De Vries and Saunders,[14] Van Mierop and Wiglesworth,[15] Shaher,[16] Rosenbaum,[17] and Van Praagh et al.[18] Most of these concepts, old and new, were based on an assumed pathogenesis.

In the last 30 years, a concept based on pure anatomy [19] has gradually evolved. This concept borrows liberally from Abbott,[20] Rokitansky,[21] and Spitzer.[22] The purpose of this concept is to simplify the task of the pathologist in diagnosing the myriad of complexes facing him at the autopsy table in which transposition may be said to be present. The present work is an attempt to present this concept as it pertains to a certain grouping of hearts which are said to be in *levocardia*.

Semantics

Transposition of the arterial trunks, as defined here, is an anomaly in which the arterial trunks or their remnants are abnormally placed with respect to each other and/or with respect to the chambers from which they emerge. In most hearts with transposition, the two points converge. However, in some complex anomalies an exact statement as to the emergence from chambers may not be possible, while

* This investigation was supported by Grant HE–07605–04 from the National Heart Institute, National Institutes of Health, Betheseda, Maryland.

the position of the vessels with respect to each other pertains. In other cases, the situation is vice versa.

It is self-evident that statements as to position of vessels are made with respect to the normal position of such vessels. Since the normal position of such vessels differs according to the position of the base-apex axis of the heart, transposition of the arterial trunks is best discussed separately in various positions of the base-apex axis. We say a heart is in levocardia when its position corresponds to the normal position of the heart, or the base-apex axis points to the left and downward. This position has also been called situs solitus. The term situs solitus is confusing, since it does not state whether the reference is to the entire heart or to the atria or ventricles. The term mesocardia is used when the base-apex axis points anteriorly or ventrally. The term dextrocardia implies that the base-apex axis points to the right and down. In this paper, transposition will be discussed only in hearts having the levocardia position, where the normal position of arterial trunks is not subject to controversy.

Since there are hearts in levocardia, mesocardia, and dextrocardia in which the atria and ventricles either correspond or do not correspond, it is necessary to make a further distinction in nomenclature. Pure levocardia, mesocardia, or dextrocardia implies that the atria and ventricles correspond. Mixed levocardia, mesocardia, or dextrocardia implies that the atria and ventricles do not correspond, ie, the right atrium leads into the left ventricle and vice versa. Here there is an inversion of chambers, either atria or ventricles. Inversion implies that there is a disturbance in laterality of structures pursuant to the longitudinal axis involved. Thus the present paper concerns itself with the anatomy of transposition of the arterial trunks in the two types of levocardia, pure levocardia and mixed levocardia.

This method of considering pathological changes has certain advantages; it is not based on an assumed pathogenesis, since pathogenesis of transposition is yet unknown, and the anatomy can be translated directly into surgical phenomena and with some modifications into physiological phenomena. In addition, it leaves uncluttered the vast majority of cases of transposition which are in hearts in pure levocardia. Transposition in mixed levocardia, mesocardia, and dextrocardia presents difficult semantic problems which need not confuse the simple concepts possible in pure levocardia.

Further concepts need be defined in order to render statements in the pathology of congenital heart disease intelligible. This disease is typified by the reactions of tissue to hemodynamic stress. Thus in discussing an entity we need discuss not only the anomalies present, but also the hemodynamic effects of these anomalies on the endocardium, myocardium, valves, conduction system, and even epicardium, if known. The data so accumulated are what we designate as the complex. The reaction of the endocardium we call endocardial hypertrophy and sclerosis, and we refer to the changes in the valves as hemodynamic changes of valves. In discussing individual entities we will have occasion to discuss both the anomaly and the complex concerned with these various reactions. It is self-evident that such reactions are judged in contrast with the normal hemodynamic reaction according to age and whenever possible by weight and height of the individual. Since reactions in the endocardium and valves are related to pressure and flow, these reactions will be mentioned only at the beginning, and will be inferred later on, where the hemo-dynamics are known.

The Normal Position of the Arterial Trunks

In an individual pathological case, it is best to know the exact position of the heart in the chest, and to make statements as to the position of various chambers and arterial trunks with relation to the chest. This makes possible a better correlation with angiocardiography. However, hearts are often presented when the exact orientation in the chest is not given. Under these circumstances this observer has found it convenient to consider position of structures vis-à-vis the ventral surface of the heart as removed from the body. The right atrium and ventricle are anterior and slightly to the right, and the left atrium and ventricle are posterior and slightly to the left. The annulus of the aortic valve is posterior and to the right, while the annulus of the pulmonary valve is anterior and to the left. These normal positions will be used in this paper in describing the various abnormal positions of chambers and vessels.

Basic Classification of Transposition in Pure Levocardia

There are four types of transposition in pure levocardia: overriding aorta, partial transposition, Taussig-Bing, and complete transposition. In an overriding aorta complex, the aorta straddles the ventricular septum over a defect emerging to a varying degree from both ventricles, while the pulmonary trunk emerges from the right ventricle. In partial transposition, both the aorta and pulmonary trunk emerge from the right ventricle with the aorta related to the defect. In Taussig-Bing, the aorta emerges completely from the right ventricle, while the pulmonary trunk emerges in a varying position, but is related to the ventricular septal defect. In complete transposition, the aorta emerges from the right ventricle or right component of a common ventricle, while the pulmonary trunk emerges from the left ventricle or left component of a common ventricle. Since in overriding aorta complex, the physiological presence or absence of pulmonary stenosis is more important than the fact of overriding, we will not use the term "overriding aorta complex" but instead "tetralogy of Fallot," and "anatomic Eisenmenger complex." Since I consider truncus arteriosus communis persistens a transposition complex, it will be included in the discussion.

Tetralogy of Fallot Complexes

Tetralogy of Fallot from the morphological standpoint consists basically of ventricular septal defect, overriding aorta, and pulmonary tract stenosis.

In this complex, the aorta and pulmonary trunk are in normal position, or the aorta is slightly more anterior, being in the same frontal plane as the pulmonary trunk. At the same time the aorta is on a caudal plane as compared to the pulmonary trunk. The aortic annulus is usually related to the mitral annulus.

Tetralogy of Fallot may be classified as follows:
1. Simple tetralogy of Fallot
2. Tetralogy with
    A. Pulmonary atresia
    B. Common A-V orifice or persistent ostium primum
    C. Absence of the pulmonary valve
    D. Tricuspid stenosis
    E. Mitral stenosis
    F. Atrial septal defect
    G. Aortic regurgitation
    H. Widely patent ductus arteriosus

Simple Tetralogy of Fallot (Fig. 1)

Ventricular Septal Defect. The defect is situated at the base of the aorta and is confluent with the mouth of the aorta. It is almost always large and is usually situated in the anterior muscular septum adjacent to the pars membranacea and involves the pars membranacea in part. It lies beneath the right aortic cusp and the adjacent part of the posterior aortic cusp. The defect may however be situated more anteriorly and not involve the pars membranacea. It sometimes lies specifically within the pars membranacea. In some cases it lies in the pars membranacea and the muscle posterior to it (posterior or common AV canal type of ventricular septal defect). In an occasional case it involves the entire base of the ventricular septum.

These defects open into the right ventricle in several ways. Usually the defect opens into the lower part of the conus below the deviated parietal band. It may lie higher in the conus and either deviate or excavate the parietal band. When it lies more posteriorly, it enters the right ventricle at the junction of the sinus and conus of the right ventricle. In the posterior type of ventricular septal defect, the defect may open into the sinus of the right ventricle adjacent to the medial leaflet of the tricuspid valve.

Overriding Aorta. In all cases the aorta rides over the ventricular septal defect in tetralogy. There is no tetralogy without this finding. The amount of overriding varies. In the largest number of autopsy cases, the aorta emerges mostly from the left ventricle, about equally from both ventricles in the next largest group, and mostly from the right ventricle in a further sizeable number of cases. The concept promulgated in some quarters that the overriding aorta is an unimportant finding in tetralogy is fallacious. The greater the overriding the greater the architectural change in the right ventricle, and the more difficult the surgical repair. It must not be overlooked that the surgeon does not close the ventricular septal defect in tetralogy, but he closes that part of the mouth of the aorta emanating from the right ventricle.

Pulmonary Tract Stenosis. The morphology of the stenosis of the pulmonary tract is related to the morphology of the muscle bundles of the conus of the right ventricle.

In 1937, Lev and Saphir [1] studied the morphology of the conal musculature in the normal heart. They coined the terms septal and parietal bands (Fig. 2). The septal band group consists of several muscles which lie on the left lateral

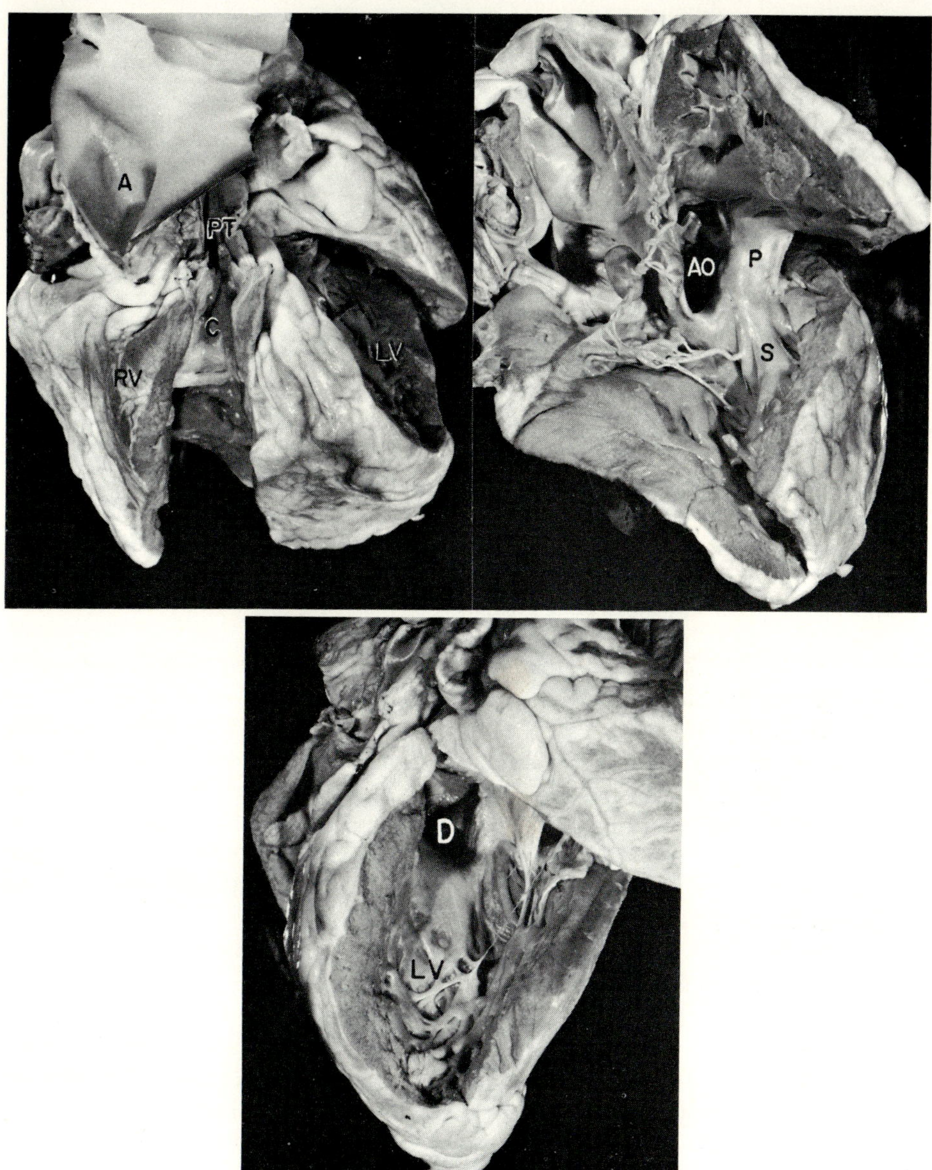

Fig. 1. Simple tetralogy of Fallot. Top left, right ventricular view showing the conus. Top right, right atrial and ventricular view. Bottom, left ventricular view. C, conus; PT, pulmonary trunk; A, aorta; RV, right ventricle; LV, left ventricle; S, septal band group; P, parietal band group; AO, aortic outflow tract; D, ventricular septal defect. (From Gasul, Arcilla, and Lev. Heart Disease in Children; Diagnosis and Treatment. Courtesy of J. B. Lippincott Co.)

margin of the right side of the septum. They originate in the region of the antero-lateral papillary muscle and proceed to the base of the pulmonary trunk. The moderator band takes off from the septal band at a varying distance from the left

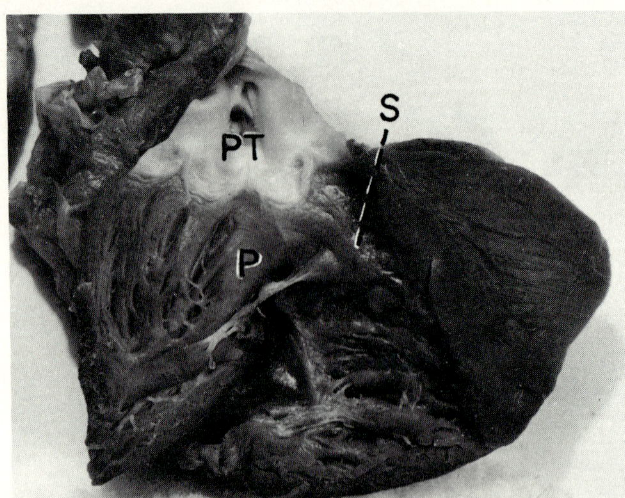

Fig. 2. Septal and parietal band group in normal child's heart. Right ventricular view. S, septal band group; P, parietal band group; PT, pulmonary trunk.

lateral wall. The parietal band group consists of several muscles which originate at the base of the pulmonic valve on the septum. It then proceeds along the right lateral margin of the anterior wall of the right ventricle in intimate contact with the base of the antero-lateral leaflet of the tricuspid valve and peters out in the vicinity of the junction of the anterior and inferior leaflets of the tricuspid valve. Beneath the pulmonary trunk, the septal and parietal bands fuse to form what I call the arch. This arch may be called the crista supraventricularis, although I have abandoned this term because of its controversial use. A raphé may demarcate the junctional line of the septal and parietal bands.

In tetralogy of Fallot, the parietal band group becomes split. The unit forming the arch (first parietal band) is deviated over the anterior wall of the right ventricle, and a second parietal band fills in the gap between the first parietal band and the antero-lateral leaflet of the tricuspid valve. This deviation of the first parietal band narrows the outflow tract of the pulmonary trunk, resulting in infundibular stenosis.

The most common form of pulmonary tract stenosis in tetralogy is diffuse infundibular stenosis. However, the deviated parietal band may combine with the septal band to narrow mostly the mouth of the infundibulum. Under these circumstances, the infundibulum becomes a separate chamber enlarged from its mouth to the pulmonary orifice. In an exceptional case a narrow conus may be further narrowed by endocardial thickening or endocardial spur formation anywhere along its course. A further narrowing at the pulmonic orifice may occur.

Rarely there is no narrowing of the conus in tetralogy but only at the pulmonic orifice. In the cases seen by me, this has occurred when the defect was located more posteriorly.

It has not been possible to differentiate cyanotic from noncyanotic tetralogy except by the complex to be described below. In other words there is no morphological type, related to the ventricular septal defect, the overriding aorta, or the pulmonary tract stenosis, which clearly demarcates an acyanotic type.

THE SIMPLE TETRALOGY OF FALLOT COMPLEX. A distinction must be made between the findings at birth or very shortly thereafter and those findings after about one month of age, which may be called the mature form. There is however generally less pulmonary tract stenosis in the acyanotic type.

In the mature cyanotic form, the right atrium is hypertrophied, with or without enlargement. The right ventricle is hypertrophied, and its size varies from smaller than normal to normal or to larger than normal. The left atrium is atrophied and smaller than normal, while the left ventricle is normal or atrophied with a smaller than normal lumen. The tricuspid orifice may be normal or smaller than normal. The pulmonic orifice is almost always smaller than normal. The mitral orifice is smaller than normal, while the aortic orifice is enlarged. The tricuspid and aortic valves show increased hemodynamic change. The pulmonic valve will be described below. The endocardium of the right atrium and ventricle shows focal hypertrophy and sclerosis.

We are dealing with the cardiac effects of increased pulmonic tract resistance, right to left shunt at the ventricular and aortic areas, and decreased pulmonary flow. Hence there is pressure hypertrophy of the right atrium and ventricle, volume atrophy of the left atrium and ventricle, and hemodynamic changes in the endocardium and valves.

In the mature acyanotic form, the left atrium and left ventricle may show volume hypertrophy due to left to right shunt at the ventricular level. The mitral orifice is then either normal or enlarged, and the valve may show increased hemodynamic change. The left atrium and left ventricle may show endocardial hypertrophy.

At birth the complex is quite different; the left atrium and left ventricle may be normal or even hypertrophied and enlarged, while the right atrium and right ventricle are not hypertrophied. It is understandable that the right side of the heart would not be hypertrophied in fetal life, since it is contracting against normal peripheral resistance by way of the aorta. It is not clear, however, why in some cases the left atrium and left ventricle are hypertrophied. This might be related to more blood going into the left than the right side in fetal life.

ASSOCIATED ABNORMALITIES. Very often associated with tetralogy of Fallot is a bicuspid pulmonic valve. These cusps are usually thickened, irregular, and often defective. A left superior vena cava entering the coronary sinus is often present in addition to a right aortic arch (Corvisart's disease). Narrowing or absence of one of the pulmonary arteries is not often seen. A variant of this occurs when one of the pulmonary arteries originates from the aorta (tetralogy with hemitruncus). The tricuspid valve has a tendency to be mitralized, ie, the inferior and medial leaflets are not sharply demarcated from each other. In addition I have seen the following anomalies in tetralogy: straddling coronary sinus opening, two coronary sinus openings—one for each atrium, left-sided coronary sinus opening, abnormal mitral valve, mitral insufficiency, calcification of the pulmonic valve, bicuspid aortic valve associated with bicuspid pulmonic valve, unicuspid pulmonic valve, aneurysm of the fossa ovalis, stenosis of the pulmonic veins, abnormal left ventricular architecture, post-stenotic dilatation of the pulmonary trunk, bifid apex, and subaortic stenosis.

THE CORONARY ARTERIES IN TETRALOGY. The coronary ostia are rotated counterclockwise about 45° to 90° as one looks downward from the aorta into the left ventricle. The left coronary ostium has a tendency to be high. In most cases the coronary artery distribution is normal. However, there may be a single coronary artery supplying the entire coronary circulation. It appears to me that a single coronary artery is more common in tetralogy than in the normal population. The right coronary ostium may take over the anterior descending coronary artery. Under these circumstances, the anterior descending artery may journey in front of the pulmonary artery and constitute a hazard in right ventriculotomies. There is also a more than normal tendency for the left coronary ostium to take over the posterior descending artery. The conal artery is almost always very prominent. I have seen one case in tetralogy where the right coronary artery originated from the pulmonary artery.

Complicated Tetralogies

TETRALOGY WITH PULMONARY ATRESIA (FIG. 3). In this anomaly, the main pulmonary trunk is represented by a small vessel which proceeds to the base of the heart without entering the chamber. The pulmonary trunk is fed by a ductus arteriosus from the aorta. The architecture of the conal musculature is somewhat different from that in tetralogy. The septal band group may proceed to the base of the pulmonary trunk where it terminates abruptly or forms an arch with a parietal band passing on to the anterior wall of the right ventricle. This divides off a small blind

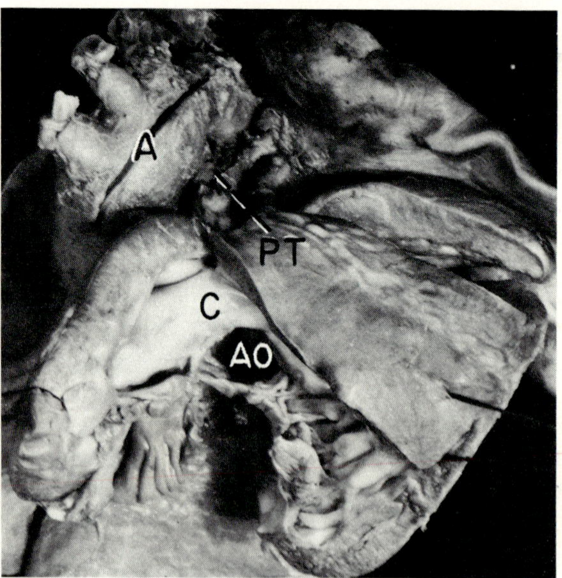

Fig. 3. Tetralogy of Fallot with pulmonary atresia. Right ventricular view. C, blind conus of pulmonary trunk; A, aorta; PT, pulmonary trunk; AO, outflow tract of aorta from right ventricle. (From Lev and Eckner. Dis. Chest., 45:251, 1964.)

conus for the pulmonary trunk, or there is no conus for the pulmonary trunk. A parietal band separated from the septal band is related to the antero-lateral leaflet of the tricuspid.

The Tetralogy with Pulmonary Atresia Complex.   The right atrium and the right ventricle are more hypertrophied than in simple tetralogy. The left atrium and left ventricle may be more atrophied than in tetralogy, but occasionally the left ventricle is normal or hypertrophied. This may be related to obstruction to the outflow from this chamber.

TETRALOGY WITH COMMON A-V ORIFICE (FIG. 4).   Instead of a ventricular septal defect, this complex contains a common A-V orifice. Because of the latter the left ventricle may be hypertrophied and enlarged, and the right atrium has a greater tendency to be hypertrophied and enlarged than in tetralogy. In one case the valvular component of the right side of the common A-V orifice was displaced downward as in Ebstein's anomaly.

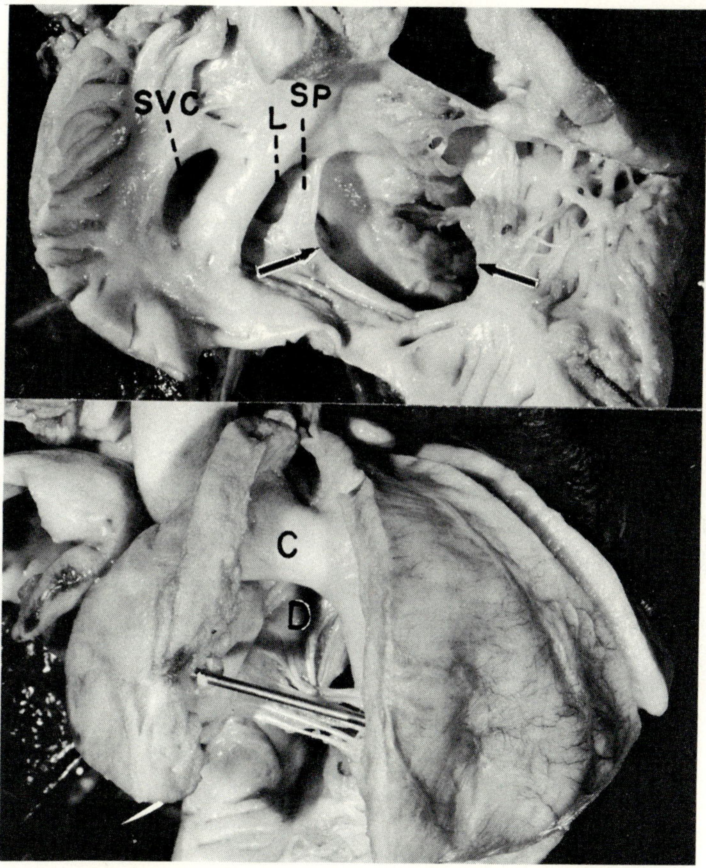

Fig. 4. Tetralogy of Fallot with common A-V orifice (canal). Top, right atrial and right ventricular view. Bottom, right ventricular view. SVC, superior vena cava; L, limbus; SP, septum primum; C, conus; D, ventricular septal defect. Arrows point to the common A-V orifice. (From Lev et al. Amer. J. Clin. Path., 36:408, 1961.)

Tetralogy with Absence of the Pulmonary Valve (Fig. 5).   Here no distinct pulmonary valve is present. Instead there are nubbins of valvular tissue where the valve should be. This is associated with pulmonary insufficiency, and hence there is aneurysmal dilatation of the pulmonary trunk and the right ventricle may be larger than in the usual tetralogy.

Tetralogy with Tricuspid Stenosis.   The tricuspid orifice has a tendency to be smaller in tetralogy than in the normal heart. This may be due to the position of the aorta that renders impossible the full expansion of the tricuspid. The tricuspid stenosis is usually of an anatomic and not of a physiological nature, since no disproportionate smallness of the right ventricle and enlargement of the left ventricle are noted.

Tetralogy with Mitral Stenosis (Fig. 6).   This may be seen when the ventricular septal defect is situated posteriorly. There is then a tendency for the

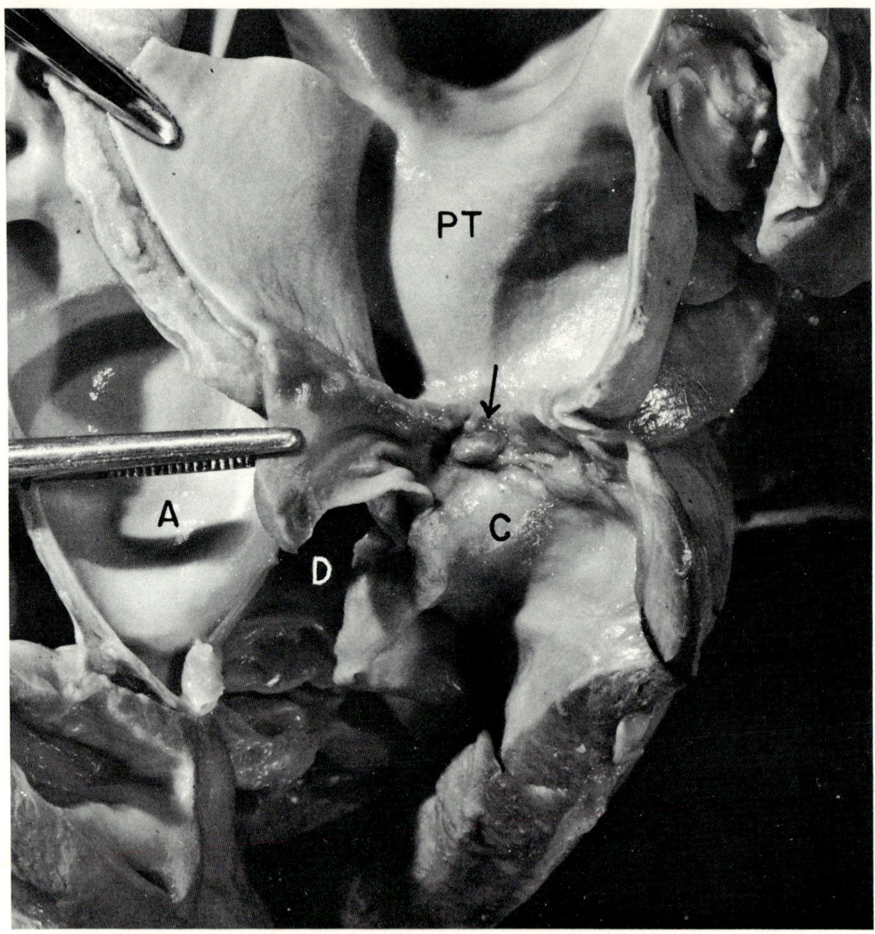

Fig. 5. Tetralogy of Fallot with absence of the pulmonary valve. Right ventricular and pulmonary trunk view. C, conus; A, aorta; PT, pulmonary trunk; D, ventricular septal defect. Arrow points to the absent pulmonary valve. (From Miller et al. Circulation, 26:266, 1962.)

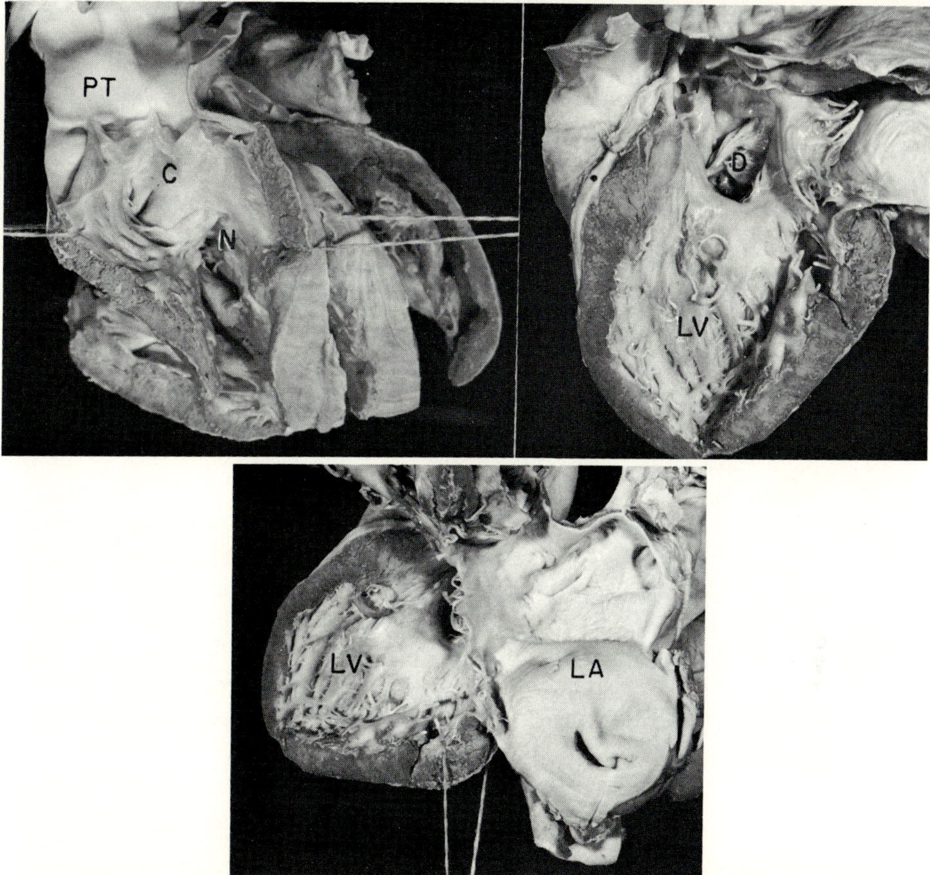

Fig. 6. Tetralogy with mitral stenosis. Top left, right ventricular view. Top right, left ventricular view. Bottom, left atrial and left ventricular view. C, conus; N, narrowing at mouth of conus; PT, pulmonary trunk; D, ventricular septal defect; LA, left atrium; LV, left ventricle.

mitral orifice to be moved somewhat toward the left and to be smaller than normal. Continuity between the mitral and tricuspid valves may be present through the defect. The left atrium is hypertrophied and enlarged, while the remainder of the complex is similar to tetralogy.

TETRALOGY WITH ATRIAL SEPTAL DEFECT. In this complex there is a true atrial septal defect of the fossa ovalis type. This is to be distinguished from the small foramen ovale seen in about half the cases of tetralogy. Despite the presence of the defect, there is no evidence of functional change on either the right or the left side.

TETRALOGY WITH AORTIC INSUFFICIENCY. In this complex, the right aortic cusp is redundant and herniated through the defect into the outflow tract of the right ventricle. This may result in left atrial and left ventricular hypertrophy and enlargement.

Tetralogy with Widely Patent Ductus Arteriosus.   A small ductus is often found in tetralogy. This is insufficient to change the physiological arrangements in this complex. Rarely, however, a large ductus arteriosus with sizeable left to right shunt may be present, producing an acyanotic type of tetralogy.

Surgical Effects

When a Blalock-Taussig procedure is performed, the proximal part of the left or right subclavian is anastomosed to the side of the left or right pulmonary artery, respectively. This vessel has a tendency to close with time. In a Potts procedure (Fig. 7) a direct anastomosis is made between the aorta distal to the ductus arteriosus and the left pulmonary artery close to the left lung. The size of the orifice so produced is important in the evaluation of secondary pathological change. In general there is enlargement of the left pulmonary artery with sclerotic changes in its lining. When the Potts anastomosis is large, there may be aneurysmal dilatation of the main pulmonary trunk and both arteries, in some cases with rupture of the aneurysm. Secondary pulmonary hypertension may ensue, and rarely infundibular atresia may eventuate. Occasionally a supravalvular pulmonic ridge may develop. In longstanding Potts procedures subacute bacterial endocarditis may be engrafted on the aortic valve. In a Brock procedure, the pulmonary valve is fractured, and the infundibulum is widened. Pulmonary insufficiency may ensue, but this is relatively innocuous. In all of these situations the left atrium and ventricle may show volume hypertrophy, which is most common and marked in Potts procedures.

In a complete repair or reconstruction procedure, the pathologist is interested in the ventriculotomy wound, the closure of the outflow tract of the right ventricle

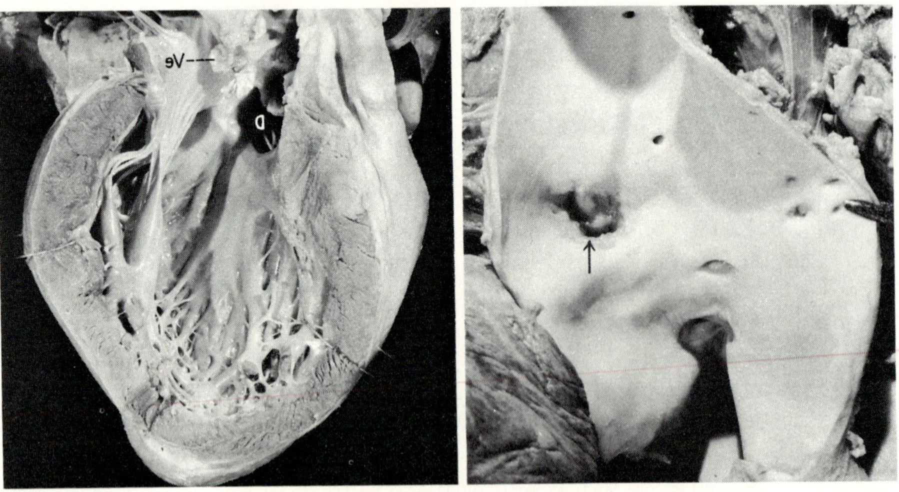

Fig. 7. Tetralogy of Fallot, with Potts procedure, and subacute bacterial endocarditis. Left, aortic view, showing Potts procedure opening. Arrow points to the aortic opening of the Potts anastomosis. Right, left ventricular view. Note the enlarged left ventricle. Ve, vegetation on the aortic valve; D, ventricular septal defect.

into the aorta, and the widening of the infundibulum. A ventriculotomy wound may cut an aberrant anterior descending coronary artery, or the normal anterior descending. It may also cut the anterolateral papillary muscle of the right ventricle. The conal artery is usually cut at its periphery, but sometimes more proximally. The outflow tract of the right ventricle into the aorta is usually closed by a prosthesis. Residual openings are often seen. The prosthesis may obstruct the tricuspid orifice. Rarely a prosthesis may detach itself completely and form an embolus in one of the pulmonary arteries. If A-V block has ensued, it is important to look carefully at the sutures, and a histological examination of the conduction system may be performed. The aortic valve may be involved in a suture to produce aortic insufficiency or later a fistula. In the excavation of the muscle of the pulmonary infundibulum, it is usually the parietal band which is mostly excavated. In some cases however the septal band is also excavated, and here it is important to look for ruptured anterior perforating arteries. The amount of residual infundibular stenosis, if any, is important. Rupture of a prosthesis in the anterior wall of the right ventricle may be found, and acute or subacute bacterial endocarditis may be engrafted on the tricuspid or pulmonic valves.

Anatomic Eisenmenger Complex

This term is used to denote the presence of a ventricular septal defect with overriding aorta, without pulmonary stenosis (Fig. 8). The term anatomic is used to distinguish the entity from the Eisenmenger complex of the clinicians. The Eisenmenger complex of the clinicians usually means any left to right shunt which has progressed to the development of severe pulmonary hypertension and resultant

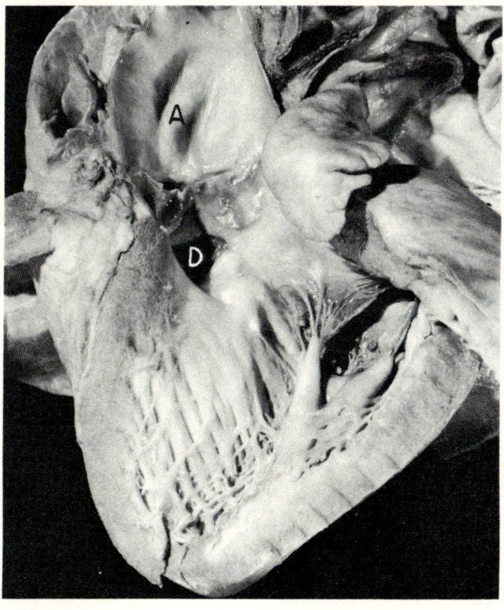

Fig. 8. The anatomic Eisenmenger complex. Left ventricular view. D, ventricular septal defect; A, aorta.

right to left shunt. The appellation Anatomic Eisenmenger Complex does not imply what the physiology is.

It is important to separate out such an entity from ordinary ventricular septal defect because the presence of appreciable overriding of the aorta changes the architecture of the right ventricle and hence the problem of surgical repair. In the anatomic Eisenmenger complex the parietal band may be deviated as in tetralogy, but not to such an extent as to narrow the outflow tract of the pulmonary trunk. In some cases the parietal band may be excavated.

If there is no pulmonary hypertension, we are dealing with the effects of left to right shunt at the ventricular level. There is thus volume hypertrophy of the ventricles and left atrium. If there is hyperkinetic pulmonary hypertension, then a vector of pressure hypertrophy appears in the right ventricle and right atrium. If there is a marked increase in pulmonary resistance with equalized pressures in the two chambers or reversal of shunts, then the left atrium and ventricle may be normal or atrophied.

Surgical Effects

In the anatomic Eisenmenger complex surgical closure of the outflow tract of the right ventricle into the aorta may be attempted. Residual defects may be present because of the obliquity of the prosthesis, and death may ensue due to obstruction of the left ventricle by the ventricular septal defect. A banding procedure may be performed. It is important for the pathologist to estimate the amount of narrowing of the pulmonic trunk so produced, and the possible effects on the right ventricle.

Partial Transposition (Double Outlet Right Ventricle of the Partial Transposition Type)

As indicated above, in partial transposition the aorta and pulmonary trunk both arise from the right ventricle with the aorta related to the defect. The aortic annulus is situated to the right, and the pulmonary annulus to the left. Uncommonly the former is anterior and to the right, and the latter is posterior and to the left. Rarely the aortic annulus is posterior and to the right, and the pulmonary annulus anterior and to the left. The aortic annulus is usually caudal to the pulmonary annulus. Partial transposition complexes may be classified as follows:

With pulmonary stenosis
Without pulmonary stenosis
With pulmonary atresia
With common A-V orifice
With partial or total anomalous pulmonary venous drainage
With mitral stenosis or atresia
With mitral stenosis or atresia or with common A-V orifice and partial or total
   anomalous pulmonary venous drainage
With Ebstein's anomaly

PARTIAL TRANSPOSITION WITH PULMONARY STENOSIS. This is an extension of simple tetralogy and cannot be separated sharply from tetralogy with marked overriding of the aorta (Fig. 9). For as long as the aorta is related to the defect

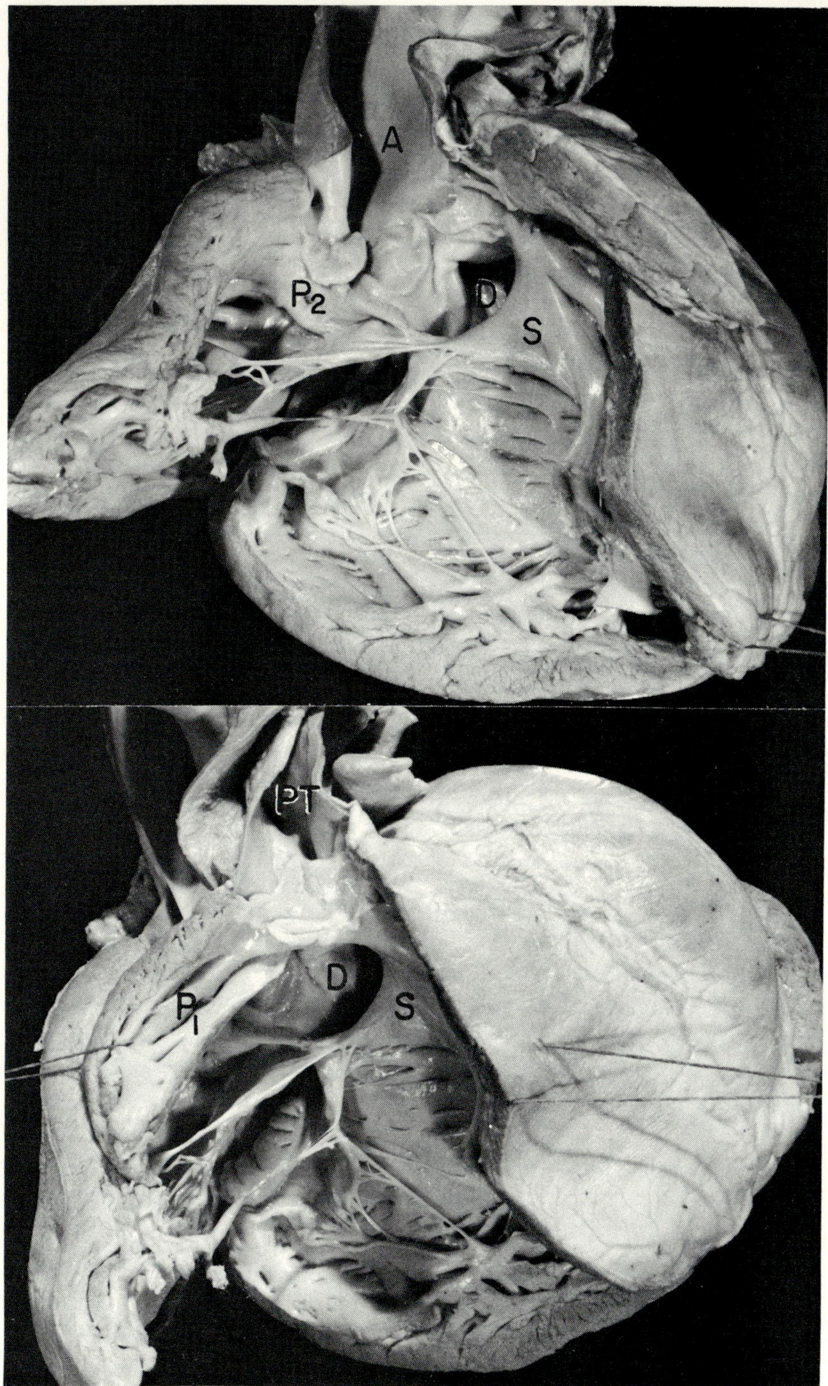

Fig. 9. Partial transposition with pulmonary stenosis. Top, right ventricular view at the outflow of the aorta. Bottom, right ventricular view at the outflow of the pulmonary trunk. A, aorta; PT, pulmonary trunk; S, septal band group; P_1, first parietal band; P_2, second parietal band; D, ventricular septal defect.

there may be said to be slight emergence from the left ventricle. Yet, with the shift of the aorta almost completely into the right ventricle, the anatomic and hence the surgical problem is altered.

Ventricular Septal Defect.   The ventricular septal defect is usually large, but not necessarily large enough to be sufficient as the only outflow from the left ventricle. It is most always situated in the anterior part of the ventricular septum at the base, but rarely it may be present posteriorly. The left side of the aortic annulus is in most cases confluent with the mitral annulus, although occasionally a muscle band separates the two structures.

Pulmonary Tract Stenosis.   This is related to the altered architecture of the muscle bundles of the conus. The septal band group proceeds to the base and bifurcates to house the ventricular septal defect. The upper prong may end at the junction of the aortic and pulmonary annuli, or it may form an arch between the aorta and pulmonary trunk with a parietal band which is markedly deviated onto the anterior wall of the right ventricle. The lower prong of the septal band may end at the defect or meet a second parietal band which proceeds from the aorta downward and is related to the anterolateral leaflet of the tricuspid valve.

This marked deviation of the arch in general narrows the infundibulum of the pulmonary trunk. There is also a tendency toward shortening of the infundibulum. As in tetralogy, the infundibulum may be narrowed at its mouth to produce a separate little conus chamber from the pulmonary trunk. The pulmonary orifice is of course small.

The Partial Transposition with Pulmonary Stenosis Complex.   There is pressure hypertrophy of the right atrium and right ventricle and a tendency toward left atrial and left ventricular atrophy. In some cases, however, the left ventricle is normal or hypertrophied. This is considered to be due to obstruction at the ventricular septal defect. The tricuspid orifice is enlarged, the mitral orifice small, and the aortic orifice large. There is focal endocardial hypertrophy of the right atrium and ventricle. We are dealing with the effects of systemic resistance acting on the right ventricle, with decreased pulmonary flow.

Associated Abnormalities.   A patent foramen ovale or an atrial septal defect of the fossa ovalis type is almost always present. This may be so large as to result in a common atrium. Bicuspid pulmonic valve, left superior vena cava entering the coronary sinus, and right aortic arch may all be found in partial transposition with pulmonary stenosis. Mitralization of the tricuspid valve is frequent, as in tetralogy. The ductus arteriosus may or may not be patent. Absence of the pulmonic valve is a frequent variant. I have also seen the following in partial transposition: tricuspid stenosis, entry of the coronary sinus into the left atrium, abnormal architecture of the left ventricle, which occasionally may be small, thick walled with fibroelastosis, aneurysm of the fossa ovalis, fetal coarctation, double tricuspid orifice, abnormal origin of the right pulmonary artery, and small left pulmonary artery.

PARTIAL TRANSPOSITION WITHOUT PULMONARY STENOSIS.   In these cases, despite the altered architecture of the conal region of the right ventricle, there is no pulmonary tract stenosis, or it is very mild and of no physiological import (Fig. 10). The physiology of this complex is thus that of ventricular septal defect. The altered anatomy of the right ventricle and the altered surgical problem, in addition

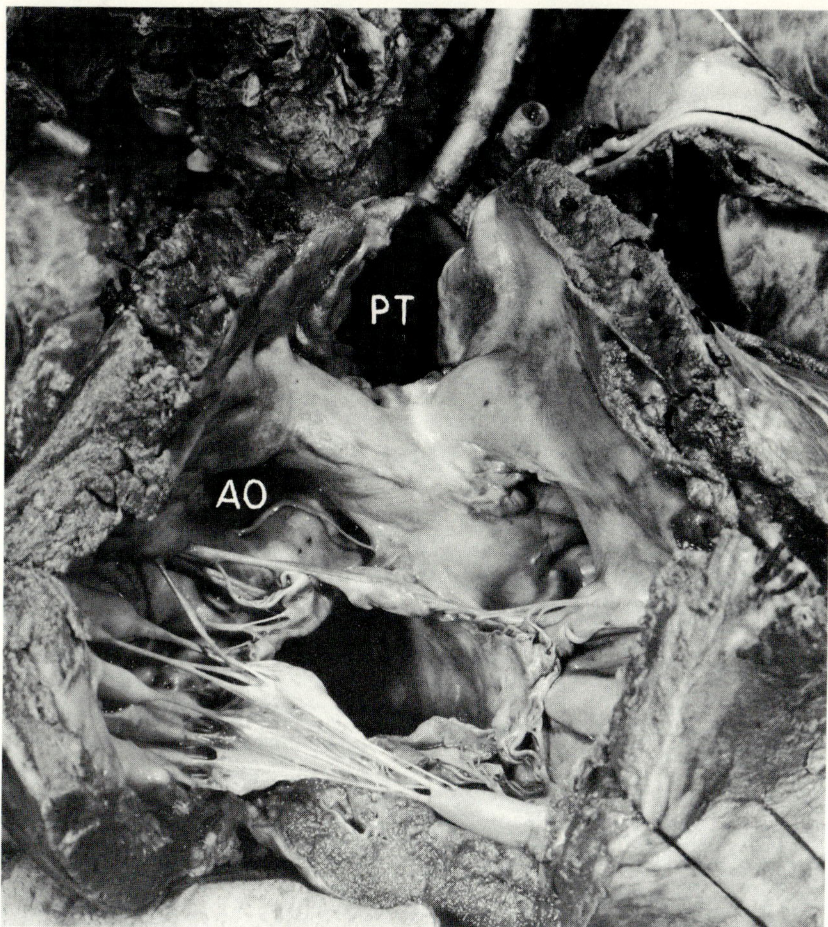

Fig. 10. Partial transposition without pulmonary stenosis. Right ventricular view. AO, out-flow tract of aorta; PT, pulmonary trunk.

to the possible obstructive effects of the ventricular septal defect on the left ventricle, warrant the separation of this entity from ventricular septal defect.

PARTIAL TRANSPOSITION WITH PULMONARY ATRESIA (FIG. 11).   Pulmonary atresia is more common in partial transposition than it is in tetralogy. The term pseudotruncus has been used for tetralogy with pulmonary atresia, partial transposition with pulmonary atresia, and complete transposition with pulmonary atresia.

In partial transposition with pulmonary atresia, the pulmonary trunk proceeds to the base of the heart without opening up into the ventricle. A vestigial valve may be present at the base. The pulmonary tree is fed via a ductus arteriosus in most cases. The architecture of the muscle bundles of the conus of the right ventricle is as follows: the septal group proceeds to the base of the aorta and bifurcates, housing the ventricular septal defect in its two limbs as in partial transposition with pulmonary stenosis. The upper prong may stop at the aortic ring or it may proceed

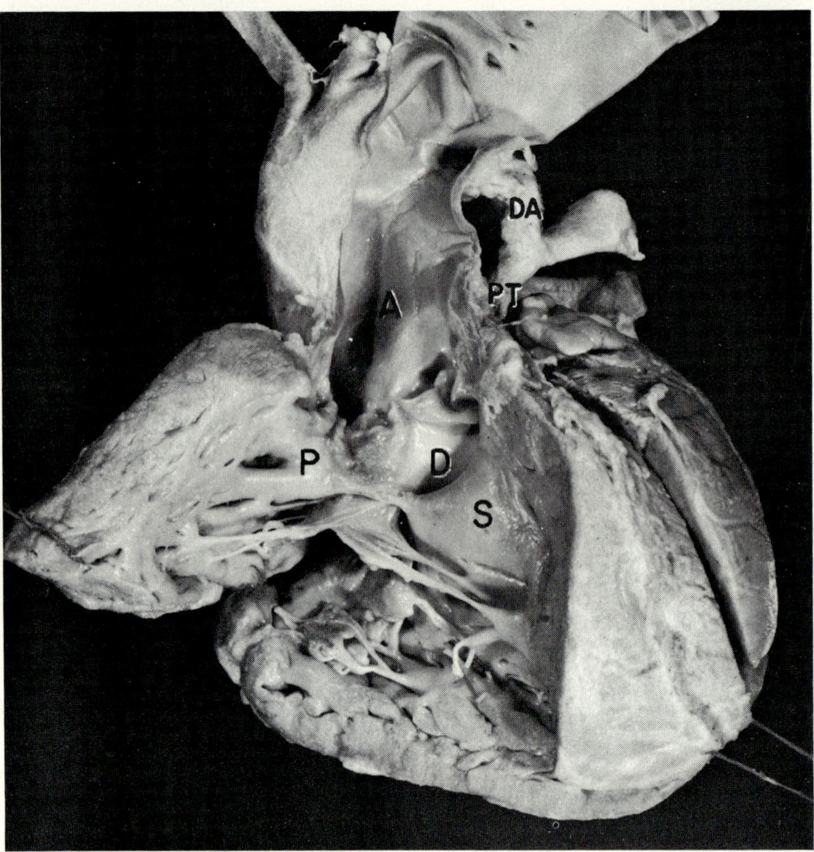

Fig. 11. Partial transposition with pulmonary atresia. Right ventricular view. A, aorta; D, ventricular septal defect; DA, ductus arteriosus; PT, pulmonary trunk; S, septal band group; P, parietal band group.

to form an arch separating off a blind little conus from the pulmonary trunk. The lower smaller prong may end at the base or may be continuous with the parietal band proceeding downward from the aorta related to the anterior leaflet of the tricuspid valve. This parietal band may extend beneath the aorta into the left ventricle separating the aortic annulus from the mitral annulus, or these annuli may be continuous. The ventricular septal defect resembles that in partial transposition with pulmonary stenosis.

Associated Abnormalities. In almost all cases a patent foramen ovale or a large atrial septal defect of the fossa ovalis type is included in the complex. This may be so large as to produce a common atrium. A still further variant is absence of the ductus arteriosus with markedly enlarged bronchial arteries. The reactions of the myocardium, endocardium, and valves resemble those of partial transposition with pulmonary stenosis.

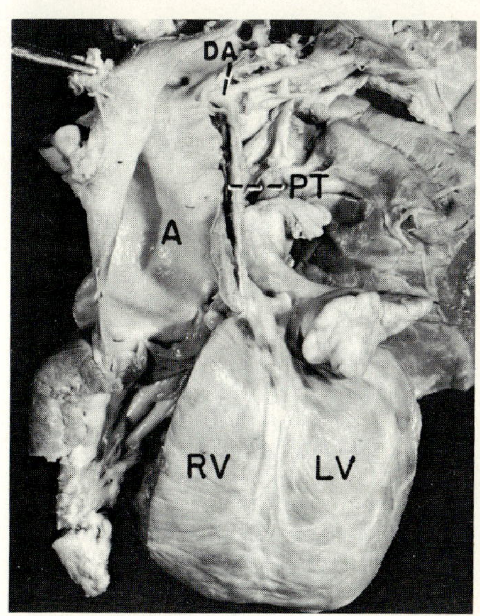

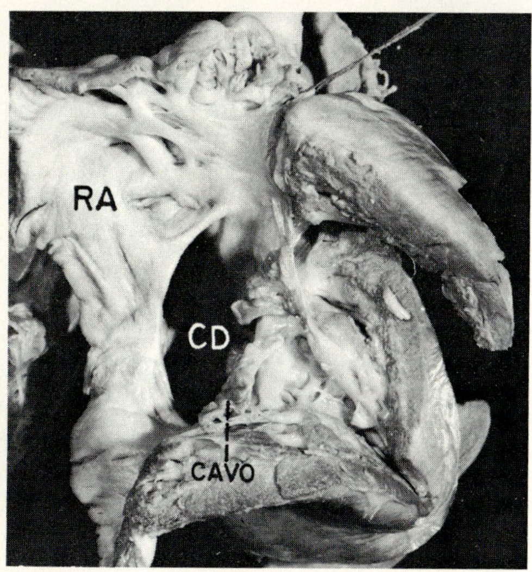

Fig. 12. Partial transposition, with common A-V orifice and pulmonary atresia. Left, anterior view. Right, right atrial and right ventricular view. A, aorta; PT, pulmonary trunk; DA, ductus arteriosus; RV, right ventricle; LV, left ventricle; RA, right atrium; CAVO, common A-V orifice; CD, combined septal defect.

PARTIAL TRANSPOSITION WITH COMMON A-V ORIFICE (FIG. 12). In this uncommon type, both arterial trunks come from the right ventricle accompanied by common A-V orifice. The ventricular septal defect portion of the combined septal defect is related to the aorta. In all cases I have seen there was either pulmonary tract stenosis or atresia.

There is pressure hypertrophy of the right ventricle and right atrium. However the left ventricle is variable, as in isolated common A-V orifice. Focal endocardial thickening is present in all chambers.

We are dealing with the effects of systemic resistance acting on the right ventricle, decreased pulmonary flow, and a varying amount of filling of the left ventricle from both atria.

PARTIAL TRANSPOSITION WITH PARTIAL OR TOTAL ANOMALOUS PULMONARY VENOUS DRAINAGE (FIG. 13). In this group the aorta and pulmonary trunk emanate from the right ventricle with all or some of the veins taking any of the usual pathways to enter the systemic circuit. There is also an atrial septal defect of the fossa ovalis type. The ventricular septal defect is the usual type found in partial transposition.

Volume and pressure hypertrophy of the right atrium and ventricle is found, with volume atrophy of the left atrium and left ventricle. The tricuspid and pulmonic orifices are enlarged, the mitral orifice is small, and the aortic orifice normal.

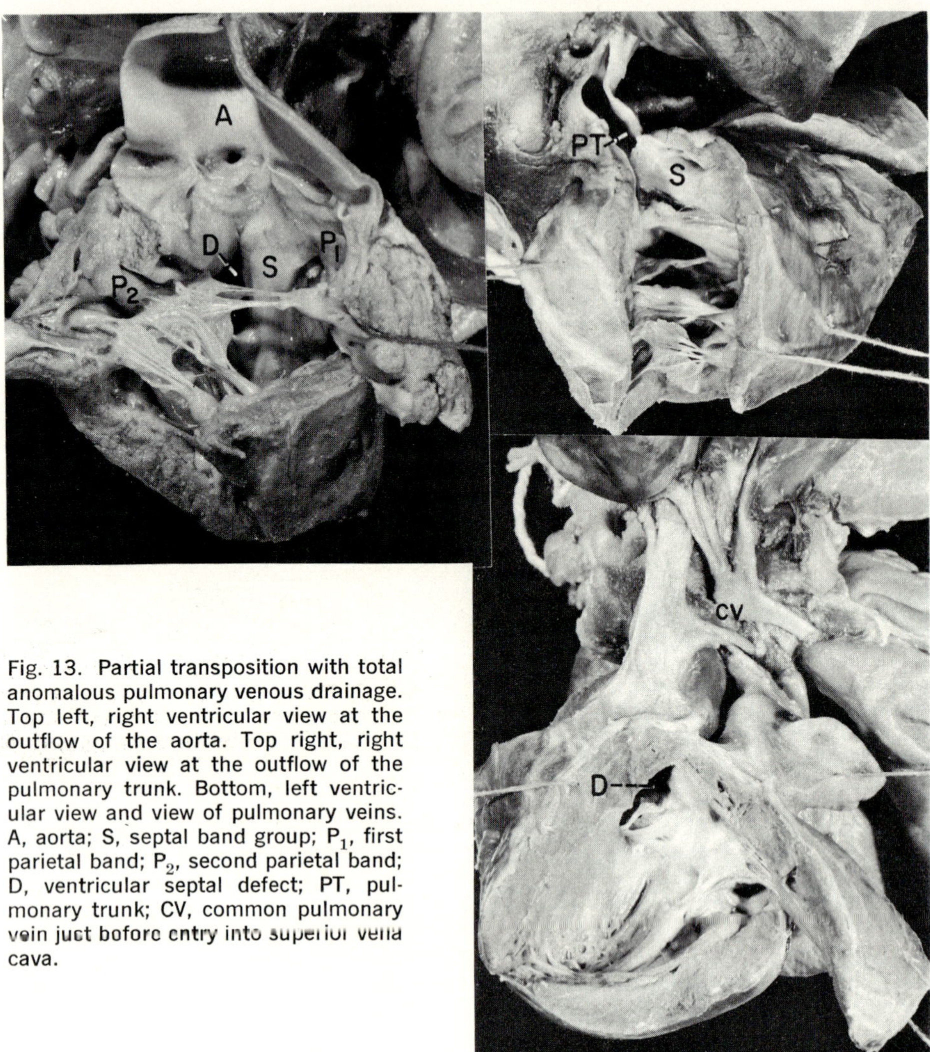

Fig. 13. Partial transposition with total anomalous pulmonary venous drainage. Top left, right ventricular view at the outflow of the aorta. Top right, right ventricular view at the outflow of the pulmonary trunk. Bottom, left ventricular view and view of pulmonary veins. A, aorta; S, septal band group; P₁, first parietal band; P₂, second parietal band; D, ventricular septal defect; PT, pulmonary trunk; CV, common pulmonary vein just before entry into superior vena cava.

PARTIAL TRANSPOSITION WITH MITRAL STENOSIS OR ATRESIA (FIG. 14).   In the few cases I have seen, the left ventricle was atrophied, and its only outlet was a ventricular septal defect. Some cases were associated with pulmonary stenosis or atresia, and others with aortic stenosis or atresia. Where there was mitral stenosis, the left atrium was enlarged. A variant of this complex is mitral stenosis or atresia, with both vessels coming from the right ventricle without ventricular septal defect. Here the left ventricle may not be seen grossly. In view of the absence of the ventricular septal defect, this is best called double outlet right ventricle with mitral stenosis or atresia.

PARTIAL TRANSPOSITION WITH MITRAL STENOSIS OR ATRESIA AND PARTIAL OR TOTAL ANOMALOUS PULMONARY VENOUS DRAINAGE.   These rare types of hearts represent the combined effects of all three component entities.

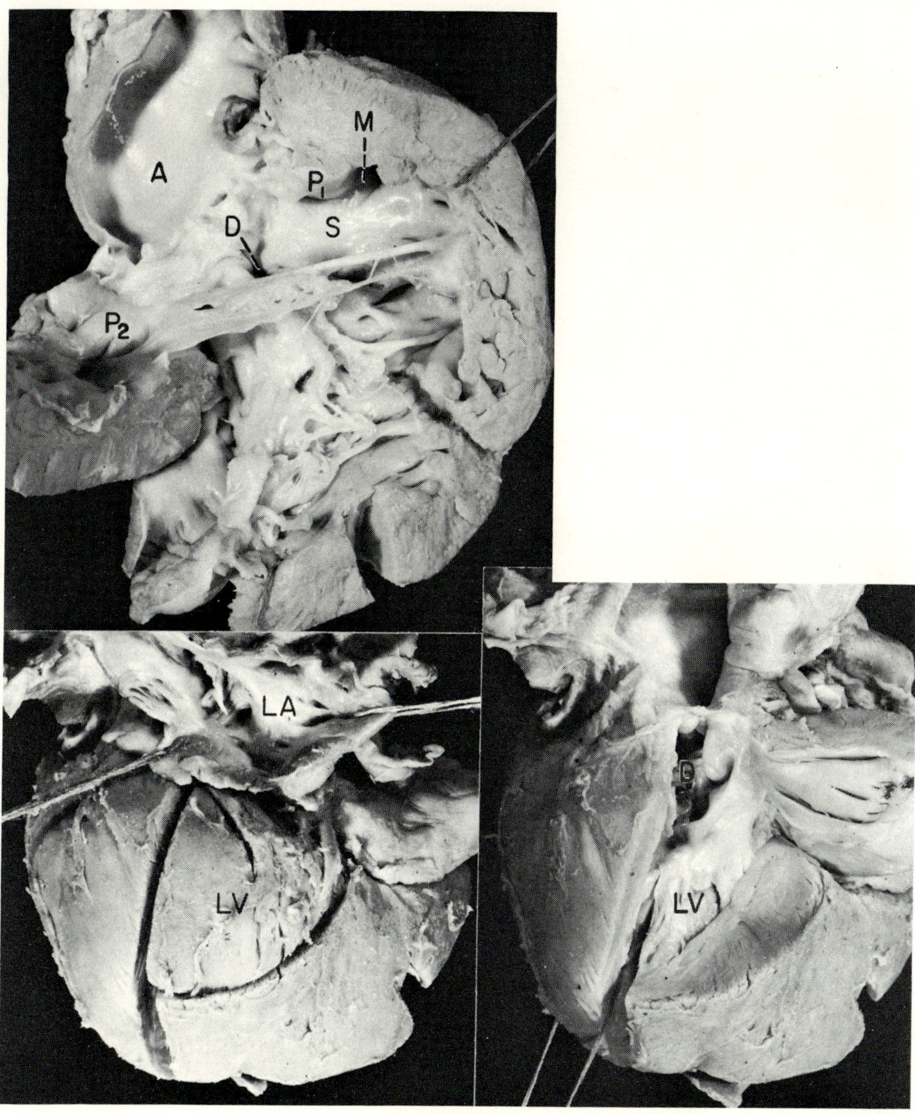

Fig. 14. Partial transposition with mitral atresia. Top, right ventricular view. Bottom left, left atrial and left ventricular view. Bottom right, left ventricular view. A, aorta; D, ventricular septal defect; M, mouth of conus into pulmonary trunk; S, septal band group; P₁, first parietal band; P₂, second parietal band; LA, left atrium; LV, left ventricle.

PARTIAL TRANSPOSITION WITH EBSTEIN'S ANOMALY (FIG. 15). There is a true downward displacement of the medial and inferior leaflets of the tricuspid valve combined with the features of a partial transposition.

THE CORONARY ARTERIES IN PARTIAL TRANSPOSITION. The coronary ostia are rotated counterclockwise when one looks toward the ventricle from the aorta, as in tetralogy. In most cases, the coronary distribution is normal. However, occasionally a single coronary artery and the origin of the anterior descending artery

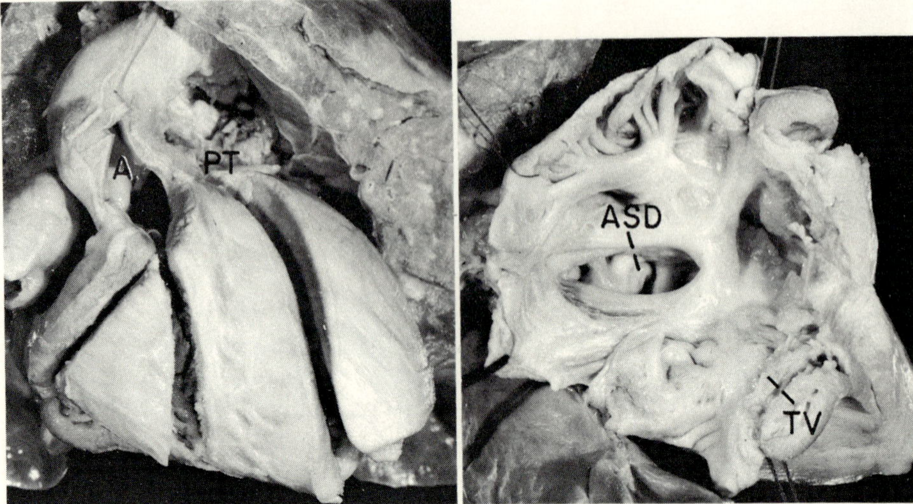

Fig. 15. Partial transposition with Ebstein's anomaly. Left, anterior view. Right, right atrial and right ventricular view. A, aorta; PT, outflow region into pulmonary trunk; ASD, atrial septal defect, fossa ovalis type; TV, displaced tricuspid valve.

from the right coronary are seen, as in tetralogy. In an occasional case the embryological left coronary ostium takes over the right circumflex. In complicated types of partial transposition, there is an occasional complete exchange of vessels between the two coronary arteries, as in Taussig-Bing and complete transposition type.

Surgical Effects

Shunting procedures and occasionally total repairs are seen in partial transposition with pulmonary stenosis. Shunting procedures can also be seen in partial transposition with pulmonary atresia. In an attempted total repair in partial transposition with or without stenosis it is common to see residual defects, since the hammock-like prosthesis has great angularity. The pathologist must also judge the size of the ventricular septal defect, to determine whether it constitutes an obstruction to the left ventricle.

Truncus Arteriosus Communis

A truncus communis is an arterial trunk from which the coronary arteries, the pulmonary trunk, and the systemic trunk arise. Such a vessel arises either in a straddling position over a defect or from the right ventricle. Therefore it is always an overriding aorta or partial transposition complex.

There are various ways of considering truncus communis; the position of exit of the truncus, the extent of the aortico-pulmonary septum, the relative size of the aortic and pulmonary trunk components of the common truncus, the size of the pulmonary arteries, and the extent of pulmonary flow are all determining factors.

As stated above the truncus emerges either from both ventricles over a defect

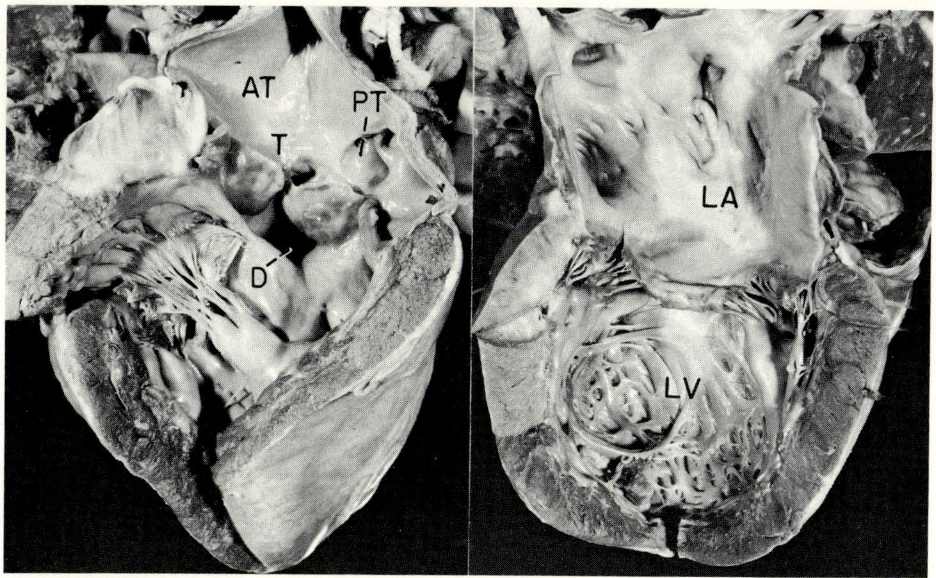

Fig. 16. Truncus communis in overriding position, with increased pulmonary flow. Left, right ventricular view. Right, left atrial and left ventricular view, showing enlargement of chambers. T, truncus communis; D, ventricular septal defect; AT, aortic tree; PT, pulmonary tree; LA, left atrium; LV, left ventricle.

of the ventricular septum (Fig. 16), or it emerges from the right ventricle (Fig. 17). The defect is in the anterior septum, and the architecture of the musculature of the right ventricle resembles that seen in partial transposition. The aortico-

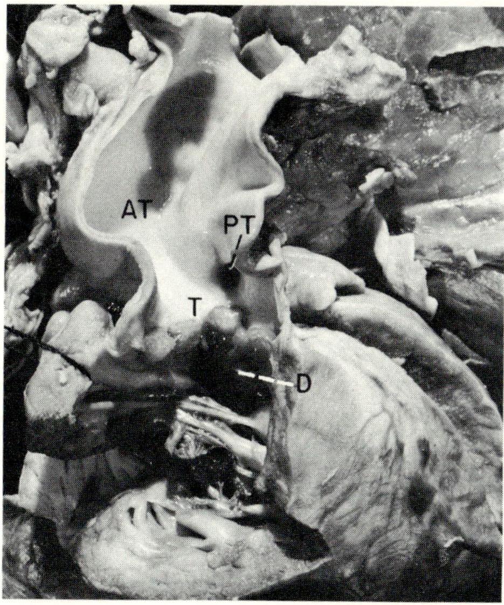

Fig. 17. Truncus communis from right ventricle. T, truncus communis; AT, aortic tree; PT, pulmonary tree; D, ventricular septal defect.

pulmonary septum may be of good size (Fig. 16), so that a distinct pulmonary trunk can be seen emerging from the common truncus. Or it may be abbreviated or absent, so that the two pulmonary arteries emerge directly from the common truncus.

From the standpoint of the relative size of the pulmonary and aortic portions of the truncus, there are two types. The more common type accentuates the aortic portion (Fig. 17), although the pulmonary portion is also of considerable size. In this type the ductus arteriosus is absent. In the less common type the pulmonary portion is accentuated and the aortic portion is small, proceeding into a hypoplastic ascending aorta with or without the presence of a transverse aorta (Fig. 18). The pulmonary portion forms the descending aorta through a widely patent ductus arteriosus. Relative to the amount of pulmonary flow, the pulmonary arteries are usually large, with increased pulmonary flow (Fig. 16). Only occasionally are the pulmonary arteries small, with decreased pulmonary flow (Fig. 19).

THE TRUNCUS ARTERIOSUS COMMUNIS COMPLEX.   Accordingly, there is always pressure hypertrophy of the right ventricle, and there is usually volume hypertrophy of the left atrium and ventricle. When there is decreased pulmonary flow, there is volume atrophy of the left atrium and ventricle. When the aorta emerges from the right ventricle, there may be stenosis at the ventricular septal defect with pressure hypertrophy of the left ventricle. The truncus valve usually consists of two, three, or four cusps.

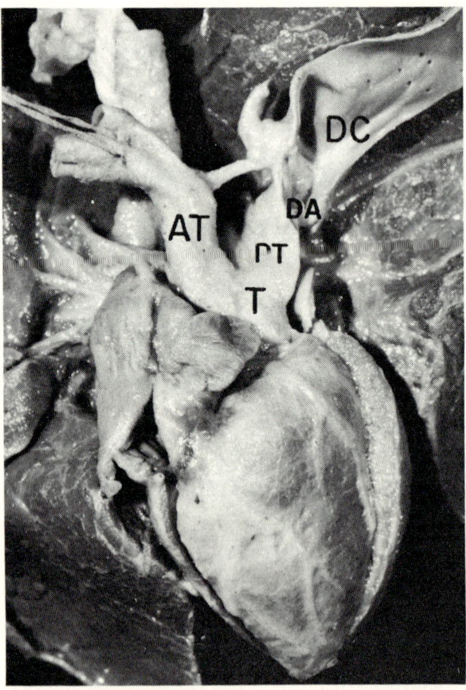

Fig. 18. Truncus communis with hypoplastic aortic tree. Anterior view. T, truncus communis; AT, aortic tree; PT, pulmonary tree; DA, ductus arteriosus; DC, descending aorta.

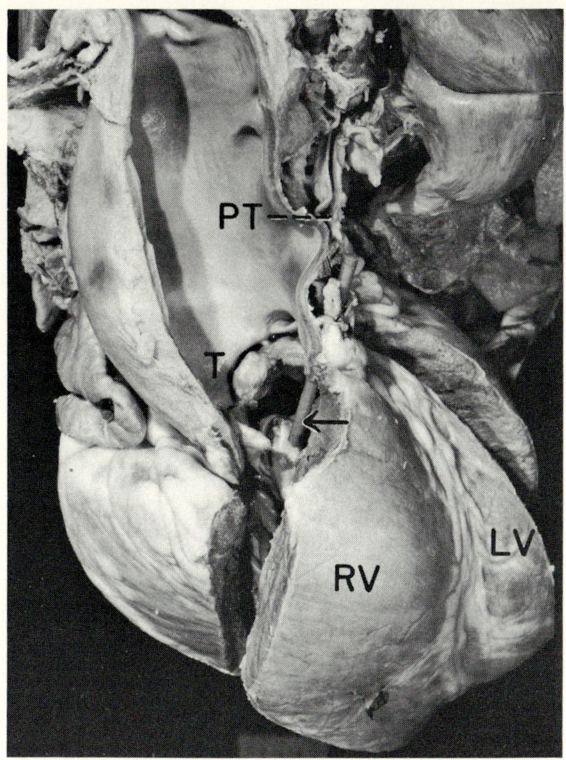

Fig. 19. Truncus communis with decreased pulmonary flow. T, truncus communis; PT, pulmonary tree; RV, right ventricle; LV, left ventricle. Arrow points to rod passing through opening of pulmonary tree into common truncus.

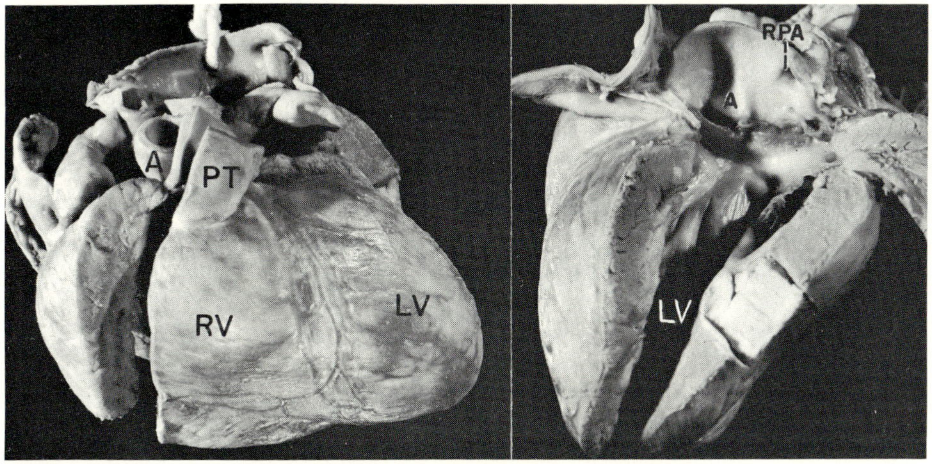

Fig. 20. Origin of right pulmonary artery from aorta (hemitruncus). Left, anterior view. Right, left ventricular view. A, aorta; PT, Pulmonary trunk leading into left pulmonary artery; RPA, origin of right pulmonary artery in aorta; RV, right ventricle; LV, left ventricle.

In some types of so called truncus communis, the pulmonary trunk and its branches are absent. Here the bronchial arteries carry the pulmonary circulation. In the so-called hemitruncus (Fig. 20), one of the pulmonary arteries emerges from the aorta, while the other emerges by way of a pulmonary trunk from the right ventricle. This may be associated with infundibular stenosis.

ASSOCIATED ABNORMALITIES. Truncus communis may be associated with common A-V orifice, mitral atresia with persistent ostium primum, stenosis of the truncus orifice with aneurysmal dilatation of the truncus, tricuspid stenosis or insufficiency, right aortic arch, atypical origin of the pulmonary arteries, various abnormalities of the subclavian artery, left superior vena cava entering the coronary sinus, single coronary artery, and aneurysm of the fossa ovalis.

The Taussig-Bing Heart (Double Outlet Right Ventricle of the Taussig-Bing Type)

As stated above, in this anomaly the aorta emerges completely from the right ventricle, unrelated to the ventricular septal defect, while the pulmonary trunk emerges to a varying extent from both ventricles related to the ventricular septal defect. In addition, the architecture of the right ventricle presents certain specific features to be discussed.

Taussig-Bing complexes may be classified as follows:

Right-sided type, without overriding pulmonary trunk
Right-sided type, with overriding pulmonary trunk
   without pulmonary stenosis
   with pulmonary stenosis
Intermediate type
Left-sided type

RIGHT-SIDED TYPE WITHOUT OVERRIDING PULMONARY TRUNK (FIG. 21). Here the pulmonary trunk emerges completely from the right ventricle, lying adjacent to the ventricular septal defect. The aorta also arises completely from the right ventricle removed from the ventricular septal defect. The vessels are situated side by side, or the aortic annulus lies anterior and to the right, and the pulmonary annulus posterior and to the left.

Ventricular Septal Defect. This defect is situated in the posterior part of the anterior septum involving part or all of the pars membranacea, with or without involvement of the anterior part of the anterior and the posterior septum.

Muscle Bundles of the Conus. The basic pattern is as follows. A septal band group proceeds to the base of the pulmonary trunk; here it divides into two prongs. The left upper prong circles around the anterior margin of the defect to meet the end of the first parietal band to be described. The right lower prong forms the floor of the defect and communicates with the first parietal band to be described. The right wall of the defect consists of musculature which passes into the left ventricle and is continuous with the first parietal band to be described. Thus what we are calling the first parietal band consists of muscle which separates the base of the aorta from the base of the pulmonic trunk, and proceeds over the anterior wall of the right ventricle. Continuous with the first parietal band there is a second

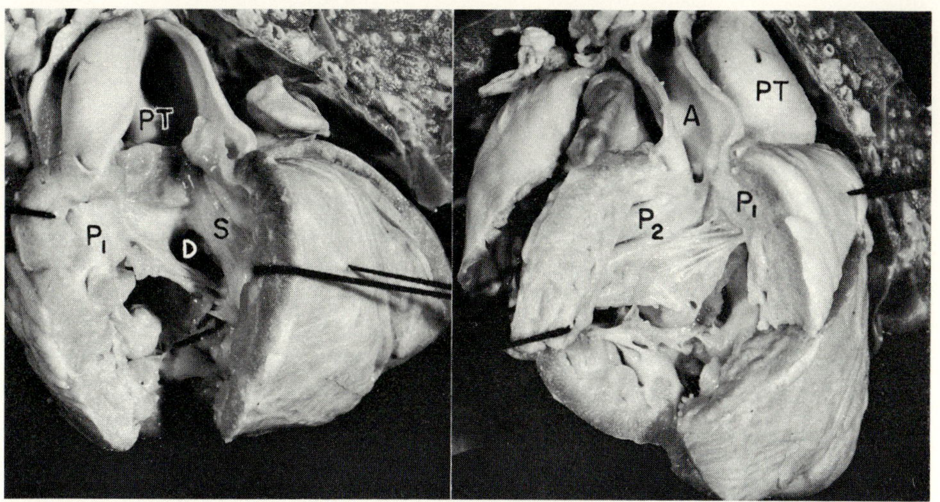

Fig. 21. Right-sided Taussig-Bing heart without overriding pulmonary trunk. Left, right ventricular view at outflow tract of pulmonary trunk. Right, right ventricular view at outflow tract of aorta. A, aorta; PT, pulmonary trunk; D, ventricular septal defect; S, septal band group; P_1, first parietal band; P_2, second parietal band.

parietal band lying beneath the aorta and related to the antero-lateral leaflet of the tricuspid valve. Thus a baffle-like structure lies beneath the aorta separating it from the ventricular septal defect.

The aorta and pulmonary trunk emerge at the same horizontal level. Neither vessel is related to the mitral valve.

THE RIGHT-SIDED TAUSSIG-BING COMPLEX.   The right atrium shows pressure hypertrophy and the right ventricle pressure and volume hypertrophy, while the left atrium and ventricle show volume hypertrophy. The tricuspid orifice is in some cases enlarged and in some cases smaller than normal. The pulmonic and mitral orifices are always enlarged; the aortic orifice may or may not be enlarged. All chambers may show focal endocardial hypertrophy. The tricuspid and pulmonic valves always show increased hemodynamic change, while the mitral valve may show such changes. We are dealing with the effects upon the heart of the right ventricle being related to peripheral and pulmonary resistance, and the left ventricle to pulmonary resistance, with bi-directional shunt at the ventricular level, and pulmonary hypertension.

RIGHT-SIDED TYPE WITH OVERRIDING PULMONARY TRUNK (FIG. 22).   Here there is no muscular rim on the top of the ventricular septal defect so that the pulmonary trunk straddles the ventricular septal defect but emerges mostly from the right ventricle. Thus the pulmonary trunk is at a somewhat lower (caudal) level than the aorta, and its annulus is partly or completely related to the mitral valve. Other findings are as in the previous type.

TAUSSIG-BING HEART WITH PULMONARY STENOSIS (FIG. 23).   In the four cases that I have seen these belong to the category of right-sided Taussig-Bing type. The infundibulum is compressed between the septal and first parietal bands producing infundibular stenosis with a small pulmonary trunk. With the decreased pulmo-

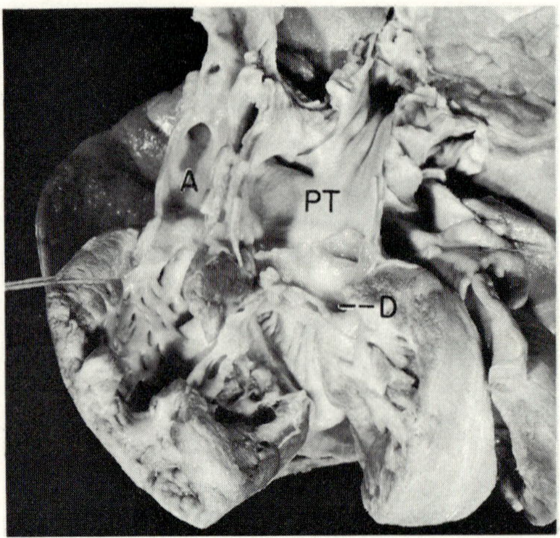

Fig. 22. Right-sided Taussig-Bing heart with overriding pulmonary trunk. Right ventricular view. Pt, pulmonary trunk; A, aorta; D, ventricular septal defect.

nary flow, the left side of the heart is atrophied. In one case there was an abnormal pulmonic valve with pulmonary valvular stenosis.

INTERMEDIATE TYPE. Here the pulmonary trunk straddles the ventricular septum, and it is difficult to say whether it emerges more from one side or the other.

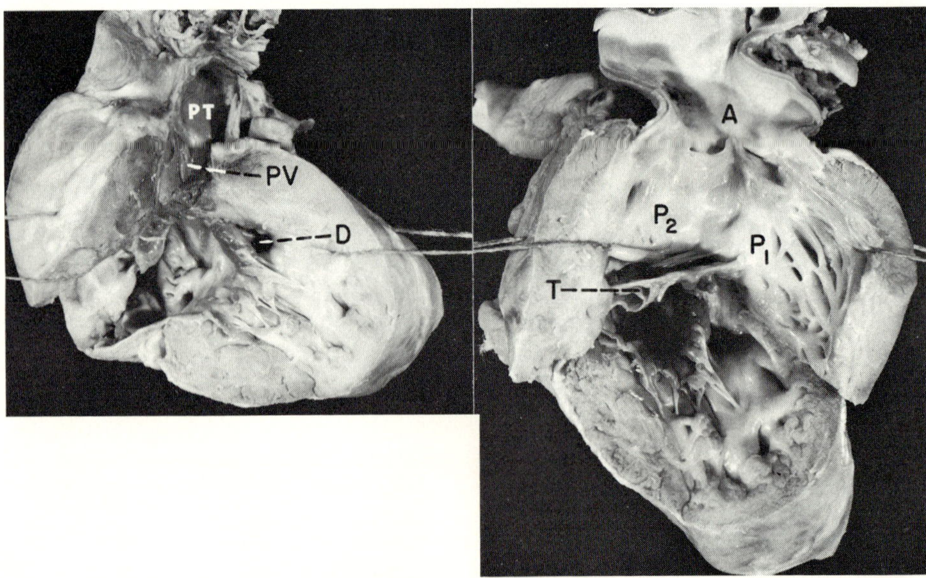

Fig. 23. Right-sided Taussig-Bing heart with pulmonary stenosis. Left, right ventricular view at outflow tract of pulmonary trunk. Right, right-sided Taussig-Bing anomaly at outflow tract of aorta. PT, pulmonary trunk; PV, pulmonary valve; D, ventricular septal defect; A, aorta; P_1, first parietal band; P_2, second parietal band; T, tricuspid valve.

The architecture of the musculature of the conus differs somewhat from the right-sided type. The first parietal band is more frontal and deviates somewhat toward the left lateral wall. The annulus of the pulmonary trunk is in all cases related to the mitral annulus, and it lies at a lower (more caudal) level compared to the aortic annulus. The other findings are like the previous types.

LEFT-SIDED TYPE (FIG. 24).   Here the pulmonary trunk emerges distinctly more from the left ventricle than from the right.

The architecture of the muscle bundles of the right ventricle differs somewhat from the intermediate type. The first parietal band is now almost in the same plane as the ventricular septum, but yet separated from it. It thus now resembles a septal band. The pulmonary annulus is now situated further downward in the left ventricle and occupies a lower level, compared to the aortic annulus. Otherwise this anomaly resembles the previous type. Quantitation of chambers reveals that the more the pulmonary trunk is shifted into the left ventricle, the greater is the ratio of muscle masses of $\frac{LV}{RV}$.

ASSOCIATED ABNORMALITIES IN TAUSSIG-BING COMPLEXES.   An atrial septal defect of the fossa ovalis type and a patent ductus arteriosus are frequently present. In some cases coarctation is found, and in others abnormalities in the mitral valve are apparent, consisting of clefting, or abnormal connections of the anterior leaflet on the septum, in some cases associated with mitral insufficiency. Also common is left superior vena cava entering the coronary sinus.

This author has also seen the following in Taussig-Bing complexes: bicuspid pulmonic valve, right aortic arch, tricuspid stenosis, straddling mitral orifice, and displaced right atrial appendage.

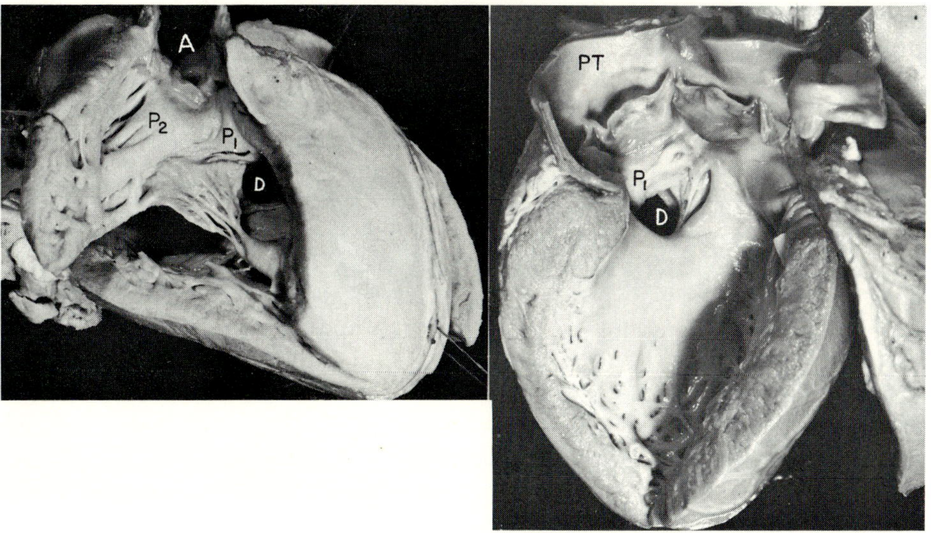

Fig. 24. Left-sided Taussig-Bing heart. Left, right ventricular view. Right, left ventricular view. PT, pulmonary trunk; P_1, first parietal band; P_2, second parietal band; D, ventricular septal defect; A, aorta.

THE CORONARY CIRCULATION IN TAUSSIG-BING HEART.   The right-sided type with overriding pulmonary trunk, the intermediate, and the left-sided types have a similar coronary artery distribution. The coronary ostia are rotated in a counterclockwise direction looking toward the ventricle from the aorta to a greater extent than in partial transposition. Thus the original embryological left coronary ostium is now situated in the posterior or right posterior sinus of Valsalva, while the original embryological right coronary ostium is situated in the left or left posterior sinus of Valsalva. In the majority of cases there is complete transfer of arteries between the two coronary arteries, as in complete transposition. Thus the embryological left (right-sided) ostium gives off the right circumflex, while the embryological right (left-sided) ostium gives off the anterior descending and left circumflex. In a minority of cases the transfer is not complete. However, in the right-sided type without overriding pulmonary trunk, the coronary circulation is either normal, as in partial transposition, or the left (right-sided) coronary ostium takes over the right circumflex.

Surgical Effects

A venous switch procedure, or banding of the pulmonary trunk, or excision of coarctation are performed in Taussig-Bing complexes without pulmonary stenosis, and shunting procedures in the complexes with pulmonary stenosis. Venous switch procedures will be discussed under complete transposition. The extent of the residual narrowing in operated coarctations should be noted.

Controversial Complexes

There is a group of complexes in which both vessels emerge from the right ventricle, but it is difficult to say anatomically which vessel is more related to the defect. Both vessels may be related to the defect, or neither may have such relationship. Since in our semantics the mutual positions of the defect and the vessels yield the terminology partial transposition and Taussig-Bing heart, it is clear that this terminology cannot be used in referring to those hearts. As alluded to above this is also true when no ventricular septal defect is present. Under these circumstances the appelation "double outlet right ventricle" might be more appropriate. One might then use the general terminology "double outlet right ventricle of the partial transposition type" or "double outlet right ventricle of the Taussig-Bing type" to designate the two distinct groups. For simplicity we prefer the terms partial transposition and Taussig-Bing where they pertain.

Complete Transposition

Complete transposition is a condition in which the aorta or its remnant emerges from the right ventricle and the pulmonary trunk or its remnant from the left. Complete transposition may be classified according to the presence or absence of ventricular septal defects, pulmonary stenosis, and abnormalities in the A-V orifices. Thus the classification might be as follows:

    I. With normal A-V orifices
        A. Simple with normal architecture
           1. Without ventricular septal defect
           2. With ventricular septal defect
           3. With pulmonary stenosis
           4. With pulmonary atresia (pseudotruncus)
        B. With common ventricle
        C. With single ventricle and small outlet chamber
    II. With abnormal A-V orifices
        A. With tricuspid stenosis or atresia
        B. With mitral stenosis or atresia
        C. With common A-V orifice (canal)

With Normal A-V Orifices

SIMPLE WITH NORMAL ARCHITECTURE. *Without Ventricular Septal Defect* (*Fig. 25*). In this complex, the architecture of the heart is the closest to the normal. The aorta emerges from the right ventricle, but not in the usual position of the pulmonary trunk. It emerges more toward the right of the right ventricle and at times is angulated toward the right. The pulmonary trunk emerges from the left ventricle, but not exactly in the position of the normal aorta. When the latter vessel emerges from the left ventricle it is usually angulated toward the right. In this complex, the pulmonary trunk emerges almost directly from this chamber. The two vessels in their upward course do not twist around each other, but are more or less parallel to each other. Usually the base of the aorta is situated anteriorly and to the right, and that of the pulmonary trunk posteriorly and to the left. Occasionally the aortic annulus is anterior and the pulmonary annulus posterior, or the aortic annulus is to the right and the pulmonary annulus to the left. The pulmonary annulus is

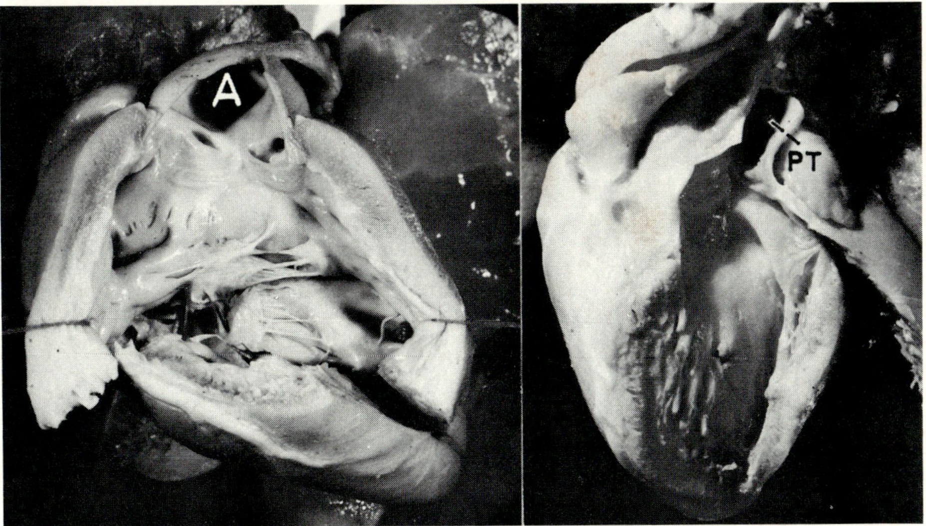

Fig. 25. Simple complete transposition without ventricular septal defect. Left, right ventricular view. Right, left ventricular view. A, aorta; PT, pulmonary trunk.

almost always related to the mitral annulus, while the aortic annulus is unrelated to either A-V annulus.

The architecture of the conus of the right ventricle resembles but is not identical with the architecture of the normal right ventricle. The septal and parietal bands form an arch which may be very similar to the normal, or often it has the following specific architecture. The septal band is in normal position but is more accentuated than the normal. The parietal band is in normal position but as it joins the septal band it forms most of the arch. Likewise the conus of the left ventricle varies somewhat from the normal. Whereas the conus of the normal left ventricle is somewhat angulated toward the right, in simple complete transposition without ventricular septal defect, the conus is more or less straight.

In almost all cases there is either a probe-patent or widely patent foramen ovale, and in most cases the ductus arteriosus is patent. The pulmonary trunk is larger than, equal to, or smaller than the aorta. There is usually hypertrophy and enlargement of all chambers.

Associated Abnormalities.   There may be a bicuspid or otherwise abnormal pulmonic valve, fetal coarctation, left superior vena cava entering the coronary sinus, abnormal tricuspid or mitral valves, and abnormal eustachian and thebesian valves. This author has also seen the following: abnormal aortic valve, aneurysm of the fossa ovalis, rete chiari, right aortic arch, tricuspid stenosis, and displaced right atrial appendage.

With Ventricular Septal Defect (Fig. 26).   The relationship of the arterial trunks to each other is the same as in the previous type. The architecture of the ventricles is more disturbed than in the previous complex, related to the presence of the ventricular septal defect. This defect may be situated in various spots. It may be found in the anterior septum, the posterior septum at the base, or in any part of the septum more apicalward. It may therefore enter the right ventricle without disturbing the arch, or it may alter the latter in various ways. When the defect is in the anterior septum, it opens into the right ventricle beneath the arch, or the arch may be mildly excavated or altered to the point of complete separation of the septal

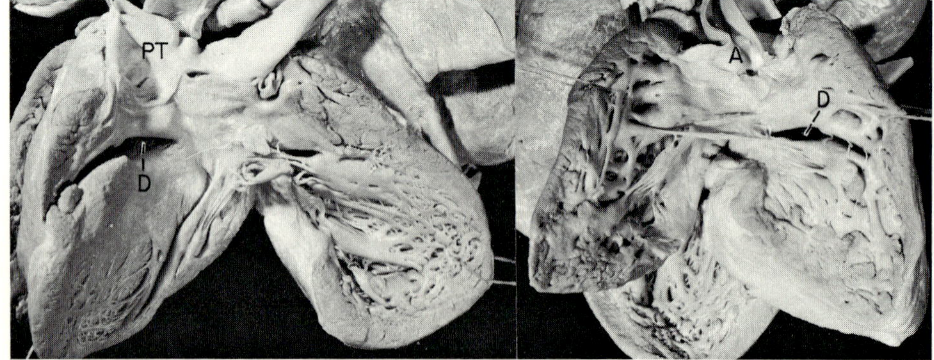

Fig. 26. Simple complete transposition with ventricular septal defect. Left, right ventricular view. Right, left ventricular view. A, aorta; PT, pulmonary trunk; D, ventricular septal defect.

and parietal bands. When the defect is more posteriorly at the base, it may alter the septal band. Frequently the defect is not related either to the aorta or to the pulmonary trunk. But it is more frequently related to the pulmonary trunk than to the aorta. Occasionally it may be related to both. When the defect is related to the pulmonary trunk, the complex must be differentiated from the left-sided Taussig-Bing complex. This is done by observing the architecture of the muscle bundles of the conus of the right ventricle. In complete transposition with ventricular septal defect there is a distinct septal band, whereas in the left-sided Taussig-Bing complex the first parietal band resembles a septal band, but in its migration (discussed above) it has not reached the septal band region. The foramen ovale is usually open, but the ductus arteriosus is often closed. A few cases show closure of both. There is hypertrophy and enlargement of all chambers.

Associated Abnormalities.   Fetal coarctation, displaced right atrial appendage, right aortic arch, and tricuspid stenosis may be present. This author has also seen the following in this complex: bicuspid aortic valve, bicuspid pulmonic valve, cleft aortic leaflet of the mitral valve, congenital aneurysm of the pars membranacea associated with the defect, double aortic arch, double mitral orifice, entry of coronary sinus into left atrium, aneurysm of the fossa ovalis, double ventricular septal defect, cirsoid aneurysm of origin of the coronary arteries, supraventricular ridge in left atrium, and straddling tricuspid orifice.

With Pulmonary Stenosis (Fig. 27).   The position of arterial trunks is more or less the same as in the previous types. In this complex, there is usually a ventricular septal defect which lies either in the anterior septum or between the anterior and posterior septum and separates off a separate conus-like chamber in

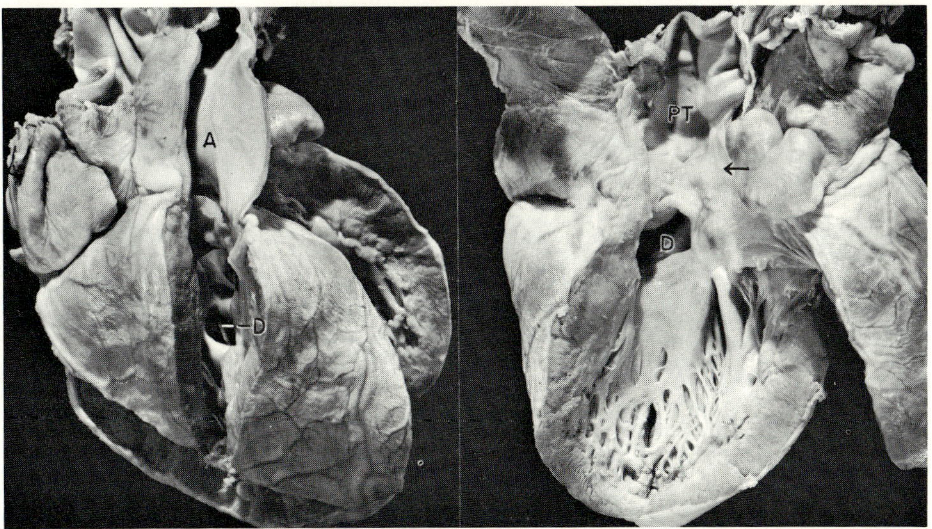

Fig. 27. Simple complete transposition with pulmonary stenosis. Left, right ventricular view. Right, left ventricular view. A, aorta; PT, pulmonary trunk; D, ventricular septal defect. Arrow points to the left infundibular stenosis. (From Lev et al. Pediatrics, 28:293, 1961.)

the left ventricle with fibroelastosis. This region is narrowed, and thus there is left infundibular stenosis. However, aside from this region, the basic architecture of the chambers is retained. The defect in general excavates the arch.

The pulmonary orifice is narrowed or normal, and the pulmonary trunk is smaller than or the same size as the aorta. Hypertrophy and enlargement of all chambers are present as in the previous types. However the muscle mass of the left ventricle is more increased than in the other types. The pulmonic valve is in some cases bicuspid or otherwise abnormally formed. An atrial septal defect may be present, but the ductus is usually closed.

Associated Abnormalities. A displaced right atrial appendage, aneurysm of the fossa ovalis, tricuspid stenosis, pulmonary valvular stenosis, and right aortic arch may be present.

COMPLETE TRANSPOSITION WITH COMMON VENTRICLE (FIG. 28). In this complex, there is almost complete absence of the posterior part of the ventricular septum, so that only a ridge remains carrying the conduction system. The anterior septum is represented by musculature reminiscent of the septal and parietal bands. Thus this common chamber receives both the mitral and tricuspid orifices, or it has a right or left entry component and gives rise to both the aorta and pulmonary trunk. The aortic annulus is situated anterior and to the right and the pulmonary posterior and to the left, or the two vessels are anterior-posterior. The aorta is smaller than the pulmonary trunk, unless there is pulmonary stenosis. The aorta is surrounded by the septal and parietal bands. This, in a sense, may limit the outflow tract into the aorta.

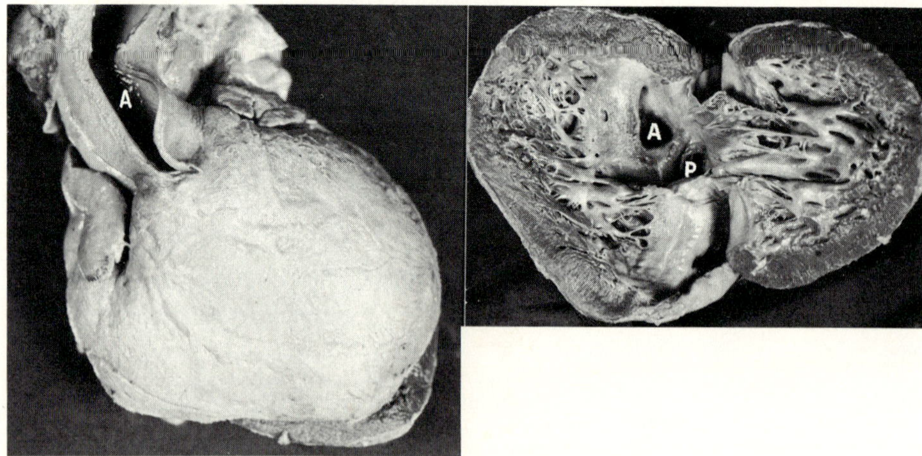

Fig. 28. Complete transposition with common ventricle. Left, anterior view. Right, common ventricular view. A, aorta; P, pulmonary trunk. (From Lev. Autopsy Diagnosis of Congenitally Malformed Hearts. 1953. Courtesy Charles C Thomas.)

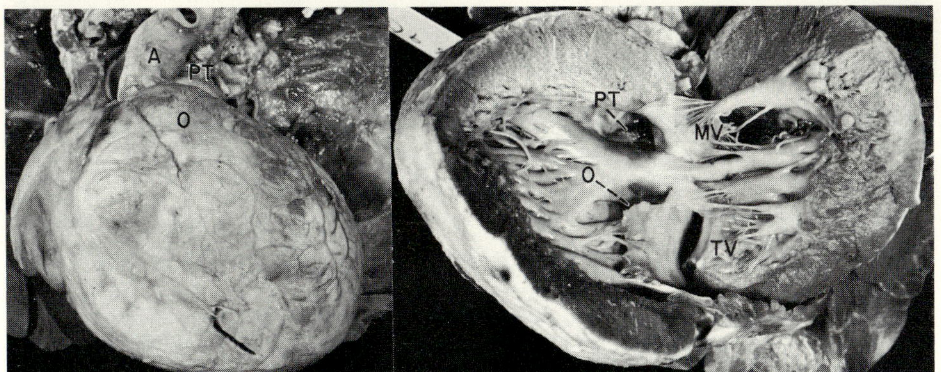

Fig. 29. Complete transposition with single ventricle and small outlet chamber. Left, anterior view. Right, view from single ventricle. A, aorta; PT, pulmonary trunk; O, small outlet chamber; TV, tricuspid orifice; MV, mitral orifice.

COMPLETE TRANSPOSITION WITH SINGLE VENTRICLE AND SMALL OUTLET CHAMBER (FIG. 29). In a previous publication, in discussing this anomaly no distinction was made between that with and that without bulbo-truncal inversion. This was a mistake. The entity now being described is without inverted transposition.

The heart here resembles the previous type except that the conal musculature separates off a small chamber, which communicates with the main chamber by way of a relatively small opening surrounded by conal musculature. This small chamber is situated anteriorly and to the right, and it gives rise to the aorta, while the large chamber receives both the mitral and tricuspid orifices, or has entry components related to the latter, and gives rise to the pulmonary trunk. The aortic annulus is situated anteriorly or anteriorly and to the right, while the pulmonary annulus is situated posteriorly or posteriorly and to the left. The inflow tracts of both the mitral and tricuspid valves are altered so that it is often difficult to decide which is mitral and which is tricuspid.

ASSOCIATED ABNORMALITIES. With common ventricle and with single ventricle and small outlet chamber, there may be tricuspid stenosis, double mitral orifice, and fetal coarctation.

With Abnormal A-V Orifices

Complete Transposition with Tricuspid Atresia or Stenosis (Fig. 30). It is possible to have mild tricuspid stenosis in simple complete transposition. This differs from complete transposition with severe stenosis or atresia. In the latter, the right ventricle consists of a conus structure with a small atrophic sinus. The conus structure gives rise to the aorta, while the pulmonary trunk arises from the

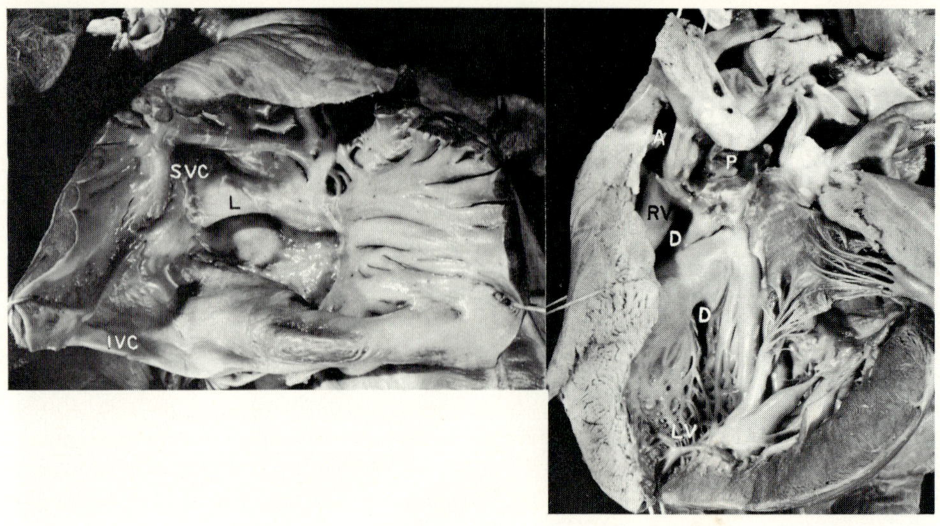

Fig. 30. Complete transposition with tricuspid atresia. Left, right atrial view. Right, left ventricular view. SVC, superior vena cava; L, limbus; ICV, inferior vena cava; A, aorta; P, pulmonary trunk; RV, right ventricle; D, ventricular septal defect; LV, left ventricle. (From Riker et al. J. Thor. & Cardiovas. Surg., 45:423, 1963.)

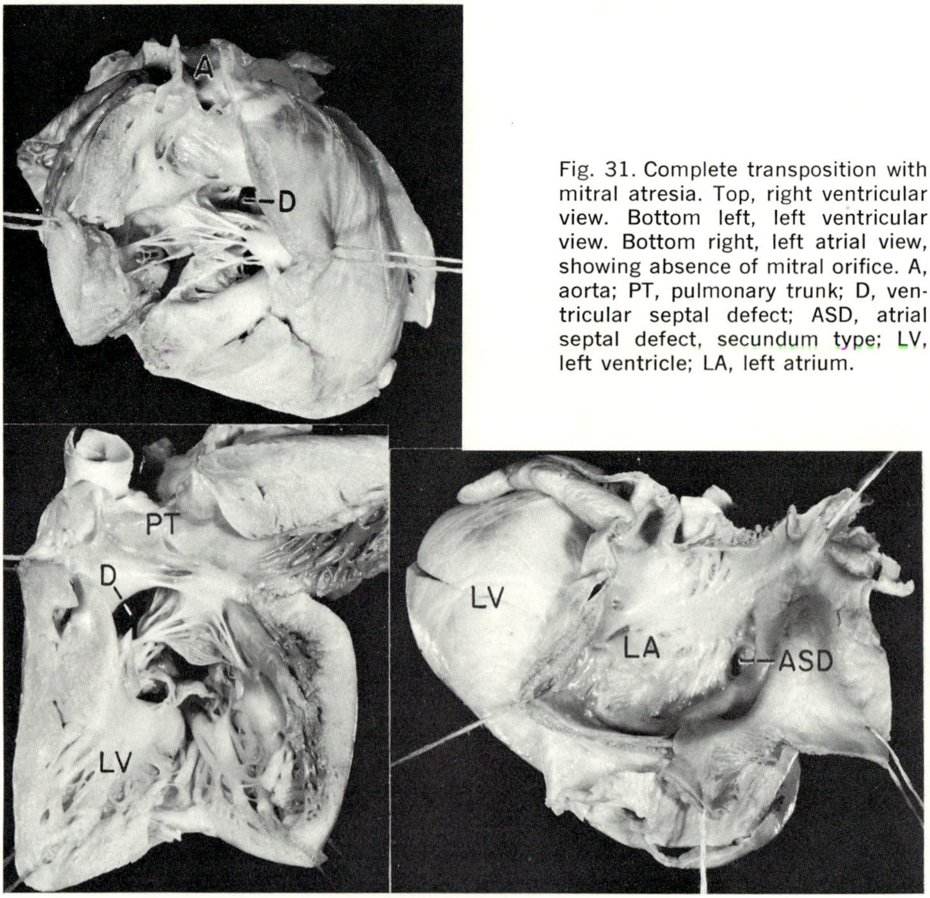

Fig. 31. Complete transposition with mitral atresia. Top, right ventricular view. Bottom left, left ventricular view. Bottom right, left atrial view, showing absence of mitral orifice. A, aorta; PT, pulmonary trunk; D, ventricular septal defect; ASD, atrial septal defect, secundum type; LV, left ventricle; LA, left atrium.

left ventricle. The aortic and pulmonary annuli are situated antero-posteriorly, or the aortic annulus is anterior and slightly to the left and the pulmonary annulus posterior and slightly to the right, or the aortic annulus is anterior and to the right and the pulmonary annulus posterior and to the left. There is an atrial septal defect of the fossa ovalis type, and usually one or more ventricular septal defects. The aorta is usually smaller than the pulmonary trunk. A rare variant of this is complete transposition with tricuspid and aortic atresia. In contrast to these types it is possible to have complete transposition with tricuspid and pulmonic atresia. In these latter cases, the ventricular septal defect is very large.

Associated Abnormalities.   There may be fetal coarctation, aneurysm of the fossa ovalis, displaced right atrial appendage, and right aortic arch. I have seen the following other abnormalities: cleft aortic leaflet of the mitral valve, persistent ostium primum, and straddling conus.

Complete Transposition with Mitral Stenosis or Atresia (Fig. 31).   In these cases there is usually a common ventricle or single ventricle with small outlet chamber and with pulmonary stenosis or atresia. A fossa ovalis defect is always present. Other abnormalities found are right aortic arch, left superior vena cava entering the coronary sinus, and straddling tricuspid orifice.

Complete Transposition with Common A-V Orifice (Fig. 32).   Here there may be separate right or left ventricles or a common ventricle, or single ventricle with small outlet chamber. Pulmonary stenosis or atresia has been present in all cases that I have seen, and total anomalous pulmonary venous drainage is a frequent concomitant. Other anomalies found are: right aortic arch, left superior vena cava entering the coronary sinus or the left atrium.

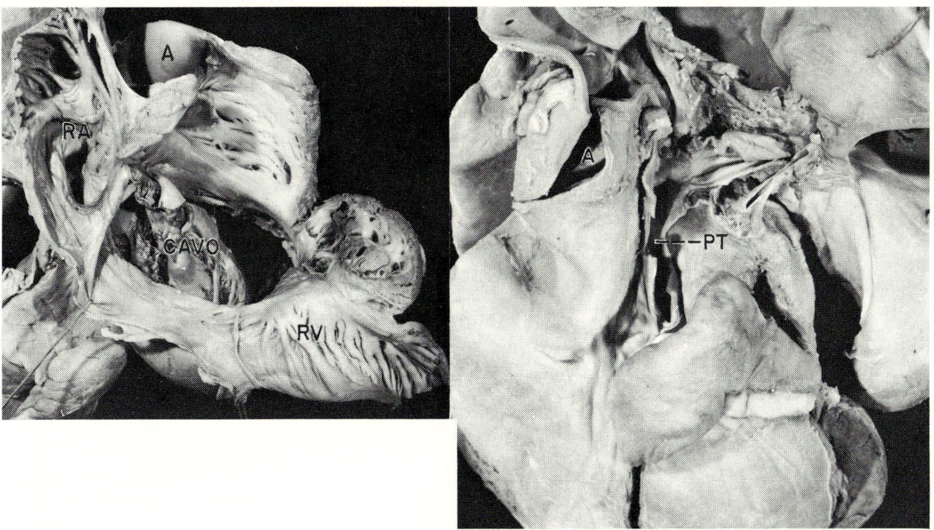

Fig. 32. Complete transposition with common A-V orifice with pulmonary atresia. Left, right atrial and right ventricular view. Right, view of aorta and pulmonary trunk anteriorly. RA, right atrium; RV, right ventricle; CAVO, common A-V canal with combined septal defect; A, aorta; PT, pulmonary trunk. (From Lev et al. Pediatrics, 28:293, 1961.)

The Coronary Arteries in Complete Transposition. The coronary ostia emerge from the posterior sinuses of Valsalva. The original embryological left coronary ostium emerges from the right posterior sinus of Valsalva and the original right coronary ostium from the left posterior sinus of Valsalva. In simple complete transposition in the majority of cases there is complete transfer of vessels from the embryological ostium to its fellow. In a minority of cases incomplete transfer occurs. A single coronary artery is again seen, probably with greater frequency than in the average population. In complete transposition with common ventricle, again there is this complete transfer, but no anterior and posterior descending coronary arteries may be present. In single ventricle and small outlet chamber, complete transfer of vessels is again seen. In addition the conus-like chamber is outlined by delimiting arteries. Complete transposition with abnormal A-V orifices has shown a coronary distribution system identical to simple complete transposition.

Surgical Effects

In simple complete transposition without pulmonary stenosis various venous switch procedures may be attempted. In the Baffes procedure the two right pulmonary veins are anastomosed to the right atrium, while the inferior vena cava is transferred to the left atrium by means of a prosthesis. The pathologist should note any obstruction to the outflow of these veins. With the lapse of time, the inferior vena cava may have a tendency to become obstructed. In the Mustard procedure, the proximal two thirds of the atrial septum is removed, and a pericardial graft is sewn in the resulting common atrium. Consequently all the pulmonary veins enter the right atrium, while the inferior and superior venae cavae enter into the left atrium. It is possible to find obstruction of the superior vena cava in this procedure. In the Blalock-Hanlon procedure, the proximal portion of the atrial septum is excised. A variant of this is the widening of a previous atrial septal defect. However, if there is pulmonary stenosis, shunting procedures may be done.

Inverted Transposition

Inverted transposition represents a disturbance in laterality as well as in anterior-posteriority. In all types of inverted transposition the arterial trunks are in mirror-image position as compared to a usual type of transposition. The most common type of inverted transposition is complete inverted transposition. I have also seen an instance of partial inverted transposition and inverted Taussig-Bing heart.

Complete inverted transposition may be associated with mixed levocardia with ventricular inversion, or with single ventricle and small outlet chamber with bulbotruncal inversion. In the first instance the entire ventricles, inlet and outlet, are inverted, while in the latter the inlet is normally placed or cannot be adequately diagnosed, and only the outlet and the arterial trunks are definitely inverted.

COMPLETE INVERTED TRANSPOSITION ASSOCIATED WITH MIXED LEVOCARDIA WITH VENTRICULAR INVERSION (FIG. 33). In these cases the aorta is situated distinctly to the left anterior, while the pulmonary trunk is situated to the right posterior. The trunks do not wind about each other but are more or less parallel to

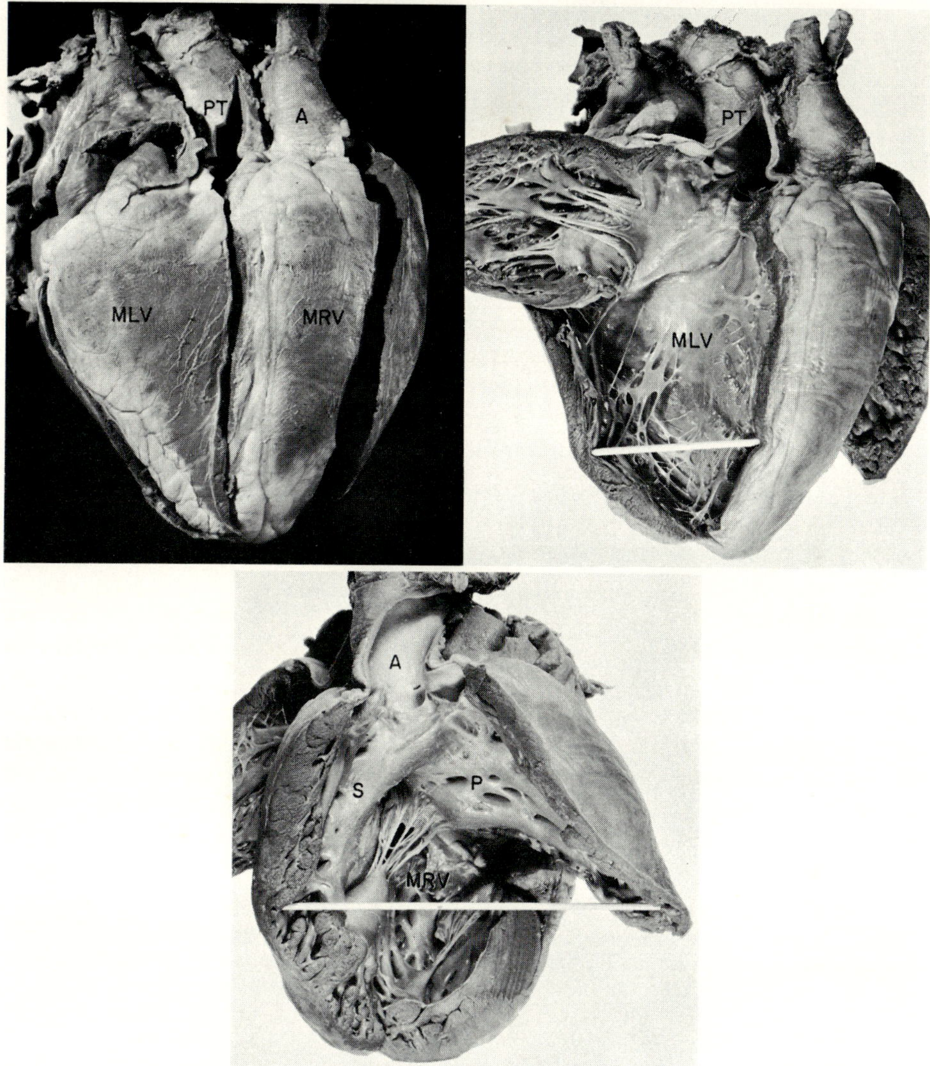

Fig. 33. Mixed levocardia with ventricular inversion, with complete, inverted transposition (corrected transposition). Top left, anterior view. Top right, morphological left (right-sided) ventricular view. Bottom, morphological right (left-sided) ventricular view. A, aorta; PT, pulmonary trunk; MLV, morphological left ventricle; MRV, morphological right ventricle; S, septal band group; P, parietal band group. (Top left, from Lev and Rowlatt. Amer. J. Cardiol., 8:216, 1961.)

each other. The right atrium is connected to the morphological left ventricle by way of a mitral orifice. The pulmonary trunk emerges from the morphological left ventricle. The left atrium is connected to a morphological right ventricle, and the aorta emerges from the latter chamber. The usual abnormalities which accompany this arrangement of chambers are: pulmonary stenosis with ventricular septal defect complex, left A-V valve (tricuspid) insufficiency complex, ventricular septal defect complex, tricuspid stenosis complex, and left-sided Ebstein's complex. Rarely the heart may show no functional abnormality.

COMPLETE INVERTED TRANSPOSITION ASSOCIATED WITH SINGLE VENTRICLE WITH SMALL OUTLET CHAMBER (FIG. 34).   The arterial trunks are related as in the previous type. The right atrium is either correctly connected by way of a tricuspid orifice with the right ventricular inlet, and likewise the left atrium with the left ventricular inlet, or the inlets cannot be adequately diagnosed. Only a small ridge which bears the conduction system demarcates off the two inlets. From the outlet of this single ventricle emerges the pulmonary trunk. A small conus chamber which gives rise to the aorta is situated to the left, anteriorly and superiorly. A defect communicates between the single ventricle and the small outlet chamber. A frequent variant of this is complete inverted transposition with single ventricle and small outlet chamber with left A-V valve stenosis or atresia (Fig. 35). It must be stressed that it is possible to have mixed levocardia with atrial or ventricular inversion with complete noninverted transposition.

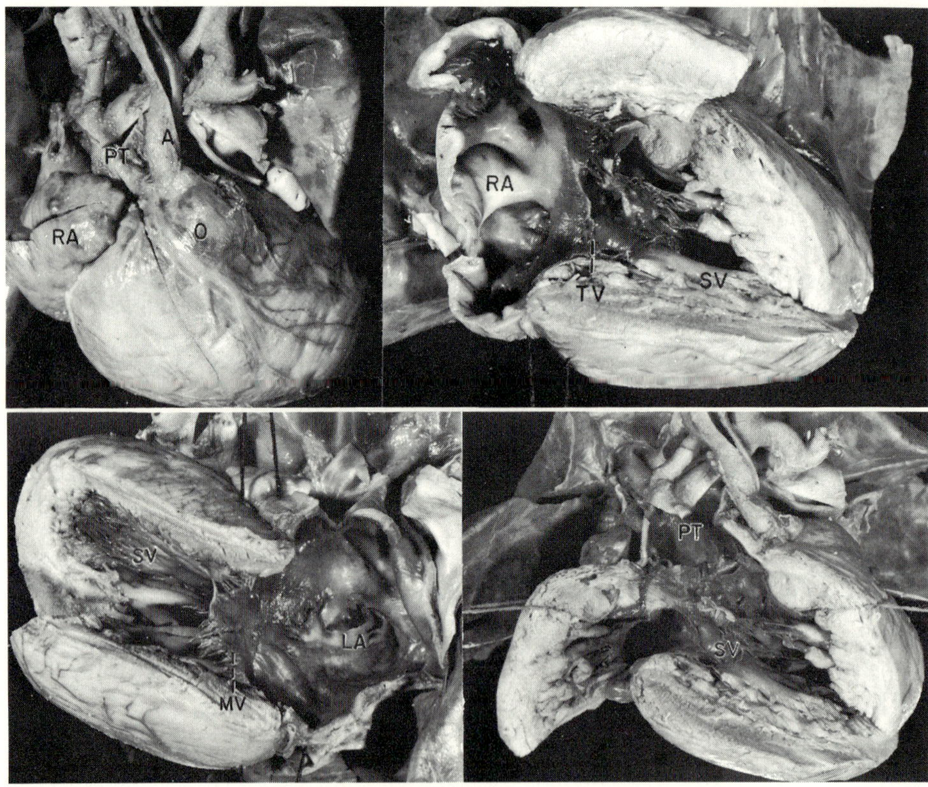

Fig. 34. Single ventricle and small outlet chamber with trunco-conal inversion. Top left, anterior view. Top right, right atrial and single ventricle view. Bottom left, left atrium and single ventricle view. Bottom right, single ventricle view. A, aorta; PT, pulmonary trunk; O, small outlet chamber; RA, right atrium; SV, single ventricle; TV, tricuspid valve; MV, mitral valve; LA, left atrium.

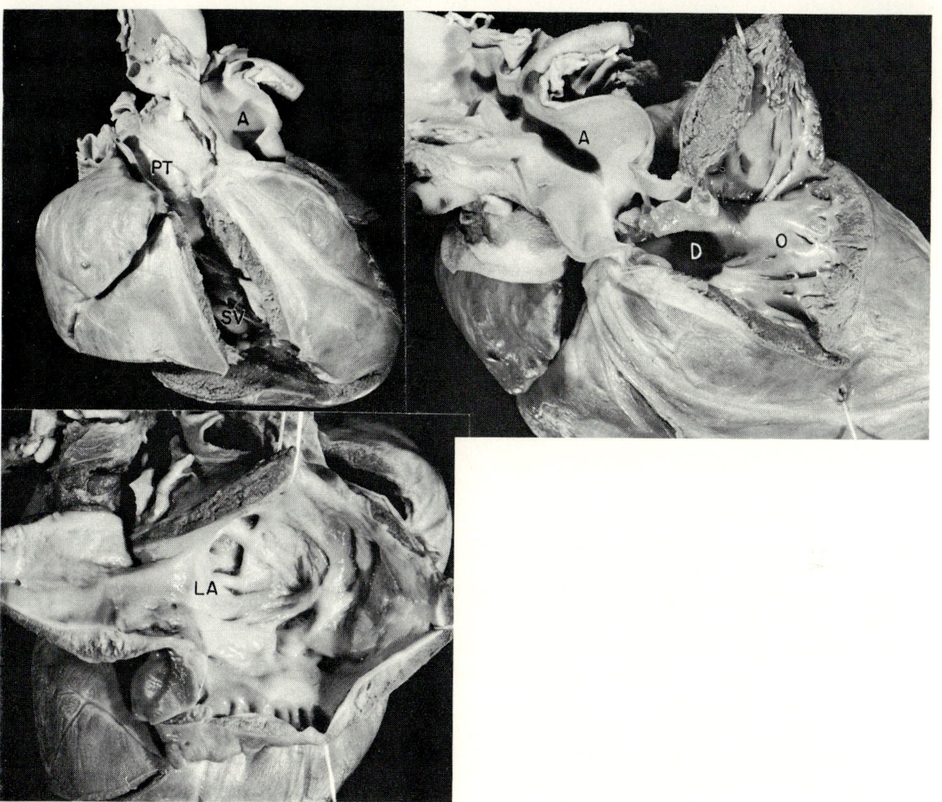

Fig. 35. Single ventricle and small outlet chamber with complete inverted transposition and left A-V valve atresia. Top left, anterior view. Top right, view of small outlet chamber. Bottom, left atrial view showing absence of left A-V valve. A, aorta; PT, pulmonary trunk; SV, single ventricle; D, ventricular septal defect; O, small outlet chamber; LA, left atrium.

THE CORONARY ARTERIES IN INVERTED TRANSPOSITION. The left-sided coronary artery emerges from the posterior sinus and the right-sided coronary artery emerges from the right anterior sinus of Valsalva. The anterior descending coronary artery is given off from the right side of the aorta, from the right-sided coronary artery.

Horizons

The purpose of a classification is to identify an entity by similarity and difference. In each discipline, an attempt at classification is made from the vantage point of the data offered by that discipline. At the same time there is the necessity of dialogue between disciplines.

The present classification is offered basically to aid the pathologist. At the same time it has been modified in various ways to make it useful to clinicians and surgeons. This is the reason why an anatomic base rather than an embryological or pathogenetic one is used. Anatomic data are easily translatable into clinical and surgical data. Although a knowledge of the pathogenesis helps to understand the anatomy of an anomaly, yet similar anatomies may have different pathogenesis. Furthermore, in the case of transposition of the arterial trunks, the pathogenesis is shrouded in controversy. In my opinion, pathogenesis should not be used as a basis of classification of transposition complexes.

At the present time, in this group of complexes, there are numerous classifications. It would be most useful if the nomenclature were standardized, in order to make dialogue possible between all disciplines. The presently offered classification is an attempt in this direction.

References

1. Lev, M., and Saphir, O. Transposition of the large vessels. J. Tech. Meth., 17:126, 1937.
2. Harris, J. S., and Farber, S. Transposition of the great cardiac vessels with special reference to the phylogenetic theory of Spitzer. Arch. Path. (Chicago), 28:427, 1939.
3. Lev, M., and Saphir, O. A theory of transposition of the arterial trunks based on the phylogenetic and ontogenetic development of the heart. Arch. Path. (Chicago), 39:172, 1945.
4. Taussig, H. B. Congenital malformations of the heart. The Commonwealth Fund, New York, 1947.
5. Shaner, R. F. Malformation of the atrioventricular endocardial cushion of the embryo pig and its relation to defects of the conus and truncus arteriosus. Amer. J. Anat., 84:431, 1949.
——— Complete and corrected transposition of the aorta, pulmonary artery and ventricles in pig embryos, and a case of corrected transposition in a child. Amer. J. Anat., 88:35, 1951.
6. Doerr, W. Die angeborenen Herzfehler. Pathologische Anatomie typischer Grundformen angeborener Herzfehler. Mschr. Kinderheilk., 100:107, 1952.
7. Goerttler, K. Hämodynamische Untersuchungen über die Entstehung der Missbildungen des arteriellen Herzendes. Virchow Arch. Path. Anat., 328:391, 1956.
——— Die Missbildungen des Herzens und der grossen Gefässe. *In* Das Herz des Menschen. Bargmann, W., and Doerr, W., eds., Stuttgart, Georg Thieme Verlag, 1963, Vol. 1.
8. Cardell, B. S. Corrected transposition of the great vessels. Brit. Heart J., 18:186, 1956.
9. De la Cruz, M. V., and Da Rocha, J. P. An ontogenetic theory for the explanation of congenital malformations involving the truncus and conus. Amer. Heart J., 51:782, 1956.
——— Anselmi, G., Cisneros, F., Reinhold, M., Portillo, B., and Espino-Vela, J. An embryologic explanation for the corrected transposition of the great vessels: Additional description of the main anatomic features of the malformation and its varieties. Amer. Heart J., 57:104, 1959.
10. Witham, A. C. Double outlet right ventricle; a partial transposition complex. Amer. Heart J., 53:928, 1957.
11. Edwards, J. E. Congenital malformations of the heart and great vessels. *In* Pathology of the Heart, 2nd ed. Gould, S. E., ed., 1960, p. 260.
12. Neufeld, H. N., DuShane, J. W., Wood, E. H., Kirklin, J. W., and Edwards, J. E. Origin of both great vessels from the right ventricle. I. Without pulmonary stenosis. Circulation, 23:399, 1961.
——— DuShane, J. W., and Edwards, J. E. Origin of both great vessels from the right ventricle. II. With pulmonary stenosis. Circulation, 23:603, 1961.

13. Grant, R. P. The morphogenesis of transposition of the great vessels. Circulation, 26:819, 1962.
    ———— The morphogenesis of corrected transposition and other anomalies of cardiac polarity. Circulation, 29:71, 1964.
14. De Vries, P. A., and Saunders, J. B. de C. M. Development of the ventricles and spiral outflow tract in the human heart. Contributions to Embryology, No. 256, Carnegie Institute of Washington, 37:84, 1962.
15. Van Mierop, L. H. S., and Wiglesworth, F. W. Pathogenesis of transposition complexes. II. Anomalies due to faulty transfer of the posterior great artery. Amer. J. Cardiol., 12:226, 1963.
    ———— Pathogenesis of transposition complexes. III. True transposition of the great vessels. Amer. J. Cardiol., 12:233, 1963.
16. Shaher, R. M. The syndromes of corrected transposition of the great vessels. Brit. Heart J., 25:431, 1963.
    ———— Complete and inverted transposition of the great vessels. Brit. Heart J., 26:51, 1964.
17. Rosenbaum, H. D. A simplified basic classification of spatial alignments of the heart, its chambers, and the great vessels. Circulation, 30:194, 1964.
18. Van Praagh, R., Ongley, P. A., and Swan, H. J. C. Anatomic types of single or common ventricle in man. Morphologic and geometric aspects of sixty autopsied cases. Amer. J. Cardiol., 13:367, 1964.
    ———— Van Praagh, S., Vlad, P., and Keith, J. D. Anatomic types of congenital dextrocardia. Diagnostic and embryologic implications. Amer. J. Cardiol., 13:510, 1964.
    ———— and Van Praagh, S. The anatomy of common aorticopulmonary trunk (Truncus arteriosus communis) and its embryologic implications. A study of 57 necropsied cases. Amer. J. Cardiol., 16:406, 1965.
19. Lev, M., and Saphir, O. Congenital aneurysm of the membranous septum. Arch. Path. (Chicago), 25:819, 1938.
    Saphir, O., and Lev, M. Tetralogy of Eisenmenger. Amer. Heart J., 21:31, 1941.
    Lev, M., and Saphir, O. Truncus arteriosus communis persistens. J. Pediat., 20:74, 1943.
    ———— and Volk, B. W. The pathologic anatomy of the Taussig-Bing heart: Riding pulmonary artery. Report of a case. Bull. Internat. Am. Med. Mus., 31:54, 1950.
    ———— Autopsy Diagnosis of Congenitally Malformed Hearts. Springfield, Ill., Charles C Thomas, 1953.
    ———— The pathologic anatomy of cardiac complexes associated with transposition of arterial trunks. Lab. Invest., 2:296, 1953.
    ———— The pathologic diagnosis of positional variations in cardiac chambers in congenital heart disease. Lab. Invest., 3:71, 1954.
    ———— Congenital heart disease. *In* Systemic Pathology. Saphir, O., ed., New York, Grune & Stratton, 1958, Vol. 1, p. 127.
    ———— Pathology of congenital heart disease. *In* Cardiology. Clinical Cardiology. Luisada, A. A., ed., McGraw-Hill Book Co., Inc., New York, 1959, Vol. 3, p. 15.
    ———— Alcalde, V. M., and Baffes, T. G. Pathologic anatomy of complete transposition of the arterial trunks. Pediatrics, 28:293, 1961.
    ———— and Rowlatt, U. F. The pathologic anatomy of mixed levocardia. A review of thirteen cases of atrial or ventricular inversion with or without corrected transposition. Amer. J. Cardiol., 8:216, 1961.
    ———— Agustsson, M. H., and Arcilla, R. The pathologic anatomy of a common atrioventricular orifice associated with tetralogy of Fallot. Amer. J. Clin. Path., 36:408, 1961.
    Riker, W. L., Potts, W. J., Grana, L., Miller, R. A., and Lev, M. Tricuspid stenosis or atresia complexes: A surgical-pathologic analysis. J. Thor. Cardiov. Surg., 45:423, 1963.

Lev, M., and Eckner, F. A. O. The pathologic anatomy of tetralogy of Fallot and its variations. Dis. Chest, 45:251, 1964.

———— Rimoldi, H. J. A., and Rowlatt, U. F. The quantitative anatomy of cyanotic tetralogy of Fallot. Circulation, 30:531, 1964.

Gasul, B. M., Arcilla, R. A., and Lev, M. Heart Disease in Children; Diagnosis and Treatment. Philadelphia, J. B. Lippincott Co., 1966.

Meng, C. C. L., Eckner, F. A. O., and Lev, M. The coronary artery distribution in tetralogy of Fallot. Arch. Surg. (Chicago), 90:363, 1965.

Lev, M., Eckner, F. A. O., Meng, C. C. L., and Rimoldi, H. J. A. Partial transposition complexes (Abstract). Amer. J. Cardiol., 15:136, 1965.

———— Rimoldi, H. J. A., Eckner, F. A. O., Melhuish, B. P., Meng, C. C. L., and Paul, M. H. The Taussig-Bing heart; qualitative and quantitative anatomy. Arch. Path. (Chicago), 81:24, 1966.

Navarro Lopez, F., Dobben, G. G., Rabinowitz, M., Ferguson, L. A., Reisler, H., Cassels, D. E., and Lev, M. Taussig-Bing complex with pulmonary stenosis. Dis. Chest., 50:1, 1966.

20. Abbott, M. E. Congenital heart disease. *In* Osler's Modern Medicine. Philadelphia, Lea and Febiger, 1927.

21. Rokitansky, C. V. Die Defecte der Scheidewände des Herzens. Wien, W. Braumüller, 1875.

22. Spitzer, A. Über den Bauplan des normalen und missbildeten Herzens. Versuch einer phylogenetischen Theorie. Virchow Arch. Path. Anat., 243:81, 1923. Translated by Lev, M., and Vass, A. Springfield, Ill., Charles C Thomas, 1951.

Addendum

Since the preceding article was written we have studied more fully double outlet right ventricle,[1,2] truncus communis,[3] and pseudotruncus.[4] This slightly alters the concept of transposition as given above.

We have enlarged the definition of transposition of the arterial trunks to be as follows: Transposition is that condition in which the arterial trunks are abnormally placed vis-à-vis each other, and/or vis-à-vis the chambers from which they emerge, and/or vis-à-vis the atrioventricular (AV) orifices. The purpose of the last addition is to make more full the concept of single ventricle with transposition.

Double Outlet Right Ventricle

We look upon double outlet right ventricle as that condition in which both arterial trunks emerge completely or almost completely from the right ventricle, and there may or may not be mitral-aortic or mitral-pulmonic continuity. From this point of view, there is a spectrum of heart entities, commencing with ventricular septal defect (VSD) and overriding aorta with or without pulmonary stenosis, which gradually enter into the realm of double outlet right ventricle, proceed from there into the Taussig-Bing heart, and finally become complete transposition.

Double outlet right ventricle is then classified as follows:

With subaortic VSD
  Without pulmonary stenosis
  With pulmonary stenosis
With subpulmonic VSD
  Without pulmonary stenosis
  With pulmonary stenosis
With doubly committed VSD
With noncommitted VSD
Complicated types
  With total anomalous pulmonary venous drainage
  With common AV orifice or ostium primum defect
    With pulmonary stenosis
    With aortic hypoplasia
  With mitral atresia or stenosis
    With pulmonary stenosis
      Without VSD
      With VSD
    With aortic stenosis or hypoplasia
      Without VSD
      With VSD
Combined complicated type

This conception implies that some Taussig-Bing hearts such as the right ventricular type are also examples of double outlet right ventricle, while others such as the intermediate and left ventricular types are transitional hearts which may be grouped separately and represent a transition to complete transposition. The term doubly committed implies that the VSD is related to both the aorta and the pulmonary trunk, and the term noncommitted implies that the defect is related to neither vessel.

Truncus Arteriosus Communis

In our recent studies we have enlarged our concept of this entity. In addition to the factors we dealt with in our original consideration in this study we now consider more fully the nature of the truncus valve, the presence or absence of truncal stenosis or insufficiency, and the presence or absence of VSD stenosis.

The truncal valve was in a majority of cases tricuspid, less commonly quadricuspid, and still less commonly bicuspid. The bicuspid and quadricuspid valves were more thickened and nodular than the tricuspid valves. Truncus stenosis and insufficiency were occasionally noted, as was VSD stenosis.

Pseudotruncus

We have recently expanded the concept of pseudotruncus. Pseudotruncus is basically pulmonary atresia with ventricular septal defect, with the aorta emerging in an overriding position or completely from the right ventricle Pseudotruncus may be simple or complex in levocardia. In the complex form there may be complete transposition with common atrioventricular orifice and pulmonary atresia, or the pseudotruncus may be associated with tricuspid or mitral atresia or single or common ventricle. In all forms of pseudotruncus, the pathologist should note: (1) the size of the right and left pulmonary arteries, (2) the origin of the aorta, (3) the bronchial circulation, and (4) the size of the left heart.

Single Ventricle

The statement made above about the conduction system being in the posterior ridge is erroneous. Recent work has shown that the AV node is situated anteriorly adjacent to the pulmonary annulus.[5] The bundle of His passes through the annulus to be on the septum between the small outlet chamber and the main chamber. There it divides into left and right bundle branches.

References

1. Lev M, Bharati S, Meng CCL, Liberthson RR, Paul MH, et al: A concept of double-outlet right ventricle. J Thorac Cardiovasc Surg 64:271, 1972
2. Lev M, Bharati S· Double outlet right ventricle associated with other cardiovascular anomalies. AMA Arch Path 95:117, 1973
3. Bharati S, McAllister HA, Jr, Rosenquist GC, Miller RA, Tatooles CJ, et al: The surgical anatomy of truncus arteriosus communis. J Thorac Cardiovasc Surg 67:501, 1974
4. Bharati S, Paul MH, Idriss FS, Potkin RT, Lev M: The surgical anatomy of pulmonary atresia with ventricular septal defect — pseudotruncus. J Thorac Cardiovasc Surg, 69:713, 1975
5. Bharati S, Lev M: The course of the conduction system in single ventricle with inverted (L-) Loop and inverted (L-) transposition. Circulation 51:723, 1975

IDIOPATHIC ARTERIAL CALCIFICATION OF INFANCY: A CLINICOPATHOLOGIC STUDY

JOHN J. MORAN

Idiopathic arterial calcification of infancy is a rare disease of undetermined etiology characterized by deposition of calcific material along the internal elastic membrane of arteries and accompanied by simultaneous proliferation of the fibrous tissue of the intima resulting in luminal narrowing. These arterial changes are widespread throughout the arteries of the body with the exception of those of the brain. Despite generalized involvement of the arterial tree, the salient clinical features and the patient's death are invariably due to involvement of the coronary arteries with resultant myocardial ischemia.

This idiopathic group of calcific arterial disease of infancy was clearly described by Stryker in 1946 [52] when, in reviewing the literature, he found a total of 15 cases, to which he added five cases from his own experience. To date, about 62 examples of this disease have been recorded in the literature (Table 1).

Age. The age of patients dying of calcific arterial disease of infancy has ranged from 3 days to 28 months, with 85 percent of patients dying within the first 6 months of life. Only three cases have been reported beyond 11 months of age (Table 1). There are three instances in which this disease occurred in premature infants.[25, 33, 52]

Sex. Idiopathic arterial calcification of infancy appears to involve both sexes equally: 27 reported cases are males and 27 are females (Table 1).

Race. Two cases of idiopathic arterial calcification of infancy were reported in the Negro race;[44, 60] the remainder were Caucasians.

Heredity. Four reports of idiopathic calcific arterial disease have been recorded in siblings.[24, 34, 38, 55] Several other authors [8, 14, 24, 37, 52] reported the sudden death of a sibling infant but autopsies were not performed. In one such case, Meurman and coauthors [37] recorded the death of a sibling at the age of 6 weeks of symptoms similar to those of their reported case of idiopathic calcific arterial disease of infancy. These two siblings are of further interest since definite consanguinity was found in this family. The mother's maternal grandfather and father's father

TABLE 1. Review of Findings in Cases from the Literature

Case No.	Author	Age	Sex	Organs Having Arterial Calcification	Changes in Other Organs	Clinical Findings
1	Surbeck[53]	3 days	M	Heart	Pericarditis, visceral calcification, splenomegaly, "focal glomerulonephritis"	Sudden death
2	Verocay[62]	5 3/4 mo	F	Heart, "abdominal organs"	"Hydrocephalus?" No evidence of syphilis	Wassermann 1+
3	Hughes and Perry[22]	7 wk	F	Heart		Sudden respiratory distress and death
4	Forrer[14]	3 mo	M	Heart	Fatty change of myocardium, low-grade glomerulonephritis	Navel granuloma, splenomegaly
5	Ramsay and Crumrine[47]	9 wk	F	None	Myocardial infarct, cardiac enlargement	Previous respiratory infection, sudden death
6	Iff[25]	1 day	M	Heart, viscera	Anasarca, abnormal aorta	
7	Oppenheimer, I[43]	6 mo	F	Heart	Cardiac enlargement, myocardial fibrosis	Sudden death
8	Oppenheimer, II[43]	4 mo	F	Heart	Myocardial fibrosis, slight cardiac enlargement	Heart failure of 24-hr duration
9	Baggenstoss and Keith[2]	5 wk	F	Heart, kidney, mesentery adrenal	Cardiac enlargement, myocardial necrosis and fibrosis	Vomiting, abdominal distention, dehydration
10	van Creveld[11]	6 wk	F	Heart	Cardiac enlargement, thrombosis of coronary artery, fatty change of myocardium, focal glomerular changes	Respiratory distress of 4-wk duration
11	Brown and Richter[5]	3½ mo	M	Heart	"Swelling of glomeruli and tubular epithelium"	Vomiting, illness of 24-hr duration

12	Scott and Miller[50]	11 mo	M	Heart, kidney, pancreas	Thrombosis of coronary artery, myocardial infarct, and fibrosis	Respiratory distress and vomiting of 2-day duration
13	Field[13]	10 wk	F	Heart, kidney, spleen, pancreas, mesentery, adrenal, lung		Debility and wasting of 1-wk duration
14	Stryker, I[52]	3 mo	M	Heart, kidney, lung, spleen	Thrombosis of splenic vein	"Pneumonia" of 3-day duration
15	Stryker, II[52]	4 mo	F	Heart, spleen	Bronchopneumonia, no anatomic evidence of syphilis	Kahn 4+, fever, diarrhea
16	Stryker, III[52]	6 mo	M	Heart, spleen, peri-adrenal fibrous tissue	Pneumonia	Feeding problem, jaundice, weakness
17	Stryker, V[52]	7 mo	F	Heart, kidney, lung, pancreas, periadrenal fibrous tissue	Cardiac enlargement, pneumonia, pulmonary edema	"Chronic cold," sudden death
18	Donat[12]	8 wk	F	Mesentery, spleen, kidney, thyroid	Cardiac enlargement, myocardial infarction	Respiratory distress
19	Hause and Antell[20]	4 mo	M	Heart, kidney, mesentery, spleen, periadrenal and parathyroidal fibrous tissue	Thrombosis of coronary artery	Respiratory distress of 2-day duration
20	Menten and Fetterman I[34]	54 days	M	Heart, kidney, lung, mesentery	Cardiac enlargement, occasional fibrosed glomeruli	Sudden respiratory distress and death
21	Menten and Fetterman, II[34]	53 days	M	Heart	Cardiac enlargement, occasional fibrosed glomeruli	Low-grade fever and dyspnea of 3-day duration
22	Menten and Fetterman, III[34]	70 days	M	Heart, kidney, lung	Myocardial infarct	Sudden respiratory distress and death
23	Prior and Bergstrom, I[46]	4 wk	F	Heart, lung, spleen, uterus, periadrenal fibrous tissue	Slight cardiac enlargement, myocardial fibrosis	Regurgitation, intermittent respiratory distress

TABLE 1. (*cont.*)

Case No.	Author	Age	Sex	Organs Having Arierial Calcification	Changes in Other Organs	Clinical Findings
24	Prior and Bergstrom, II[46]	3 mo	F	Heart, pancreas, peri-adrenal fibrous tissue	Myocardial infarct, some glomerular reaction	Sudden respiratory distress and death
25	Lipman et al [31]	5 mo	M	Heart, lung, periadrenal fibrous tissue	Myocardial infarct, endocardial fibrosis	Poor nutrition, cough, fever, weight loss
26	Wahlgren[59]	41 days	F	Heart, mesentery, spleen, adrenal	Moderate cardiac enlargement, myocardial myelomalacia, acute pericarditis, endocardial fibrosis	Illness of 2-day duration, tachycardia
27	Sladden, I[51]	18 mo	M	Heart, kidney, tongue, pancreas	Cardiac enlargement, infarct of kidney	Slight respiratory distress edema of feet, fever, vomiting, 4-mo illness
28	Sladden, II[51]	3 mo	M	Heart, kidney, mesentery spleen, pancreas, adrenal, extremities	Myocardial infarct	Sudden respiratory distress acute abdominal crisis (?), negative celiotomy
29	Mant et al[33]	8 mo	F	Heart	Cardiac enlargement myocardial infarct and fibrosis, pulmonary edema	Anorexia and weight loss of 2-mo duration, sudden respiratory distress
30	Cochrane and Bowden, I[10]	7 mo	?	Heart, kidney	Cardiac enlargement	Respiratory distress, 5-day illness
31	Cochrane and Bowden, II[10]	3 mo	?	Heart	Cardiac enlargement, pulmonary edema	Respiratory distress of 12-hr duration
32	Cochrane and Bowden, III[10]	1 mo	?	Heart, kidney	Cardiac enlargement	Respiratory distress of 1-day duration
33	Cochrane and Bowden, IV[10]	3 mo	?	Heart	Cardiac enlargement, few scarred glomeruli	Respiratory distress of 3-day duration
34	Cochrane and Bowden, V[10]	4 days	?	Heart	Cardiac enlargement	Respiratory distress of 4-day duration
35	Cochrane and Bowden, VI[10]	5 mo	?	Heart	Cardiac enlargement, slight interstitial and glomerular fibrosis	Respiratory distress for (?) 3 mo

36	Leach[29]	9 mo	M	Heart, kidney, periadrenal fat, spleen	Myocardial infarct, bronchopneumonia	Respiratory distress, mild fever, anorexia of 36-hr duration
37	Zischka[63]	4 mo	M	Aorta, lung, carotid and lingual arteries		Fever
38	Weens and Marin, I[60]	16 mo	M	Heart, kidney, spleen, adrenal	Cardiac enlargement, myocardial fibrosis	
39	Weens and Marin, II[60]	25 days	M	Heart, kidney, pancreas, adrenal, thyroid	Cardiac enlargement, myocardial fibrosis, infarct of kidney	Subarachnoid hemorrhage, illness of several days' duration
40	Traisman et al[57]	8 wk	F	Heart, thyroid, adrenal		Vomiting, cough, dehydration
41	Thomas et al[55]	2 mo	M	Heart, pancreas, skeleton	Cardiac enlargement, myocardial infarct	Heart failure for 2 wk
42	Thomas et al[55]	3 mo	M	Heart	Cardiac enlargement, myocardial infarct	Respiratory distress for 12 hr
43	Holm[23]	28 mo	M	Heart	Cardiac enlargement, myocardial fibrosis,	Poor appetite, attacks of dyspnea, ECG changes, hypertension
44	Hunt and Leys, I[24]	1 mo	M	Heart, perithyroidal fibrous tissue, adrenal, pancreas, thymus	Myocardial fibrosis	Respiratory distress, fever
45	Hunt and Leys, II[24]	4 wk	F	Heart	Myocardial infarct	Anorexia, loose stools, sudden death
46	Moran and Becker, I[38]	5 wk	F	Heart, lung, periadrenal, peripancreatic, perithyroidal, and perirenal connective tissue	Cardiac enlargement, coronary artery thrombosis, myocardial infarct	Respiratory distress, tachycardia, 24 hr illness
47	Moran and Becker, II[38]	2 mo	F	Lung, kidney	Interstitial pneumonia	"Fulminating pneumonia"

TABLE 1. (*cont.*)

Case No.	Author	Age	Sex	Organs Having Arterial Calcification	Changes in Other Organs	Clinical Findings
48	Chipman[8]	2 mo	M	Spleen, kidney, lung, heart	Cardiac enlargement, fibroelastosis of endocardium, recent myocardial infarct, scattered hyalinized glomeruli	Fever, respiratory distress
49	Newton and Misugi[41]	5½ wk	F	Lung, heart	Cardiac enlargement, myocardial fibrosis	Cyanosis, ECG changes, congestive heart failure
50	Nielsen, I[42]	5 mo	M	Mesentery, small intestine, spleen, pancreas, heart	Cardiac enlargement, fibroelastosis of endocardium, ulceration and stenosis of small intestine	Intestinal obstruction requiring resection
51	Nielsen, II[42]	8 wk	F	Thyroid, heart	Cardiac enlargement, acute myocardial infarction	Respiratory distress
52	Hilgenberg[21]	5 wk	?	Heart		Listlessness, congestive heart failure, cyanosis
53	Bickel and Janssen, I[3]	6 wk	F	Heart, lung	Calcium in Bowman's capsule	Cyanosis, vomiting
54	Bickel and Janssen, II[3]	6 wk	F	Lung, pancreas, kidney, heart	Cardiac enlargement	Respiratory distress, ECG changes
55	Gower and Pinkerton, I[16]	9 wk	M	Mediastinum, heart	Cardiac enlargement, myocardial infarction	Vomiting, refused feeding, cough, cyanosis
56	Gower and Pinkerton, II[16]	7 wk	M	Heart	Slight cardiac enlargement, myocardial infarction	Respiratory distress
57	Meurman et al[37]	6 wk	F	Lung, kidney, heart	Cardiac enlargement	Hyperpnea, screaming attacks
58	Paine and Grafton[44]	3 mo	F	Mesentery, pancreas, kidney, periadrenal tissues, spleen, heart	Myocardial infarction	Dead on arrival

59	Parker et al[45]	24 days	M	Lung, upper and lower extremities, kidney, adrenal, pancreas, thymus, thyroid, heart	Cardiac enlargement, left hydronephrosis and hydroureter	Respiratory problem at birth and later, fever, congestive failure, hypertension, diagnosed radiologically ECG abnormality
60	Bird, I[4]	11 mo	M	Heart, pancreas, periadrenal tissues, perithyroid, mesentery	Cardiac enlargement, myocardial fibrosis	Pallor, refusal to feed, lethargy, fever
61	Bird, II[4]	3 mo	F	Heart	Cardiac enlargement, myocardial fibrosis	Sweating, vomiting, refusal to eat, abnormal ECG
62	Moran and Erickson[39]	6 wk	M	Lung, adrenal, periadrenal tissues, thyroid, aorta, heart	Cardiac enlargement, myocardial fibrosis, scattered calcification of glomeruli and renal tubules.	Feeding difficulties, congestive failure, abnormal ECG diagnosed radiographically

were brothers. No other instance of infant mortality was present in over 80 descendants from the siblings of the patient's parents. In a proven instance of idiopathic calcific arterial disease of infancy in siblings, a review of the three generations of lineage on the maternal and paternal lines failed to reveal any other instance of this disease.[38]

Clinical Features

The clinical diagnosis of idiopathic calcific arterial disease of infancy offers a tremendous challenge to even the most astute clinician, and only two of the published cases were diagnosed prior to autopsy.[39, 45] Many cases were clinically diagnosed as myocarditis and respiratory tract infection.

The most common presenting symptom in about 50 percent of the reported cases was respiratory distress of varying type (Table 1). Symptoms involving the gastrointestinal tract, including refusal to feed and vomiting, are frequently noted. Fever was noted in at least ten patients. Other clinical findings were cyanosis, pallor, listlessness, hypertension, congestive heart failure, lethargy, tachycardia, sweating, diarrhea, hypernea, and "screaming attacks." A single patient, described by Nielsen,[42] presented with the findings of intestinal obstruction owing to ulceration and stenosis of the small intestine, which required bowel resection. Calcific arterial lesions were found in the mesentery, which were probably responsible for the ischemic lesions of the bowel. This patient also had similar vascular lesions of the coronary, splenic, and pancreatic arteries.

The length of illness or symptomatic period noted in patients with idiopathic arterial calcification of infancy is usually relatively short, with most ranging from 4 hours to 5 weeks. Holm [23] described one patient who survived 26 months following the initial symptoms.

Abnormal changes were noted in ECGs of seven patients. Most of these changes were compatible with ischemia of the myocardium.[3, 4, 23, 39, 41, 45] Cardiac enlargement was a frequent observation in the radiographic studies of the chests of these patients.

Laboratory Findings

Extensive laboratory studies are lacking in most of these reported cases of idiopathic arterial calcification of infancy. In view of the resemblance of these lesions to those of metastatic calcification secondary to hypercalcemia, considerable interest has centered around the serum calcium levels. A number of reports [4, 39, 45, 46, 51, 57, 59] of antemortem serum calcium levels show no abnormal values. Serum phosphates were within normal limits in two cases.[35, 45] Serum alkaline phosphatase was within normal range in three cases.[39, 45, 46] Serum electrolytes and blood glucose were within normal limits in two reports.[39, 45] Investigation of the serum proteins and lipids [39, 45] failed to show any abnormalities. None of the authors recorded evidence of uremia. Screening tests of urine for inborn errors of metabolism were negative in two patients.[39, 45] Urine amino acid chromatography showed a normal pattern in one patient [45] and normal urine mucopolysaccharides in these same patients. Serologic tests for syphilis were recorded in six reported cases and were positive in two instances.[52, 62] Neither of these patients revealed anatomic evidence of congenital syphilis.

Although the laboratory evaluation of idiopathic calcific arterial disease of infancy has been limited, all the available results show that in none of the cases were there defects of calcium metabolism, electrolyte balance, renal function or lipid metabolism, or inborn metabolic defects.

Radiographic Diagnosis

In 1954 Cochrane and Bowden [10] suggested that soft tissue radiography of the neck and the limbs may be of diagnostic value in the diagnosis of idiopathic calcific arterial disease of infancy. Two years later, Weens and Marin [60] used retrospective radiologic findings to confirm the existence of calcification of the arteries of the upper arms and forearms. In the same study, roentgenograms of the chest and abdomen failed to disclose calcification of visceral structures. It was not until 1971 that Parker and coworkers [45] used radiography to demonstrate calcification of coronary arteries, thoracic and abdominal aorta, and femoral, carotid, axillary, brachial, radial, and ulnar arteries in a 4-day-old male infant who survived 20 days following the initial diagnosis. In 1974 Moran and Erickson [39] reported similar arterial calcifications in the four extremities (Figs. 1 and 2) of a 3-week-old male

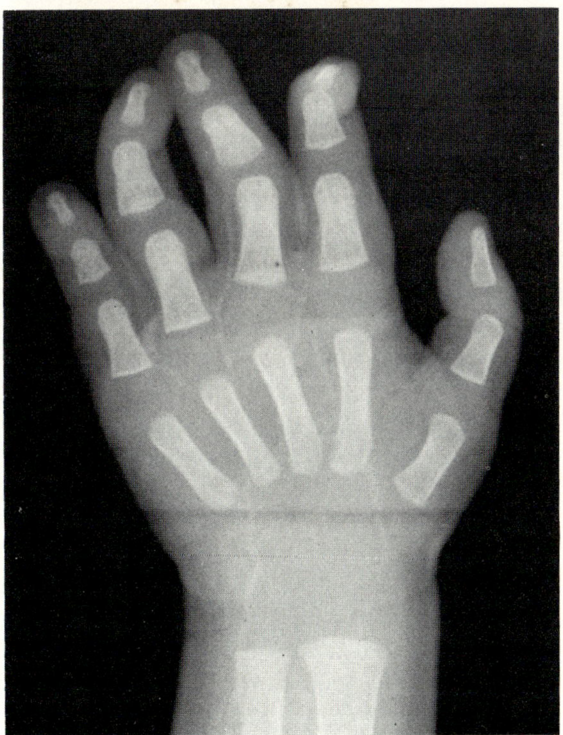

Fig. 1. Infant's hand showing linear calcification of ulnar, radial, and digital arteries (case 62).

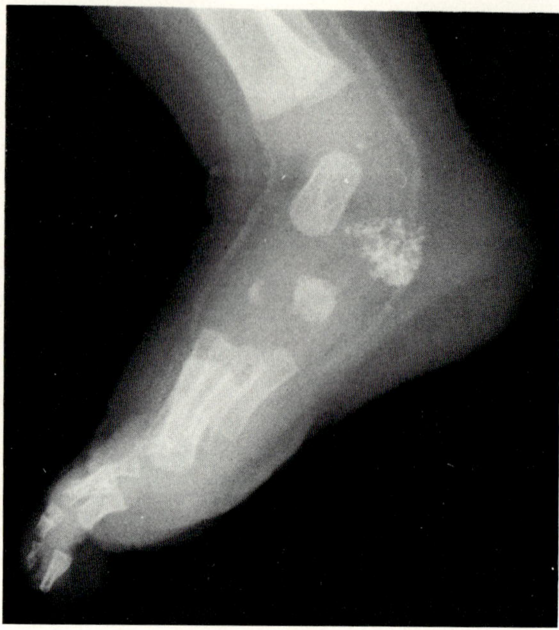

Fig. 2. Foot showing linear calcification of dorsalis pedis and posterior tibial arteries. Stippled calcifications are present in the epiphysis or synovia below ankle (case 62).

infant who was followed for 4-week period until his demise. In both cases the early diagnosis allowed time for more extensive biochemical investigation of this disease.

A second group of radiographic findings has been noted in two cases of idiopathic arterial calcification of infancy, in which stippled calcifications of the zone of the epiphyseal cartilage were noted independently by two observers.[39, 45] In the first patient, stippled calcifications were seen in epiphyseal cartilage just beyond the right ulnar distal metaphysis. In the second patient, similar stippled calcifications were noted about both hip joints (Fig. 3), both knee joints, and the region of the tarsal bone (Fig. 2). These stippled calcifications about the joints are radiographically similar to chondrodystrophia calcificans congenita, or Conradis disease, which is a rare autosomal recessive disorder of infancy.[27, 54] In Conradis disease many other abnormalities may accompany the punctate epiphyseal calcification, including saddle-nose deformity, congenital cataracts, optic atrophy, contractures, numerous dermatoses, and shortening of the proximal long bones. About 115 cases of this disease have been reported. Most of these children die within the first year of life. Thus far, no calcific arterial lesions have been reported in this disease.[27, 54]

Roentgenograms of organs removed at autopsy serve to demonstrate the extensive arterial calcific lesions which are obscured on the usual chest and abdominal films (Fig. 4). Thus radiographic studies of the head, neck, and extremities for calcified arteries offer the only practical method by which a clinical diagnosis of idiopathic calcific arterial disease of infancy can be made. The diagnostic significance of stippled epiphyses requires further investigation.

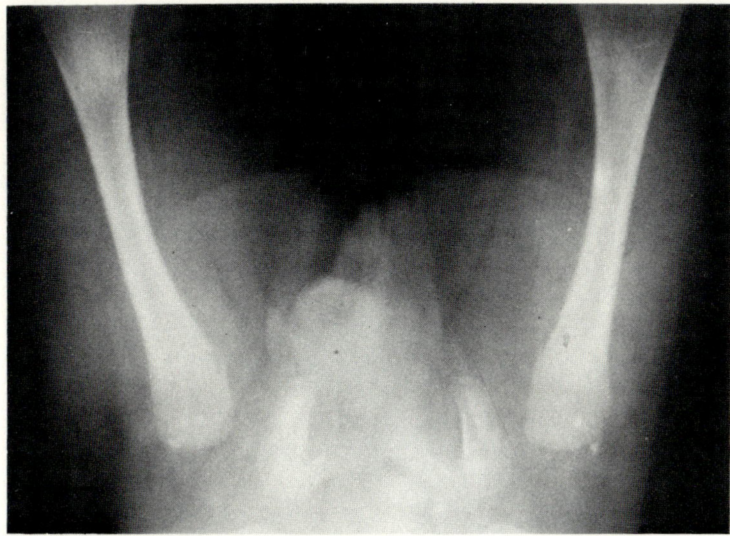

Fig. 3. Stippled foci of calcification present in region of both hip joints (case 62).

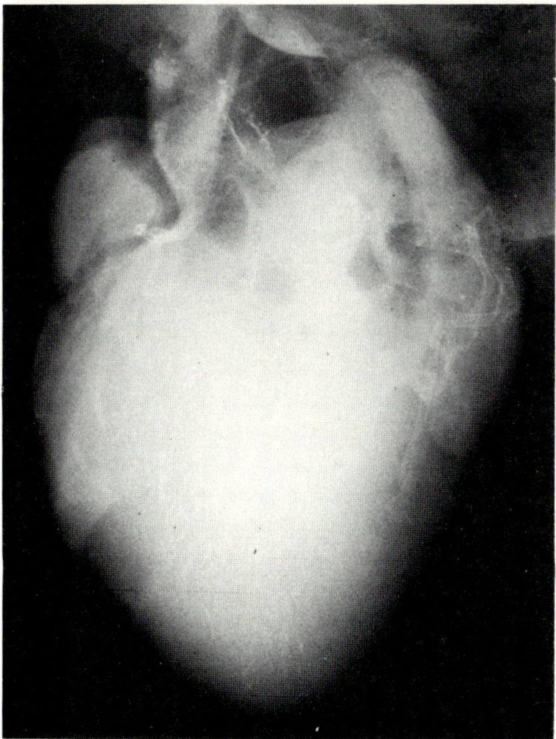

Fig. 4. Radiograph of heart following removal at necropsy shows calcification of coronary arteries and aorta (case 62).

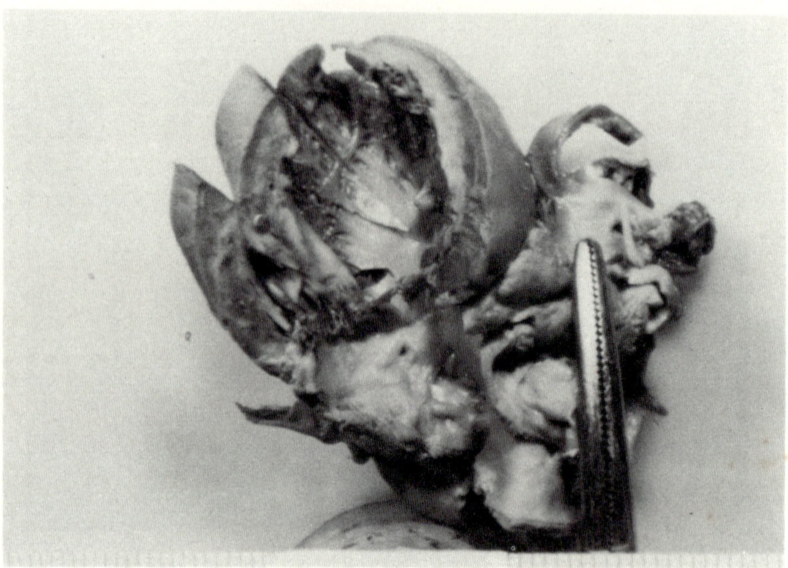

Fig. 5. Gross appearance of left ventricle showing myocardial hypertrophy, focal opacity of endocardium overlying septum, and a pale infarcted area of myocardium (case 46).

Gross Pathology

Most authors state that the heart is markedly enlarged (Table 1) in idiopathic arterial calcification of infancy. The enlargement has most commonly been described as biventricular or left ventricular. The coronary arteries are sometimes described as being firm, thickened and tortuous,[38, 59] but some authors note no gross abnormality.[60] Many describe varying size areas of opacity of the endocardium, usually of the left ventricle. Abnormalities of the myocardium of the left ventricle are usually seen as pale or mottled areas (Fig. 5) or other color changes indicative of infarction.

Other organs, including the aorta, fail to show any distinctive gross changes.

Microscopic Findings

The arterial lesions of idiopathic arterial calcification of infancy are distinctly different than atherosclerosis insofar as no observers have noted any lipid deposits in the intima. These lesions also differ from Monckeberg's sclerosis, since the initial calcium deposits are along the internal elastic membrane (Fig. 6) and are accompanied by fibrous proliferation of the intima (Figs. 5 to 8).

The deposition of calcium along the internal elastic membrane is not by any means unique. In 1924 Jores [26] reported isolated calcification of the internal elastic membrane accompanied by mild subintimal fibrous proliferation, particularly in the region of the pericapsular arteries of the thyroid gland seen mainly in middle age. This change has been confirmed by other observers; [4] it does not correlate

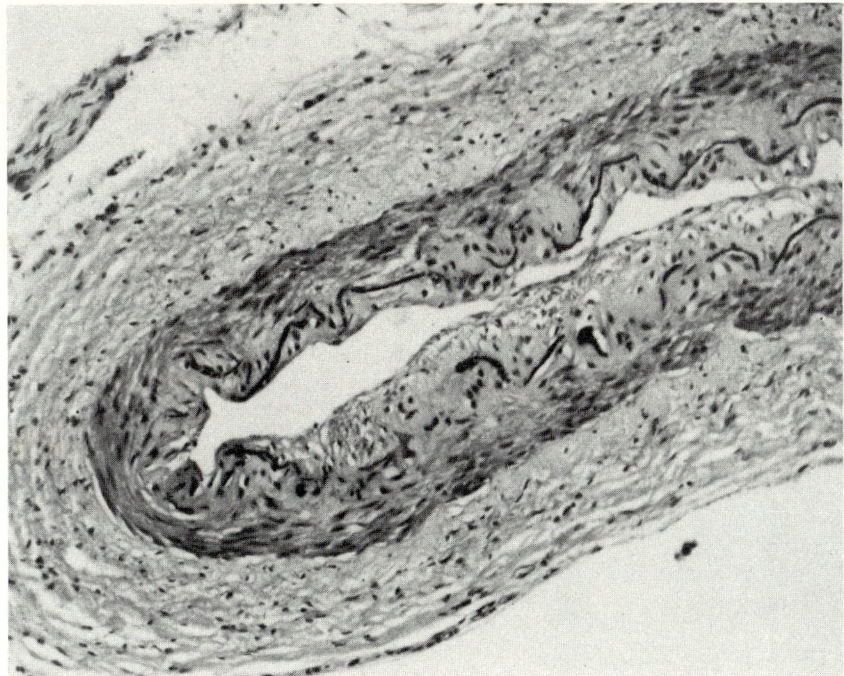

Fig. 6. Coronary artery (case 62) showing relatively mild calcific deposition along the internal elastic membrane and minimal fibrous thickening of intima. H & E × 100.

with atherosclerosis and is of no clinical significance. Meyer and Lind [36] reported the calcific incrustation of common and internal iliac arteries of 50 percent of a series of newborn infants in first four weeks of life and in almost all cases after one year. They reported [35] similar changes in the carotid siphon of normal infants and children 1 to 16 years of age.

The usual changes of idiopathic arterial calcification of infancy are devoid of inflammatory reaction, with the exception of an occasional focus of foreign body reaction [8, 38, 42] around the calcific deposition.

Throughout this chapter the terms "calcification" and "calcific deposits" are used with the understanding that this process is not a simple deposition of a single mineral but rather a more complex compound. The term "calcification" has been used throughout the literature undoubtedly because of the appearance of the deposit as a deeply basophilic substance as seen with the usual hematoxylin-and-eosin-stained sections. The same lesions, when stained with periodic acid Schiff procedure, were shown to be PAS positive.[38] These same areas are also positive when stained with Hales colloidal iron stain. These lesions take a positive von Kossa and alizarin red stain,[38] indicating the presence of calcium. These staining features suggest that the basophilic deposit is an acid mucopolysaccharide containing iron and calcium.

In five patients, in addition to the usual calcific changes, the coronary arteries were thrombosed.[11, 20, 38, 47, 50] Sections of the myocardium showed the character-

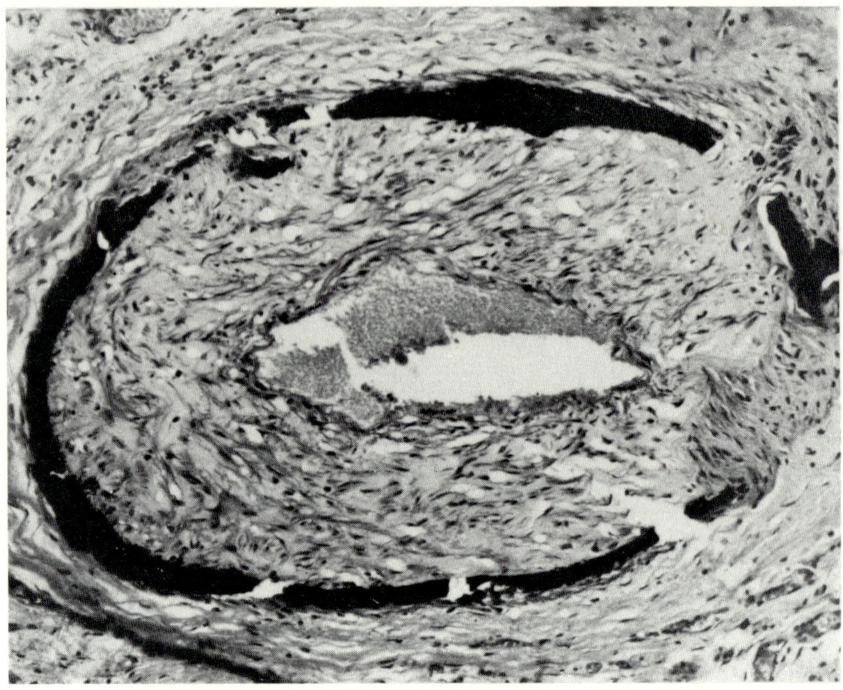

Fig. 7. Coronary artery (case 62) showing heavy deposition of calcific material that obliterates details of internal elastic membrane and marked fibrous thickening of intima. H & E × 100.

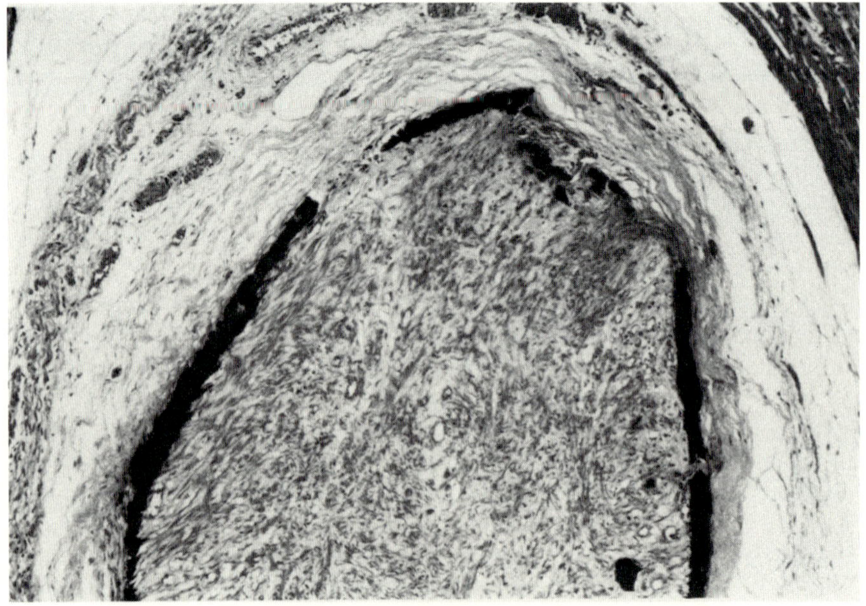

Fig. 8. Coronary artery (case 62) showing heavy calcific deposits along internal elastic membrane and obliteration of lumen by fibrous proliferation of intima. H & E × 100.

istic changes that would be expected with myocardial infarctions of varying duration. Many authors reported early myocardial changes of degeneration or necrosis
(Fig. 9). Some have noted the presence of focal areas of calcification in either
myocardial fibers or connective tissue (Fig. 10). Almost all cases show varying
degrees of fibrosis (Fig. 11). Myocardial infarction or fibrosis was diagnosed pathologically in 32 of the recorded cases.

Some authors [3] use the term "fibroelastosis" to describe the opacity or thickening of the endocardium. Thomas and coworkers [54] have reported endocardial
fibroelastosis to be associated with similar calcific arterial lesions. The arterial
lesions were not present in another review of 20 cases of fibroelastosis by the
same senior authors.[55] Therefore it is believed that the subendocardial fibrosis
commonly noted in the idiopathic arterial calcific group reflects the same ischemic
changes as noted in the myocardium rather than representing changes of true endocardial fibroelastosis.

Similar calcific arterial lesions are found throughout the body (Figs. 12 to
15) with the exception of the brain and spinal cord. The other organs most

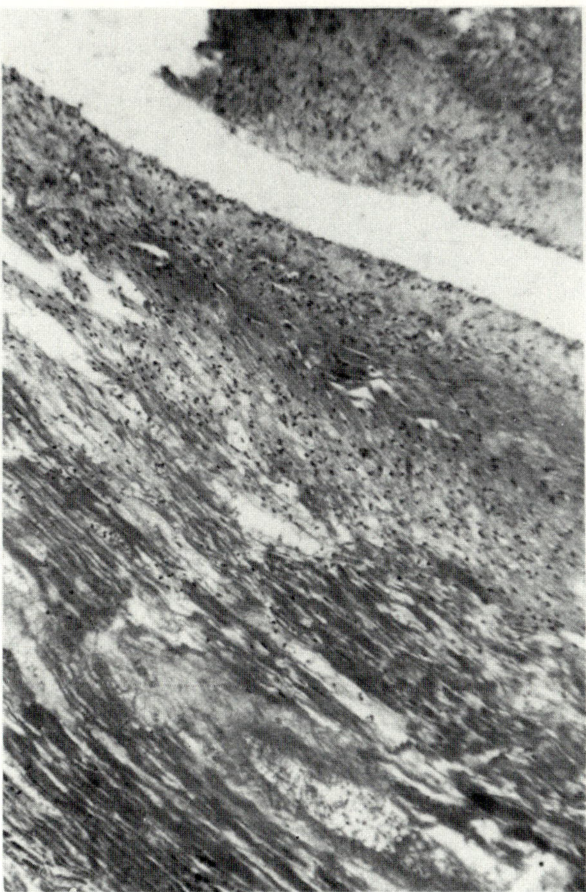

Fig. 9. Area of recent myocardial necrosis (case 62) of left ventricle. H & E × 100.

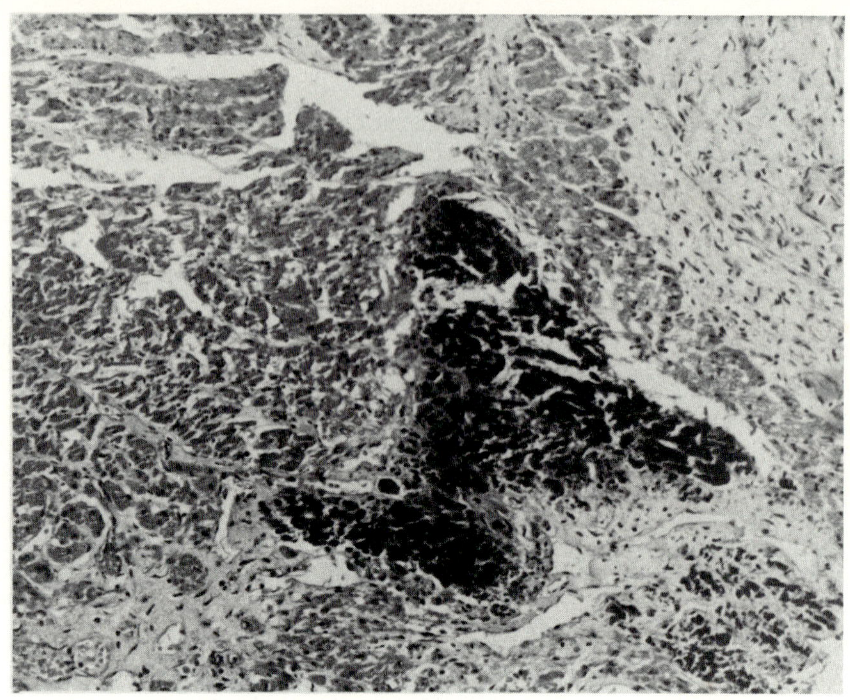

Fig. 10. Myocardial fibrosis of left ventricle (case 62) with focal area of calcium deposition in myocardial fibers. H & E × 100.

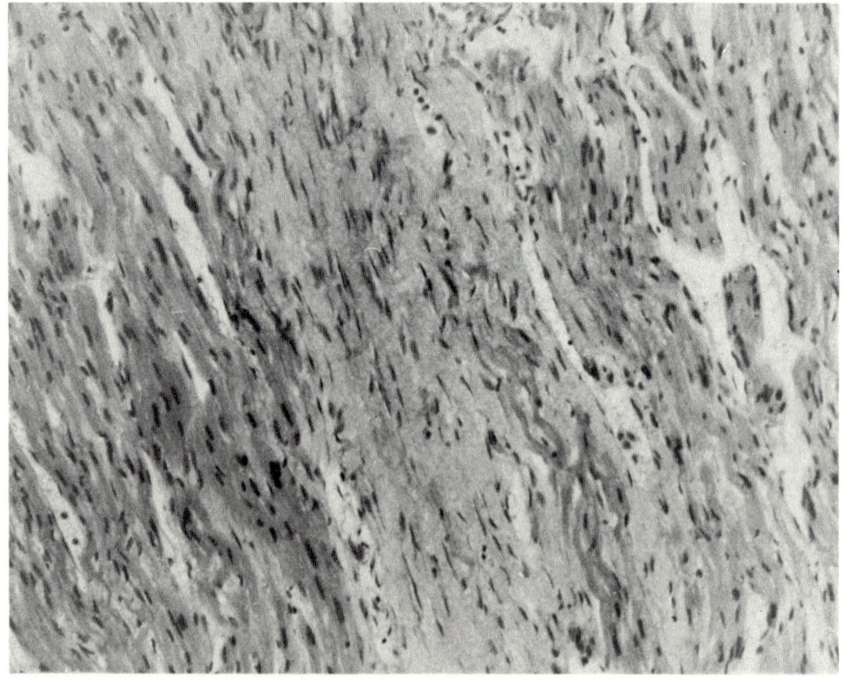

Fig. 11. Area of mature fibrosis of left ventricle (case 62). H & E × 100.

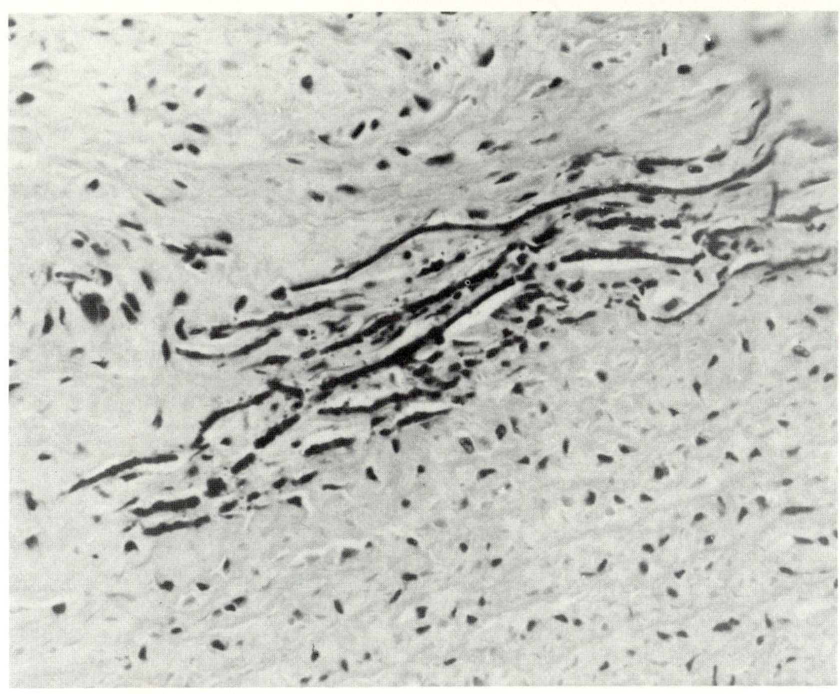

Fig. 12. Calcific deposits along elastic fibers of aorta (case 62). H & E × 250.

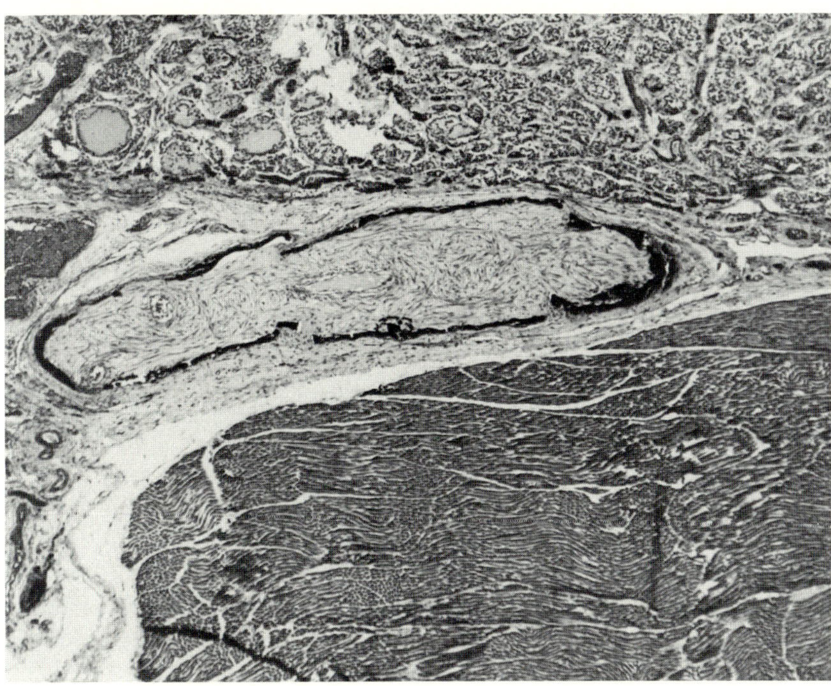

Fig. 13. Perithyroidal artery (case 62) showing calcific changes of internal elastic membrane and almost total fibrous obliteration of lumen. H & E × 100.

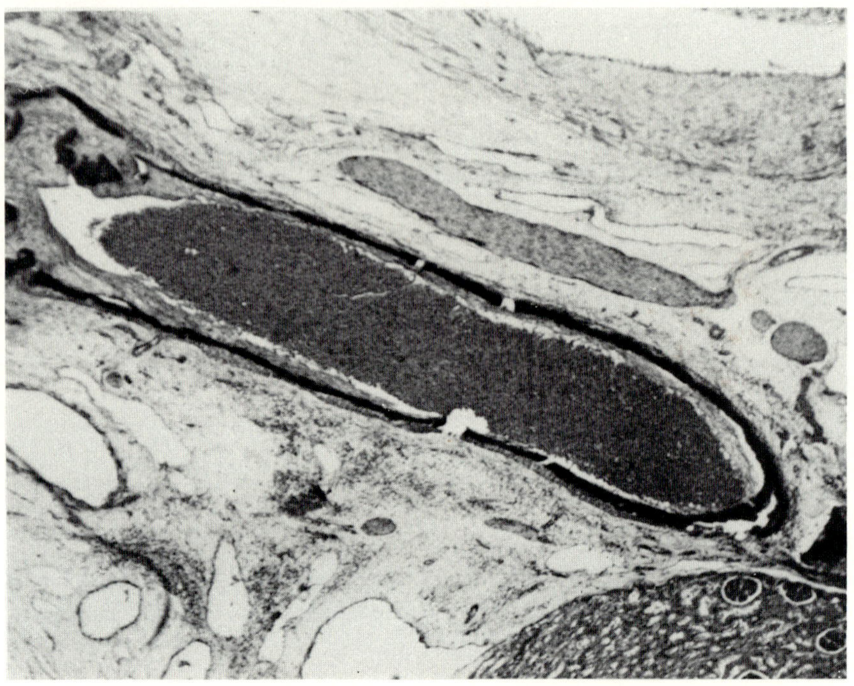

Fig. 14. Renal artery (case 62) showing heavy calcification of internal elastic membrane but only minimal intimal proliferation. H & E × 100. (From Moran and Becker: Am J Clin Pathol 31:520, 1959)

commonly cited are kidney, adrenal and periadrenal tissue, pancreas, lung, mesentery, and thyroid. It is interesting to note that morphologic evidence of ischemia produced by these arterial lesions has been limited to the heart, with the exception of the report of one of Nielsen's [42] cases who presented with an ischemic lesion of the small intestine.

Histologic examination of the parathyroid glands was reported to be normal in 12 of the patients having idiopathic arterial calcification of infancy.[4, 7, 13, 25, 28, 39, 42, 43, 45, 47]

The kidneys showed numerous instances of calcific changes of the renal arteries (Fig. 14). Other findings included occasional focal calcification of glomeruli (Fig. 16) and tubules.[8, 10, 38, 39]

No significant pathologic lesions of bone have been reported.[28, 31]

Discussion

The histologic changes in the arteries of patients having idiopathic calcific arterial disease of infancy are indistinguishable from the changes noted in metastatic calcification of arteries secondary to advanced renal disease, arterial calcification in conjunction with anomalies of the heart or great vessels, or arterial lesions

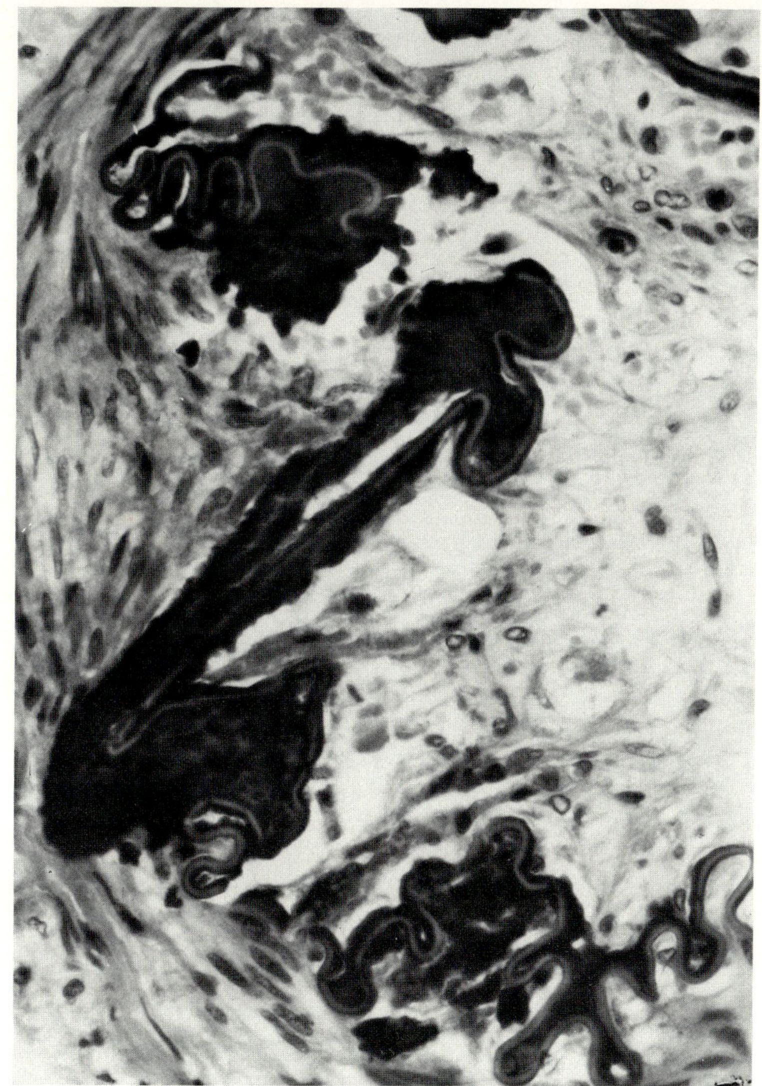

Fig. 15. Pancreatic artery (case 46) revealing heavy calcium deposition along both sides of internal elastic membrane. H & E × 250.

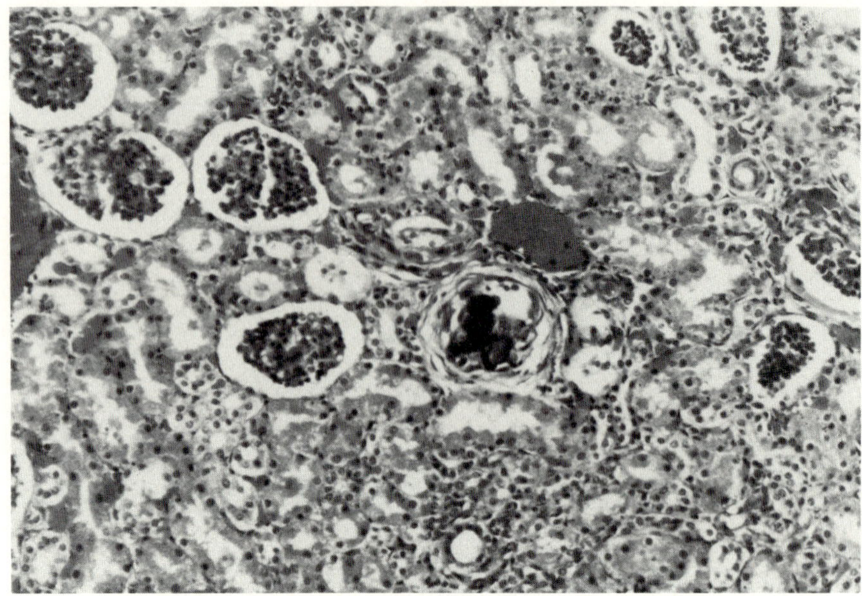

Fig. 16. Focal calcification of glomerulus (case 62). H & E × 100.

in hypervitaminosis D. Although these specific backgrounds of calcific disease have been excluded as causes in this series of cases, it is useful to examine them as clues to the pathogenesis of the idiopathic group.

Many authors have described widespread calcification of the medium-size arteries in patients with severe renal disease.[1, 6, 10, 18, 43, 53] These patients show hypercalcemia, hypophosphatemia, secondary hyperplasia of the parathyroid glands, skeletal changes, and metastatic calcification of viscera.

Calcific arterial lesions of the aorta and pulmonary arteries have been described by Oppenheimer[43] in a patient having atresia of the right pulmonary artery. Mant et al[33] described calcific arterial disease in a 4-year-old child with an anomaly of the coronary arteries. A third instance of disseminated calcific arterial disease was reported in a 5-year-old boy who died following open cardiotomy for repair of an interventricular septal defect.[40] The lesions in this latter case were indistinguishable from the arterial lesion seen in the idiopathic group (Fig. 17). It is difficult or impossible to interrelate these cases of arterial calcification, but probably they are due to changes in local hemodynamics plus degenerative changes in elastic tissues. The third case has a resemblance to a heritable disorder of elastic tissue.

Ross and Williams[49] have described hypervitaminosis D as producing arterial calcification with sudden death in patients receiving 20,000 to 40,000 USP units of vitamin D daily. In the instance in which an autopsy was performed, metastatic calcification was present in the inner media of arteries, cardiac muscle, alveoli of lungs, bronchi, muscularis mucosae of stomach, and renal tubules. A similar distribution of lesions was reported in experimental studies by Hass and associates.[19]

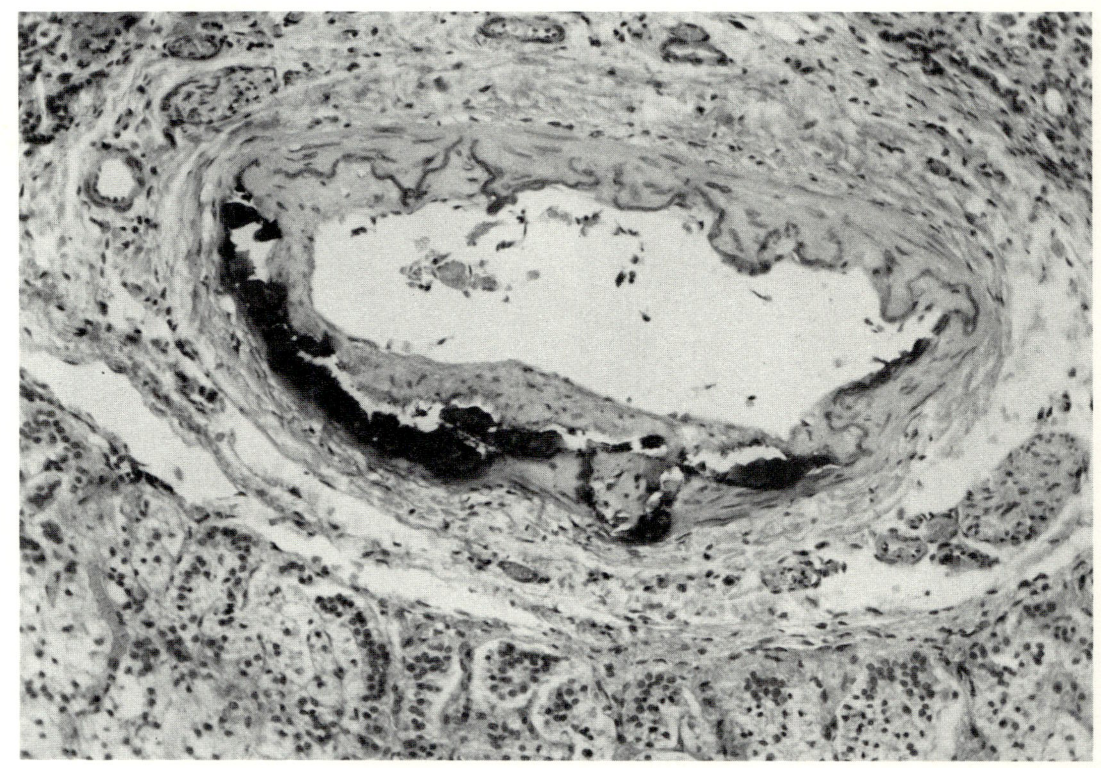

Fig. 17. Periadrenal artery showing calcification of internal elastic membrane and fibrous thickening of intima from 5-year-old boy who died following repair of interventricular septal defect.[39] H & E × 225. (From Moran and Steiner: Am J Clin Pathol 73:523, 1962)

Wolf [61] described a patient who received 3,500,000 units of vitamin D administered over a two-week period. At autopsy, calcium deposits were observed in the renal tubules only. Bird [4] stated that, in the 1950s, more than 200 cases of hypercalcemia were reported in Britain and were probably due to overdosage of vitamin D. In this group the deposition of calcium salts was mainly in the kidneys and soft tissues. Arteries were rarely affected and then only in the late stages. Thus, despite occasional calcific vascular lesions occurring in hypervitaminosis D, the distribution of calcium in other tissues is quite different. A history of normal vitamin D intake was recorded in 12 cases of idiopathic calcific arterial disease of infancy.[4, 5, 13, 16, 20, 29, 31, 34, 37, 45, 51, 52, 60] There are no instances recorded of abnormally high intake of vitamins in this same group.

Opinions vary greatly as to the role of the elastic tissue in the causation of the lesion of idiopathic arterial calcification of infancy. In 1946 Field [13] described calcium deposition in the media adjacent to the internal elastic lamina. Gower and Pinkerton [16] also stated that the changes in the muscular arteries consist of a calcification of the media immediately adjacent to the internal elastic membrane but no demonstrable calcification of the elastica itself, which acts as a limiting membrane preventing the spread of calcium into the subintimal tissue. The elastic membrane remains undamaged, retaining its normal acidophil-staining properties. They further stated that the change in the elastic vessels, such as aorta, pulmonary arteries, and proximal common carotid, consist of loss of outline with basophilia in individual elastic fibers, but showing no calcification. Other authors [38, 51, 52] believe that the calcium deposits are laid down along the internal elastic membrane.

Bird [4] states "there may be an embryonal dystrophy, perhaps hereditary of the elastic fibers making them more sensitive to toxic agents of which one might be vitamin D." Interesting experimental work by Grasso and Selye [17] showed that in rats sensitized by a single oral dose of dihydrotachysterol, subsequent intravenous injection of ferric oxide saccharate induced massive necrosis irregularly distributed throughout the myocardium along with calcification of all branches of the coronary arterial system. The calcium deposits formed plaques surrounded by proliferating fibrous tissue. This fibrous proliferation contained Prussian-blue-positive granules. The authors thought such changes to be reminiscent of the changes of Monckeberg's medial sclerosis and atherosclerosis. In animals sensitized by pretreatment with agents that promote calcification, there develops a state of altered tissue reactivity of calciphylaxis.[17] This condition is manifest only during a brief critical period after the systemic administration of the calcifying agent. It is characterized by sudden attraction of calcium to regions challenged by "vital mordants for calcium."[17]

Walford and Kaplan [58] described 12 cases in which the lungs showed pulmonary fibrosis and giant cell reaction with altered elastic tissue. This alteration of the elastic tissue was accompanied by degeneration of the elastic tissue and deposition of iron compounds, while stains for calcium were negative.

Perhaps this state of altered reactivity of elastic tissue has been neglected because the conspicuous calcium deposits have received too much attention. As Gower and Pinkerton [16] pointed out, surprisingly little attention has been paid to the somewhat less conspicuous subintimal fibrosis, which in most cases of idiopathic arterial calcification of infancy is the immediate cause of the luminal occlusion and resultant myocardial ischemia. Possibly three separate reports of myocardial infarction of early infancy [9, 15, 32] owing to fibrous thickening of the intima of the coronary arteries but lacking calcification of the internal elastic membrane belong to the same general idiopathic group of occlusive coronary artery disease.

In 1974 Rosenberg [48] published a report of five infants who died of chronic arsenic poisoning. Pathologic examination showed intimal thickening in the small- and medium-size arteries of the heart, gastrointestinal tract, skin, and pancreas. Two of the infants suffered myocardial infarctions, while one presented as an acute abdomen.

Thus it can be seen through examination of these other causes of arterial calcification and intimal proliferation that many mechanisms can be operative in the production of similar arterial lesions.

Summary

The clinical and pathologic features of a group of 62 infants dying of idiopathic calcific arterial disease were reviewed. The disease most commonly occurs in infants less than 6 months of age. Pathologically, it is characterized by calcific deposits along the internal elastic membrane of arteries accompanied by fibrous thickening of the intima which causes luminal narrowing. The arterial lesions are widespread but the resultant luminal narrowing invariably promotes myocardial ischemia, causing the infants' deaths. A definite tendency of the disease to occur in siblings has been noted, but additional patterns of inheritance are not yet apparent. Clinical diagnosis is feasible with radiologic study of arteries of the head, neck, and extremities. There is a similarity of idiopathic calcific arterial disease of infancy to the arterial lesions of metastatic calcification in severe renal disease, calcific arterial lesions noted in conjunction with certain cardiovascular anomalies, and hypervitaminosis D. Certain experimental situations and toxic states can also produce calcific and proliferative vascular lesions.

References

1. Andersen DH, Schlesinger ER: Renal hyperparathyroidism with calcification of the arteries in infancy. Am J Dis Child 63:102–125, 1942
2. Baggenstoss AH, Keith HM: Calcification of the arteries of an infant. J Pediatr 18:95–102, 1941
3. Bickel E, Janssen W: Arteriopathia calcificans infantum. Arch Kinderheilk 169: 274–285, 1963
4. Bird T: Idiopathic arterial calcification in infancy. Arch Dis Child 49:82–89, 1974
5. Brown CE, Richter IM: Medial coronary sclerosis in infancy. Arch Pathol 31:449–457, 1941
6. Bryant JH, White WH: A case of calcification of arteries and obliterative endarteritis associated with hydronephrosis in a child aged 6 months. Guy's Hosp Rep 55:17–28, 1891
7. Bunting H: Histochemical analysis of pathological mineral deposits at various sites with discussion of methods used. Arch Pathol 52:458–469, 1951
8. Chipman CD: Calcific sclerosis of coronary arteries in an infant. Can Med Assoc J 83:955–957, 1960
9. Clapp JF III, Naeye RL: Intra-uterine myocardial infarction. JAMA 178:1039–1040, 1961

10. Cochrane WA, Bowden DH: Calcification of the arteries in infancy and childhood. Pediatrics 14:222–231, 1954

11. van Creveld S: Coronary calcification and thrombosis in an infant. Ann Pediatr (Paris) 157:84–92, 1941

12. Donat R: Zum Vorkommen von Mediaverkalkungen in Säuglingsalter. Z Gesamte Inn Med 1:68–77, 1946

13. Field MH: Medial calcification of arteries of infants. Arch Pathol 42:607–618, 1946

14. Forrer H: Ausgedehnte Gefässverkalkung in frühen Kindesalter. As quoted by J. H. Meier in inaugural dissertation. Zurich, 1930

15. Gault MH, Usher R: Coronary thrombosis with myocardial infarction in a newborn infant. Clinical, electrocardiographic and post-morten findings. N Engl J Med 263:379–382, 1960

16. Gower ND, Pinkerton JRH: Idiopathic arterial calcification in infancy. Arch Dis Child 38:408–411, 1963

17. Grasso S, Selye H: Calciphylaxis in relation to the humoral production of occlusive coronary lesion with infarction. J Pathol and Bacteriol 83:495–500, 1962

18. Greenstein NM, Kramer L: Metastatic calcification in newborn. Am J Dis Child 82:37–42, 1951

19. Hass GM, Trueheart RE, Taylor CB, Stumpe M: An experimental histologic study of hypervitaminosis D. Am J Pathol 34:395–431, 1958

20. Hause WA, Antell GJ: Arteriosclerosis in infancy. Arch Pathol 44:82–86, 1947

21. Hilgenberg F: Coronary arteriosclerosis in an infant. Monatsschr Kinderheilkd 109:200–202, 1961

22. Hughes FWT, and Perry CB: Senile arterial changes in a child aged 7 weeks. Bristol Med Chir J 46:219–222, 1929

23. Holm V: Arteriopathia calcificans infantum. Acta Paediatr Scand, 56:537–540, 1967

24. Hunt AC, Leys DG: Generalized arterial calcification of infancy. Br M J 1:385–386, 1957

25. Iff W: Über angeborne Verkalkungen besonders der Arterien. Arch Pathol Anat 281:377–395, 1931

26. Jores L: In Henke I, Lubarsch O (eds): Handbuch der Speziellen Pathologischen Anatomie and Histologie. Berlin, Springer, 1924, p 631

27. Josephson BM, Oriatti MD: Chondrodystrophia calcificans congenita. Report of a case and review of the literature. Pediatrics 28.425–435, 1961

28. Kent SP, Vawter GF, Dowben RM, Benson RE: Hypervitaminosis D in monkeys. Am J Pathol 34:37–59, 1958

29. Leach WB: Calcific arteriosclerosis of infancy. Can Med Assoc J 73:733–735, 1955

30. Lightwood R: A case of dwarfism and calcinosis associated with widespread arterial degeneration. Arch Dis Child 7: 193–208, 1932

31. Lipman BL, Rosenthal IM, Lowenburg H Jr: Arteriosclerosis in infancy. Am J Dis Child 82:561–566, 1951

32. MacMahon HE, Dickinson PCT: Occlusive fibroelastosis of coronary arteries in the newborn. Circulation 35:3–9, 1967

33. Mant AK, Trounce JR, Vulliamy DG: Disease of the coronary arteries as a cause of death in infancy and childhood. Guy's Hosp Rep 101:115–125, 1952

34. Menten ML, Fetterman GH: Coronary sclerosis in infancy. Am J Clin Pathol 18:805–810, 1948

35. Meyer WW, Lind J: Calcification of the carotid siphon-common findings in infancy and childhood. Arch Dis Child 47:355–363, 1972

36. Meyer WW, Lind J: Calcification of the iliac arteries in newborn and infants. Arch Dis Child 47:364–372, 1972

37. Meurman L, Somersalo O, Tuuteri L: Sudden death in infancy caused by idopathic arterial calcification. Ann Paediat Fenn 11:19–24, 1965

38. Moran JJ, Becker SM: Idiopathic arterial calcification of infancy. Report of 2 cases occurring in siblings and review of literature. Am J Clin Pathol 31:517–529, 1959

39. Moran JJ, Erickson W: Arterial calcification of infancy. Bull Geisinger Med Center 26:76, 1974

40. Moran JJ, Steiner GL: Idiopathic arterial calcification in a 5 year old child. Am J Clin Pathol 73:521–526, 1962

41. Newton WA, Misugi K: Partial obliteration of coronary arteries in a newborn infant. Yokohama Med Bull 11:59–68, 1960

42. Nielsen K: Infantile arterial calcification. Acta Pathol Microbiol Scand 51:67–69, 1961

43. Oppenheimer EH: Partial atresia of the main branches of the pumonary artery occurring in infancy and accompanied by calcification of the pulmonary artery and aorta. Bull Johns Hopkins Hosp 63:261–277, 1938

44. Paine TD, Grafton WD: Calcification of the arteries in infancy: report of a case. J La State Med Soc 122:344–345, 1970

45. Parker RJ, Smith EH, Stoneman MER: Generalised arterial calcification of infancy. Clin Radiol 22:69–73, 1971

46. Prior JT, Bergstrom VW: Generalized arterial calcification in infants. Am J Dis Child 76:91–101, 1948

47. Ramsay RE, Crumrine RM: Coronary thrombosis in an infant aged 4 months. Am J Dis Child 42:107–110, 1931

48. Rosenberg HG: Systemic arterial disease and chronic arsenism in infants. Arch Pathol 97:360–365, 1974

49. Ross SG, Williams WE: Vitamin D intoxication in infancy. Am J Dis Child 58:1142, 1939

50. Scott EP, Miller AJ: Coronary thrombosis—report of a case in an infant 11 months of age. J Pediatr 28:478–480, 1946

51. Sladden RA: Coronary arteriosclerosis and calcification in infancy. J Clin Pathol 5:175–182, 1952

52. Stryker WA: Arterial calcification in infancy with special reference to the coronary arteries. Am J Pathol 22:1007–1031, 1946.

53. Surbeck K: Über einer Fall von kongenitaler Verkalkung. mit vorwiegender Beteiligung der Arterien. Z Allg Pathol 28:25–39, 1917

54. Tasker WG, Mastri AR, Gold AP: Chondrodystrophia calcificans congenita (dysplasia epiphysalis punctata). Recognition of the clinical picture. Am J Dis Child 119:122–126, 1970

55. Thomas WA, Lee KT, McGavran MH, Rabin ER: Endocardial fibroelastosis in infants associated with thrombosis and calcification of arteries and myocardial infarcts. N Engl J Med 255:464–468, 1956

56. Thomas WA, Randall RV, Bland EF, Castleman B: Endocardial fibroelastosis: factor in heart disease of obscure etiology: study of 20 autopsied cases in children and adults. N Engl J Med 251:327–338, 1954

57. Traisman HD, Limperis NM, Traisman AS: Myocardial infarction due to calcification of arteries in infant. Am J Dis Child 91:34–37, 1956

58. Walford RL, Kaplan L: Pulmonary fibrosis and giant cell reaction with altered elastic tissue. Arch Pathol 63:75–90, 1957

59. Wahlgren F: Arteriosclerosis-like arterial disease with myocardial infarcts in infant. Cardiologia 21:373–379, 1952

60. Weens HS, Marin CA: Infantile arteriosclerosis. Radiology 67:168–174, 1956

61. Wolf IJ: Safety of large doses of vitamin D in the prevention and treatment of rickets in infancy. J Pediatr 22:707–718, 1943

62. Verocay J: Arterienverkalkung bei angeborener Lues. Frankfurt Z Pathol 24:109–135, 1920

63. Zischka W: Uber eine eigenartige Arterioenerkrankung beim Neugeborenen und Kleinstkind ("Arteriopathia calcificans infantum"). Beitr Pathol Anat 115:586–598, 1955

SIGNIFICANCE OF THE EXTRACELLULAR HYALINE SUBSTANCES*

BERNARD M. WAGNER
SHIRLEY SIEW

Virchow and others referred to the material which served to connect cells as the intercellular cement. This material also filled the spaces between extracellular fibers and was called "ground substance." The biological functions of the connective tissues are many. By virtue of location between the cells and capillaries, the connective tissue serves to regulate the transfer of important metabolites. Regulation of extracellular water and ions by the ground substance serves to maintain the pericellular environment. Thus, the connective tissue is a dynamic system which helps other homeostatic mechanisms to support the host's steady state. This makes the connective tissues peculiarly vulnerable to a variety of changes. The loss of thyroid hormone because of disease or surgery leads to a marked increase in water binding in the subcutaneous connective tissue leading to myxedema. Administration of thyroid hormone reverses the process. Circulating antibodies frequently meet their reactive antigens in the extracellular connective tissue, resulting in immunopathology. When abnormal proteins are deposited in basement membranes, ground substance, or vascular walls, the connective tissue function is rendered more static with resultant deleterious effects on cells.

The transport of metabolites between capillary and cell in establishing and maintaining a given order of homeostasis requires the active participation of the intercellular and extravascular ground substance. The connective tissue ground substance is interfibrillar material and may range from a well defined basement membrane or pericapillary mesenchyme to an amorphous loose type of connective tissue.

* Supported by AAUW International Fellowship and Training Program NIH-AM5382.

Thus, the ground substance of the umbilical cord is gelatinous while in bone it is extremely dense and hard. Routine staining techniques demonstrate the collagen, elastic, and reticulin fibers of connective tissue and the apparent fibrillar nature of basement membranes. Hematoxylin and eosin (H&E) stained sections show the ground substance as an acellular, amorphous, homogenous mass of variable staining intensity. The strategic location of the connective tissue in one form or another in between the cell membrane and the capillary wall must of necessity predict an active, dynamic role in regulating cellular activity and vascular function.

A variety of descriptive terms have been applied to structural alterations of the intercellular materials and vascular walls. *Mucoid degeneration* (Fig. 1) or mucinous alteration of the ground substance refers to a pale, faintly eosinophilic, acellular increase in ground substance noted in myxedema. When the connective tissue is altered due to unusual protein deposits or degeneration of fibers or cells, such changes may be visualized as an amorphous, acellular, smoothly eosinophilic substance in clumps or bands obscuring normal morphology. Because of the refractile nature of this material when viewed by light microscopy, the term *hyalin* has been

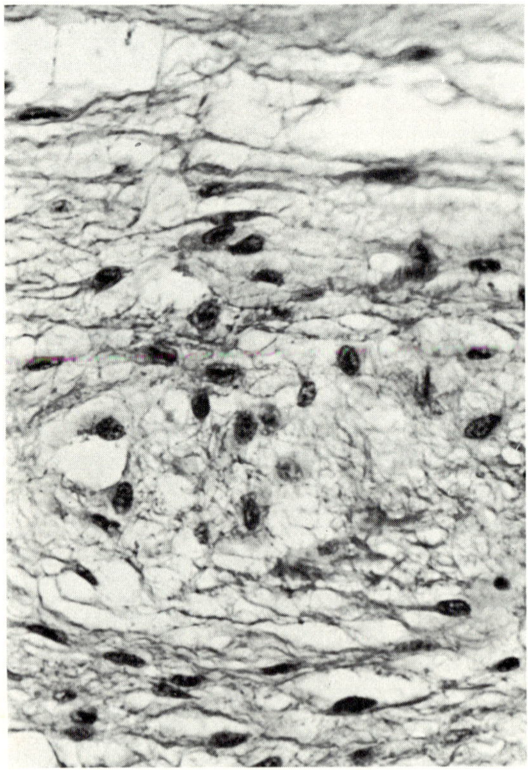

Fig. 1. Mucoid swelling of the connective tissue ground substance. Mitral valve leaflet from rabbit treated with streptococcal proteinase. Note the loose, "watery" appearance of the stroma. Carnoy fixed, paraffin section. H&E. × 500.

used to describe this change. Hyaline arteriolar change is the commonest vascular pathology observed in man and is most frequently present in the spleen and kidneys. The end stage of repair in many sites results in hyalinization of the fibrous tissue and is commonly seen in scars. Under certain pathological conditions in the same areas where hyalin may develop, a different type of alteration known as fibrinoid degeneration may occur. In order to understand the possible mechanisms responsible for mucoid, hyaline, and fibrinoid degeneration, it is necessary to review briefly the pertinent biochemical and physical properties of the connective tissue.

The terms generally used to denote the ground substance are descriptive and imply a simplicity of chemical composition. Ground substance includes a large variety of chemical materials; many of which are unknown. Some of these substances arise locally while others are derived from circulating blood. Gersh and Catchpole [1] define ground substance as a place name for macromolecular aggregates. Some of these aggregates occur as very thin (10 to 30 Å), highly elongate (1,000 to 5,000 Å) particles which may polymerize end to end and laterally to firm fibrillar structures. These macromolecular systems may be studied by physicochemical, crystallographic, and electron microscopic techniques. In addition, the methods of tissue culture, cytochemistry, and histochemistry have been of value in the localization of the ground substance components.

Basement Membranes

These structures have been studied intensively by electron microscopy. Such micrographs reveal a dense osmiophilic layer with diffuse outlines immediately adjacent to the basal cell membrane of all epithelial surfaces. This layer varies in thickness in different tissues from 150 to 800 Å. If filamentous structures are observed, they are separated by a very narrow space, filled with homogeneous substance from the adjacent cell membrane. At the base of epithelial surfaces a delicate meshwork of reticular fibrils is associated with this ground substance, and this combination of fibrillar and nonfibrillar elements constitutes the basement membrane. In most instances, the nonfibrillar ground substance of the basement membrane can be identified by its mucopolysaccharide reactions while the fine reticular fibrils are localized by their argyrophilia. The exact chemical nature of the homogeneous component of the basement membrane is unknown. However, protein-bound SH and alpha-NH_2 groups may be determined by histochemical methods. It is thought that the mucopolysaccharide constituents are protein bound.

The Dynamic State of the Ground Substance

Progress in the structural analysis of mucopolysaccharides has been slow. Considerable difficulty is encountered in separating the mucopolysaccharide from noncarbohydrate material and then obtaining a homogeneous polysaccharide preparation. Frequently, it is necessary to break covalent linkages or use proteolytic enzymes. Chemical analyses utilizing hydrolysis, methylation, and periodate oxidation are complicated by the presence of amino sugars or uronic acid residues. Also,

Table 1. Major Chemical Constituents of Connective Tissue

Ground Substance

I. Mucopolysaccharides
    A. Acid   Hyaluronic Acid, Chondroitin Sulfate A,
                             B, and C, Chondroitin, Keratosulfate,
                             Heparitin Sulfate.
    B. Neutral
II. Proteins—locally synthesized including soluble collagen
III. Derivatives from plasma
    A. Water and electrolytes
    B. Serum proteins including antibodies
    C. Enzymes
    D. Hormones and vitamins
    E. Products of cellular metabolism

the occurrence of acetyl or sulphate groups renders these studies more difficult. The general molecular structure of the simpler mucopolysaccharides is sharply limited.

The acid mucopolysaccharides (AMP), listed in Table 1, all contain alternating sequences of two monosaccharide residues. Hyaluronic acid is a polymer of a disaccharide N-acetylhyalobiuronic acid and has an estimated molecular weight of eight million. Dense tissue such as cartilage concentrates ions while the electrolytes of loose connective tissue may not differ greatly from plasma. Enzymatically depolymerized hyaluronate exhibits an increased water-binding capacity probably due to the increased number of particles. Gersh and Catchpole [1] have studied the interaction of sodium, potassium, and other ions in connective tissue by an electrometric method. A colloid-rich and water-rich two phase system was evaluated. Loose connective tissues (water-rich) contain small amounts of insoluble, highly aggregated colloids binding potassium and calcium in concentrations similar to those of blood, while in cartilage (colloid-rich), potassium concentration is more than ten times that of blood. The values obtained were in agreement with the Gibbs-Donnan equilibrium.

In a total system, ground substance is an important regulating device of interstitial water and electrolytes. The swelling of connective tissue is primarily caused by an increase in water binding by the mucopolysaccharide-protein complexes, reflecting ion shifts. Collagen fibers in such areas are secondarily hydrated. Since the immediate environment of most cells is the ground substance and not the blood plasma, these considerations directly affect cellular homeostasis. The ionic environment of cells is maintained constant by thermodynamic principles determining the equilibrium between the density of colloidal charges in plasma and ground substance, the Gibbs-Donnan effect and the free energies of formation of ground substance complexes. Finally a variety of hormones and vitamins act on the ground substance. Thus, despite vigorous investigative efforts certain basic information remains unknown.

The shape of large molecules in solution is a random coil model of a flexible chain of small light-scattering units within a large, approximately spherical domain of solution producing spheres 2,100 Å in diameter. These individual spheres overlap, and the chains interpenetrate effecting certain properties, viscosity, elasticity, and structural rigidity. Such solutions when at rest can act as a continuous meshwork through which solvent flows with difficulty, but through which small molecules pass without difficulty.

The various chondroitin sulfates appear to be polymers of N-acetyl-chondrosamine, glucouronic acid, and sulfate. These acid mucopolysaccharides are bound to protein in the tissues much more firmly than hyaluronic acid. Chondroitin and keratosulfates have been isolated from bovine cornea. Recent studies have shown that connective tissue also contains significant amounts of polysaccharides which do not contain hexuronic acids as constituents. These have been referred to by some as neutral heteropolysaccharides and are strongly combined to proteins. A review of current studies concerned with synthesis of the carbohydrate chains, incorporation of $S^{35}O_4$, and proteins associated with the acid mucopolysaccharides is beyond the scope of this paper. However, the acid mucopolysaccharides as a group possess unique molecular configurations and spatial relationships.

Acid mucopolysaccharides have a capacity for binding various cations and basic residues in an ion exchange reaction. The total concentration of base-binding groups (colloidal negative charge) in the ground substance determines distribution of water and electrolytes between the blood and the ground substance. The origin and exact chemical nature of ground substance has been revealed in part. The detailed interrelationships between hormones, vitamins, enzymes, and trace metals in maintaining the homeostasis of ground substance are under intense study. This lack of fundamental information obscures attempts to understand the structural changes noted under abnormal homeostatic conditions.

Connective Tissue Fibers

Numerous reviews concerning the properties of the connective tissue fibers are available. Collagen occurs in dense fibrous tissue of high tensile strength, eg, tendons, or in less compactly woven tissue such as skin and loose connective tissue in a scattered fiber form. This class of fibrous proteins is uniquely characterized by its amino acid composition, x-ray diffraction pattern, and banded appearance under the electron microscope. The collagen macromolecule is a three stranded helix called a protofibril when arranged in a column. The lateral association of these protofibrils forms the collagen fibril which constitutes the characteristic collagen fiber observed under the light microscope.

Mature adult collagen fibers show the presence of bands at regular intervals of 650 Å with asymmetrical subspacing while embryonal and newly formed fibers show a prominent pattern of 210 Å. Characteristically, collagen contains considerable glycine, protein, and hydroxyproline in addition to 19 other identifiable amino acids. The nature of collagen's nonfibrous precursor has not been fully elucidated. Collagen may be rendered soluble by appropriate acid or alkali solutions. Solubilization[2, 3] begins with the breaking of the hydrogen bonds which stabilize the polypeptide chains as insoluble collagen. The addition of certain salts, mucopolysaccharides, and/or proteins to preparations of soluble collagen results in fiber formation with long spacings. Studies reveal that soluble collagen proteins obtained by any process are nearly identical and should be considered as a group of connective tissue proteins in a continuous spectrum of aggregation. Russian investigators have termed these aggregates "procollagens," indicating that they are the soluble precursors of insoluble collagen.

The fundamental building block of collagen, the tropocollagen molecule, contains extrahelix peptide chains. These telopeptides, of unknown number, are susceptible to digestion by a variety of noncollagenase proteases. Such proteolysis changes the properties of the tropocollagen but not its main structural features. Most of the intra- and intermolecular cross-links found in collagen occur through the telopeptides.

A long debated problem concerns the relationship of the ground substance constituents to collagen fiber formation. In amphibia and reptiles, collagen fibers are produced in the absence of mesenchymal cells and may develop from cellular materials of nonmesenchymal origin. These observations suggest that in these animals collagen fiber formation results from the interaction of macromolecular colloids. In the human, collagen fibers have been regarded as being derived from fibroblasts. Nevertheless, the possibility that collagen fibers may be formed in vivo in the absence of obvious cellular activity deserves serious consideration in human biology.

It has been postulated that fibroblasts elaborate a globular protein and mucopolysaccharides. A shift in the local pH to the acid range causes the protein to precipitate on the polysaccharide, and fibers are built up on the template, formed by regularly spaced acidic groups of the polysaccharide. Subsequent enzymatic digestion removes the polysaccharide sheath about the fibrils. Other observations suggest that collagen is crystallized out of the gel structure by the elimination of polysaccharide from the proteins of the collagen precursors. These findings are ample evidence to support the thesis concerning the mutually reciprocal roles of the fibroblast and the ground substance in collagen fiber formation. However, fibroblastic proliferation need not be related to collagen fiber formation, and collagen fiber production need not depend on fibroplasia. This concept helps to explain certain observations in pathology.

Reticulin refers to the fine extracellular fibrillary substances. These fibers branch and unite with each other to form a network or reticulum. The protein of reticulin appears to be similar to collagen and suggests an evolutionary relationship.

The nature of the elastic fiber is even less satisfactorily understood. Elastin is a polypeptide containing glycine, valine, alanine, and a small number of polar residues. X-ray diffractions of stretched elastic fibers show alternating, oriented and disoriented, long chains, a characteristic property of elastic proteins. Some analyses have revealed the presence of unsaturated fatty acids.

In addition to fibroblasts, normal connective tissue may contain mast cells, histiocytes, and occasional lymphocytes. Mast cell granules in the rat have been shown to contain heparin, serotonin, and histamine. These substances possess strong biological properties. The chemical composition of human mast cell granules is not clear. In addition, mast cells and histiocytes contain proteolytic enzymes. Histiocytes, like other cell members of the reticuloendothelial system, are rich in cytoplasmic acid phosphatase and esterases. The presence of lymphocytes in a random or focal collection may be related to the overall immune status of the host. Recent studies indicate that lymphocytes may have genetic importance.

Regulators

Extensive literature exists demonstrating the hormonal regulation of connective tissue. Hormones may influence basic synthetic mechanisms, cellular metabolism, integrity of fibers, and ground substance. In addition, the complex interactions of multiple hormones may produce profound systemic alterations of connective tissue with secondary changes in organ function. Cortisone, thyroxin, estrogen, testosterone, relaxin, insulin, deoxycorticosterone (DOCA), ACTH, TSH, and growth hormone may be concerned with the functional state of connective tissue.

Selected examples of hormonal influence would include the decrease of AMP by cortisone, while estrogen and testosterone stimulate an increase. In thyroidectomized guinea pigs, administration of TSH causes depletion of normal fat with replacement by a mucinous material rich in AMP. On the other hand, thyroxin opposes the effects of TSH. It is important to remember that measurable hormonally induced connective tissue changes are dependent on the age, sex, and species studied. Inferring such changes in man requires careful consideration.

Hyaluronidases are enzymes capable of hydrolyzing hyaluronic acid and have been isolated from Group A streptococci and testicular tissue. Collagenases are enzymes which degrade reticulin and collagen and are extracted from Clostridia organisms. The enzyme elastase has been derived from the pancreas and acts on elastin. These enzymes are difficult to purify and separate from contaminating enzymes. Thus, many preparations of hyaluronidase from bull testis contain chondromucinase and proteases. While there are normal (post-partum uterus) and experimental situations (dietary cirrhosis in the rat) associated with collagen absorption, no collagenase system has been identified to account satisfactorily for the reabsorption. In a similar manner, the significance of an elastase system in biological homeostasis has not been demonstrated.

Of the various vitamins, ascorbic acid is the most important in regulating the metabolic function of fibroblasts and the formation of collagen. Recent studies by Ross and Benditt,[4] utilizing proline-H^3 in assessing wound healing in normal and scorbutic guinea pigs, have demonstrated differences in rates of uptake and release of the label by fibroblasts. However, filamentous nonbanded material in the extracellular space is noted in the scorbutic animal at a time when fibril aggregation occurs in the normal. In addition, these workers have shown that scorbutic fibroblasts have an altered endoplasmic reticulum and lack intracytoplasmic collagen fibrils. It would seem that vitamin C is essential to the protein synthetic activities of the fibroblast and the ultimate formation of collagen. The role of other vitamins and trace metals in maintaining connective tissue function is largely unknown.

All biological systems are determined or regulated by genetic factors. A brief consideration of inborn errors of connective tissue metabolism must include Hurler's disease or gargoylism, Marfan's syndrome, and the Ehlers-Danlos syndrome.

Hurler's disease refers to a defect in either the formation or utilization of chondroitin sulfate C or heparitin sulfate. This material is excreted in the urine of

Hurler's patients in large amounts. Demonstration of heparitin sulfate in the urine has made careful genetic analysis of families and the detection of subtle cases or "formes frustes" possible. Typical patients present with retarded growth and mental abilities. In addition, there are serious complications in the eye and heart. Usually the structural alterations occur in tissues rich in chondroitin sulfate C.

Marfan's syndrome is a genetically determined defect in elastic fiber stability. In contrast to Hurler's disease, patients with Marfan's syndrome are tall, thin, with unusually long upper extremities, and long, tapered fingers. The root of the aorta dilates and may result in an intimal tear with subsequent hemorrhage into the aortic wall and fatal rupture. Microscopically, the aorta shows a disorganization of the normal elastic lamellar pattern with fragmentation of the fibers. There is preliminary evidence to suggest that the urinary excretion of hydroxyproline increases in Marfan's disease. Since this amino acid is primarily associated with the collagen fiber, Marfan's syndrome demonstrates the close relationship between collagen and elastin proteins.

Ehlers-Danlos syndrome, an inherited disorder, results in an unusual degree of elasticity of the connective tissue. These patients show hyperextensibility of joints and unusual stretch properties of skin.

The molecular defect is defined in Hurler's disease, so that the term mucopolysaccharidosis has been advocated. However, the molecular abnormalities in other heritable disorders of connective tissue remain unknown. Research is now in progress to ascertain the molecular defects which serve as chemical fingerprints in tracing the familial distribution of these diseases.

The Extracellular Hyaline Substance

Mucoid degeneration or mucinous alteration of connective tissue appears to be a reversible condition.[5] Apparently, local changes resulting in increased water binding by ground substance constituents account for the noted swelling. However, this particular change is not considered as a hyaline change. The extracellular hyaline substances are those materials observed in vascular walls or spaces and connective tissue. They include hyalin, fibrinoid, and amyloid.

Splenic arteriolar hyalinization is the most common vascular change observed. Hyalin is an amorphous, homogeneous, refractile material characteristically staining with eosin. The frequency, intensity, and distribution of arteriolar hyalin is increased by the presence of diabetes mellitus and/or hypertension in age-matched populations. However, vascular hyalinization in so-called normal individuals over the age of 70 years is present in 95 percent of the cases.[6] The relationship between aging and hyalinization of vessels and connective tissue in all mammals studied is remarkable. Yet the reasons for this relationship remain obscure.

Hyalin represents a particular phase in the shifting steady-state of connective tissue. Depending on the specific pathogenetic factors operating, hyalin varies in its physico-chemical properties. Hyalin is a generic, descriptive term limited by the subjective, qualitative character of the criteria used in the definition. Thus, hyalin has been reported to contain fibrin, platelets, glycoproteins, mucopolysaccharides, fragments of basement membranes, and products of degenerated cells. There are the hematogeneous and nohematogeneous theories of hyalin.[6] Both theories contain valid observations and it is possible that, depending on the state of the host, one or both are correct. The definition of hyalin should be regarded as encompassing a broad spectrum of biological materials.

We are indebted to Neumann (1880) for the introduction of "fibrinoid" into medical terminology. He used this term to describe an eosinophilic, acellular, homogeneous, and refractile material, which he has observed in a variety of inflammatory processes. Neumann considered that this substance was "fibrin-like" as it had tinctorial properties of fibrin. However, he distinguished it from fibrin and believed that its development had followed the degeneration of collagenous fibers, which had acquired the staining characteristics of fibrin.

In 1933 Klinge [7] postulated that fibrinoid was the pathognomonic lesion of hyperergic reactions. On the basis of fibrinoid presence, he maintained that it was justifiable to group such diseases as polyarteritis nodosa, malignant arteriosclerosis, Buerger's disease, some cases of nephritis, dermatomyositis, rheumatic fever, and chronic cardiovascular conditions, all of which could be regarded as immune biological reactions. He thought that the hyperergic mechanism allowed a melting together of cellular pathology with the modern humoral pathology, bacteriological, and serological theories.

Klemperer [8] disagreed with the sweeping generalizations of Klinge but felt that credit should be given to him for having been the first to recognize that fibrinoid was of significance in the pathogenesis of the lesions in which it was found.

Klinge focused attention upon the ground substance and said that the process began as a swelling or turgescence of the interfibrillar ground or cementing substance as well as the swelling of the delicate fibers of collagen. Gradually a "hyaline, fibrinoid-waxy refractile mass" was formed which showed the partial tinctorial reactions of fibrin. There were no cells in the center of this area, but towards the periphery monocytes, histiocytes, and even giant cells were often present. Granulation tissue was formed around the edges and led to the gradual encapsulation of the area with replacement of the cells. This interpretation of the development of the experimental lesion has formed the basis of the concept of the pathogenesis of the collagen diseases.

In 1942 while studying the lesions of disseminated lupus erythematosus and diffuse scleroderma, Klemperer, Pollack and Baehr [9] observed a fundamental widespread alteration of collagenous tissue; fibrinoid degeneration was the most prominent change. The term "diffuse collagen disease" was suggested by these authors in a representative sense. They wondered whether it would be justifiable to assume that a widespread derangement could exist, if it could not be demonstrated by ordinary histological methods. The collagenous system could be identified as the seat of certain diseases, but Klemperer et al [9] warned that this should not lead one to identify these diseases with one another or even to assume that they were related. Although widespread involvement of the collagenous tissue and fibrinoid degeneration were found in rheumatic fever, disseminated lupus erythematosus (S.L.E.), and diffuse scleroderma, they stressed the clearcut differences in the localization and evolution of the characteristic lesions and thought that these diseases should be strictly separated.

The term "diffuse mesenchymal diseases" has been reintroduced in recent times by Good et al [10] who were impressed by the "inordinate frequency" with which rheumatoid arthritis and other representatives of the so-called group of collagen diseases occurred in cases of agammaglobulinemia. They suggested that there was a common basis of mesenchymal tissue dysfunction in such instances. The presence of agammaglobulinemia would not rule out the operation of an immunological mechanism, since such patients retain specific immunological capacities of certain types.

The familial incidence of the collagen diseases has been studied and stressed as a possible etiological factor in rheumatic fever, rheumatoid arthritis, and lupus erythematosus. Good et al [10] contend that certain families have a high incidence of mesenchymal disease because of inherited predisposition. This may be manifested either by alteration of the immune mechanism or through another variation of the organization of the primitive mesenchymal system.

Venters and Good [11] prefer the term "mesenchymal" diseases to "connective tissue" diseases since it avoids confusion with the connective tissue disorders in which heritable disturbances of mucopolysaccharide metabolism are present, such as the Hurlers, Ehlers-Danlos, and Marfan syndromes.

A variety of terms have been proposed to replace "collagen diseases." However, like the original designation, the newer ones offer no insights into pathogenesis. In 1962, Klemperer [12] was satisfied to have "collagen diseases" replaced by the less controversial term "connective tissue diseases."

The evolution of fibrinoid as a manifestation of immunological phenomena was given impetus by the application of immunofluorescent techniques. Localization of gamma globulin in fibrinoid was regarded as evidence of antigen-antibody interaction. Since the antigen in most cases could not be identified, the assumption was made that the deposition of gamma globulin resulted from an immune precipitate. There is little doubt that in certain experimental situations, such as the Arthus reaction, antibody gamma globulin can be identified in the vascular fibrinoid.

Exactly how antigen-antibody interaction elicits tissue injury is not completely understood. In addition to the identification of gamma globulin (7S), complement (βlc-globulin) has been localized in the fibrinoid of vasculitis. Table 2 indicates

Table 2. Localization of Fluorescein-Labeled Protein Antibodies in Fibrinoid

	RHEUM. CARDITIS	SCLERODERMA	S.L.E.	EXP. FIBRINOID
Rabbit anti-human albumin	+	—	—	—
Rabbit anti-human γ globulin	+++	+	++	—
Rabbit anti-human fibrinogen	++	—	—	—
Horse anti-rabbit γ globulin	—	—	—	+++

Key: — no localization; + to ++++, slight to intense fluorescence

some of the proteins identified by the authors in human fibrinoid from fatal cases of rheumatic carditis (Aschoff body), generalized scleroderma (renal arterioles), systemic lupus erythematosus (S.L.E.) (glomerular "wire-loops"), and experimental vasculitis in the rabbit.

Table 3. Susceptibility of Fibrinoid to Enzyme Action

Enzyme	Rheum. Carditis	Scleroderma	S.L.E.	Exp. Fibrinoid
Trypsin	++++	—	++	++++
Pepsin	++++	++++	++++	++++
Fibrinolysin	+	—	—	+++
Strep. Hyaluronidase	—	—	—	—
Test. Hyaluronidase	++++	—	—	++
β-Glucuronidase	—	—	—	—
Diastase	—	—	—	—

Key: — no effect; + to ++++ slight to complete digestion

The theory that a spectrum of fibrinoids exists is further supported by Table 3. Here, a variety of enzymes was used to act on the fibrinoid substrate. Using carefully controlled conditions, the only variable was the fibrinoid itself. Obviously, the fibrinoid in each case reflected the intensity and duration of the host's response and the influence of potent drug therapy. In spite of this, the results have been amazingly reproducible and a pattern emerges for each disease. Figure 2 is a tangential section of a renal arteriole from the case of scleroderma. Fibrinoid appears as broad lakes or pools. By contrast, Figure 3 is from the myocardium of a rabbit immunized with bovine serum albumin (BSA). The fibrinoid appears as dense clumps or bands sharply delineated from surrounding structures. Figure 4 shows a glomerulus

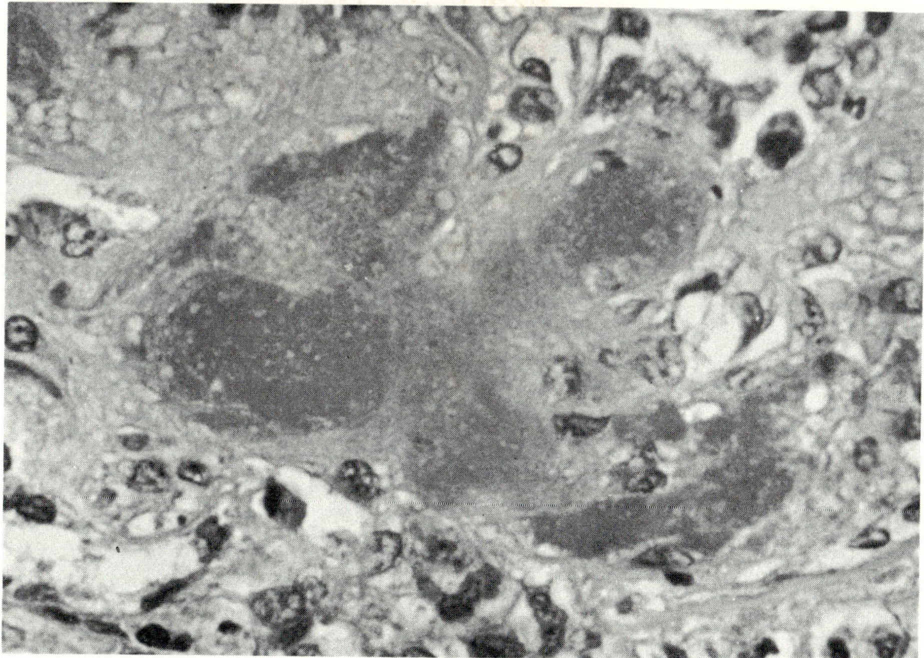

Fig. 2. Tangential section of renal arteriole from a fatal case of generalized scleroderma. Fibrinoid is present in lakes or pools with a fine vacuolated appearance. Formalin fixed, paraffin section. H&E. × 800.

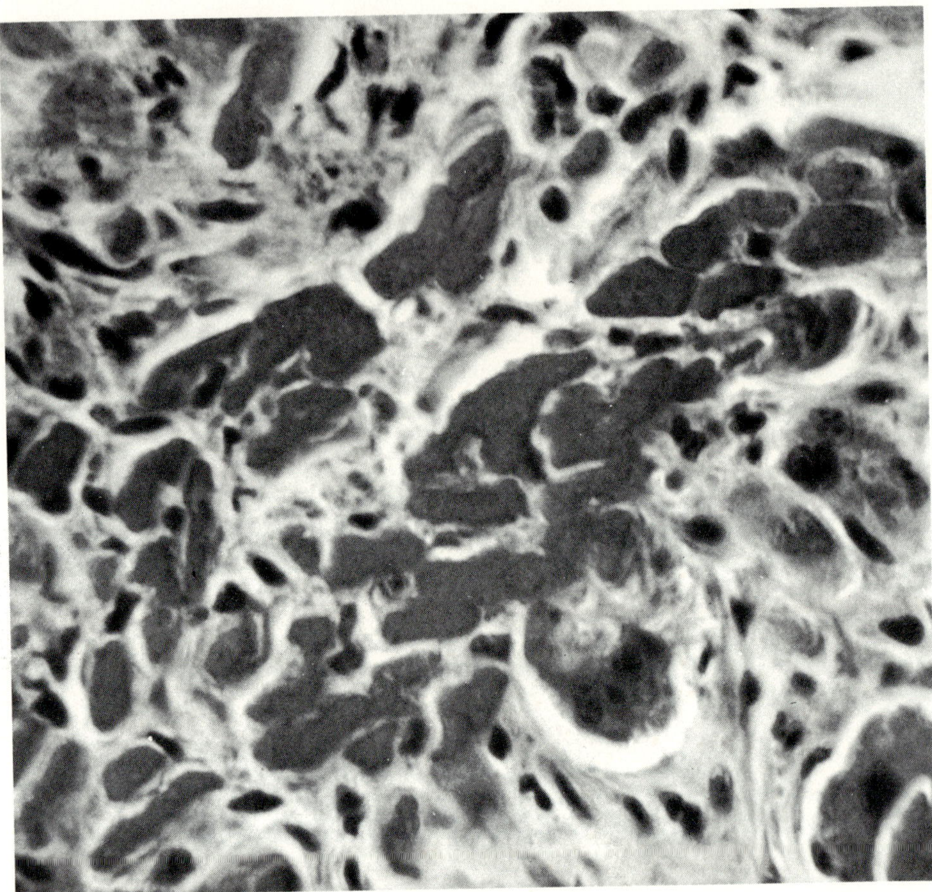

Fig. 3. Adult male New Zealand rabbit immunized with BSA. Section of myocardium reveals fibrinoid in the connective tissue stroma. Formalin fixed, paraffin section. H&E. × 800.

from an S.L.E. case after treatment with trypsin. The fibrinoid has been removed from a wire-loop lesion and only the outer wall of the loop is visible. When intravascular coagulation takes place in a glomerulus, as in Figure 5, one may frequently see the agglutination of red cells and thrombus formation. This is fibrin and clearly not fibrinoid.

One should not regard fibrinoid as a broad, descriptive term. It should be used always with a particular spontaneous disease or experimentally induced condition. Scleroderma fibrinoid is quite different from rheumatic fibrinoid, which is different from experimental Arthus fibrinoid. The aim of modern pathology should be to elucidate the mechanisms involved in fibrinoid production for clearly identifiable disease states. Experimental models are helpful but remain limited by the nature of the manipulations involved. Spontaneous diseases of animals associated with

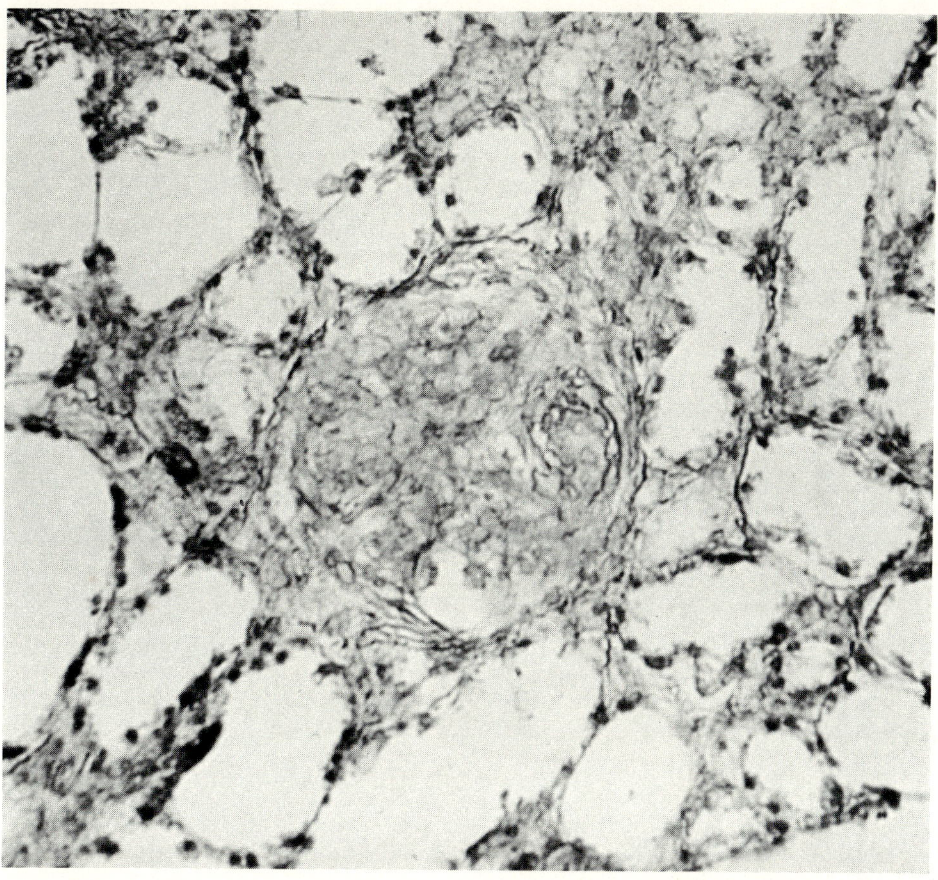

Fig. 4. Section of kidney from fatal case of S.L.E. treated with trypsin (lmg/ml, 2 hours at 37°C) to digest fibrinoid in the "wire loops" of glomeruli. Glomerulus in the center shows the outlines of capillaries which originally were typical thickened fibrinoid bands. Frozen section, unfixed. H&E. × 460.

fibrinoid alterations would offer a more fruitful source of material. Aleutian disease of mink, equine infectious anemia, polyarteritis of rats, and amyloidosis of mice are examples of naturally occurring disease states with extracellular hyaline substances present.

The nature and pathogenesis of amyloid have recently been reviewed in an excellent paper by Cohen.[13] Amyloid is unique among the hyaline substances in its characteristic fibrillar appearance by electron microscopy. There is abundant evidence to suggest that the reticuloendothelial cell is primarily involved in the genesis of the amyloid fibril. Unlike the fibrinoids, amyloids are strikingly resistant to proteolytic enzyme digestion. Amyloid shares with hyalin the propensity to occur spontaneously in man and other species as a function of age.

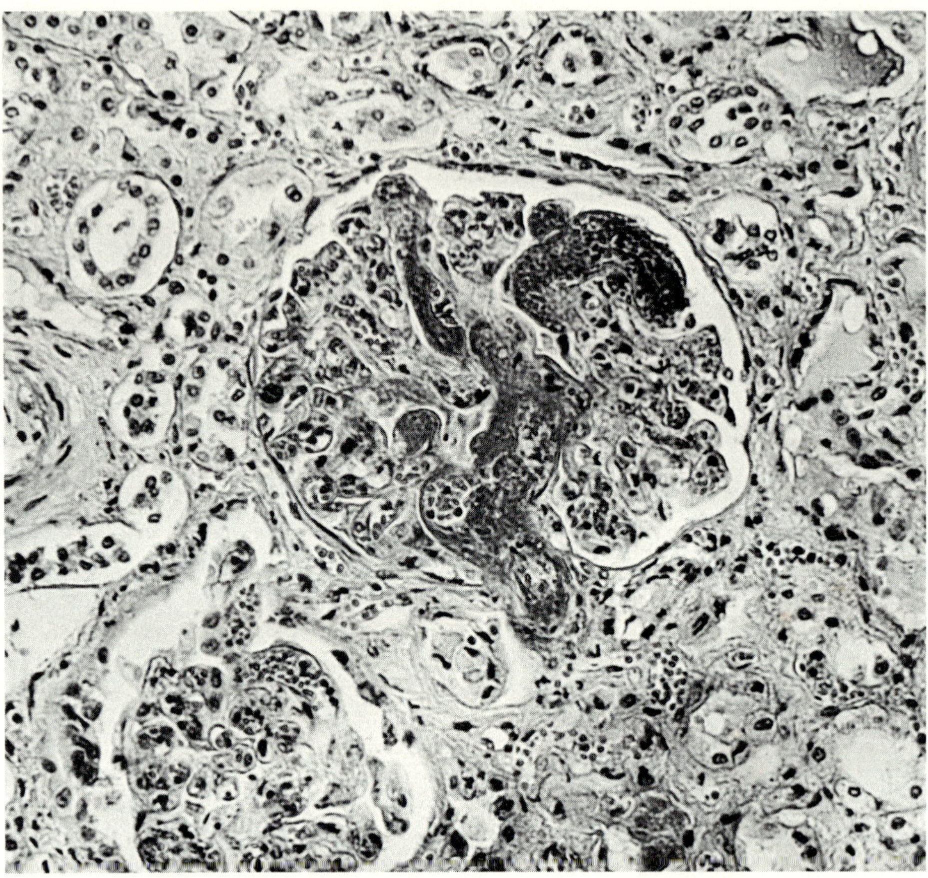

Fig. 5. Renal tissue from rabbit treated with endotoxin to elicit the generalized Shwartz-man reaction. A glomerulus in the center with intracapillary coagulation and fibrinoid appearing material. Note the aggregation of red cells and incorporation into the amorphous mass. Formalin fixed, paraffin section. H&E. × 460.

Summary

The abnormal deposition of material in the extracellular ground substance creates a barrier to the effective transport of materials between the cell and its nutrient supplying capillary. As this state intensifies a variety of changes occur in the function of tissues and organs. "Systemic connective tissue disease" is currently most acceptable as a conceptual term. Classical pathology has given us the terms hyalin, fibrinoid, and amyloid, which may be grouped as extracellular hyaline substances. Until these materials are identified and their evolution understood, it serves no useful purpose to propose other terms. A spectrum of hyalins, fibrinoids, and amyloids exists. The study of these substances in spontaneous diseases of man and animals continues to be an important function of modern biology.

References

1. Gersh, I., and Catchpole, H. R. The nature of the ground substance of connective tissue. Perspect. Biol. Med. (Paris), 3:282, 1960.
2. Drake, M. P., Davison, P. F., Bump, S., and Schmitt, F. O. Action of proteolytic enzymes on tropocollagen and insoluble collagen. Biochemistry (Wash.), 5:301, 1966.
3. Bornstein, P., Kang, A. H., and Piez, K. A. The nature and location of intramolecular cross-links in collagen. Proc. Nat. Acad. Sci., 55:417, 1966.
4. Ross, R., and Benditt, E. P. Wound healing and collagen formation: III. J. Cell Biol., 15:99, 1962.
5. Wagner, B. M. Hypersensitivity, The role of the connective tissue. *In* Analytical Pathology, Mellors, R., ed., New York, McGraw-Hill Book Company, Inc., 1957, pp. 429–470.
6. McKinney, B. The pathogenesis of hyaline arteriosclerosis. J. Path. Bact., 83:449, 1962.
7. Klinge, F. Der Rheumatismus. Ergebn. Allg. Path., 27:1, 1933.
8. Klemperer, P. Über fibrinoide Substanzen. Wien, Klin. Wochen., 36:713, 1953.
9. Klemperer, P., Pollack, A., and Baehr, G. Concept of the collagen diseases. J.A.M.A., 119:331, 1942.
10. Good, R. A., Venters, H. D., Jr., Page, A. R., and Good, T. A. Diffuse connective tissue diseases in childhood. Lancet, 81:192, 1961.
11. Venters, H. D., Jr., and Good, R. A. Current concepts of the pathogenesis of the so-called collagen diseases. Pediat. Clin. N. Amer., 10:1017, 1963.
12. Klemperer, P. Personal communication, 1962.
13. Cohen, A. The Nature of Amyloid. *In* Connective Tissue Monograph, Wagner, B., and Smith, D., eds., Philadelphia, The Williams & Wilkins Co. In Press.

Addendum

Continuing analysis of fibrinoid as it occurs in arterial walls and extravascular sites has demonstrated that immunologic reactants are almost invariably present at some time These reactants include immunoglobulins, complement factors, and immune complexes. However. other plasma proteins, especially fibrinogen frequently can be identified. The method commonly employed for localization and identification of these proteins is immunofluorescence Reagents are readily available and the procedure is now as routine as staining with hematoxylin and eosin. Immunofluorescent staining is a histochemical procedure, not a general staining reaction, and requires stringent controls if results are to be considered valid. Careful attention must be directed to the "materials and methods" sections of all reports claiming to show protein moieties in fibrinoid.

Nonspecific staining (NSS) with fluorescein-labeled antibodies is based on electrostatic adsorption of labeled IgG by more positively charged tissue proteins. Globulins with a high dye content give a strong NSS. The labeling of IgG with fluorescein isothiocyanate results in heterogeneous conjugates. Recently, Arnold and Mayersbach have carefully studied the solubility of immunoglobulins after fluorescent labeling and its influence on immunofluorescent techniques.[1] They clearly establish the need to control the precipitation of IgG conjugates in the precipitation-purification method by determining the appropriate conditions either for avoiding heavy losses of IgG or for increasing the precipitation in order to eliminate NSS. It is now apparent that much of the conflicting data as to the protein constituents in fibrinoid—while influenced by the nature, duration, and intensity of the disease process—are due to discrepancies in immunofluorescent techniques.

The recent interest in organ transplants has led to additional interesting observations on vascular fibrinoid. Sinclair et al studied the arterial lesions in rat cardiac allografts.[2] There was strong evidence relating graft arterial fibrinoid to antibody mediated damage and subsequent rejection. Immunofluorescence showed that the fibrinoid contained complement (C3) and IgG. However, in a series of long-surviving treated human renal allografts, IgM was common in arteries with fibrinoid and obliterative lesions.[3] A most important observation made by Sinclair et al was the presence of mononuclear cells marginating against arterial endothelium and within the subendothelial space before C3 and IgG were frequently present. This implies that mononuclear cells can accumulate in the absence of antibody and complement. Healing of vessels with fibrinoid is by intimal thickening. Since endothelial vacuolation and edema are common findings in vessels of rejecting allografts, mononuclear cells producing cytotoxic effects may be responsible. These changes may precede the intramural deposition of immunologic reactants recognized by light microscopy as fibrinoid.

Amyloid is a highly organized substance composed of fibrils having a characteristic appearance in the electron microscope. Glenner has shown that the major constituent of amyloid is a protein related to the light chain of immunoglobulins.[4] This protein consists of either the whole light chain or of a variable fragment. Glenner's patients had plasma-cell neoplasms or primary amyloidosis. Most of them had in their serum or urine a light chain or myeloma protein closely related or identical in structure to that in the tissue. Glenner also showed that some Bence-Jones proteins can develop the typical fibrillar appearance of amyloid in vitro after proteolytic digestion. It seems likely that this type of amyloid results from the degradation of certain L chains and their deposition in tissues. Amyloid related to heavy chains has not been observed to date.

In contrast, other investigators have reported that the major component of secondary amyloid and amyloid associated with familial Mediterranean fever is a unique protein not related to immunoglobulin or any known sequenced protein.[5] Heterogeneity at the amino terminus suggests a possible origin by proteolysis of a precursor. Some L chain-related proteins in these amyloids have been demonstrated recently.[6] It now appears likely that the chemical and immunologic studies in progress will provide a more rational basis for the classification of amyloid. More attention must be given to the amyloid of aging since it has been observed widely in diverse mammalian species.

Advances in understanding the nature of mucoid swelling of the ground substance and extracellular hyalin have not kept pace with studies of the various fibrinoids and amyloids. However. a model is now available for study and may yield significant information concerning the dynamic nature of the extracellular connective tissue ground substance.

Spontaneous, canine mitral valvular fibrosis is a disease of unknown origin. It is most frequently seen in smaller breeds and can lead to mitral insufficiency and cardiac failure The earliest change noted in the mitral valve leaflets is mucoid swelling.[7] This is followed by a slow, progressive deposition of collagen. In time the collagen is converted to an amorphous hyaline mass. Inflammatory cells are rarely observed. The natural history of the valvular changes clearly demonstrates that ground substance swelling precedes eventual hyalinization of the area. The intermediate role of collagen formation is not clear and may represent a response to hemodynamic stresses.[8] Histochemical studies of the early mucoid changes suggest that there is increased water-binding by the acid mucopolysaccharides.

In experimental immune damage of the rabbit cornea,[9] mucoid swelling or edema precedes the degradation of collagen produced by leukocytic lysosomal enzymes. The relationship between the protein–AMP complexes and the collagen fibers they invest is critical in order to maintain the integrity of the connective tissue.[10] It would seem that alterations in AMP can set off either a proliferative or degradative collagen response. Factors controlling the steady state of the ground substance are under investigation.

References

1. Arnold W, Mayersbach H: Changes in the solubility of immunoglobulins after fluorescent labeling and its influence on immunofluorescent techniques. J Histochem Cytochem 20:975, 1972
2. Sinclair RA, Andres G A, Hsu KC: Immunofluorescent studies of the arterial lesions in rat cardiac allografts. Arch Pathol 94·331, 1972
3 Busch JG, Galvanek EG, Reynolds ES: Human renal allografts: analysis of lesions in long-term survivors. Hum Pathol 2:253, 1971
4. Glenner GG, Terry WD, Isersky C: Amyloidosis: its nature and pathogenesis. Semin Hematol 10:65, 1973
5. Levin M, Pras M, Franklin EC: Immunologic studies of the major nonimmunoglobulin protein of amyloid. J Exp Med 138:373, 1973
6. Franklin EC: The complexity of amyloid. N Engl J Med 290:512 1974
7. Wagner BM: Myocardial disease in man and dog. Ann NY Acad Sci 147:354, 1968
8. Fenoglio JJ, Jr, Wagner BM: Current concepts of acquired valvular heart disease. J Mt Sinai Hosp (NY) 41:341, 1974
9. Mohos S, Wagner BM: Immune precipitate induced corneal damage Arch Pathol 3:20, 1969
10. Fenoglio JJ, Jr, Wagner BM: Studies in rheumatic fever. VI. Ultrastructure of chronic carditis. Am J Pathol 73:623, 1974

VEGETATIVE ENDOCARDITIS*

ALFRED ANGRIST

MASAMICHI OKA

KOMEI NAKAO

This presentation will not attempt to review the subject of human endocarditis but will offer the authors' experience with valvular vegetations in an extensive series of autopsies, and discuss the theoretical implications. Many excellent informative and analytical pathological and clinical surveys with bacteriological data and their correlations are available.[1-21] A survey of the history of endocarditis is given because the evolution of our knowledge of the valvular vegetation helps with the appreciation of the separate morphological forms and their interrelationships and is pertinent for the understanding of the many transitional forms encountered. The early mechanisms and the related fundamental biological background of endocarditis will be the focus of discussion.

Why such a pathological entity as endocarditis exists at all is of primary interest. Why do not the equivalent lesions occur with equal frequency in the endothelium and in the veins and arteries? Why the high incidence and the peculiar character of the valvular vegetation? How do these unique lesions of the valve take on their characteristic forms? We believe that valvular vegetative endocarditis occurs as an entity because of a peculiarity of valve tissue. This connective tissue is unique; it remains labile and reactive throughout life and is prone to respond to local allergy. It remains responsive to specific hormonal influences and general stress stimulations. The heart valve is rich in mucopolysaccharides (Boström et al)[22, 23] and has a high uptake of tritiated L-proline.[24] Valves originate from the valve cushions, the mesenchyme. The unique reactivity of this tissue, "persistent mesenchyme," has been

* Work supported by NIH Grant 5 R01 HE 02190—1 to 11.

stressed by von Albertini,[25] Dietrich,[26] and Siegmund,[27] its susceptibility to allergic reactions by Böhmig [28, 29] and Böhmig and Klein.[30]

History of Vegetative Endocarditis

The historical development of the subject of endocarditis is of interest. At first no distinction between bacterial and nonbacterial vegetations was made, and the vegetations were confused with postmortem staining and clots, the so-called polypi. Description, subdivision, and classification are the general rules applied for the historical evolution of all pathology. Only recently because of the ambiguous transitional forms has the problem of interrelationship of the individual forms of endocarditis come into focus. Now with antibiotic therapy, the transitional forms have become more frequent than ever. These concepts originated from the transitional instances of endocarditis encountered at autopsy.[31-33] Classical lesions and transitions were then experimentally verified.[35-38]

The entity of endocarditis has been a source of confusion for many years, since postmortem clots were not distinguished from vegetations. In addition ambiguous terms like "polyps," "carbuncles," "tubercles," and "ulcerations" were used. In 1630 Bartoletti [39] described an "ulceration of the heart"; in 1646 Riverius [40] made the clinical diagnosis of "obstruction of the vessels by soft tubercles" and found at autopsy "carbuncles like the substance of the lungs, the larger of which resembled hazelnuts and blocked the aorta." Morgagni [41] described "carbuncles" of the heart valve and considered them the result of venereal disease, since the vegetations were similar to venereal warts. The latter idea prevailed until Laennec, and in 1707 Lancisi [42] recorded a case that was probably subacute bacterial endocarditis. Baillie [43] in 1797 described valves in a state of "inflammation" with a layer of "coagulated lymph."

Many years later, in 1813, Kreysig [44] read a paper on "Pulposa Carditis," which stressed inflammation in the formation of the polyps, significantly intimating that "they grew out from the valves and heart wall and were not deposited from the blood." He considered these lesions a product of illness and not its main cause; he also recognized the possibility of their role in endocarditis as a cause of embolism and of death. In the same year Hodgeson [45] described several examples of aortic endocarditis. Bertini [46] described valvular vegetations in 1824.

In 1819, three years after his invention of the stethoscope, Laennec [47] turned his attention to endocarditis; he diagnosed stenosis or "ossification" of the mitral valve and described warty excrescences which looked like venereal warts. He did not believe the lesions to be venereal in origin, as did his teacher Corvisart,[48] who coined the word "vegetation." Laennec felt that the warty excrescences were due to "coagulation without inflammation" of the blood. He also described ruptured chordae.

Though others had related rheumatism to heart disease, Bouillaud [49] is credited with this association, for in 1835 he emphasized the relation of rheumatic fever to valvular disease. Bouillaud gave us the term "endocarditis"; he also disposed of the myths of postmortem clots and postmortem staining. Most of his contemporaries disagreed with Bouillaud. However Bright [50] did note a relationship between chorea and endocarditis, and thus supported Bouillaud, as did Paget.[51] Paget also described a case of endocarditis in a patient who had gonorrhea.

Embolism as a consequence of vegetations was intimated by Kreysig,[44] but the concept was clearly established by Kirkes,[52] who in 1852 noted large fibrinous masses on heart valves with the equivalent of infarcts in the spleen and kidney. Wilks[53] described "vegetations of fibrous coagula" as a focus of infection with "pyemia." Ormerod[54] in 1851 clearly differentiated between rheumatic and ulcerative endocarditis.

The modern view of endocarditis, including embolization, was the result of the work of Virchow.[55, 56] This was based on human autopsy experience and experimental work. In 1870 Winge,[57, 58] a student of Virchow, found in a case of endocarditis and thrombosis organisms in the form of "threads" on smear, "which were not fibrin and were rod-shaped, round bodies, branched in places" resembling bacteria. Winge considered the lesion to be due to a parasitic disorder and tried unsuccessfully to reproduce the lesion. Rokitansky[59] demonstrated, in a single microscopic study, microorganisms in a vegetation.

In 1872 Heiberg[60] found microorganisms in a case of ulcerative endocarditis in puerpural fever, and his observation was confirmed at least in part by Virchow. Heiberg tried but failed to produce endocarditis in the dog by introducing portions of the vegetations subcutaneously, intraperitoneally, and intravenously. Klebs[61] in 1878 differentiated the "ulcerative form with cocci" or "monads" from the "verrucous form without bacteria." Jaccoud[62] in 1885 noted the value of blood culture, and gave a rather clear clinical description of bacterial endocarditis (BE). In 1886, Wyssokowitsch[63] isolated *Staphylococcus aureus* from ulcerative endocarditis and produced this disease in animals by trauma to the valve followed by injection of the bacterium.

Thus infectious bacterial endocarditis was the first to be recognized and produced experimentally; only later were the nonbacterial lesions recognized. Königer[64] related bacterial infection of a previously nonbacterial vegetation. Harbitz[65] actuated the present classification of endocarditis in 1861 with a description of "chronic and acute" forms. Only later did Lenhartz,[66] Schottmüller,[67] Libman and Celler,[68] Libman,[69] Osler,[70, 71] and others[1] separate subacute bacterial endocarditis (SBE) from the acute form (ABE) as a clinical entity and pathological lesion. Lenhartz[66] clearly demarcated the chronic form of endocarditis in 1901. Nonbacterial vegetations included rheumatic, thrombotic, terminal or marantic forms, and only later, the Libman-Sacks or atypical verrucous lesions.

Most clinicians and pathologists stressed the acute form of the disease with the dramatic clinical picture. Different terms were used, such as "embolic endocarditis" by Koester[72] in 1878, "malignant endocarditis" by Osler[70] in 1885, "septic endocarditis" by Lenhartz[66] in 1901, and "infectious endocarditis" by Horder[1] in 1908. Thayer[7] favored the last term, for now in addition to bacteria, rickettsia, histoplasma, and fungi were also found.

It was Schottmüller[67] and Libman and Celler[68] who emphasized the association of viridans streptococci with the subacute form of the disease. Osler[71] ultimately accepted the subacute type as a distinctive entity in 1909. Clawson et al[3, 4] studied 220 cases of endocarditis and maintained that rheumatic and bacterial endocarditis are reactions of different intensity to the same organism; he thought viridans streptococci were responsible for both rheumatic (RE) and subacute bacterial endocarditis.

Osler,[71, 72] Libman,[69] Blumer,[2] Thayer,[7] Laws and Levine,[65] David and Weiss,[74] Perry,[8] Gross and Friedberg,[75] Von Glahn and Pappenheimer,[76] Ribbert,[77] and others [78] emphasized the fact that bacterial endocarditis was often associated with a previous valvular deformity, particularly with old rheumatic heart disease and congenital heart lesions.[79-83]

Valvular Distortions and Nonbacterial Thrombotic Endocarditis (NBTE)

Nonbacterial thrombotic endocarditis (NBTE) occurs frequently on a damaged valve, but can occur on the normal valve, particularly in the older patient, in a terminal cachectic individual or in severe sepsis in the young. The clinical significance of NBTE is based on its tendency to become infected or to be dislodged as a bland embolus, and to become organized and distort valves.

It is well known that patients develop valvular distortion long after the first attack of rheumatic fever, often never again experiencing another incident of frank rheumatic disease; yet the stenosis evolves progressively over the years. What happens during the long silent interval from the first attack to the manifest valvular distortion, stenosis, or insufficiency is a critical question. It is our contention that infections (other than RE) and/or nonspecific stress can affect the valve.[31-38] Endocrine factors can also promote valvular changes.[82, 83] Recently, Vaisman et al [84] concluded that "penicillin could not alter the course of acute rheumatic valvulitis" and further, that "once rheumatic fever developed, streptococci had nothing to do with it." It is suggested that rheumatic fever is not the only causative factor for valvular distortion, as in stenosis. Experimental studies indicate that many forms of nonspecific stress, including parabiosis, physical cold, high altitude,[35] different hormones,[38] and arteriovenous shunts [82] are capable of producing valvular distortion (Table 1).

Table 1. Proposed Theory for Mechanism of Endocarditis

Stress	Specific—infection, allergy Nonspecific—cold, altitude, etc
Hormonal Changes	Pituitary-adrenal, axis, ACTH Deoxycorticosterone acetate, growth, etc
Interstitial Valvulitis	Edema, cellularity, collagen changes
Vegetation—NBTE	Platelets, fibrin, fibrinoid, etc
Surface Contamination	Sterilized or progressive
Inflammation and Ulceration, etc	BE—ABE or SBE

Valvular distortions include thickening, fibrosis, hyalinization, elastification, collagen alteration, fusion with stenosis, retraction with regurgitation, cellular reaction, and vegetation formation. In many acute illnesses and in shock or uremia, edema (Fig. 1) is an initial and early valvular distortion and often appears at the edge of valves. This early change is particularly prominent in the young subject. Histologically the edematous area contains acid mucopolysaccharide and incor-

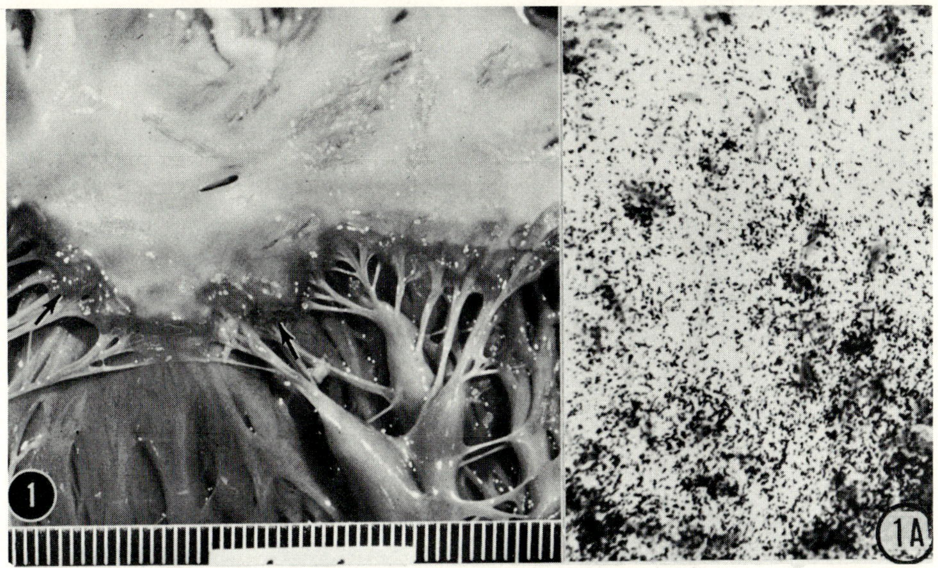

Fig. 1. Gross appearance of mitral valve in a 24 year old adult male who died of uremia due to glomerulonephritis. Note the edematous edge of the valve (arrows) which appears a bit darker because of mild hemolytic staining. Increments of such change over the years can alter and thicken the regional tissue of the valve considerably. 1A. Autoradiograph of the heart valve of Figure 1. Thin segment of the edge of the valve was incubated in 5 μc of S^{35} in 5 ml of buffer for four hours. Paraffin sections were then dipped in NTB-3 emulsion and exposed two weeks. Silver grains are increased considerably and accumulate in foci, when compared to a valve lacking the edematous change.

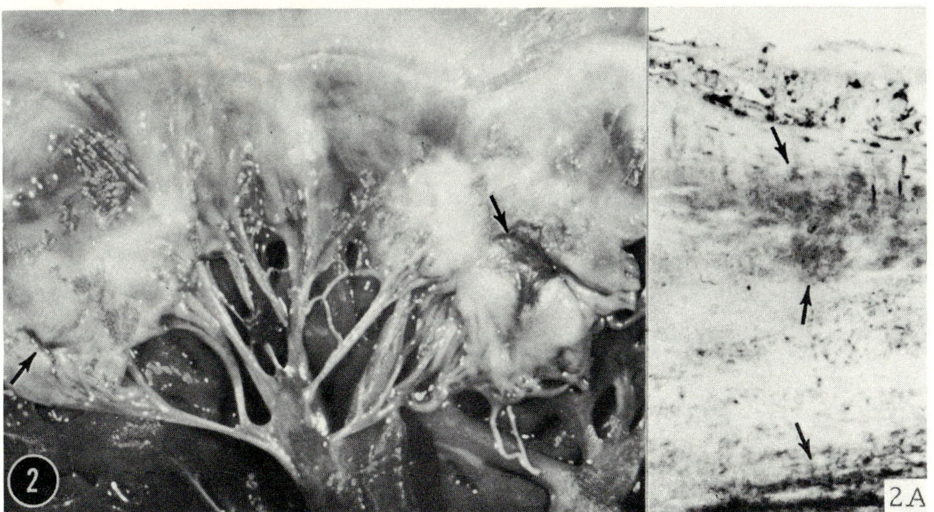

Fig. 2. A senile nonrheumatic tricuspid valve in an individual 72 years old. Note the elongated bulging appearance. Arrows point to areas of erosion of the thickened valve cusp. The chordae tendinae tend to insert into the edge of the valve and are also thickened. This so-called billowing sail distortion of the valve is the most common deformity of the valve of aged dogs with cardiac decompensation. 2A. Section through the thickened valve shows distortion of the collagen. Arrows point to the darker area of strained lipid. $\times$ 80.

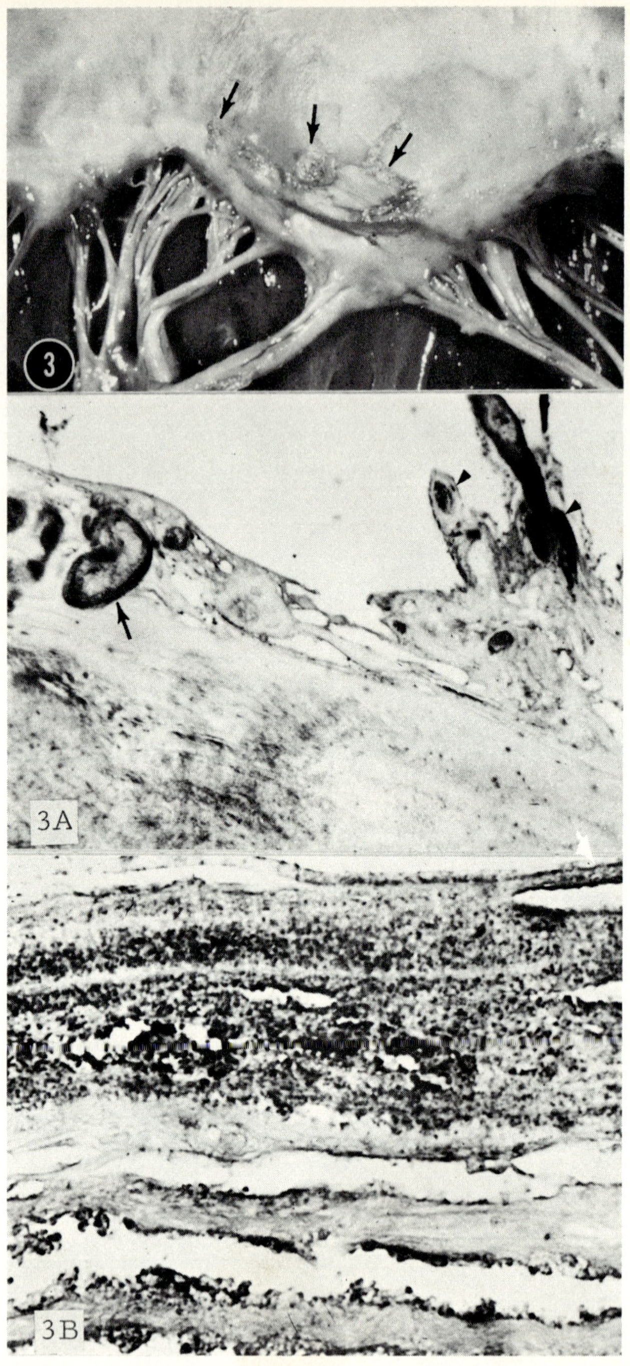

Fig. 3. Thickened mitral valve from a 72 year old male with granular irregularities indicated by arrows. Note the thickening of the chordae tendinae and their insertion into the very edge. The pearly white thickening of the valve surface proper is intimated in this photograph. 3A. Microscopic section of the valve through the region of the superficial granular distortion. Oval and circular zones of darker staining (arrow) beneath the endothelium are lipid stained with oil-red-O. This tissue also reacts positively with the elastica stain. Note also the extension of such areas above the surface of the valve (arrowheads). Fibrillation of the valve contributes to the roughened appearance. × 25. 3B. Elastica Van Gieson stain of the valve. Note globular elastin and extent of the fibrillar alteration and the depth to which it goes. Platelets often accumulate on the surface of such a valve and in the slit-like spaces. × 230.

porates S[35] (Fig. 1A) in both the experimental animal and in human valves with this change. With the edematous distortion often an interstitial cellular reaction occurs and ultimately a fibrous thickening. When thickening of the valve supervenes, the cellular reaction subsides and hyalinization of collagen fibers follows; this sclerotic region of the valve often shows lipid and is positive with oil-red-0 (Fig. 2A).

In addition, sclerosis of the valves occurs as a phenomenon of aging[34] and as a result of fibrous organization of recurrent NBTE (Table 2). In the aged group, the

Table 2. NBTE Without Infection
(Platelets, Fibrin, Fibrinoid, few RBC and WBC)

Early Lesion	No inflammation, no organization changes, bland embolization to brain, coronaries, and other viscera.
Outcome of Bland NBTE	Lysis with absorption (fibrinolysis), indolent reaction and organization (histiocyte, round cell, and fibroblasts) with fibrosis beginning at base.
Resolution or Valve Distortions	Fusion of commissures, tabs and whiskers, collagenous scarring with stenosis (thickening), rare insufficiency (dog), calcification and ossification (valve and ring).
Recurrent NBTE	Increments of fibrosis to give final variable and even marked valvular distortion.

valves tend to present these later alterations along with the so-called billowing sail distortion (Fig. 2). Very often there is an associated superficial erosion or ulceration (Fig. 2 arrow). Distortion of the staining of collagen in the form of a dense eosinophilia and oil-red-0 staining (Fig. 2A) also occurs in thickened areas of the valves. In such a valve the erosion or ulceration is often, but not always, covered with fibrin or platelets. The valve with more advanced distortion of this type shows a rough surface or even a granular appearance on the surface grossly (Fig. 3).

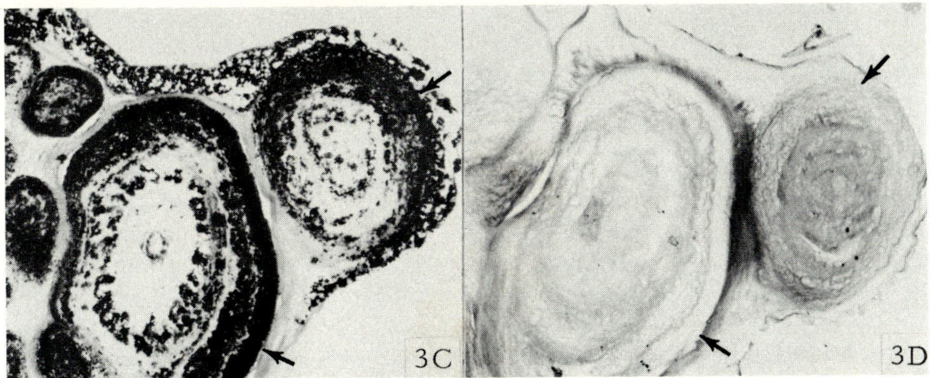

Fig. 3C. Elastica stain of some of the whiskers. Note the concentric circular arrangement of globular elastin (arrow). This pattern is common in such nodules. × 90. 3D. Next section from the same block as in Figure 3C, digested by elastase for a period of three hours. Globular elastin disappeared, leaving empty spaces (arrows). × 90.

Histologically the rough thick valve often reveals so-called buried fibrinoid nodules (Fig. 3A) [85, 86] and globular elastin with fatty change. In such a distorted valve a fibrillated appearance, like arthritic cartilage, is frequently encountered on the surface (Fig. 3B). This material is partly digested by elastase, as is the increased elastica component (Figs. 3C, 3D). The hyaline collagen is less susceptible to collagenase.

It is of interest to note that elastin often appears in the "whiskers" (Figs. 3A, 3C) or at the surface of such distorted valves and may have a granular or globular appearance, instead of the ordinary fibrillar or lamellar form (Figs. 3B, 3C). Such elastin may be more resistant to elastase digestion than the ordinary fibrillar elastin. Lansing et al [87, 88] noted that older elastin digested more readily. If Lansing's data apply to the globular valvular elastin, this globular elastin is younger even though it is more common in the aged. Some relationship may well exist between the globular elastin and platelet accumulation often found in such areas.

The DPNH diaphorase reaction often demonstrates platelets attached to the irregularities and the surface (Fig. 8), as do electron microscopic studies [89] (Figs. 7, 7A, 29).

NBTE and Its Varying Morphology and Sequences

Siegmund [27] considered the vegetation a thromboendocarditic process based on an indifferent mesenchymal reaction in the endothelial layer, and described a lesion beneath the endothelium which then established a nidus by an alteration of the overlying endothelium. Pfuhl,[90] Königer,[63] Coombs,[85, 86] De Vecchi,[91] Cziner,[92] Holsti,[93] Semsroth and Koch,[94] Klinge and Vaubel,[95] Leary,[96] Gross and Friedberg,[75] Böhmig,[30] and Clawson [3] all stressed that the lesion beneath the endothelium is the primary one. Miller et al [97] stressed the interstitial changes in the valve due to lymphatic obstruction in the dog. Stetson,[98] Grant et al,[99] Nedzel,[100, 101] and others stressed the role of early accretion of platelets. We conclude that there is an early subendothelial lesion and then the endothelial change that follows with super-imposed platelets (Figs. 7, 8, 29).

Ziegler [102] in 1888 used the term "thrombo-endocarditis" to describe a noninflammatory disease similar to the marantic thrombi. Harbitz [65] (1889) used the term "cachectic endocarditis" because the vegetations were terminal, occurring toward the end of a lethal disease.

Gross and Friedberg [75] tried to ascertain whether thrombotic endocarditis occurred merely as an accidental and incidental finding in common diseases or whether such NBTE represented part of a definitive, characteristic, and specific syndrome, comparable to what prevails with rheumatic fever or with atypical verrucous endocarditis in lupus erythematosus. They concluded from their studies that nonbacterial thrombotic endocarditis is an "accidental occurrence in the course of many different fatal diseases," "without any appreciable clinical significance." Gould [103] also maintained the same view. However, Angrist [31-33] and MacDonald and Robbins [104] recognized the clinical as well as the pathological significance of NBTE, particularly as a source of bland embolism (Figs. 4, 5, 5A, 6).

Duguid,[105] Tweedy,[106] and Magarey [107] emphasized the thrombotic deposit as a cause of valvular thickening in rheumatic heart valves. In their studies of 50 cases

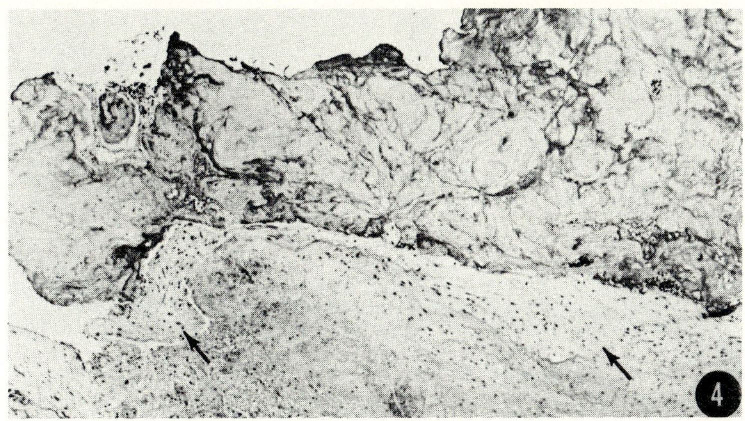

Fig. 4. Mitral valve from 72 year old white male with cerebral infarct. Below is an altered thickened valve with subendothelial myxomatous swelling (arrows) with superficially attached platelet NBTE vegetation with minimal fibrin. No inflammatory reaction in relation to the base of the platelet vegetation proper. Proliferating cells are scant and probably antedate the vegetation. Scant amount of fibrin in contrast to the platelet areas of the vegetation (pale areas). H&E. × 40.

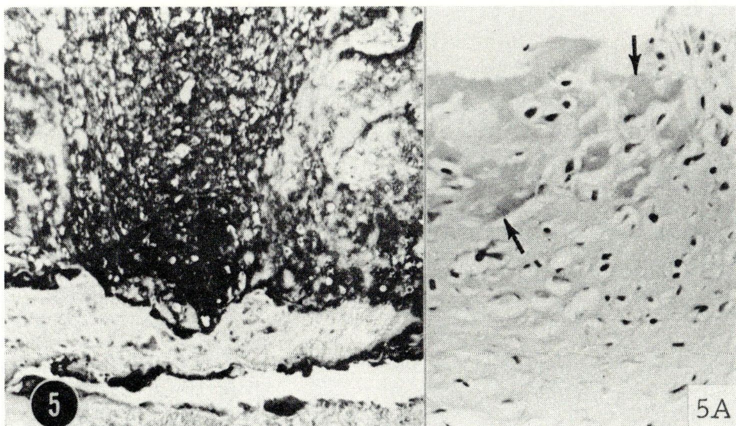

Fig. 5. Fresh NBTE vegetation shows an area with more abundant fibrin and less platelet massing. This is a phosphotungstic acid hematoxylin (PTAH) stain to identify the fibrin component. No inflammatory reaction in relation to the site of attachment of the NBTE vegetation. Some edematous swelling in relation to this site of attachment of the vegetation. × 90. 5A. Photomicrograph of a mitral valve from a 59 year old male with old rheumatic heart disease. Fibrinoid (arrows) in the valve. H&E. × 160.

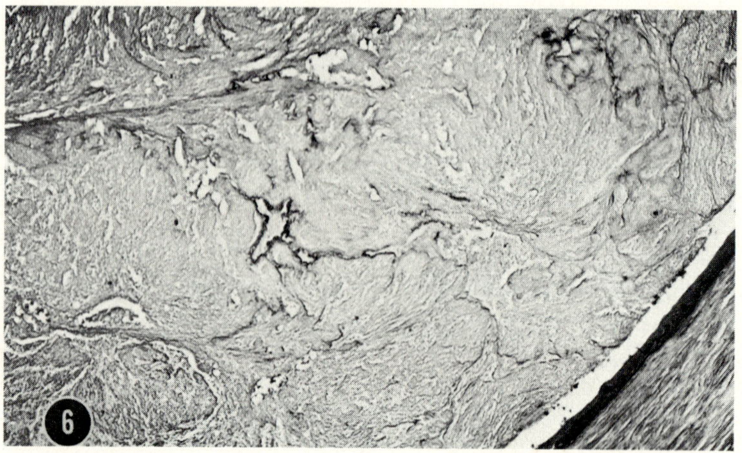

Fig. 6. Photomicrograph of actual embolus in situ in a middle cerebral artery (the wall of which is seen in a lower right hand corner) of the same case as Figures 4 and 5. The embolus had the same gross translucent granular feature as the remaining vegetations still attached to the valve surface. Microscopically the embolus also had the same appearance as the persistent attached vegetation, with the same relative components of abundant platelets and scant fibrin. PTAH. × 90.

of "degenerative verrucal endocardiosis" Allen and Sirota [108] maintained that a good many of the vegetations in "endocardiosis" (NBTE) were not thrombotic, but rather consisted of protuberant underlying altered collagen. From the morphological standpoint, Friedberg [109] noted that "the essential feature in nonbacterial thrombotic endocarditis was the presence of nonspecific valvular vegetations" which may "resemble those of rheumatic endocarditis." Friedberg stated that "valvular deformities do not result from the lesions." This is an impression easily gleaned from a study of the early lesion only in "terminal" cases. On the basis of transitions from early stages to complete scarring, actually encountered in such lesions, with and without progressive calcification (Figs. 33A, B), it is our firm conviction that valvular deformities can and frequently do follow organization and fibrosis and calcification of such NBTE lesions.

Microscopically the vegetations often consist essentially of agglutinated blood-platelets (Fig. 4) with variable and often minimal fibrin [89] (Fig. 5) or fibrinoid (Fig. 5A). It is this easily dislodged early platelet vegetation which yields an embolus (Fig. 6). The electron microscopic appearance of a fresh NBTE is seen in Figures 7, 7A. Superficially there is often a thin layer or a larger "cap" of fresh platelet thrombus superimposed upon an area of older altered mass of platelets (Fig. 8). This may cover an irregular area of valve substance, which has undergone eosinophilic or fibrinoid degeneration or myxoid swelling (Fig. 4). The precise structural relationship of the fresh vegetation to the underlying valvular changes remains obscure. Electron microscopic studies confirm that platelets are lodged in relation to ulcerated areas of value and exposed collagen (Figs. 7A, 29).

A striking feature of NBTE, which contrasts with the findings in active rheumatic endocarditis, is the paucity or total absence of an inflammatory reaction beneath the vegetation in the valve cusp (Fig. 9); this is true for some

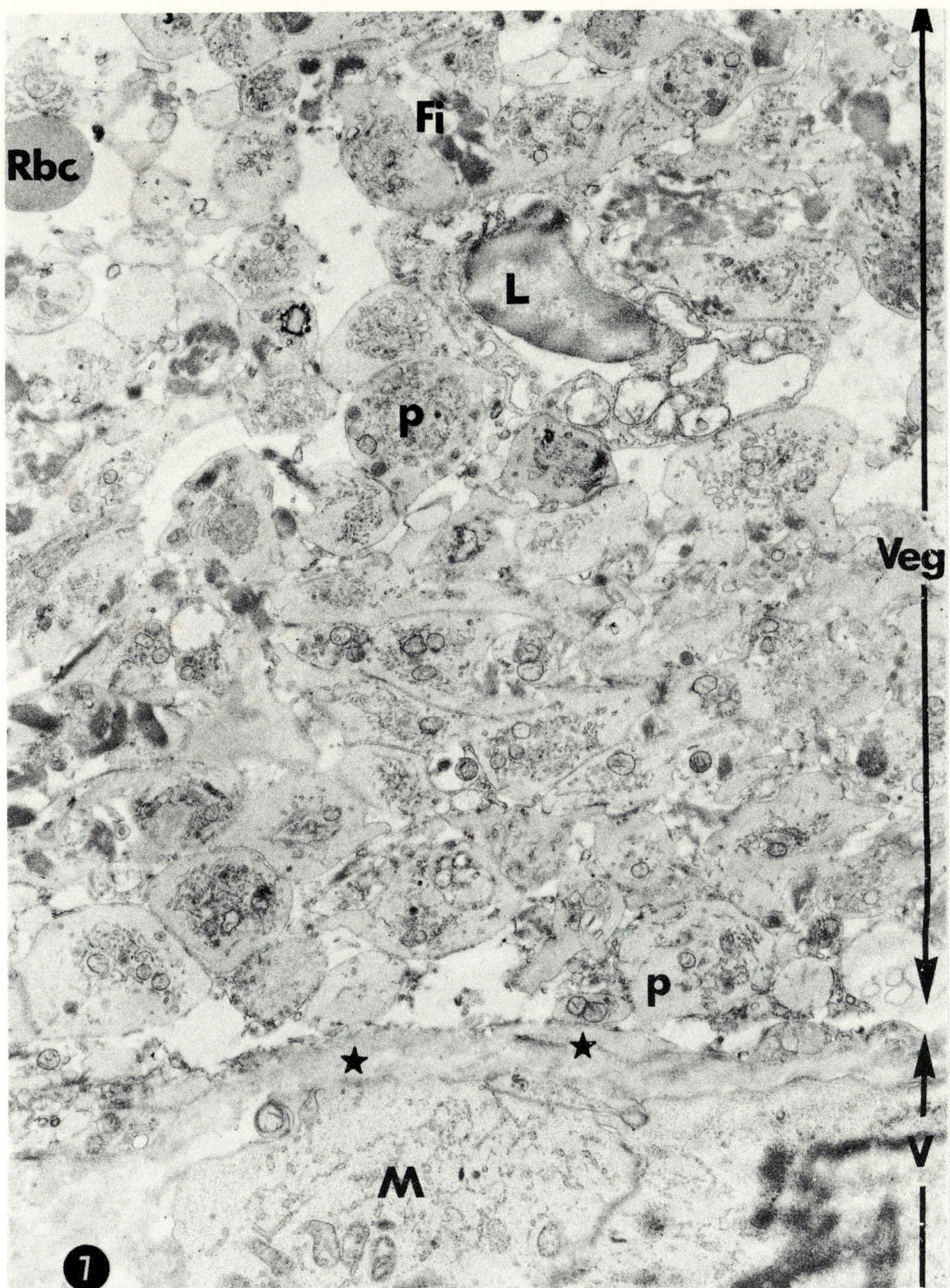

Fig. 7. An electron micrograph of a fresh platelet NBTE. Along the lower fifth of the micrograph will be found the delimitation of the valve (V) with platelet vegetation (Veg) overlying it. The vegetation consists mainly of well preserved platelets. This vegetation comes from an 80 year old female and was found incidently on the mitral valve as a terminal type of endocarditis at autopsy. The valve surface is denuded of endothelium, and the vegetation (Veg) is closely apposed to the exposed valve tissue. In this region is found some fibrillar material. The region between the two stars corresponds to the ulcerated area. An occasional red blood cell (Rbc) and some fibrin (Fi) are seen in the vegetation. The upper portion of this photograph is vegetation and consists essentially of platelets (p). Altered muscle cell (M) and part of a polymorphonuclear cell (L) are seen. $\times$ 8,400.

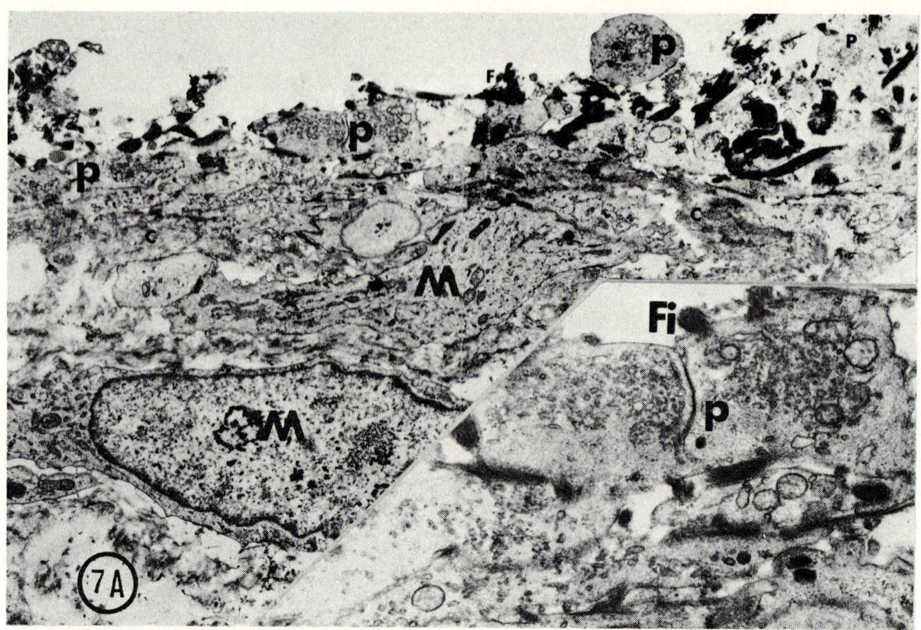

Fig. 7A. Electron micrograph of a valve showing the remnants of a nonbacterial thrombotic vegetation of an 80 year old female with a recent cerebral infarct. Along the upper surface is the probable site of a detached platelet vegetation. Here a thin layer of platelets (p) adherent to the valve in this region without an intact underlying endothelial cell layer can be seen. Altered smooth muscle (M). × 1,600. Area marked by the middle p is enlarged in the inset and shows platelets (p), fibrin (Fi). × 15,000.

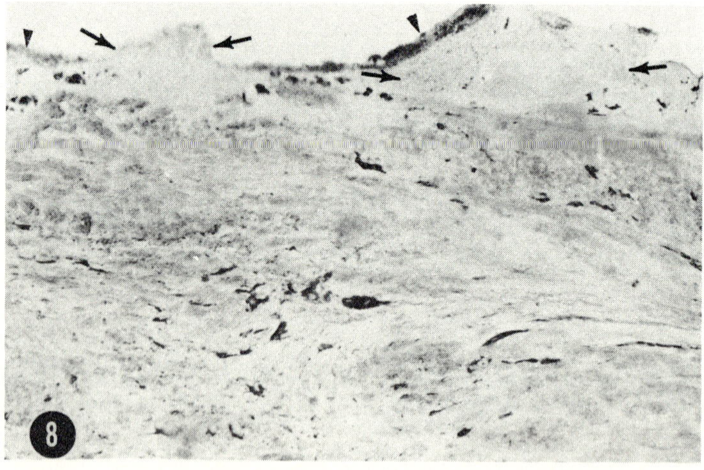

Fig. 8. DPNH diaphorase preparation of the mitral valve from a 78 year old female with old rheumatic heart disease. No NBTE could be discerned grossly. Most of the photograph shows the altered collagen in the valve. Along the surface of the valve there are some pale amorphous zones (between arrows) which represent old and much altered platelets, showing no enzyme reaction. Superficially along the surface are seen some areas stained by the formazan, corresponding to fresher platelet zones (arrowheads). Repetitive increment of platelets is very common in NBTE. × 90.

102

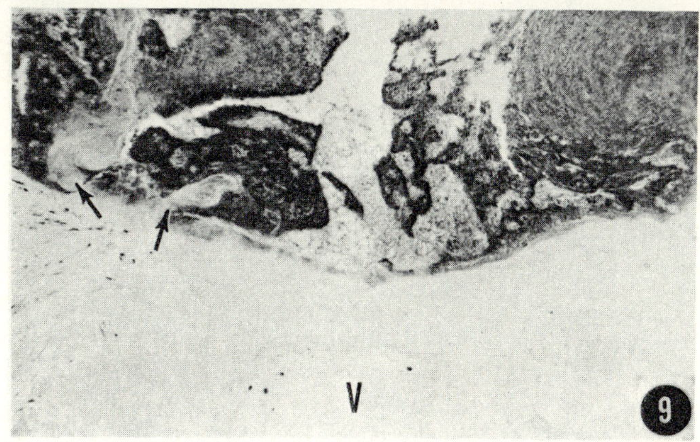

Fig. 9. Photomicrograph is taken from mitral valve of a 78 year old female with old rheumatic heart disease. It is representative of the most common type of fresh NBTE. In the lower half of the photomicrograph is seen the homogeneous hyaline collagen of the thickened valve (V). Attached to the pale staining valve is an NBTE vegetation (upper half of photograph) which stains with different intensity in different areas with the DPNH diaphorase reaction. Older areas of platelets are pale (arrows); the fresher platelet masses are more deeply stained. DPNH diaphorase reaction and PTAH stain bring out the differences in their staining features corresponding to their age. Underlying the vegetation proper no reactive inflammatory cells are seen. This is very characteristic for an early NBTE. Over to the left some organization changes in the valve proper are seen. This NBTE vegetation looked quite uniform and homogeneous in the gross and in the ordinary hematoxylin-eosin stain. $\times$ 30.

time after a fresh NBTE forms. When cells are present they are usually lymphocytes, monocytes, and fibroblasts; these participate in early organization of the base of the vegetation (Fig. 10).

The DPNH diaphorase reaction demonstrates that platelets often form the bulk of the vegetation and are clearly of different ages, occurring in superimposed irregular layers. As the platelets become older, they show less formazan precipitate, indicating a loss of overall enzymatic activities (Fig. 11).

As noted, fresh vegetations are often located on the acellular fibrotic valve surface (Fig. 9). The cellular reaction that does ultimately occur is indolent and suggests organization rather than inflammation. Organization does not ever involve the free luminal surface initially but always appears first at the base of the vegetation (Figs. 10, 11). As the process of organization goes on, the formazan precipitate is found less and less in the platelets and more and more in the mitochondria and microsomes of the cells involved in its organization (Fig. 12).

Crucial to the understanding of the nature of the classical forms of vegetative endocarditis and their transitions and variations is the full appreciation of gross features of NBTE, with its subtle differences. Attention directed to subtle, minute variations in the gross appearance of NBTE makes possible the selection of characteristic areas of the vegetation for detailed microscopic evaluation; this requires many blocks, not a single microscopic section. The single section can only give one picture, which is usually not representative of the whole, since histology varies a good deal in different areas. Each section must be selected for

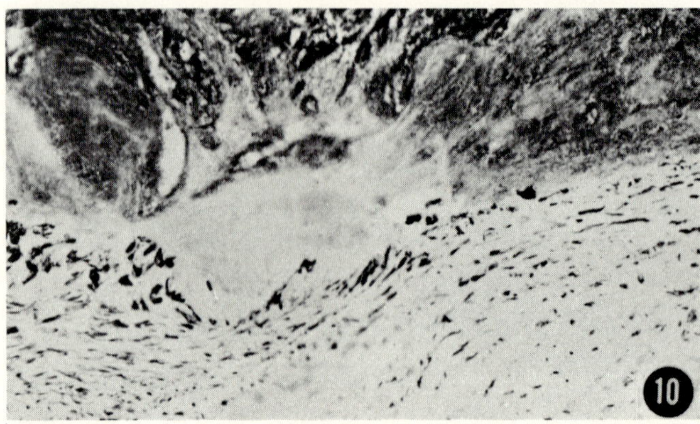

Fig. 10. Aortic valve from a 27 year old female who has had rheumatic fever previously and died with pneumonia. This platelet vegetation shows some reactive changes in the valve at the base. Above is the platelet vegetation. Note the older more deeply placed area of the platelet vegetation immediately above the valve. The surface layer of the valve proper shows some proliferating fibroblastic cells. This is more prominent toward the left where a tendency to a more perpendicular orientation, rather than the parallel arrangement else-where, is seen. DPNH diaphorase reaction. $\times$ 90.

specific gross features, and a map or diagram or a marked photograph of the valve should be kept. In many cases of endocarditis all vegetations are not alike and uniform throughout. Even in a case of advanced infectious endocarditis all areas of the valves may not be in the same stage of evolution and will not show identical features of cellular reaction or even bacterial contamination and growth.

The earliest NBTE (Fig. 13) is a translucent, somewhat irregular, protuberant vegetation which is readily detached by the slightest manipulation. It is rather uniform throughout and can be seen in depth; it is not opaque nor dense white. It may be pink with hemolytic staining (Fig. 13 arrow); it may have a red component from trapped red blood cells. On microscopic study usually very few red blood cells or white blood cells are included. No evidence of organization or inflammation is present early in the valve or in the vegetation (Fig. 9).

To appreciate how little may remain at a site of origin after an NBTE embolus has been dislodged (Fig. 7A), it is suggested that an early nonbacterial vegetation be deliberately removed from a valve and the exact site of attachment then studied histologically with a hand lens, and a binocular low power stereoscopic microscope. Such studies will point out the difficulty of finding the site of a cerebral, coronary, or other embolus a few days after the event, when the original site is already endothelialized; endothelialization can occur rapidly.

Only after an NBTE has been present for some time does organization occur at the base (Figs. 10, 11, 12). Such a healing or organizing vegetation is more granular (Fig. 14) and then more rounded with a smoother surface and more opaque (Figs. 15, 16, 17). As might be expected, it is then dislodged less readily and a larger basal portion may remain as a site of irregularity on the valve. Such gross features are soon discerned readily if an awareness of their significance exists and such detailed macroscopic features are sought. Microscopic study alone is inadequate for full understanding.

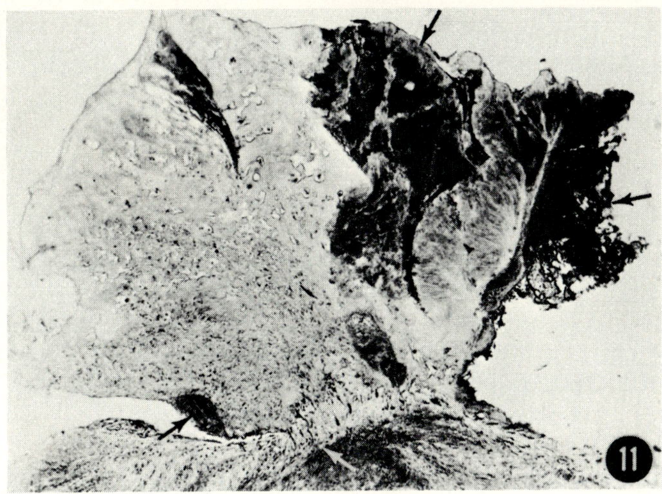

Fig. 11. Photomicrograph is taken from a mitral valve of a 76 year old female, without any stigma of rheumatic heart disease, who died with a myocardial infarct. This is an older NBTE vegetation undergoing organization. Some fresh darkly stained platelets (arrows) are seen in relation to the organizing portion of vegetation toward the surface and in clefts. The left half of the vegetation shows organization, without any formazan precipitation. Cellular reaction is seen at the base of vegetation, with a perpendicular orientation (white arrow near bottom.) × 25.

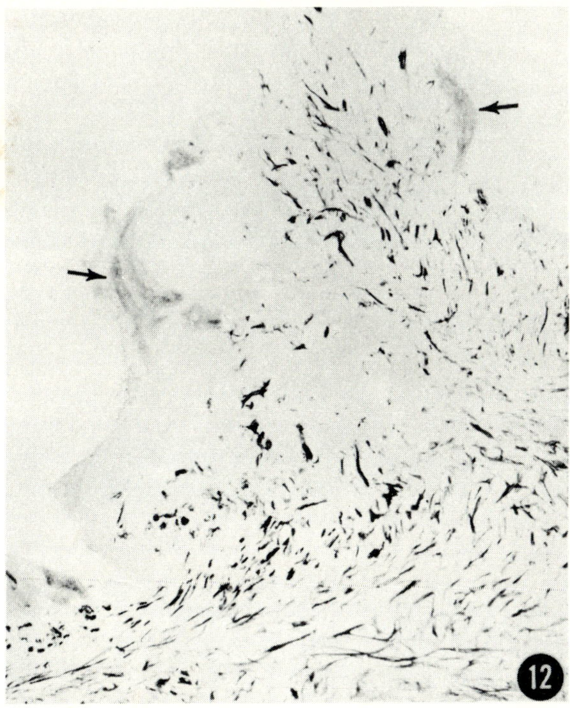

Fig. 12. Organizing NBTE vegetation from a 57 year old male with glomerulonephritis. DPNH reaction shows the organizing cells in the valve and in the vegetation proper very clearly. This is an older vegetation and so most of the platelets do not stain at all. There are zones indicated by arrows where a pale staining of the platelets still persists. × 80.

105

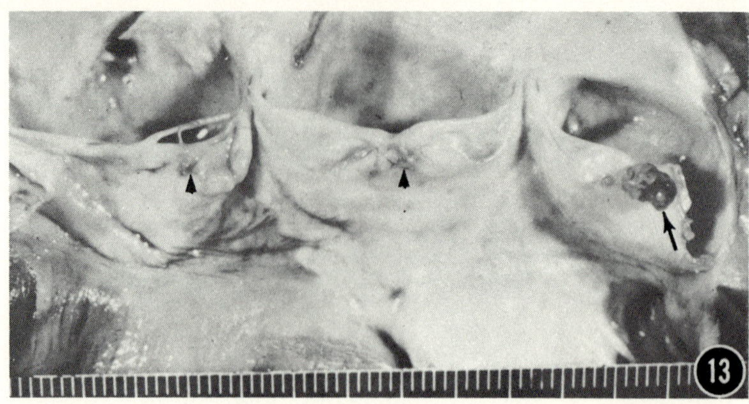

Fig. 13. Gross appearance of an aortic valve of a 78 year old female with some fresh NBTE vegetation on the cusps. Part of the larger vegetation shows some hemolytic staining; this area appears darker in the photograph (arrow). Other small areas of NBTE are found along the line of closure (arrowheads).

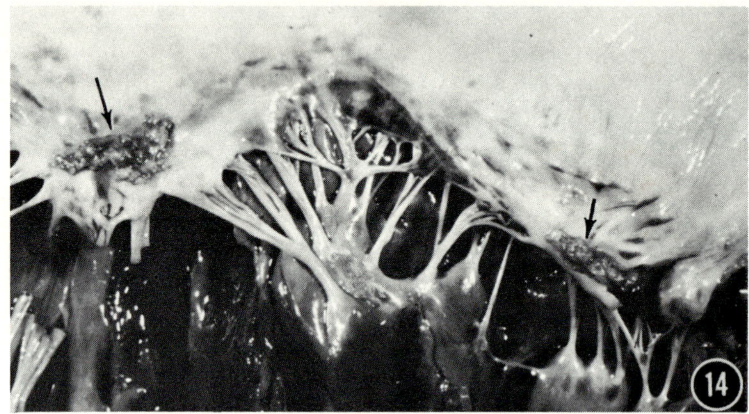

Fig. 14. Mitral valve of a 76 year old female who died of a cerebral vascular accident. Vegetations (arrows) with granular appearance are seen on the rheumatic thickened valve.

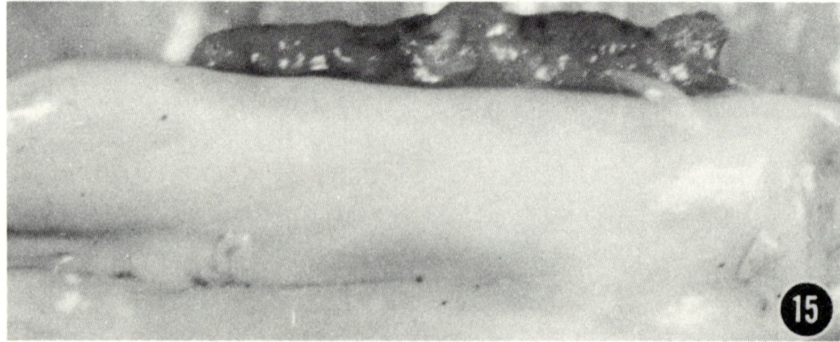

Fig. 15. An older NBTE vegetation undergoing organization on the aortic valve of a 62 year old male with cancer of the gall bladder. Note the smoothness of the surface and the merging of the vegetation with the valve tissue toward the right. Complete endothelial-ization of the NBTE has occurred. × 4.

106

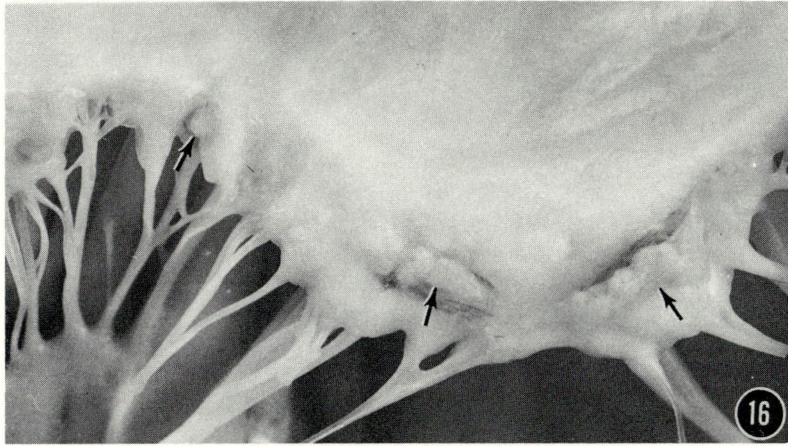

Fig. 16. Gross example of older NBTE vegetations undergoing organization and frank incorporation into the substance of the valve (arrows). Mitral valve of a 61 year old male with chronic glomerulonephritis. Background valve shows thickening and sclerosis with rather coarse chordae inserting into edge of the valve toward the right.

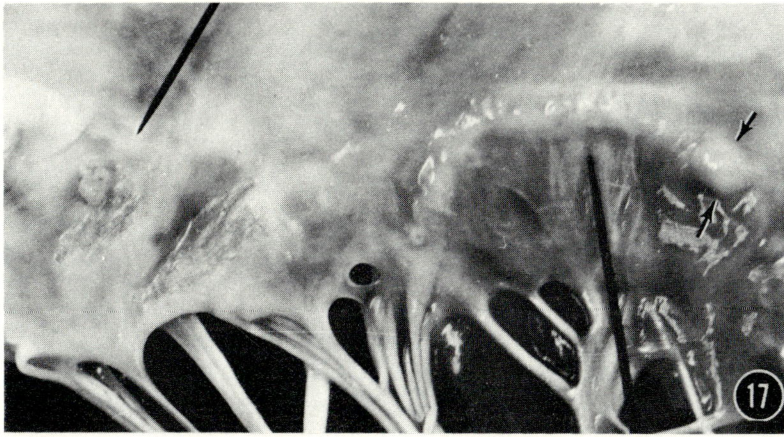

Fig. 17. Gross specimen of a mitral valve from the same patient as in Figure 15. Valve is sclerotic and shows a small NBTE undergoing organization and incorporation into the valve substance (needle points to this small vegetation). Advanced organized nodule with smooth surface (arrows) is seen on right.

With early infection, little change is discernible at first in the NBTE vegetation. Only an increase in opacity or occasionally chalky-white foci is seen. These may actually be white colonies of bacteria (Fig. 24), which are occasionally calcific with antibiotic therapy. It may be stated that the early acute bacterial lesion may be easily missed in the gross specimen (Figs. 18, 18A). The sites of infection may be very small or they may represent very small foci in a large NBTE vegetation. Bacterial colonies may be present on the surface of NBTE (Fig. 19, 19A). Such surface contamination is also seen with the electron microscope (Fig. 20).

The lesions of subacute (SBE) (Figs. 21, 21A, 22) or acute bacterial endocarditis (ABE) (Figs. 23, 23A, 24) are the result (Table 3) of contamination, persistence, and proliferation of the bacteria. With modern antibiotics, complete sterilization of even far advanced ABE and SBE vegetations can occur. Finally, only the distorting fibrosis will remain with loss of an inflammatory reaction. Whenever destructive changes in the valve occur, there will remain permanent distorting fibrosis, perforations, and bulging aneurysmal sites (Fig. 24) which affect valve function (Table 3).

Table 3. NBTE With Infection

Surface Bacterial Contamination	Initial Without inflammation
Progressive Bacterial Proliferation	With inflammation
ABE	Virulent organisms—rapidly progressive, destructive ulcerative lesions with small or large, red or yellow vegetations, mycotic aneurysm, perforation, and septic embolism.
SBE	Less virulent organisms—larger, more flat, less red-tawny, yellow spreading vegetations with ulceration, destruction of valve and chordae, mycotic aneurysm, perforation, septic and bland embolism.
Potent Treatment	Sterilization ("bacteria-free" stage) in ABE and more often in SBE with bland embolization, healed defects of valves and chordae.
Recurrent NBTE	Repetitive potential of NBTE with and without infection.

No case of endocarditis, nonbacterial or bacterial, represents a single episode. All forms of endocarditis, particularly SBE, are dynamic lesions with ebbs and flows of remission and progression, lysis and healing. Healed forms of endocarditis, both nonbacterial and bacterial, are prone to develop additional NBTE, with and without superimposed infections, which increase the distortion of valves as a result of new nonbacterial and/or recurrent bacterial endocarditis (Tables 2, 3).

Transitions Between Healing NBTE and Other Nonbacterial Forms of Endocarditis. (Rheumatic and Atypical Verrucous Lesions)

The nature and extent of the cellular reaction at the base of NBTE is determined by many factors, including: the basic underlying disease process, age of subject, constituents of vegetation, ie, the amount of platelets, the fibrin and

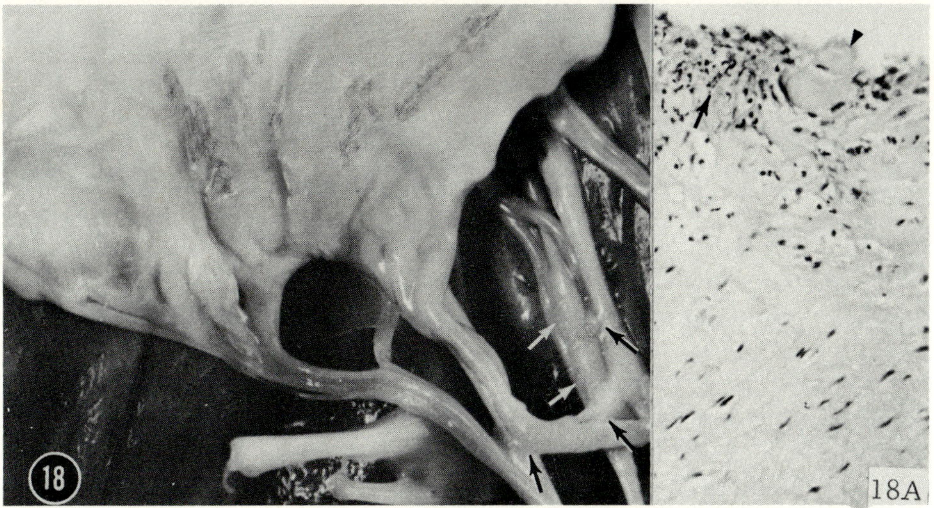

Fig. 18. Gross appearance of a mitral valve of a 59 year old male who had suffered from GU tract infection. Valve shows "billowing sail" sclerosis. Thickened chordae show an area of fusion (black arrows) and a delimited zone with granular appearance (white arrows). 18A. Microscopic section through region of white arrow in Figure 18 showing hyaline thickened collagenized tissue of chordae with superficial inflammatory reaction (arrow) and surface bacteria which were seen with bacterial staining. A small vegetation is seen (arrowhead) and corresponds to white arrows in Figure 18. H&E. × 180.

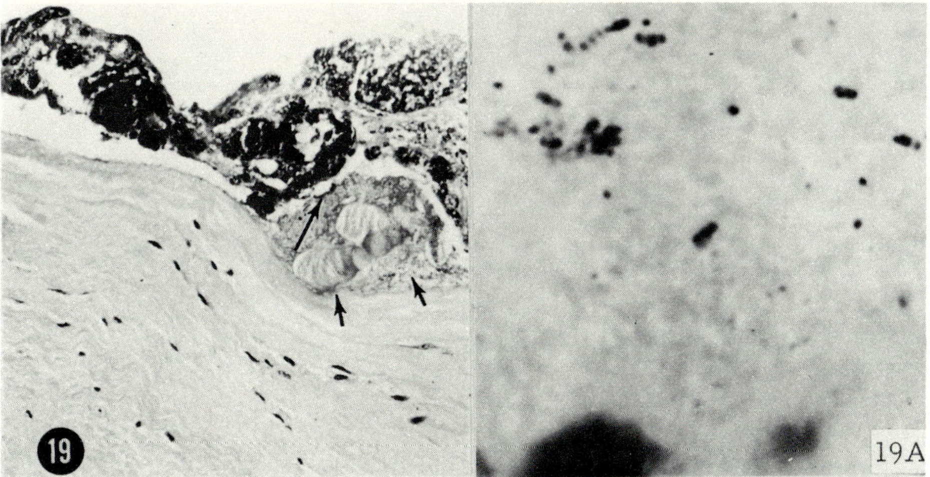

Fig. 19. Photomicrograph from a mitral valve of an 82 year old male with pneumonia. Extensive bacterial colonies (dark staining) appeared in the vegetation on the nonreacting valve. Darker stain differentiates the bacteria from the platelet vegetation below (short arrows). Long arrow indicates bacteria on top of NBTE (see Fig. 19A). Underlying tissue also shows sclerosis. Note that no inflammatory reaction is present in relation to this early bacterial vegetation. H&E. × 180. 19A. Higher magnification of the area marked with the long arrow in Figure 19, indicating bacteria in situ on the NBTE vegetation. Brown-Brenn stain. × 1,800.

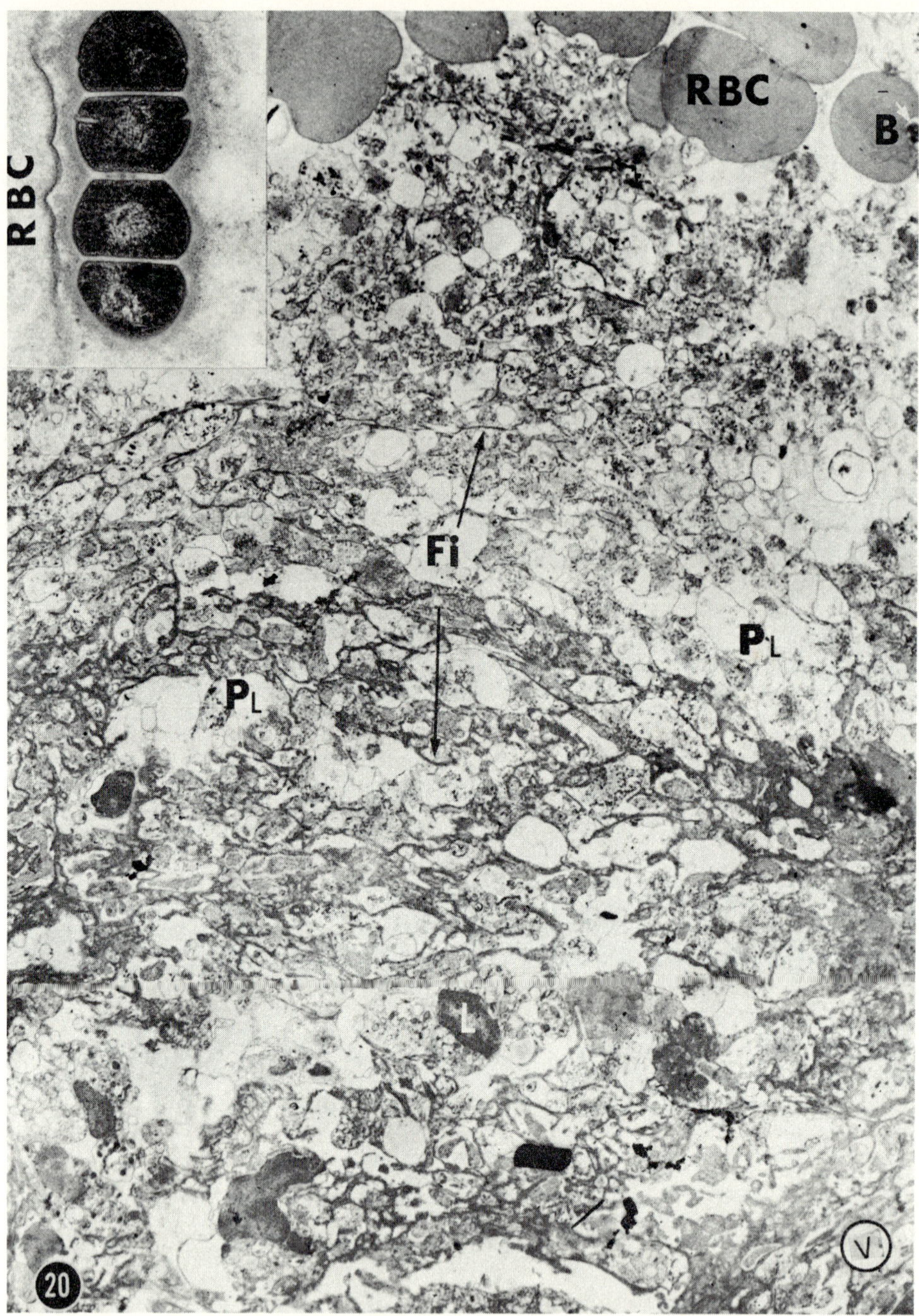

Fig. 20. A 25 year old male with a previous history of rheumatic heart disease who developed acute bacterial endocarditis of the aortic valve. Electron micrograph of an early bacterial vegetation with the base of the thrombotic vegetation in the lowermost right corner (V). Vegetation occupies nearly all of the photograph and consists mainly of altered platelet masses (PL), strands of fibrin (Fi) and a few leukocytes (L); bacteria are present in upper right (B with white arrow) on the surface layer of the vegetation where red blood cells (RBC) are found. × 3,750. The inset in the upper left corner shows the margin of a red blood cell (RBC) and some bacteria in chain formation just adjacent to it. × 25,000.

110

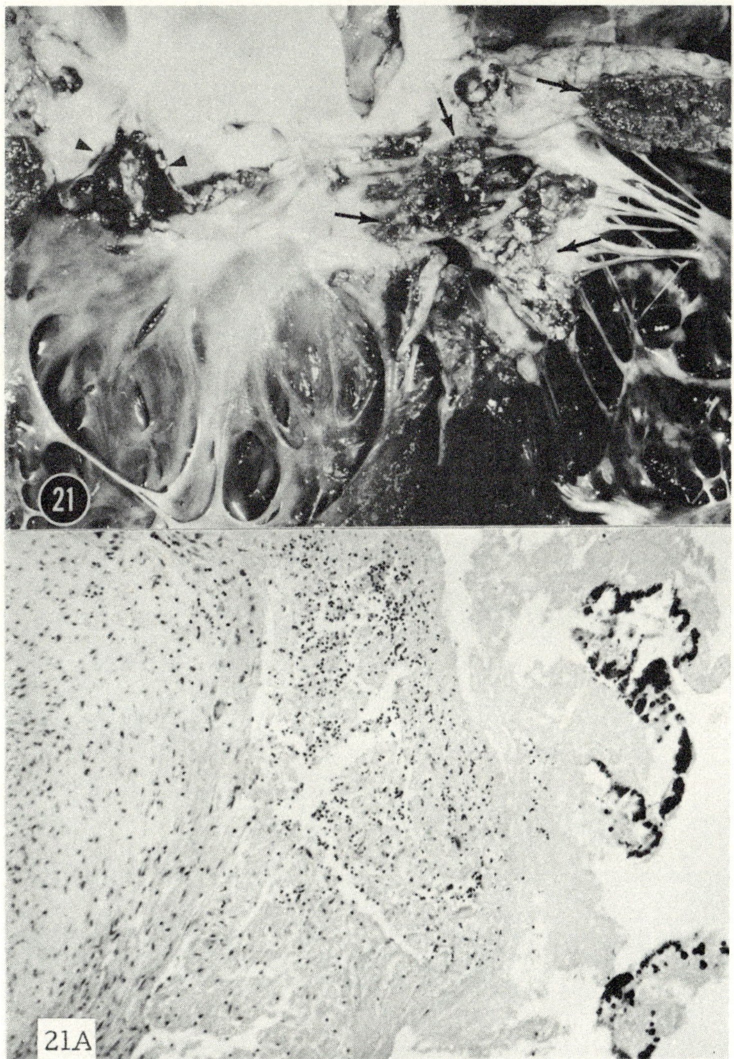

Fig. 21. Gross photograph of an aortic and ventricular aspect of mitral valves of a 29 year old male with previous rheumatic heart disease with SBE. Extensive broad flat vegetations on the mitral valve (arrows). Note particularly the "creeping" extension of the vegetation along the ventricular surface and onto the adjacent anterior cusp of the mitral valve. Bulky bulging vegetation on the aortic valve at the commissure is seen (arrowheads). Note the white sclerotic thickening of the adjacent ventricular endocardium due to previous rheumatic aortic insufficiency. 21A. Microscopic appearance of the vegetation through the area of ulceration of the mitral valve cusp in Figure 21. Note the sclerotic valve to the left, with polymorphonuclear exudation on the surface as well as fibrin and some platelets. In the superficial portion there are large bulky bacterial colonies in situ.

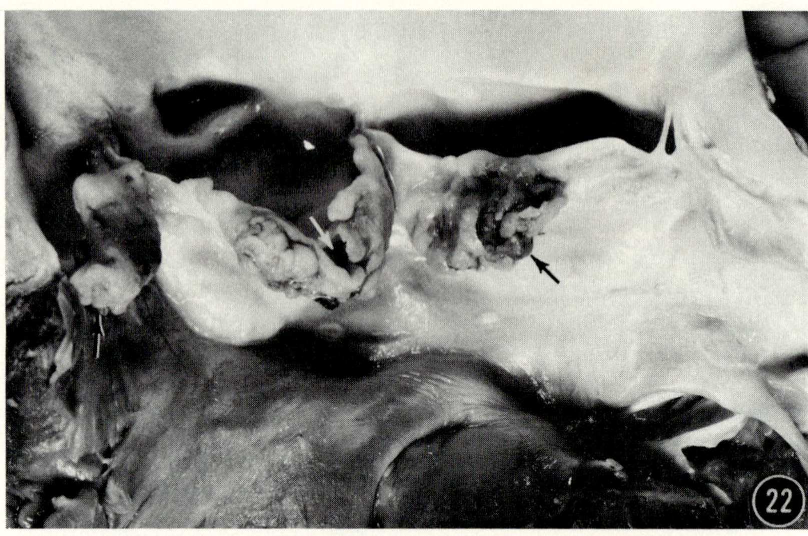

Fig. 22. Aortic cusp showing a healing SBE from a 72 year old male, with a fissure-like destructive ulceration of the valve cusp (white arrow) and a bulky vegetation on the adjacent cusps (arrows). Surface of vegetations are rather smooth.

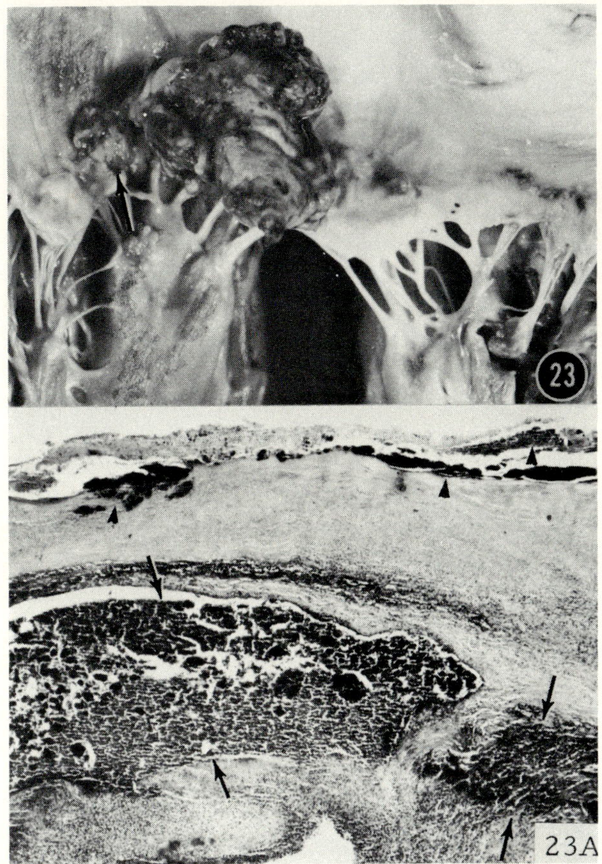

Fig. 23. ABE on the mitral valve of a 70 year old female with previous rheumatic heart disease with a large bulky vegetation on the mitral valve. This bulky vegetation consists mainly of fibrin and much altered platelets and red blood cells. 23A. Microscopic section through zone marked by arrow in Figure 23. Note bacterial colonies toward the surface (arrowheads) and extensive suppurative and phlegmonous inflammation with destruction of the valve (arrows). H&E. × 40.

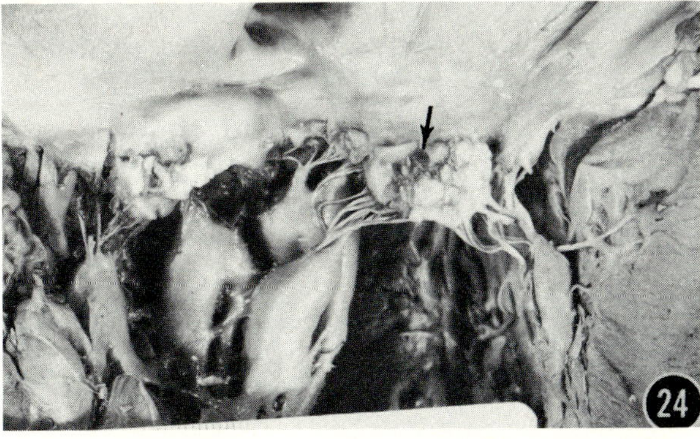

Fig. 24. Mitral valve of a 64 year old female with active florid SBE, with aneurysmal bulging, and perforation of anterior cusp (arrow). Note the chalky white superficial areas on the vegetation on both cusps. These areas have massive bacterial colonies with some calcification. Cerebral embolism occurred one week prior to death.

fibrinoid components, and the age of the vegetation. In general, with NBTE on the old sclerotic valve, the cellular reaction of organization is delayed and is not prominent when compared to the reactive changes in NBTE on the valves of young subjects.

A characteristic of rheumatic verrucae has been the palisading in the cellular reaction at the base of the vegetation; yet this is not always present (Fig. 25). In some instances no appreciable perpendicular or diffuse cellular reaction in the valve in active rheumatic fever is seen, particularly when the vegetation is still fresh. On the other hand, considerable cellular reaction may be present at the base of NBTE when the vegetation becomes older (Fig. 26). In the process of organization of the base of NBTE, the fibroblasts and some Anitschkow cells may be oriented perpendicularly and mimic rheumatic verrucae. Others have noted such transitional features.[3, 76, 109] Some vegetations have more fibrin (Fig. 5) in their bulk than platelets, or fibrinoid (Fig. 5A) may be present along the base of the vegetation and on the surface of the valve. Fibrin is lysed by fibrinolysin and other proteolytic enzymes and tends toward successful absorption or organization and fibrosis. Fibrinoid and massed platelets do not undergo lytic absorption as readily as does fibrin.

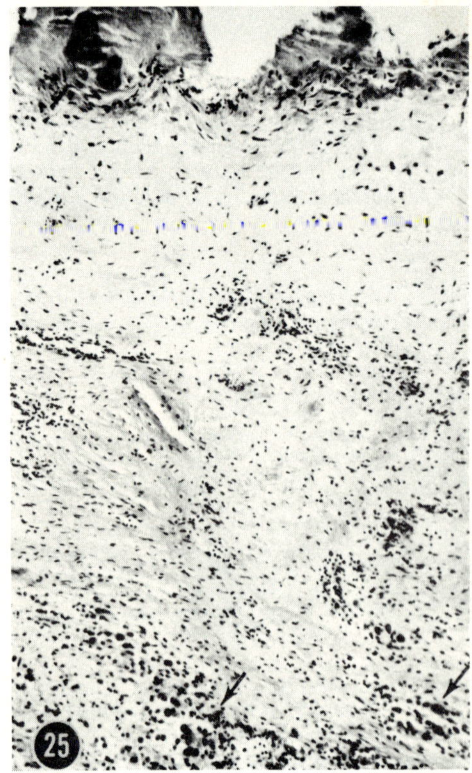

Fig. 25. Microscopic view of a valve with rheumatic verrucous endocarditis. Note the old fused platelet vegetations on the surface with reactive cells immediately beneath the verrucae. These reactive cells do not have a parallel perpendicular or palisaded arrangement. In the valve proper considerable inflammatory cell infiltration is evident. Some of the cells are grouped to form Aschoff nodules (arrows) with giant cells. Valve shows considerable edema. Clustered focal arrangement of the cellular infiltrate is evident in this micrograph. H&E. × 80.

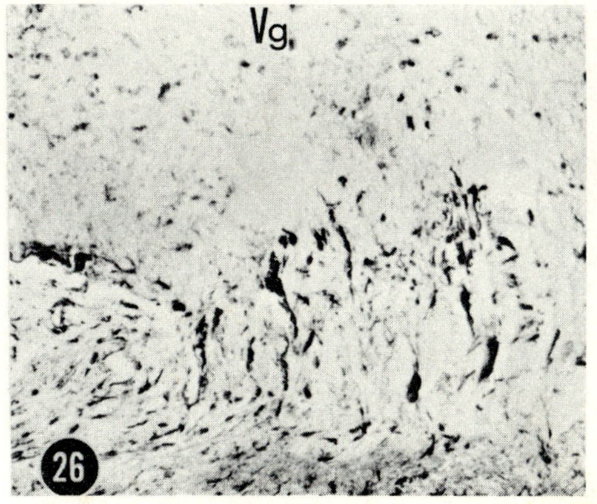

Fig. 26. Older NBTE vegetation from a 76 year old female who died of a cerebral vascular accient. Note the cellular reaction in the valve surface just beneath the vegetation (VG). Some cells tend toward a perpendicular arrangement. Patient did not have any evidence of old or recent rheumatic infection. DPNH-diaphorase reaction. × 100.

Studies of collagen synthesis utilizing tritiated L-proline revealed that the distorted valve showed more of an uptake, regardless of age of the patient (Figs. 27, 28). The fact that NBTE is usually formed on the scarred valve also suggests a significant relationship between collagen and NBTE formation. This parallels the morphologic findings at the electron microscopic level (Fig. 29). In healing bacterial vegetations the electron microscopic appearance of the fibroblastic cells with active ER suggests active protein synthesis, probably collagen (Fig. 30).

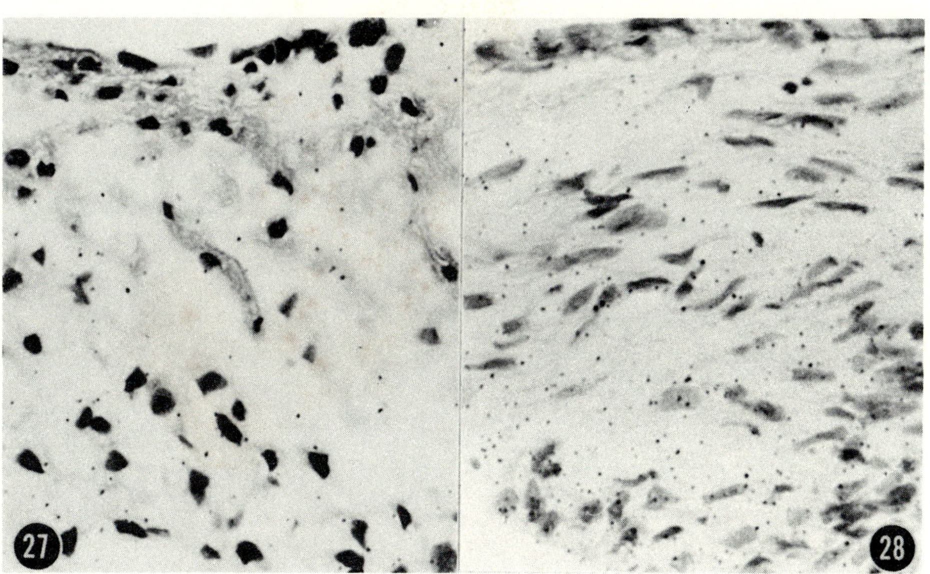

Figs. 27, 28. Autoradiographs (× 480) of sections from (Fig. 27) normal vitral valve of 11 week old rat and (Fig. 28) distorted sclerotic mitral valve with some reactive changes including increased cellularity from a 24 month old rat. Four μc of tritiated L-proline (proline H³) per gram body weight was given intraperitoneally to both rats which were sacrificed four days later. Routine dipping and exposure were done. With normal valves the young growing rat usually has a larger uptake of L-proline than the old rat. Old rats with distorted valves had an even greater uptake of L-proline than did the young adult rat with normal valves.

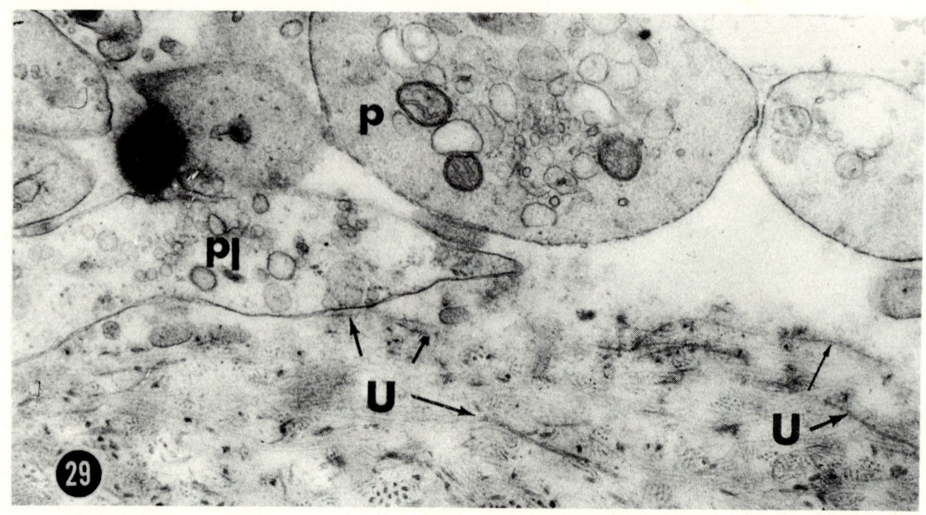

Fig. 29. Electron micrograph of a layer of platelets (p) attached to a zone of the valve denuded of endothelium. Some platelets show lysis particularly the one (pl) closest to valve surface. Note the collagenous unit fibrils at the site of platelet attachment without any intervening endothelium (U and arrows). Denser fibers of collagen are seen in the depths of the valve. × 25,000.

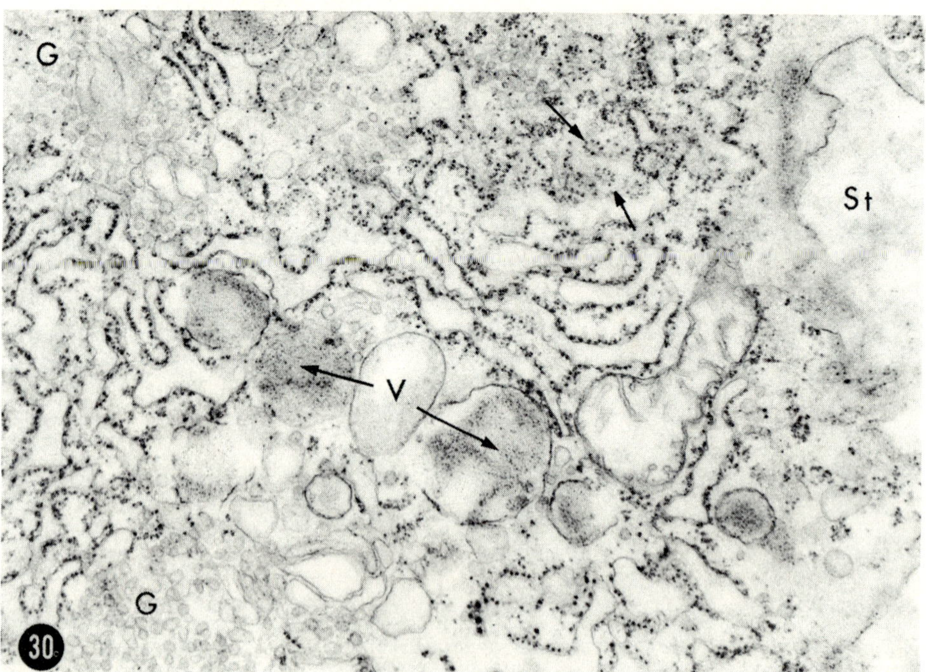

Fig. 30. Fibroblast in zona spongiosa of valve suggests active collagen synthesis. Hyperplastic and hypertrophic Golgi field (G). Golgi vacuoles containing fibrillar material (V). Extracellular matrix (St). Arrows indicate characteristic polyribosomes for this type of cell. × 20,000.

116

The modern classification of endocarditis neatly subdivides all vegetations and places all of them into individual categories. This grouping may be a bit arbitrary. The authors have had some difficulty in distinguishing, grossly and microscopically, some forms of NBTE from rheumatic verrucous endocarditis. Transitional forms between NBTE and all other forms of nonbacterial vegetations have been seen.

The vegetation of Libman-Sacks (Figs. 31, 31A) is a variant form of NBTE; it is a nonbacterial vegetation usually with some or an abundance of fibrinoid, often with considerable reactive cellular changes in valve and vegetation; the latter is the basis for the synonym, "intermediate" endocarditis. The atypical verrucous vegetation, more often than not, has no absolutely pathognomonic feature, though hematoxylin bodies may be present on occasion (Fig. 31A); this type of vegetation often cannot be distinguished as such on the basis of its own gross and microscopic features alone. The associated disease and its localization in valve pockets help determine its nature.

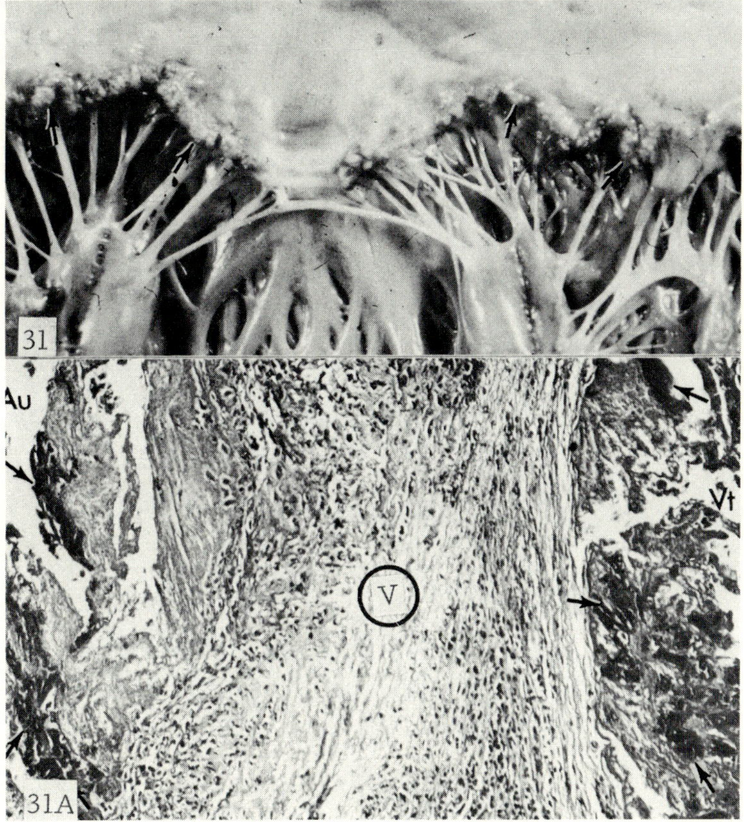

Fig. 31. Gross photograph shows mitral valve with a rather extensive atypical verrucous endocarditis (Libman-Sacks) (arrows); most of the edge of the valve is involved. Vegetations (arrows) involve both auricular and ventricular surface of the valve as can be seen on microscopic examination. 31A. Histology of valve in Figure 31 with fibrinoid and considerable cellular exudate involving the valve proper (V) and the vegetation. Both surfaces, representing the auricular (Au) and the ventricular (Vt) surfaces of the mitral valve, to the right and to the left of the central area corresponding to the valve proper (V), show vegetations. Hematoxylin bodies with darker stain are seen in the vegetations (arrows). H&E. × 100.

Rarely, rheumatoid nodules involve the heart valve, usually with contiguous myocardium, in the region of the ring (Figs. 32, 32A).[110]

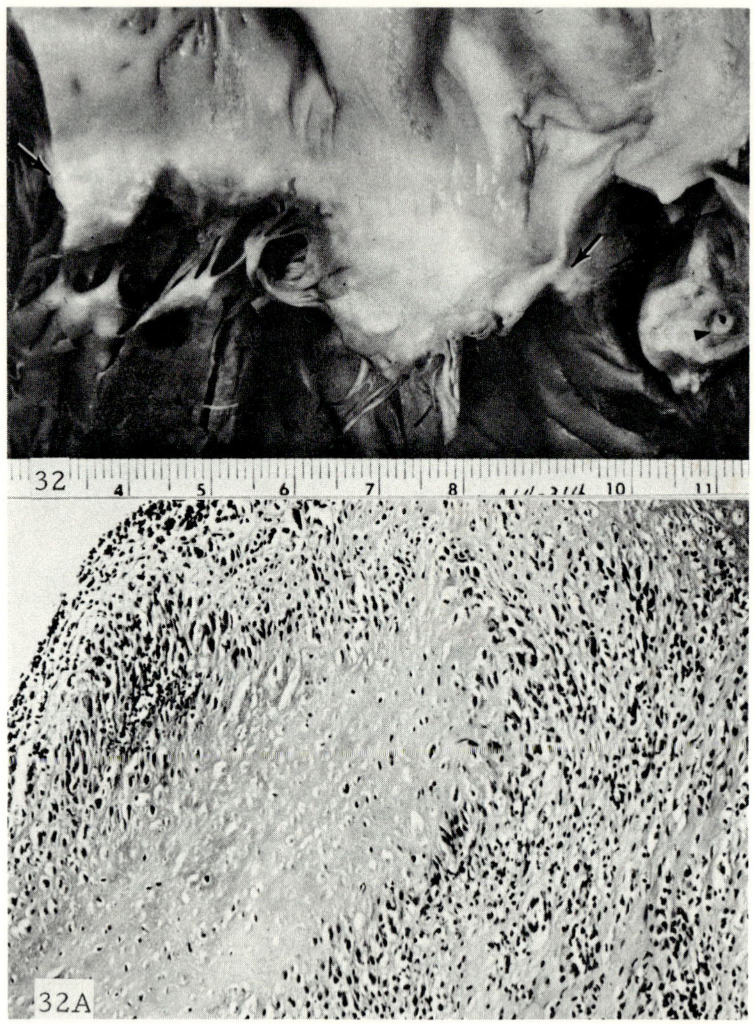

Fig. 32. Mitral valve of a 61 year old female with well-documented rheumatoid arthritis for 20 years with prolonged steroid therapy. Extensive rheumatoid disease involved joints, heart, pericardium, and even the meninges and the lung parenchyma proper. Cusps showed a rough surface and thickening. Arrows indicate a rheumatoid nodule in the ring region of the valve extending to the valve proper. Valve shows no evidence of past or present rheumatic valvular disease. Arrowhead points to coronary vessel, showing rheumatoid involvement with thickening of vessel wall. 32A. Histology of the area of the rheumatoid nodule as it extends into valve. Auricular surface is shown in the upper left hand corner. Characteristic collagen necrosis is seen centrally with a palisaded zone around it. H&E. × 100.

Mechanism of Formation of BE, ie, Transition of NBTE to BE

For the proper understanding of BE, its basic lesion and common denominator, NBTE, must be understood. One cannot categorically deny that bacteria can settle on the normal endothelium of the valve, or can be phagocytosed by its endothelial cells. This does happen in experimental bacteremia when myriads of organisms are injected directly into the circulation. MacNeil et al,[111] Nedzel,[100, 101] Siegmund,[27] Freifeld,[112] and Leschke [113] found bacteria on and in the endothelium of the valve. Whether this occurs naturally in the human is a moot question, at least based on the experience so far encountered in studying a large number of human specimens. This latter origin of a bacterial vegetation must be rare indeed, though not impossible.

Hutrya and Marek,[114] Winge,[57] Koester,[72] Haushalter,[115] and Schoene [116] believed that bacterial endocarditis was initiated by bacterial embolization of the vessels of the valve.

The more common mechanism is undoubtedly the seeding of organisms on a previously existing NBTE.[11, 31, 32, 36, 117] It is not necessary that this NBTE be a bulky one; often only a very thin layer of NBTE attaches to the surface, hardly seen grossly; yet such a small site can also be a good growth medium for attachment and proliferation of microorganisms (Figs. 18, 18A, 19, 20). This seeding has been seen in instances of atypical verrucous endocarditis too; contamination of the surface of one-third of such vegetations was reported in the original group of lupus erythematosus.[118] Cases at autopsy are often encountered at the stage of *only surface contamination* of NBTE without inflammatory changes; this stage can also be found in the experimental animal.[9, 11, 36, 117] Porrini [119] noted verrucous and bacterial vegetations in the same valve using influenza organisms. This is common in human BE.

With antibiotic therapy vegetations at this stage are often sterilized and the bacterial colonies then can go on to lysis, absorption, or calcification (Fig. 33A, 33B). The bacterial vegetation then returns quickly to the equivalent of the old "bacteria-free" stage of subacute bacterial endocarditis; subsequent healing can then ensue (Table 3).

As noted, bacterial contamination of NBTE gives rise to bacterial endocarditis (BE), either acute (ABE) or subacute (SBE), depending upon the virulence of the organism and the resistance of the host. Transitions are encountered from the earliest contamination to the fully evolved inflammatory vegetation with abundant bacterial colonies which causes destructive changes in the underlying valve structure. Some manifestations of healing may be present too. The latter healing did occur to some degree spontaneously, particularly in SBE, but healing is seen more often now in both ABE and SBE, induced by effective antibiotic therapy.[120-24]

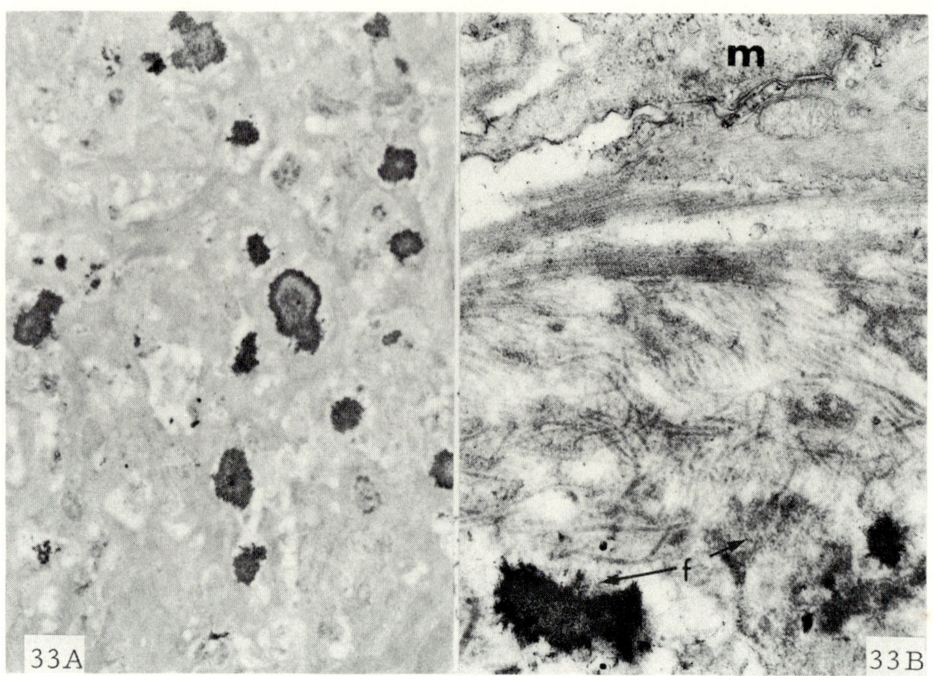

Figs. 33A. Electron micrograph of fibrinoid area of healed SBE showing calcification. Some of the latter suggested calcification of dead bacterial colonies. × 6,000. 33B. Electron micrograph showing calcification found in areas of collagen fiber formation. Calcium deposits appear associated with fine fibrils (f, with arrows). Irregular arrangement of unit collagen fibrils is evident. Monocyte (m) is present along the upper edge of micrograph. × 20,000.

Morphological Features of Bacterial Vegetations

ABE is associated clinically with extensive toxicity, high hectic fever, leukocytosis, and a rapid course often with cardiac failure, but most important is the virulence of the causative organism which affects the duration of the illness and thus the appearance of the vegetations. The SBE has a more prolonged, less violent course without severe toxicity or high fever, and cardiac failure occurs late in the course, usually from dynamic valve defects (Fig. 34).

With frank infection and proliferation of organisms, vegetations become softer, more friable, bulky, and variable in color, red but more often yellow, at least in areas. In some areas the appearance may be frankly purulent. SBE tends to be less variable in the size and height of vegetations and in general appearance (Figs. 21, 22). Contiguous inflammatory changes with edema and congestion may be evident in active BE, especially ABE. Subacute vegetations tend to be more flat, less red, more tawny-yellow, and less protuberant with more indolent inflammation and less congestive margins in the regional tissue.

The *duration of the lesion* and the *nature of the organism,* or those complex biological features which combine to give virulence, determine the appearance of BE at autopsy. For instance, pneumococcus and gonococcus yield large, bulky

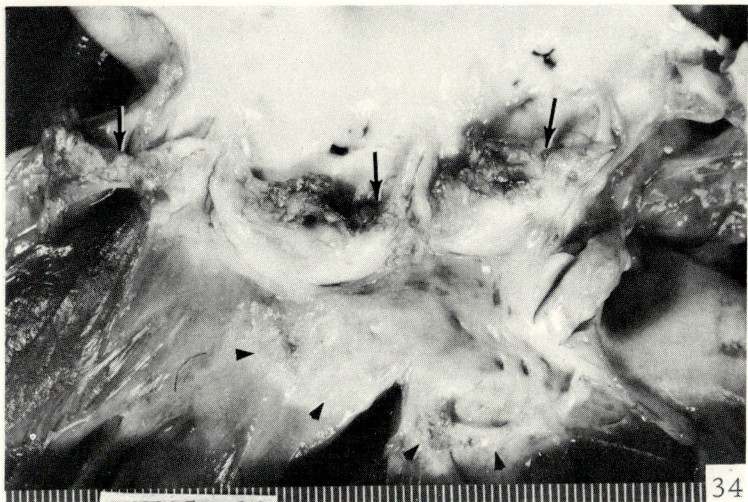

Fig. 34. Gross appearance of aortic valve with SBE, taken from a young adult male of unknown age. Note destruction of cusps (arrows) with loss of substance along the edge of
valve and the corresponding thickening of the regional ventricular endocardium due to
prior regurgitation (arrowheads). Smooth healing is seen in the vegetation proper on the
valve.

vegetations, with large bacterial colonies and abundant fibrin. Coagulase positive
staphylococcus may yield large and rapidly ulcerative and destructive lesions of the
valve in identical periods of time compared to coagulase negative organisms; exceptions however do occur. ABE is associated with virulent organisms and is more
destructive with larger vegetations for the same duration (Figs. 23, 23A). SBE
usually has a longer duration and this yields ultimately a more widespread and
extensive destructive distortion of the valve and the chordae, and more diffuse
involvement of the regional auricular and other endocardial tissue by progressive
"creeping extension" (Fig. 21).

The phenomenon of "creeping extension" with contiguous spread, so characteristic of SBE, is ascribed to the progression of primary and initial NBTE
formation adjacent to the bacterial vegetation, which then becomes repetitively contaminated from the external bathing blood stream. Bacterial growth on the surface
of such early NBTE adjacent to the bacterial lesions verifies the "creeping extension" phenomenon.

Transitions Between ABE and SBE

The classical features of distinction between ABE and SBE may be lacking; [15, 17, 18, 123, 125] the same organism can be recovered from both forms of
bacterial endocarditis. It is true that ABE tends to involve the normal valve more
frequently, but ABE also occurs, and with increasing frequency, on the previously
damaged valve. SBE, which is so commonly found on the damaged valve, can
involve the unaltered normal valve, and this is now happening more often too.
The gross, and less consistently the microscopic, findings at autopsy really reflect

the *duration* of the valve lesion; the rule of thumb subdividing the two on the basis of the clinical history of six weeks is as good as any, for the gross picture does vary accordingly. The older histological criteria for SBE, ie, the presence of an indolent type of inflammation with some round cells and granulation tissue, which prevailed in the days before the antibiotic era, are no longer applicable. Today transitional features exist during the stage of ascendency, with and without therapy, and during the stage of defervescence, spontaneously or under therapy.

With the proper understanding of the dynamic nature of the valvular vegetation, the transitions encountered in vegetative endocarditis become explicable and even expected. The failure to classify a particular lesion need not be ascribed to inadequacy on the part of the pathologist, it is due mainly to the very nature of the entity with the graded transitions that do actually occur. It is desirable to identify ABE because this form of BE requires intensive immediate therapy without delay; at autopsy the compulsion to label a known form of BE as ABE or SBE may become a pathological obsession.[123, 125]

All forms of endocarditis are never static; they are constantly changing due to additions and subtractions. Healed forms of endocarditis, both *nonbacterial and bacterial,* are prone to develop additional NBTE and additional infections to spell out additional increments of distortion on valves as a result of new nonbacterial and bacterial endocarditis (Tables 2, 3).

Healing of Endocarditis, Particularly BE

The event of healing has become a common one in all forms of endocarditis, including bacterial endocarditis. Spontaneous healing of BE occurred only very rarely, possibly in 2 to 3 percent of cases, more often in the subacute form.[120] Now healing is a common phenomenon in both ABE and SBE. The first step is, as expected, sterilization of bacteria; this is followed by subsidence of the acute inflammation with its intense polymorphonuclear reaction; then the appearance and persistence of more indolent inflammatory changes and fibroblastic proliferation. Finally, there is fibrosis and collagenization. It is the resulting fibrotic distortion of valves which causes changes in the cardiac valvular hemodynamics and may lead to cardiac failure. Late cardiac failure has become a significant factor in mortality (Figs. 21, 22, 24, 34, 35). Also cardiac failure does not occur only during the active disease process with recent destruction of the valve as heretofore, but now appears frequently some time after complete healing has taken place.[13-21]

Vascularization of a valve is often considered the residuum of rheumatic fever. However, in healing bacterial endocarditis, formation of vascular channels, including capillaries, is a striking feature (Figs. 36, 36A, 36B), particularly during the healing process. This is demonstrated best by the ATPase reaction (Fig. 37). The difference between the vascularization following rheumatic fever and BE is mainly in the thicker vascular walls and less numerous capillary loops, like granulations, in the former. On the other hand, after the healing of NBTE we encounter less vascularization and more so-called whiskers, "papillomas"[126] (Figs. 38, 38A).

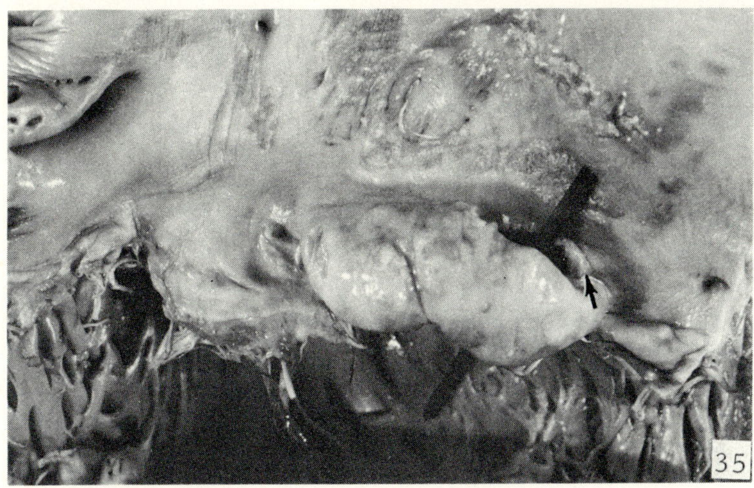

Fig. 35. Mitral valve of 47 year old female with a healed (treated) bacterial endocarditis, with bulging aneurysmal deformity of the valve and a perforation. Black stylus shows the large perforation. Note the smoothness of the surface and of the perforation (arrow) at the edge as healing proceeds.

When an organized NBTE is not incorporated into the substance of the valve, a nodular or fibrous thickening without capillary formation can occur (Fig. 39). Figure 40 shows the gross appearance of a healing bacterial vegetation and an NBTE (Figs. 40A, 40B) on the same valve.

Table 2 lists a range of changes that can occur and the various sequences and end results of NBTE without the complication of infection. Final fibrosis can lead to the gross distortions already discussed. Histologically this includes "whiskers," deposition of elastin in globular or fibrillar form, elastification of collagen proper, atheroma formation, a fibrillated appearance, and splitting of the valve collagen with deposition of plasma protein, and then also fibrin and platelets anew. Finally, calcification of the NBTE, particularly of the platelet vegetations and of the fibrinoid areas, does occur (Figs. 33A, 33B). As noted above, transitions are found between all stages, ie, between nonorganized, calcific, and otherwise altered NBTE. Table 3 lists the range of possibilities with infection of NBTE, both without and with ultimate healing.

The histoenzymatic studies on human and experimental NBTE are detailed below. In established BE the enzymatic patterns showed changes different from those which prevailed in NBTE. Experimental bacterial vegetations permitted control of the age of BE lesions by timing of the intravenous bacterial injections and of healing by timing of therapy. In such established experimental BE the DPNH diaphorase reaction was diminished (Fig. 41A), and the ADPase (Fig. 41B) or ATPase and the

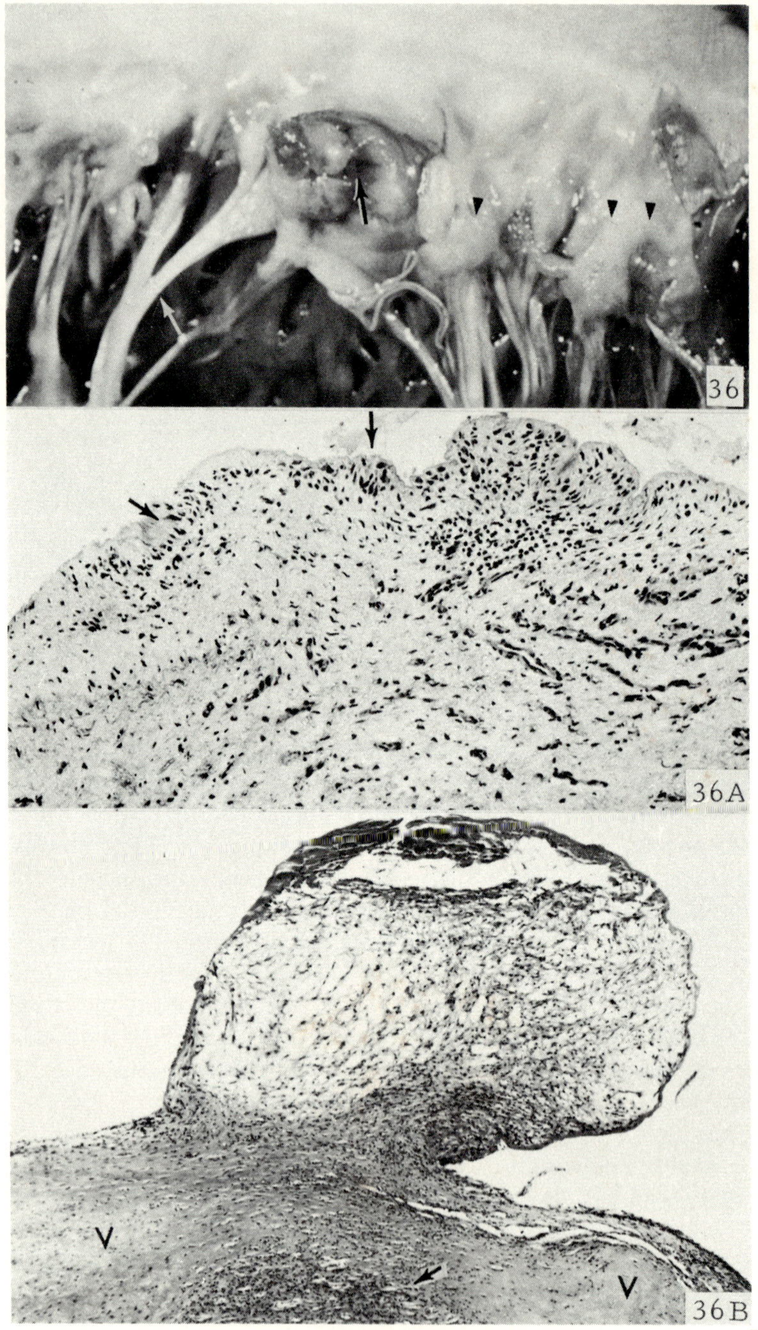

(Fig. 36. Legend on facing page.)

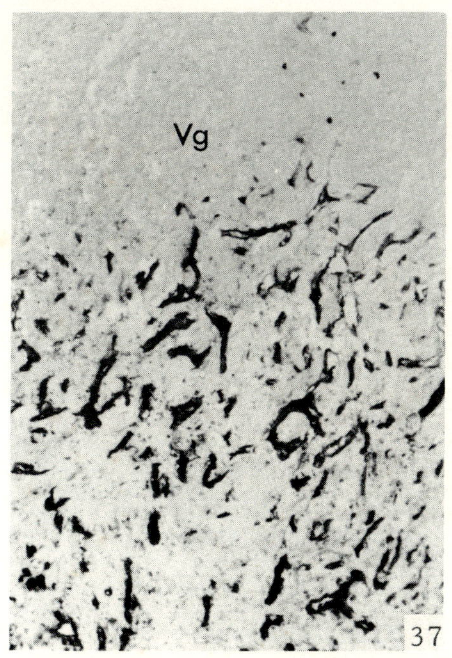

Fig. 37. ATPase study of healing SBE. Remnant of vegetation is seen in the upper third of the photograph (Vg). Below are seen numerous vascular loops and channels of the organizing vegetation and valve at the base of same. × 100.

alkaline phosphatase (Fig. 41C) reactions were also decreased, or even disappeared in the valve at the base of the BE vegetation. However, the AMPase reaction (Fig. 41D) remained strongly positive in the valve. Once a healing process supervened (Fig. 42), in the human too, then the DPNH diaphorase (Fig. 42A), the ATPase (Fig. 42B) or ADPase, and the alkaline phosphatase (Fig. 42C) reactions all again became evident, while the AMPase reaction (Fig. 42D), in contrast, remained weak or negligible.

Fig. 36. Mitral valve of 73 year old female showing a healing SBE with mycotic aneurysm of the valve and a perforation (arrow). Some older thickened chordae tendinae (white arrow) suggest a previous alteration of the valve. To the right can be seen a suggestion of the senile ectatic "billowing sail" distortion (arrowheads) of the valve. 36A. Photomicrograph of Figure 36 shows an area of the vegetation of the valve which is "rather clean" with some indolent inflammatory cells, and some with perpendicular arrangement toward the surface (arrows). Vascularization and fibrosis are prominent. Fibrin can be seen along the very edge of the valve. H&E. × 40. 36B. Section from same valve showing SBE in healing stage with a "cleaned up" vegetation, now lacking bacterial colonies and showing advanced organization. Remnant of the original vegetation seen superficially. Focus of the old inflammatory site with vascularization (arrow) can be seen within the depths of the valve. Some of the valve shows hyaline fibrosis (V) which represents an original distortion on which the SBE was engrafted. Protruding vegetation shows numerous capillary channels as well as evidence of organization and endothelialization. H&E. × 40.

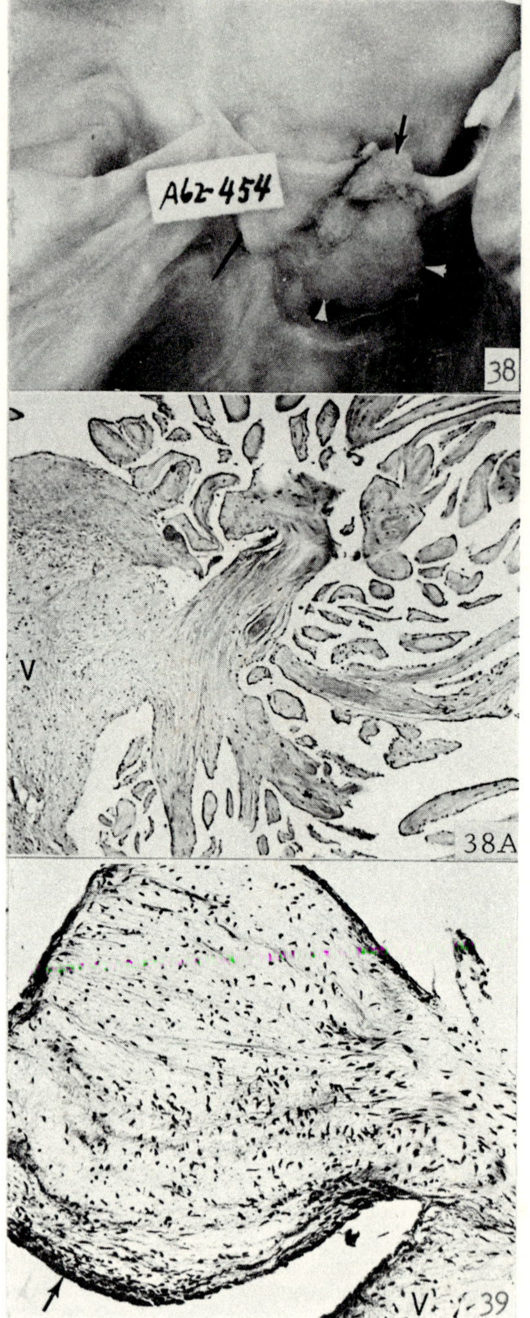

Fig. 38. Aortic valve of 72 year old male with atherosclerotic heart disease. Note the healed bulky vegetation (NBTE) at the commissure between the two aortic cusps. Papilliforous appearance of the healed vegetation can be seen in the upper portion where it is firmer (arrow), and there is a finer more filamentous appearance in the lower portion (arrowheads). 38A. Microscopic section of the "raspberry" filiform healed NBTE shown in Figure 38. Note that the stalk of the filiform extensions (arrowheads in Fig. 38) is quite avascular. No evidence of inflammation exists and few capillary channels are seen at the base of the vegetation, where it is attached to the valve structure (V). H&E. × 25.

Fig. 39. Healing NBTE showing fibrous organization with only some persistent minimal cellular reaction (arrow). No capillary formation is seen in the nodular vegetation. (Compare with Figs. 36, 36A, 36B and 37, 38). H&E. × 100.

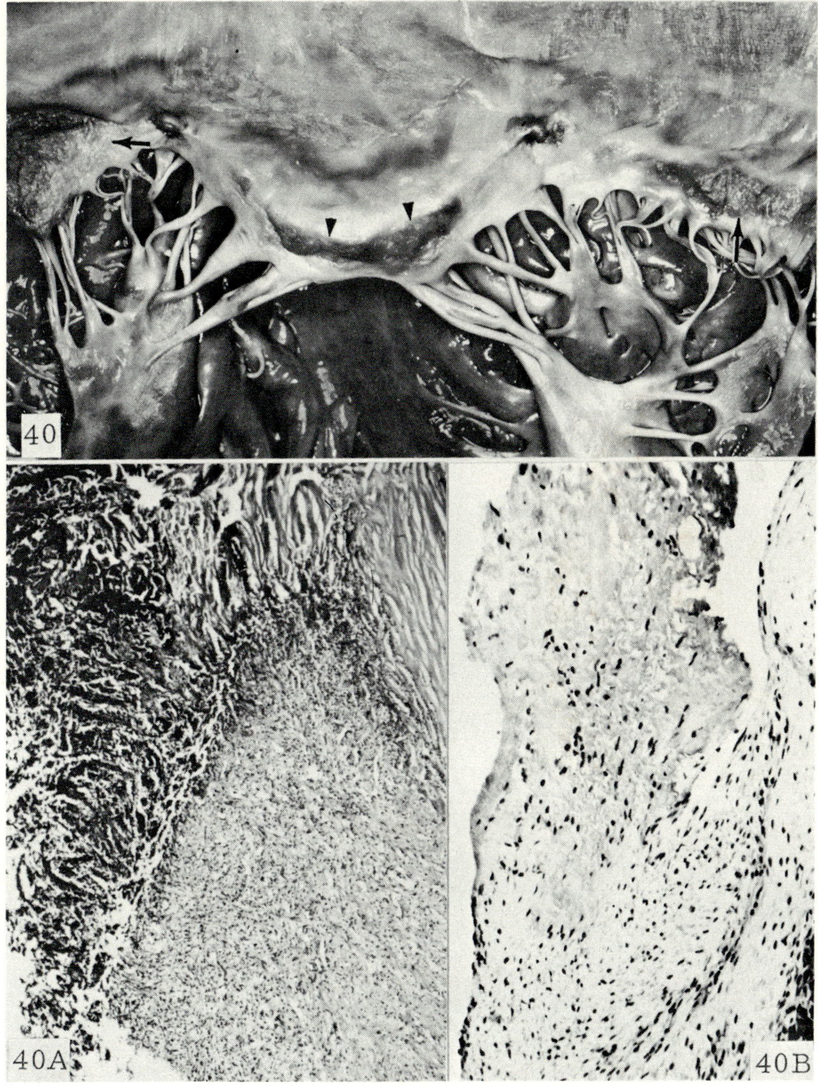

Fig. 40. Mitral valve from a 69 year old male with prostatic carcinoma, showing thickening and fusion of the free edge and chordae. Healing bacterial endocarditis (arrows) is seen on the posterior cusp and an organizing nonbacterial vegetation (arrowheads) on the anterior cusp. The two vegetations look different grossly. 40A. Healing BE with granulation tissue in right lower half of photograph, and persistent portion of sterilized vegetation (Fig. 40, arrows) above to the left. × 40. 40B. The appearance of the healing verrucous NBTE lesion (Fig. 40, arrowheads). In this instance it could not be determined whether the bacterial endocarditis was ABE or SBE. Organizing NBTE with no evidence of inflammatory exudate or bacterial contamination was found in this vegetation on multiple sections. H&E. × 40.

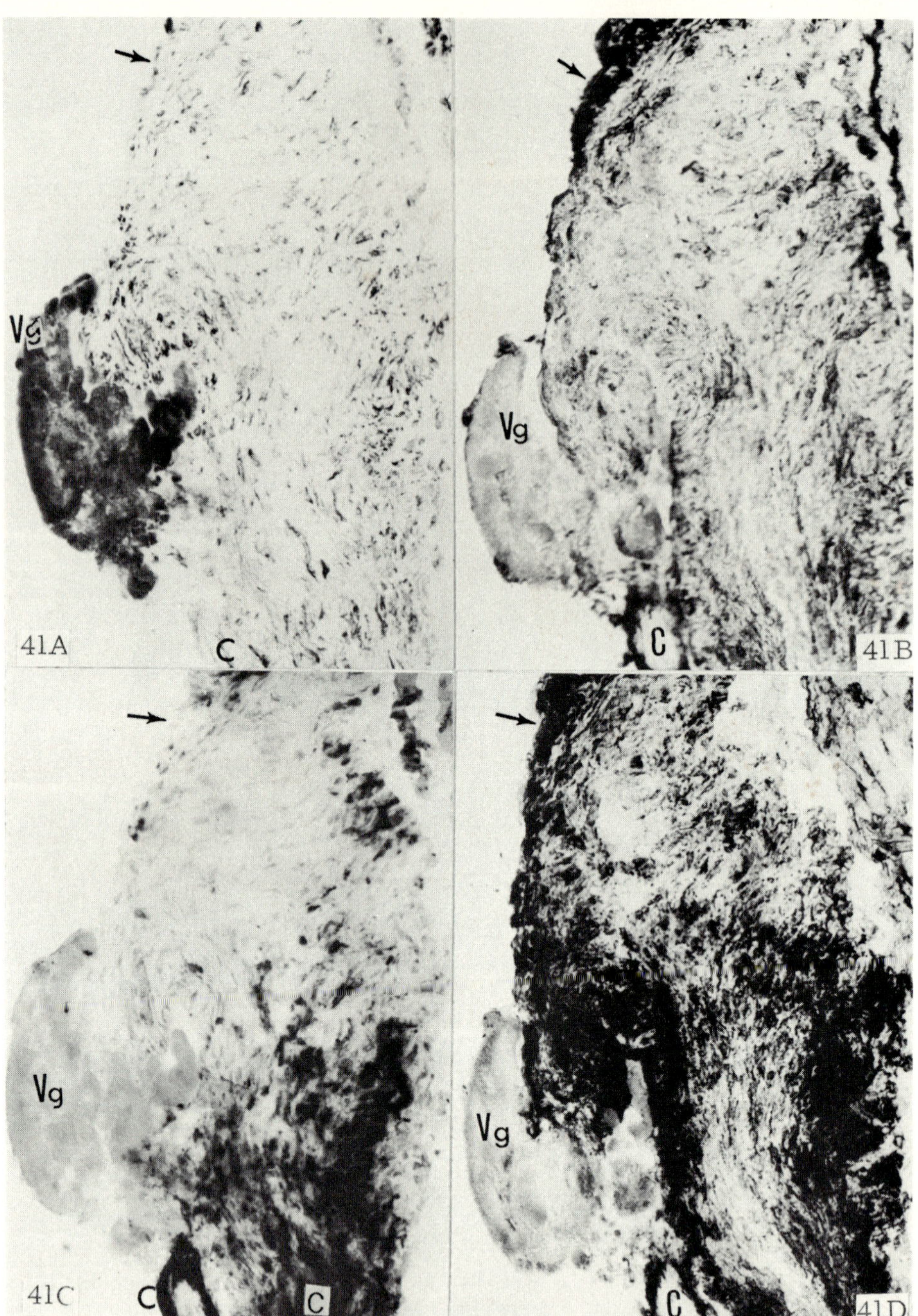

Figs. 41A, 41B, 41C, and 41D. Consecutive sections of the mitral valve of a rat who received **S. faecalis** and was sacrificed two days later. These photographs have the same magnification. (C), chorda. × 160. 41A. DPNH diaphorase reaction: vegetation (Vg) shows a strongly positive reaction in the region of bacterial contamination, confirmed by Brown-Brenn stain. Most cells in the valve at base of vegetation show minimal formazan precipitation. (Legend cont. on p. 129.)

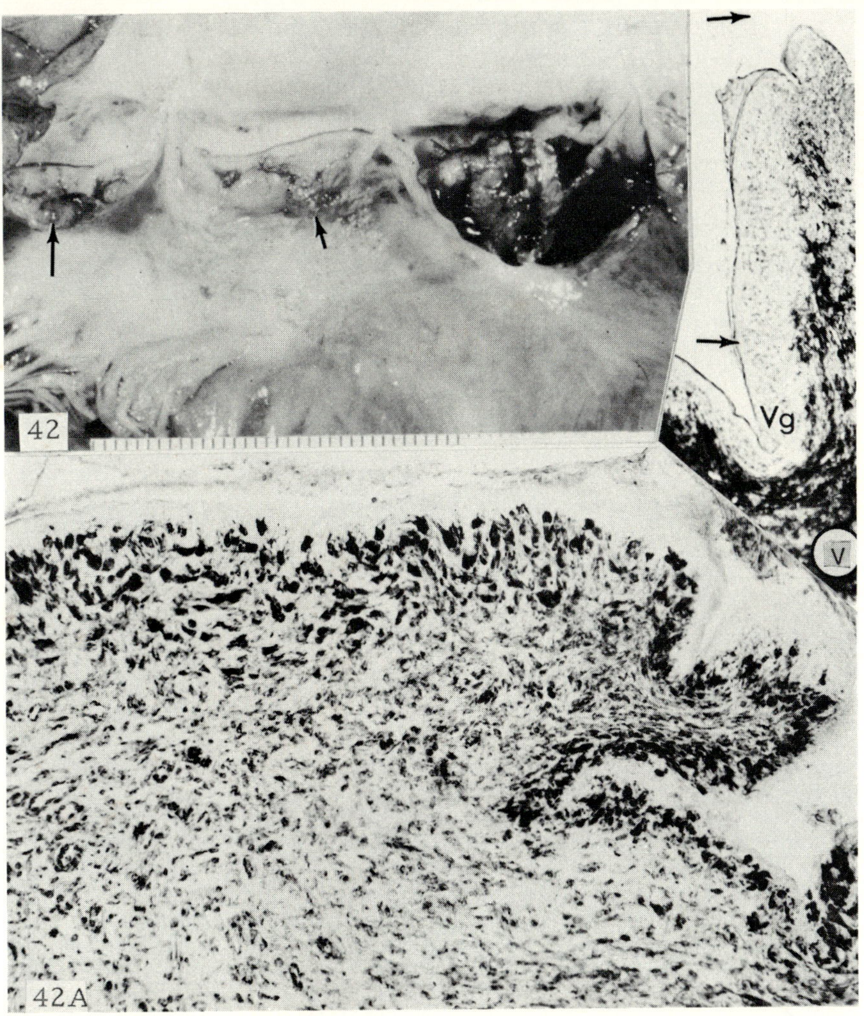

Fig. 42. This aortic valve is from a 27 year old female with SBE, treated with antibiotics for seven weeks. The two left cusps showed a healing process and deformity (arrows); yet one cusp still has severe active destruction going on. Figures 42A, 42B, 42C, and 42D are consecutive sections ($\times$ 110) through region of long arrow in Figure 42. The insert is the alkaline phosphatase reaction in low magnification, showing a part of vegetation (Vg) with the valve (V). DPNH diaphorase reaction: active cellular reaction is evident with perpendicular orientation toward the surface. DPNH diaphorase reaction is most prominent toward the surface in the reacting cells. Fibrin or platelet vegetation covers the surface.

(Fig. 41 Legend cont.)

Fig. 41B. ADPase reaction: minimal positive reaction is present at the base of vegetation, though a strongly positive reaction is present at the surface of the valve proper at some distance from the vegetation (arrow).

Fig. 41C. Alkaline phosphatase: no reaction is seen at the base of vegetation except for the area of the inserting chorda (C).

Fig. 41D. AMPase reaction: strongly positive reaction is present in the valve proper and at the base of the vegetation (Vg).

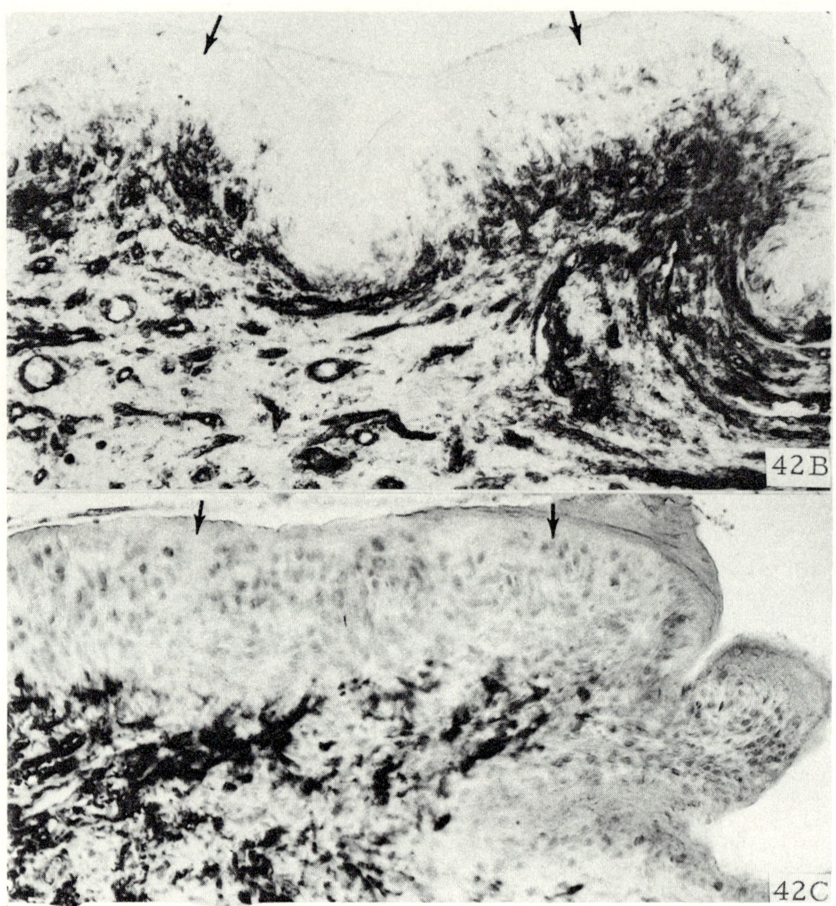

Fig. 42B. ATPase reaction: strongly positive reaction is seen in the organizing vegetation. There is no reaction product present (arrows) on the outer surface in coating vegetation. Note the active vascularization in the depth of vegetation. 42C. Alkaline phosphatase reaction. Positive reaction is present in the depth of vegetation toward the base, yet the cellular area above this shows almost no reaction product (arrows).

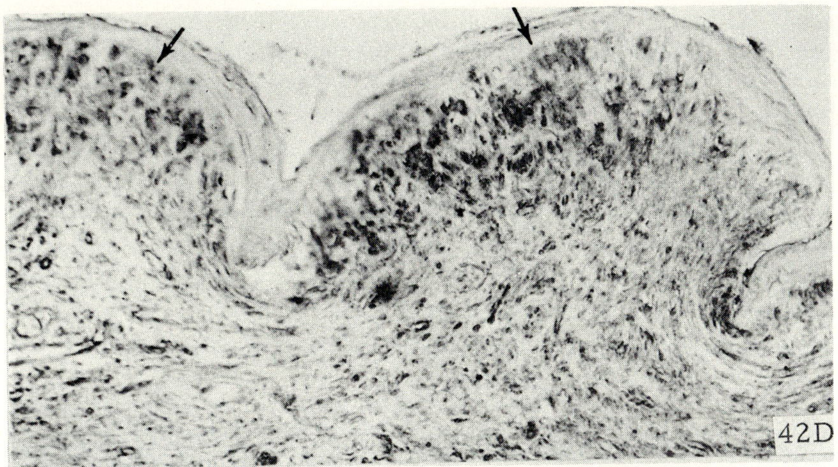

Fig. 42D. AMPase reaction: only a very weak reaction is seen at the outer cellular marginal zone (arrows), otherwise the reaction is negligible in this region where the ATPase is strongly positive (see Fig. 42B).

Postcardiotomy Endocarditis (PCE)

With the increase in cardiac surgery for the correction of congenital and acquired defects, a new form of endocarditis has appeared on the scene (PCE).[127-133] This type of endocarditis has some unique clinical and pathological features. It may be entirely lacking in dramatic clinical picture and all symptoms of sepsis may be quite subdued. Only general symptoms may prevail and these may be of a rather indolent, chronic, mild nature. It is not uncommonly discovered first at autopsy. Staphylococcus is the most common organism,[134-137] and this does account for at least some of the six-fold increase in staphylococcus endocarditis in the last decade.[138] Coagulase negative staphylococcus as well as the coagulase positive variety are recovered from such lesions. Many of these staphylococci from PCE are resistant to penicillins for at least a six week period. Also more esoteric organisms occur in PCE, including fungi [21, 129-134, 139-144] (Fig. 43).

It is also noteworthy that PCE may appear after a considerable interval of time following the surgery. No adequate explanation exists for this latent period or the frequently subdued clinical course. The infected site is often related to a suture or other foreign material. Yet cusps not tampered with during surgical manipulation can show vegetations. This is mindful of what occurs after experimental peripheral A-V shunts, with the long interval and the distant cusp involvement in the heart.[145] PCE is mindful of the first successful experiment done by Wyssokowitsch[63] to obtain valvular endocarditis, for we have in effect a combination of local trauma followed by bacterial invasion. In PCE we have the trauma and the fleeting passive, if not active, persisting bacteremia. Grant, Wood, and Jones[99] repeated the Wyssokowitsch experiment, separating the trauma to the valve from the bacterial inoculation and found platelet vegetations first, before subsequent bacteremic inoculation contaminated the same specimen to yield a bacterial vegetation. This may intimate what happens in PCE and it suggests an explanation of the unique long interval, ie, *both* the local fibrin or platelet thrombus *and* the seeding bacteremia are required with an overlapping in time relationship for a complicating BE to ensue.

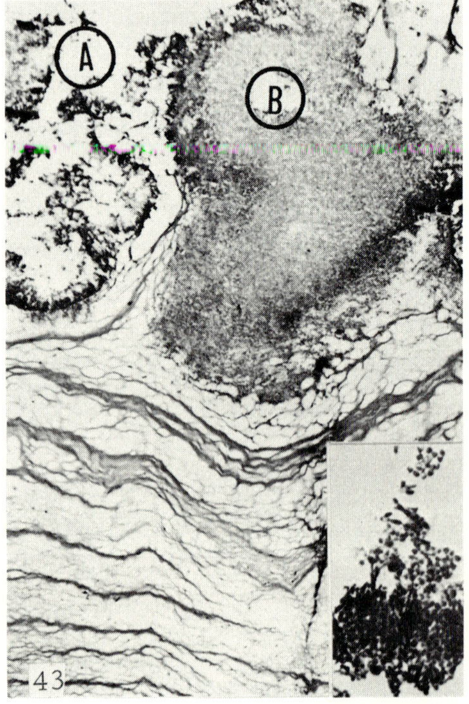

Fig. 43. This is a vegetation from a postcardiotomy endocarditis (PCE) showing overgrowth of fungi on the surface of the vegetation. The underlying inflammatory reaction was minimal below this site. This discrepancy is explained in part only by postmortem proliferation (area A), vital proliferation being present in area B. Blood cultures were positive for **Candida albicans.** PAS stain. × 100. The insertion is a DPNH diaphorase reaction and shows yeast forms. × 400.

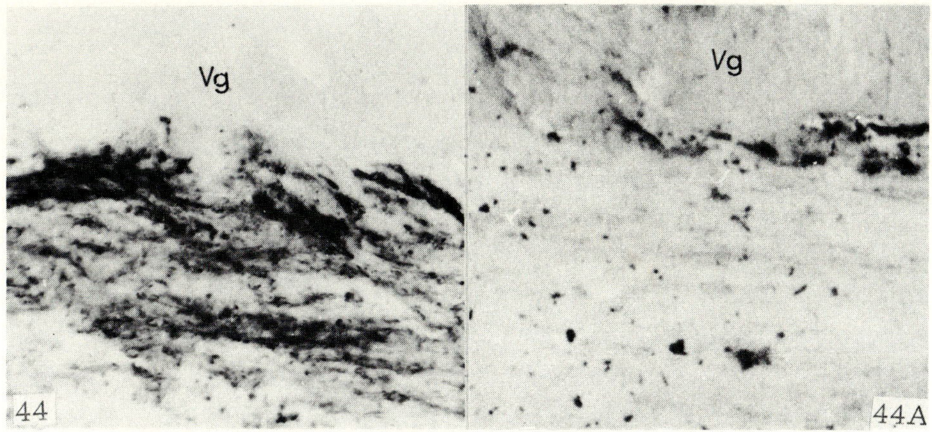

Figs. 44, 44A. AMPase and ATPase reactions, respectively, of an NBTE on the aortic valve of a 59 year old male who died of colonic carcinoma with generalized metastasis. The positive AMPase reaction is present in the valve at the base of vegetation, yet the vegetation (Vg) in the region of NBTE is pale and shows no reaction product. The ATPase reaction (Fig. 44A) appears positive only focally. This is an early NBTE. × 130.

Histoenzymatic and Electron Microscopic Studies
   of Valves and Vegetations

Histoenzymatic studies have been done on distorted human heart valves and experimental animals to understand the mechanisms of NBTE formation and enzymatic alterations in ABE and SBE.[146-148] Studies on adenosine nucleotides and their relationship to NBTE formation have been done at the histological level by utilizing the enzymes ADPase and the related enzymes, ATPase and AMPase. The AMPase and ATPase reactions were found positive at different times, in different places, and in different phases of the development of NBTE. The AMPase reaction appeared first and at the base of the vegetation (Fig. 44); then the ADPase reaction, and finally the ATPase reaction was found (Fig. 44A). As the AMPase reaction subsided (Fig. 45), the ADPase and ATPase reactions appeared (Fig. 45A). The enzymatic reactions then appeared at different, but in a rather set time sequence in relation to NBTE formation; this was parallel to the pattern of the aging of the platelets of the vegetation as revealed by the DPNH diaphorase reaction. The enzymatic changes with BE and its changes in the healing reaction are given above in the presentation of the healing process.

At the base of NBTE, alcian blue positive material, probably acid mucopolysaccharide, was present quite constantly and the uptake of S^{35} was also prominent (Fig. 46). The alkaline phosphatase studies yielded no reaction product at the base of NBTE (Fig. 47), regardless of any organizing cellular response. In contrast, alkaline phosphatase was positive at the base of vegetations in BE (Fig. 48); this was true even when the bacterial vegetation was sterile.

Platelets tend to aggregate on *exposed collagen* (Figs. 7, 7A, 29). Agglutinated platelets result in a release of ADP from the platelets, and in turn such liberated

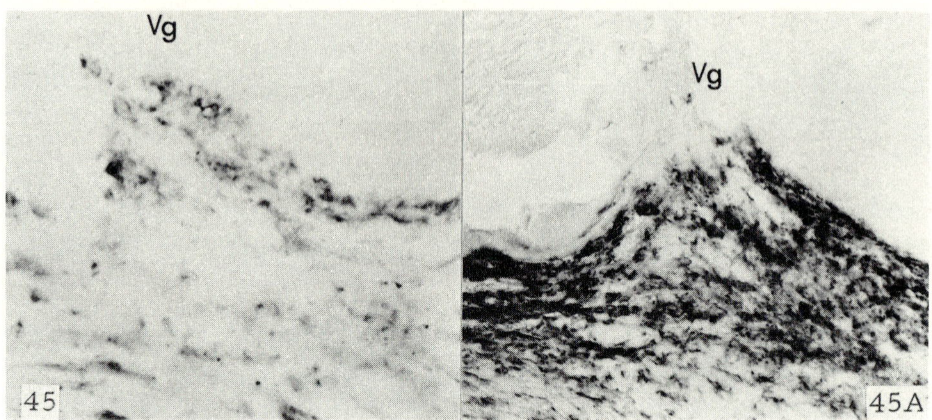

Figs. 45, 45A. AMPase and ATPase reactions, respectively, of an NBTE on the mitral valve from a 75 year old female who died of heart failure with mitral stenosis. The positive AMPase reaction is rather weak in the valve at the base of vegetation. The vegetation itself shows no positive reaction at all. The ADPase or ATPase reactions (Fig. 45A) show a strongly positive reaction product in the valve at the base of vegetation. This NBTE is older than in the previous case (Figs. 44, 44A); both show no reactions in the vegetation.

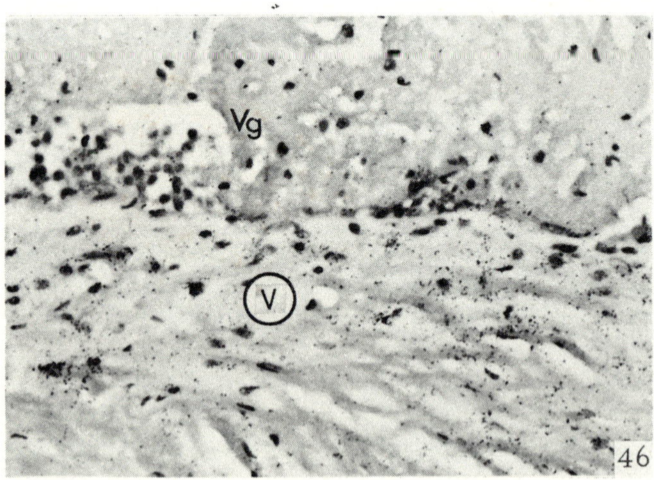

Fig. 46. Autoradiograph of NBTE obtained by the same in vitro procedure as for Figure 1A. An increased S^{35} uptake is seen at the base of vegetation. The vegetation (upper part in this photograph) (Vg) shows very little uptake. S^{35} is localized in the myxomatous area of the valve (V). $\times$ 250.

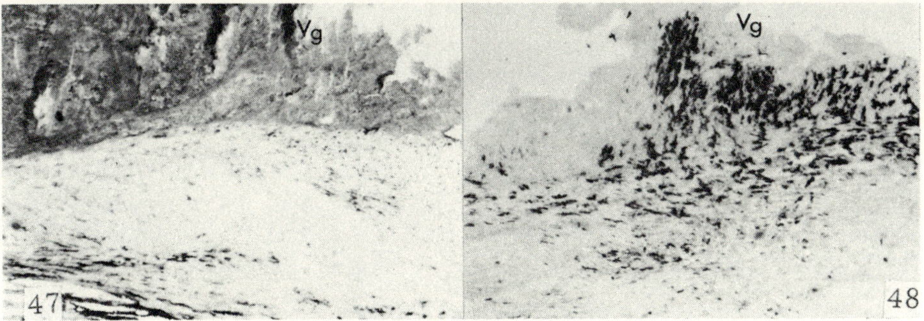

Fig. 47. Alkaline phosphatase reaction of an NBTE on the mitral valve. No alkaline phosphatase reaction in the valve at the base of vegetation (Vg), though some cellular response is present. × 32.

Fig. 48. Alkaline phosphatase reaction of a BE on the mitral valve. Note the strongly positive reaction at the base of vegetation (Vg). Such a positive alkaline phosphatase reaction is also seen after the vegetation has been sterilized by antibiotic therapy. × 32.

ADP favors further aggregation of platelets. This phenomenon has been demonstrated by Zucker and Borrelli,[149] Hovig,[150, 151] Hughes,[152] Glynn et al,[153] Borne,[154-156] and others.[157-158] It is known that when collagen, collagen of the heart valves is no exception, is exposed to the blood stream platelets stick to collagen fibers; this is probably the most common initial manifestation of NBTE. Hovig [150, 151] also demonstrated that when platelets adhered to collagen, disappearance of organelles of platelets occurred, yet this did not occur so readily in ADP-induced aggregated platelets. It is this early, undramatic NBTE vegetation which is loosely attached and easily torn off.

With human heart valves, it was found difficult to obtain a timed fresh NBTE of known age for histoenzymatic study. Fresh NBTE lesions were produced experimentally, and the enzymes AMPase, ADPase, ATPase, and alkaline phosphatase were found positive at the base of NBTE and on the surface of the valve with the pattern of distribution noted. Enzymatic findings with experimental BE are given in the discussion above on healing BE.

In electron microscopic studies the early thrombotic site on the valve consisted almost exclusively of platelets clumped closely together (Figs. 7, 7A) with other blood elements such as neutrophils, erythrocytes, or even fibrin contributing little. It was evident that unit collagen fibrils seemed to be in close approximation to the platelet cytoplasmic membrane at the bottom of the platelet thrombi (Fig. 29). Commonly, fine fibrils (100 to 200 Å wide) were found in close approximation to the massed platelets (Fig. 29). The nature of degradation in platelets following their adhesion to different structures seemed to be variable. During acute bacterial inflammation platelets found at the valve surface tended to show an incomplete or low response, in that there was a retention of the granules, often with their central condensation with other elements such as mitochondria, glycogen, and vesicles. No active violent rupture of the platelet granules occurred such as took place on contact with collagen fibrils of 640 Å periodicity. Furthermore, the actual liberation of the granules through the platelet cytoplasmic membrane was not demonstrated; such liberation was encountered in nonbacterial vegetations (Figs. 7, 7A, 29), particularly following trauma with resultant exposure of platelets to underlying unit collagen fibrils. With human material, the unit collagen fibrils in most instances were detectable in the electron microscopic studies in isolated form and in different stages of alteration depending upon the nature of the lesion in the valve.

The collagen in the altered valve and in the older valve does show some significant biological changes, including a tendency to hyaline transformation. The collagen fibers are more readily altered to stain like elastica after slight denaturation with mild heat, urea, etc, and are then more subject to digestion by elastase and collagenase.

In the distorted valves of rats, the AMPase reaction increased regardless of age,[159] and with it also occurred a change in the acid mucopolysaccharides. Kirk's [160] biochemical assay of aortas from different age groups revealed that more ground substances, ie, acid mucopolysaccharides, were found in the child than in the adult and that the acid mucopolysaccharides possessed anti-coagulant activities.[161] Torii also found variations.[162] Therefore, an increase of AMPase reaction and acid mucopolysaccharides in the distorted valve, or at the base of the very fresh NBTE, may indicate a biological protective phenomenon.

It is the platelet mass in the stage of viscous transformation which is sticky and promotes the adhesion of bacteria to contaminate the vegetation, with all that this implies, as noted (Fig. 20) (Table 3). Bacteria can also be arrested in the fibrin or fibrinoid of NBTE. It is clear that NBTE is a complex phenomenon rather than a simple and unimportant entity—the role heretofore assigned to it.

The relationships of the coagulation factors (some are enzymatic), heparin, fibrinolysin, other less specific cathepsins, and specific proteases, to the formation, persistence, and resolution of vegetations remain as yet unexplored. The prevention of vegetation formation, by the control of agglutination and transformation of platelets, and the prevention of contamination of the NBTE once it does form, should be our objectives.

Endocrine Factor in Endocarditis

For many years clinicians have noted that certain patients are prone to develop "rheumatism." They were anxious about patients with a certain endocrine status, particularly those with fine skin, red hair, the so-called status lymphaticus habitus." Such patients have thin adrenals and are prone to develop rheumatic heart disease. Lesions of the valves and the endocardium are associated with the carcinoid syndrome and excess of serotonin. Hormones from the ovary, testicle, and from the thyroid, pituitary, and adrenal glands affect connective tissue and have been utilized experimentally to produce valvulitis and vegetations.[35-38] The effect of hormones on the connective tissue, including the valve stroma, has been stressed by Klemperer,[163, 164] Gersh et al,[165] Ragan et al,[166] Layton,[167] Boström and Odelblad,[168] Jacobson and Boström,[169] and recently by Asboe-Hansen.[75] ACTH, cortisone, and many of its modifications and variants are utilized in the treatment of valvular disease. Valve lesions have been produced by pitressin, adrenalin, estrogen, growth hormone, DOCA, and ACTH.[36, 38] In our own experimental production of valvular lesions, a consistent correlation was found between the hypertrophy of the adrenals and the degree of severity of the valvular lesions.[35, 38] This hypertrophy was interpreted as due to stimulation of the adrenal by ACTH, which simultaneously may well have an affect on the valvular connective tissue.

Many have obtained valvular changes, including vegetative lesions with nonspecific stress such as high altitude, cold, or arterio-venous shunts.[30, 35] Nonspecific stress is known to affect the endocrine system, particularly the pituitary-adrenal axis, as noted by Selye [170, 171] and others. The exact mechanism of action of stress as such, or of any or all of the endocrines and their hormones, on the valve remains quite unknown. Yet some overall influence on selected connective tissue, and on the valvular connective tissue, does seem to prevail and cannot be contradicted.

Incidence Studies and Their Significance

With the advent of the antibiotic era, the incidence of bacterial endocarditis has diminished,[172-177] especially in persons under 50 years of age (Table 4). There has been a corresponding increase in NBTE on both deformed and normal valves. The ratio of BE to NBTE decreased [123] from 1 to 1 to 1 to about 5 (Table 4). The experience for a comparable period before and after chemotherapy and antibiotics has already been detailed.[123] The present data are included for comparison in Tables 4 and 5. It should be noted that many more cases of *all forms* of

Table 4. Incidence of NBTE and BE in Young and Old Before and After Antibiotic Era

	1936–1946			1956–1965		
	TOTAL	UNDER 50 YR	OVER 50 YR	TOTAL	UNDER 50 YR	OVER 50 YR
Autopsy	5035	2239	2796	6126	1799	4327
NBTE	97 1.9%	52 3.2%	45 0.8%	415 6.8%	58 3.2%	357 8.2%
ABE+SBE	94 1.9%	72 2.3%	22 1.6%	87 1.4%	28 1.6%	59 1.4%

Table 5. Incidence of Acute, Subacute Bacterial Endocarditis and NBTE Before and After Antibiotic Era

	NONBACT. ENDOCARD.	BACT. ENDOCARD.		TOTAL AUTOPSY
		ACUTE	SUBACUTE	
1936–46	97 1.92%	47 0.93%	37 0.73%	5035
1947–52	197 3.97%	10 0.20%	16 0.32%	4958
1956–65	415 6.77%	60 0.97%	28 0.45%	6126

endocarditis now occur in the aged (Table 4). This changing age incidence reflects that effective antibiotic therapy has also been more effective than expected because of population aging as a whole.

Patients on steroids, immunosuppressive drugs, or radiation, on antibiotic or chemotherapy, and patients with advanced malignancy or diabetics or cirrhotics are prone to develop NBTE, and consequently BE, too. Eger,[178] and Tiffany et al [179] noted an association of NBTE with cancer. Rohner [180] has noted the high incidence of NBTE in cases of mucinogenic cancer from many sites. A case of carcinomatous endocarditis in a primary tumor from a bronchus has been seen. By the position of the cancer tissue in the vegetation proper, this represented the end result of trapping and growth of tumor cells, rather than tumor cell emboli to the relatively avascular valve.

The ratio of ABE to SBE has also changed from a ratio of 2 to 3 for the period from 1947 to 1952 to a ratio of 2 to 1 for the decade 1956–1965.[21] Uwaydah and Weinberg [20] also noted a change in the proportion of ABE to SBE from an early ratio of less than 1 to 3 to a present ratio of less than 1 to 1. In comparing a series of autopsies seen by one of us from 1936 to 1946, before the antibiotic era, with a group from 1956 to 1965, the incidence of NBTE *increased* from 1.9 percent to 6.8 percent; in the group for those 50 years of age and over the increase was from 1.6 to 8.2 percent (Table 4). Some of this increase is undoubtedly also attributable to more careful examination of the heart valves in recent years, in part at least. Nevertheless BE *diminished* in frequency from 1.9 percent to 1.4 percent for this same period; yet for the age group above 50, BE *increased* from 0.8 percent before antibiotics to 1.4 after 1956 (Table 4). This similar tendency has been noted by Pankey,[156] Wilson,[159] and others.[181-189] As a result BE in the elderly is now considered more important.

In the young, valvular disease still occurs mainly in the rheumatic group. Normal valves no longer help distinguish ABE from SBE; this is particularly true in the aged. In the aged it is the sclerotic and calcified valve which develops both NBTE and BE, with SBE occurring more frequently than before. The ratio of NBTE in rheumatic heart disease has changed in its relation to nonrheumatic valvular distortions, from 7 to 3 before to 1 to 3 after 1956 (Table 6). For BE this ratio was 7 to 3 before and 1 to 2 after 1956. Both NBTE and BE now occur more frequently in nonrheumatic heart disease (Table 6).

Alpha hemolytic streptococcus still is the most common organism in SBE, while *Staphylococcus aureus* [190, 191] is still the most common in the acute form and as

Table 6. Incidence of NBTE and BE in RHD and in Non-RHD
Before and After Antibiotic Era

		TOTAL	WITH RHD	NON-RHD	RATIO RHD/ NON-RHD
1936–46					
	NBTE	93	65 (70%)	28 (30%)	7:3
	BE	94	68 (72%)	26 (28%)	7:3
1956–65					
	NBTE	415	103 (25%)	312 (75%)	1:3
	BE	87	28 (32%)	59 (68%)	1:2

noted, has increased in frequency [20, 124-127] from 14 percent to 23 percent.[20] Group A beta streptococci and group D enterococcus [192-196] have also become more common. A wider range of etiological organisms also is now found and many rare esoteric bacteria,[21, 139-144, 197-205] rickettsia,[206] histoplasma,[207-209] and other fungi are now included. Viral endocarditis also has been stressed recently.[210, 211]

Ninety percent of endocarditis is still due to streptococci and staphylococci. Viridans streptococci and microaerophilic organisms are found now more frequently in ABE. Viridans streptococci cause one half of all BE but about four fifths of SBE. Staphylococcus causes one quarter of all endocarditis but about half of ABE. Pneumococcus is now a rare etiology; it used to account for as much as 10 percent of the cases in some series. Table 7 gives our bacteriological experience.

Table 7. Bacterial Studies in Acute and Subacute Bact. Endocarditis Before and After Antibiotic Era

	ACUTE			SUBACUTE		
	1936–46	1947–52	1956–56	1936–46	1947–52	1956–65
Streptococci						
hemolytic	14	0	3	0	2	1
nonhemolytic	4	0	4	1	0	0
viridans	3	1	2	33	10	6
Staph. aureus	8	13	22	4	1	4
Pneumococci	11	0	2	0	0	0
E. coli	5	1	12	0	1	4
Mixed	11	7	0	3	4	1
Unknown	9	2	30	10	7	8

It is still noteworthy that gram negative bacterial endocarditis, particularly *E. coli,* is relatively rare, despite the frequency of such bacteremias.[20] This may be due to the peculiar effects of the endotoxin containing organisms on the body in general, and on the adrenals in particular. The latter finds its maximum expression in the Waterhouse-Friderichsen syndrome. The possible role of the adrenal and other endocrines in valvular changes has been discussed above (See Table 1).

Bacterial endocarditis now occurs less frequently in the young and particularly on the rheumatic valve (Table 6); this indicates a control of bacteremic seeding of the basic NBTE lesion; thus NBTE persists as such and its incidence has increased correspondingly in this group too. Acute bacterial endocarditis is commonly caused by staphylococcus and is still found in the young on relatively normal valves more frequently. All of the above findings fit well into the concept of the relationship of NBTE to BE.

Summary and Conclusion

The evolution of our knowledge of vegetative endocarditis is detailed to add a deeper understanding and significance to all valvular lesions as encountered. A large human autopsy experience is the basis for some generalizations about stages of development and interrelationships of all types of endocarditis. The classification, the mechanisms, and the sequences involved in the origin of the different forms of vegetative endocarditis are discussed. A rational basis for the morphological features of each type of vegetation and the differences found is offered; this includes an explanation for the transitions that occur between the classical forms of endocarditis. An endocrine factor in endocarditis is indicated. Histoenzymatic and electron microscopic studies and some experiments with isotopes are noted. The healing of vegetative lesions, in the past and present, is discussed. Incidence studies before and after the antibiotic era of all forms of endocarditis are given, and the significances of the prevalent changes are recorded.

References

1. Horder, T. J. Infective endocarditis: with an analysis of 150 cases and with special reference to the chronic form of the diseases. Quart. J. Med., 2:289, 1908.
2. Blumer, G. Subacute bacterial endocarditis. Medicine, 2:105, 1923.
3. Clawson, B. J. Analysis of 220 cases of endocarditis with special reference to subacute bacterial type. Arch. Intern. Med. (Chicago), 33:157, 1924.
4. ———— Etiology of acute rheumatic fever. J. Infect. Dis., 36:444, 1925.
5. ———— and Bell, E. T. A comparison of acute rheumatic and subacute bacterial endocarditis. Arch. Intern. Med. (Chicago), 37:66, 1926.
6. ———— Bell, E. T., and Hartzell, T. B. Valvular disease of the heart with special reference to the pathogenesis of old valvular defects. Amer. J. Path., 2:193, 1926.
7. Thayer, W. S. Studies on bacterial (infective) endocarditis. Johns Hopkins Hosp. Reports, 22:1, 1926.
8. Perry, C. B. Bacterial Endocarditis. London, Simpkin Marshall Ltd., 1936.
9. Middleton, W. S., and Burke, M. Streptococcus viridans endocarditis lenta: a clinicopathologic analysis of the experience in the Wisconsin General Hospital. Amer. J. M. Sci., 198:301, 1939.
10. Christian, H. A. The determinative background of subacute bacterial endocarditis. Amer. J. M. Sci., 201:34, 1941.
11. Keefer, C. S. Pathogenesis of bacterial endocarditis. Amer. Heart J., 19:352, 1940.
12. Kelson, S. R., and White, P. D. Notes on 250 cases of subacute bacterial (streptococcal) endocarditis studied and treated between 1927 and 1939. Ann. Intern. Med., 22:40, 1945.
13. Cates, J. E., and Christie, R. Subacute bacterial endocarditis. A review of 442 patients treated in 14 centers appointed by the penicillin trials committee of the Medical Research Council. Quart. J. Med., 20:93, 1951.
14. Germer, W. D. Endokarditis lenta. Pathogenese und Beziehung zwischen Verlaufsform Erregerart und Ausscheidengemöglichkeit. Ergebn. Inn. Med. Kinderheilk., 2:296, 1951.
15. Afremow, M. L. A review of 202 cases of bacterial endocarditis 1948–1952 (Cook County Hosp.). Illinois M. J., 107:67, 1955.
16. Kerr, A., Jr. In Subacute Bacterial Endocarditis. Pullen, R. L. ed., Springfield, Ill., Charles C Thomas, 1955, p. 343.
17. Morgan, W. L., and Bland, E. F. Bacterial endocarditis in the antibiotic era with special reference to the later complications. Circulation, 19:753, 1959.
18. Vogler, W., Dorney, E., Bridges, H. Bacterial endocarditis: a review of 148 cases. Amer. J. Med., 32:910, 1962.
19. Rabinovich, S., Evans, J., Smith, I. M., and January, L. E. A long-term view of bacterial endocarditis, 337 cases 1924 to 1963. Ann. Intern. Med., 63:185, 1965.
20. Uwaydah, M. M., and Weinberg, A. N. Bacterial endocarditis—a changing pattern. New Eng. J. Med., 273:1231, 1965.

21. Lerner, P. I., and Weinstein, L. Infective endocarditis in the antibiotic era. New Eng. J. Med., 274:199, 259, 323, 388, 1966.
22. Boström, H., and Odeblad, E. Autoradiographic observations on the incorporation of S^{35} labeled sodium sulfate in the rabbit fetus. Anat. Rec., 115:505, 1953.
23. ———— Moretti, A., and Whitehouse, M. W. Studies on the biochemistry of heart valves. 1. On the biosynthesis of mucopolysaccharides in bovine heart valves. Biochim. Biophys. Acta, 74:213, 1963.
24. Oka, M., and Brodie, S. Age sequence of tagged fibroblasts and collagen in the cardiac valves and aorta of rats. Fed. Proc. Part 1. 25:665 (abstract), 1966.
25. Albertini, A. Die Bedeutung der histiocytären Reaktion bei Endocarditis (Immunisatorische und allergische Phenomene bei Endocarditis). Int. Arch. Allerg. Suppl. 1., 1:12, 1950–51.
26. Dietrich, A. Versuche Über Herzklapentzündung. Ztsch. Exper. Med., 50:85, 1926.
27. Siegmund, H. Über einige Reaktionen der Gefässwände und des Endokards bei experimentellen und menschlichen Allgemeininfektionen. Zlb. Allg. Path., 36:250, 1925.
28. Boehmig, R. Pathologie und Bakteriologie der Endokarditis. Klin. Wschr., 27:417, 1949.
29. ———— Seröse Endocarditis bei Kleinkindern und Jugendlichen. Virchow. Arch. Path. Anat., 318:646, 1950.
30. ———— and Klein, P. Pathologie und Bakteriologie der Endokarditis. Berlin, Göttinger-Heidelberg, Springer Verlag, 1953.
31. Angrist, A., and Weinberg, F. The clinical and pathologic significance of so-called thrombotic non-bacterial endocarditis. Abst. Proc. N.Y. Path. Soc., 1950–51:89, 1951.
32. ———— A concept of the pathogenesis of endocarditis based on a study of transitional lesions. Proc. N.Y. State Assn. Pub. Health, 30:50, 1950.
33. ———— A concept of the origin of the cardiac valvular vegetation. J. Mount Sinai Hosp. N.Y., 24:669, 1957.
34. ———— Aging heart valves and a unitary pathological hypothesis for sclerosis. J. Geront., 19:135, 1964.
35. ———— Oka, M., Nakao, K., and Marquiss, J. Studies in experimental endocarditis. 1. Production of valvular lesions by mechanisms not involving infection or sensitivity factors. Amer. J. Path., 36:181, 1960.
36. ———— and Oka, M. Experimental endocarditis. *In* Methods and Achievements in Experimental Pathology. Bajusz, E., and Jasmin, G., eds., Basel and New York, S. Karger, 1966, Vol. 2.
37. Oka, M., Nakao, K., and Angrist, A. Nonspecific aspects of endocarditis: clinical applications of an experimental study. New York J. Med., 60:669, 1960.
38. ———— and Angrist, A. Experimental endocarditis. Rev. Canad. Biol., 22:297, 1963 (Symp. Internat. Pt. II).
39. Bartoletti, F. "Methodus in dyspnocaen" Bononiae. *Cited in* A History of the Heart and the Circulation, Willius, F. and Dry, T. J. Philadelphia, W. B. Saunders Co., 1948, p. 56.
40. Riverius, L. Opera Omnie Venice, Viezeic (case seen in 1646). 1723, p. 526.
41. Morgagni, J. B. The seats and causes of diseases investigated by anatomy. Translated by Alexander. London, 1769.
42. Lancisi, J. M. De Subitaneis Mortibus Observatio. Rome, 4:149, 1707.
43. Baillie, M. The Morbid Anatomy of Some of the Most Important Parts of the Human Body, 2nd ed. London, 1797.
44. Kreysig, F. L. Die Krankheiten des Herzens. Berlin, 1814.
45. Hodgeson, J. A Treatise on the Diseases of Arteries and Veins, Containing the Pathology and Treatment of Aneurysms and Wounded Arteries. London, T. Underwood, 1815.

46. Bertin, R. J. H. *In* A History of the Heart and Circulation. Willius, F. A., and Dry, T. J., Philadelphia, W. B. Saunders Co., 1948, p. 124.

47. Laennec, R. T. H. Traité de l'Auscultation médiate. 1819.

48. Corvisart, J. N. A treatise on the diseases and organic lesions of the heart and great vessels. 2nd ed. Translated by C. H. Webb. London, 1813.

49. Bouillaud, J. Bertin's Traité des Maladies du Coeur et des gros Vaisseaux. Paris, 1824.

50. Williams, F. A., and Dry, T. J. A History of the Heart and Circulation. Philadelphia, W. B. Saunders Co., 1948.

51. Paget, J. On white spots on the surface of the heart, and on the frequency of pericarditis. Med. Chir. Tr., 23:29, 1840.

52. Kirkes, W. S. On some of the principal effects resulting from the detachment of fibrous deposits from the interior of the heart and their mixture with the circulating blood. Med. Chir. Tr., 35:281, 1851.

53. Wilks, S. Capillary embolism or arterial pyaemia. Guy's Hosp. Rep., 15:29, 1870.

54. Ormerod, E. L. The Gulstonian lectures; pathology and treatment of disease of the heart. Lond. Med. Gaz., 47:503, 529, 573, 617, 661, 705, 793, 1851.

55. Virchow, R. Endocarditis mit besonderer Berücksichtigung der ulcerösen und thrombotischen Formen. Charité Ann., Berlin, 4:793, 1879.

56. ———— Endocarditis Ulcerosa. Charité Ann., Berlin, 5:723, 1880.

57. Winge, E. Mycocis endocardii. Nordisk med. Arkiv Bd 2, 1870.

58. ———— Mycocis endocardii. Jahresbericht über ges. Med. (abst) 2:95, 1871.

59. Rokitansky, C. Lehrbuch der Pathologischen Anatomie. ed. 3, Wien, Wilhelm Braumüller, 1855.

60. Heiberg, H. Ein fall von Endocarditis ulcerosa puerperalis mit Pilzbildungen im Herzen. Virchow Arch. Path. Anat., 56:407, 1872.

61. Klebs. Weitere Beiträge zur Entstehungsgeschichte der Endocarditis. Arch. Exper. Path. Pharm., 9:52, 1878.

62. Jaccoud, S. Sur l'endocardite infectieuse. Leçons de Clin. Med. de la Pitié (Paris), Leçon 1, 5:1, 1885–6.

63. Wyssokowitsch, W. Beiträge zur Lehre von der Endokarditis. Virchow Arch. Path. Anat., 103:301, 1886.

64. Königer, H. Histologische Untersuchungen über Endokarditis. Arb. Path. Inst. Leipzig, 2:1, 1903.

65. Harbitz, F. Studien über Endocarditis. Dtsch. Med. Wschr., 25:121, 1899.

66. Lenhartz, H. Über die septische Endocarditis. Münch. Med. Wschr., 48:1123, 1178, 1901.

67. Schottmüller, H. Endocarditis lenta; zugleich ein Beitrag zur Artunterscheidung der pathogenen Streptokokken. Münch. Med. Wschr., 57:617, 1910.

68. Libman, E., and Celler, H. L. The etiology of subacute infective endocarditis. Amer. J. Med. Sci., 140:516, 1910.

69. ———— Characterization of various forms of endocarditis. J.A.M.A., 80:813, 1923.

70. Osler, W. Gulstonian lectures: Malignant endocarditis. British Med. J., 1:467, 522, 577, 1885.

71. Osler, W. Chronic infectious endocarditis. Quart. J. Med., 2:219, 1909.

72. Koester, K. Die embolische Endocarditis. Virchow Arch. Path. Anat., 72:257, 1878.

73. Laws, C. L., and Levine, S. A. Clinical notes on rheumatic heart disease with special reference to the cause of death. Amer. J. Med. Sci., 186:833, 1933.

74. Davis, D., and Weiss, S. The relation of subacute and acute bacterial endocarditis to rheumatic endocarditis. A study of 66 cases with necropsies. New Eng. J. Med., 208:619, 1933.

75. Gross, L., and Friedberg, C. K. Nonbacterial thrombotic endocarditis classification and general description. Arch. Intern. Med. (Chicago), 58:620, 1936.

76. Von Glahn, W. C., and Pappenheimer, A. M. Relationship between rheumatic and subacute bacterial endocarditis. Arch. Intern. Med. (Chicago), 55:173, 1935.

77. Ribbert, H. Die Erkrankungen des Endokards. *In* Henke & Lubarsch. Handbuch der speziellen pathologischen Anatomie und Histologie. Berlin, Julius Springer, 1924, Vol. 2.

78. Held, I. W., and Lieberson, A. Pathogenesis of subacute bacterial endocarditis. Amer. Heart J. 25:478, 1943.

79. Abbott, M. E. On the incidence of bacterial inflammatory processes in cardiovascular defects and on malformed semilunar cusps. Ann. Clin. Med., 4:189, 1925.

80. Lewis, T., and Grant, R. T. Observations relating to subacute infective endocarditis. Heart, 10:21, 1923.

81. Gelfman, R., and Levine, S. A. The incidence of acute and subacute bacterial endocarditis in congenital heart disease. Amer. J. Med. Sci., 204:324, 1943.

82. Oka, M., Shirota, A., and Angrist, A. Experimental endocarditis-endocrine factors in valve lesions on A-V shunt rats. Arch. Path., 82:85, 1966.

83. Asboe-Hanson, G. Hormone control of connective tissue. Fed. Proc., 25:1136, 1966.

84. Vaisman, S. B., Guasch, J. L., Vignau, A. I., Correa, E. T., Schuster, A. C., Mortimer, E. A., Jr., and Rammelkamp, C. H., Jr. Failure of penicillin to alter acute rheumatic valvulitis. J.A.M.A., 194:1284, 1965.

85. Coombs, C. F. Rheumatic Heart Disease. New York, William Wood & Co., 1924.

86. ———— Streptococcal infections of the heart. Quart. J. Med., 15:114, 1922.

87. Lansing, A. I., Rosenthal, T. B., Alex, M., and Dempsey, E. W. The structure and chemical characterization of elastic fiber as revealed by elastase and by electron microscopy. Anat. Rec., 114:555, 1952.

88. ———— Aging of elastic tissue and the systemic effects of elastase. CIBA Foundation Colloquia on Aging. Vol. 1. General Aspect 88, 1954.

89. Nakao, A., Angrist, A., and Mao, P. Collagen and platelet interaction in experimental vegetative cardiac valvular lesions. Exp. Molec. Path., In press.

90. Pfuhl, W. Die Histiozyten der Herzklappen: Farbstoffspeicherung, Zellzerfall, Neubildung, Zellform, und Abstammungsfragen. Z. Mikr. Anat. Forsch., 24:237, 1931.

91. De Vecchi, B. Sur la myocardite rheumatismale, étude anatomopathologique et expérimentale. Arch. Med. Exper. Anat. Path., 24:352, 1912.

92. Czirer, L. Über die Veränderung der Herzklappen bei akuten Infektiouskrankeiten. Virchow Arch. Path. Anat., 213:272, 1913.

93. Holsti, O. Beiträge zur Kenntnis der entzündlichen Klappen affektionen mit besonderer Berücksichtigung der Pathogenese. Arb. Path. Inst. Helsingfors., 5:401, 1927–1928.

94. Semsroth, K., and Koch, R. Studies on the pathogenesis of bacterial endocarditis. Arch. Path., 8:921, 1929.

95. Klinge, F., and Vaubel, E. Das Gewebsbild des fieberhaften Rheumatismus. Die Gefässe beim Rheumatismus, in besondere die "Aortitis rheumatica" (mit Betrachtung zur Ätiologie des fieberhaften Rheumatismus von pathologisch-anatomischen Standpunkt). Virchow Arch. Path. Anat., 281:701, 1931.

96. Leary, T. Early lesions of rheumatic endocarditis. Arch. Path., 13:1, 1932.

97. Miller, A. J., Pick, R., Kline, I. K., and Katz, I. N. The susceptibility of dogs with chronic impairment of cardiac lymph flow to staphylococcal valvular endocarditis. Circulation, 30:417, 1964.

98. Stetson, C. A. The occurrence of leucocyte-platelet thrombosis in rheumatic carditis. J. Exp. Med., 94:493, 1951.

99. Grant, R. T., Wood, J. E., and Jones, T. R. Heart valve irregularities in relation to subacute bacterial endocarditis. Heart, 14:247, 1927.

100. Nedzel, A. J. Experimental endocarditis. Arch. Path., 24:143, 1937.

101. ———— The histopathology of experimentally produced endocarditis. Amer. J. Path., 13:627, 1937.

102. Ziegler. Über den Bau und die Entstehung der endocarditischen Efflorescenzen. Verhand. Congress Inn. Med., 7:339, 1888.
103. Gould, S. E., ed. Pathology of the Heart. 2nd ed. Springfield, Ill., Charles C Thomas, 1960.
104. MacDonald, R. A., and Robbins, S. L. Significance of nonbacterial thrombotic endocarditis: autopsy and clinical study of 78 cases. Ann. Intern. Med., 46:255, 1957.
105. Duguid, J. B. The role of the connective tissues in arterial disease. In Connective Tissue, Thrombosis, and Atherosclerosis. Page, I. H., ed., New York and London, Academic Press, 1959, p. 13.
106. Tweedy, P. S. Pathogenesis of valvular thickening in rheumatic heart disease. Brit. Heart J., 48:173, 1956.
107. Magarey, F. R. On the mode of formation of Lambl's excrescences and their relation to chronic thickening of the mitral valve. J. Path. Bact., 61:203, 1949.
108. Allen, A. C., and Sirota, J. M. The morphogenesis and significance of degenerative verrucal endocarditis (terminal endocarditis, endocarditis simplex, nonbacterial thrombotic endocarditis). Amer. J. Path., 20:1025, 1944.
109. Friedberg, C. K. Diseases of the Heart. Philadelphia, W. B. Saunders Co., 1956.
110. Contin, J., and Oka, M. Unusual cardiac, pulmonary and meningeal involvement in rheumatoid arthritis. Report of a case. Dis. Chest, 49:552, 1966.
111. MacNeil, W. J., Spence, M. J., and Slavkin, A. E. Early lesions of experimental endocarditis lenta. Amer. J. Path., 19:735, 1943.
112. Freifeld, H. Vaccination und Endokarditis. Klin. Wchschr. 7:1645, 1948.
113. Leschke, E. Endokarditis. Berlin & Wien, Spec. Path. Therapeu. Krakh., 4:579, 1924.
114. Hutyra, F., and Marek, J. Special pathology and therapeutics of the diseases of domestic animals. Mohler, J. R., and Eichhorn, A., eds., London, Bailliere, Tindall & Cox, 1912, Vol. 1.
115. Haushalter. Endocardite à pneumocoques. Rev. Méd. Paris, 8:328, 1888.
116. Schöne, C. Endocarditis lenta. Deutsch. Med. Wschr., 38:579, 1912.
117. Angrist, A., and Oka, M. Pathogenesis of bacterial endocarditis. J.A.M.A., 183:249, 1963.
118. Klemperer, P., Pollak, A., and Baehr, G. Pathology of disseminated lupus erythematosus. Arch. Path., 32:569, 1941.
119. Porrini, A. Untersuchungen über die mit dem Influenzabacillus erzungte Endokarditis. Virchow Arch. Path. Anat., 204:169, 1911.
120. Libman, E. A study of the endocardial lesions of subacute bacterial endocarditis, with particular reference to healing or healed lesions: with clinical notes. Amer. J. Med. Sci., 144:313, 1912.
121. Weiss, S., and Rhodes, C. P. Healing and healed vegetative (subacute bacterial) endocarditis. New Eng. J. Med. 199:70, 1928.
122. Robinson, M. J., and Ruedy, J. Sequelae of bacterial endocarditis. Amer. J. Med., 32:922, 1962.
123. Angrist, A., and Marquiss, J. The changing morphologic picture of endocarditis since the advent of chemotherapy and antibiotic agents. Amer. J. Path., 30:39, 1954.
124. More, R. A. Cellular mechanism of recovery after treatment with penicillin: subacute endocarditis. J. Lab. & Clin. Med., 31:1279, 1946.
125. Friedberg, C. K., Goldman, H. M., and Field, L. E. Study of bacterial endocarditis. Comparisons in ninety-five cases. Arch. Intern. Med. (Chicago), 107:6, 1961.
126. Albertini, A. Pathologie des Endokard. In Das Herz der Menschen, Band II. Bargmann, W., and Doero, W., eds., Stuttgart, Georg Thieme Verlag, 1963, p. 603.
127. Koiwai, E. K., and Nahas, H. C. Subacute bacterial endocarditis following cardiac surgery. Arch. Surg., 73:272, 1956.

128. Denton, C., Pappas, E. G., Uricchio, J. G., Goldberg, H., and Likoff, W. Bacterial endocarditis following surgery. Circulation, 15:525, 1957.
129. Hoffman, F. G., Zimmerman, S. L., Bradley, E. A., and Lapidus, B. Bacterial endocarditis after surgery for acquired heart disease. New Eng. J. Med., 260:152, 1959.
130. Heins, H. L., Jr., and Linde, L. M. Bacterial endocarditis after surgery for congenital heart disease. New Eng. J. Med., 263:65, 1960.
131. Linde, L. M., and Heins, H. L. Bacterial endocarditis following surgery for congenital heart disease. New Eng. J. Med., 263:65, 1960.
132. Kelch, J. V., and Thomson, N. B., Jr. Bacterial endocarditis complicating repair of a ventricular septal defect. New Eng. J. Med., 265:1245, 1961.
133. Lord, J. W., Jr., Imparato, A. M., Hackel, A., and Doyle, E. F. Endocarditis complicating open-heart surgery. Circulation, 23:489, 1961.
134. Fleming, H. A., and Seal, R. M. E. Staphylococcal infection following cardiac surgery. Thorax, 10:327, 1955.
135. Cohen, S. Staphylococcal infections of the heart. Circulation, 20:96, 1959.
136. Lisan, P., Uricchio, J. F., Marino, D. J., Deshmukh, M., and Likoff, W. Staphylococcal endocarditis. Amer. Heart J., 59:184, 1960.
137. Quinn, E. L., and Cox, F., Jr. Staphylococcus albus (epidermidis) endocarditis: report of 16 cases seen between 1953–1962. Antimicrobial Agents & Chemotherapy. (Proceedings of the Third InterScience Conference on Antimicrobial Agents and Chemotherapy.) Washington, D.C., Am. Soc. Microbiology, 1963, p. 635.
138. ———— Cox, F., and Drake, E. H. Staphylococcic endocarditis; a disease of increasing importance. J.A.M.A., 196:815, 1966.
139. Merchant, R. K., Louria, D. B., Geisler, P. H., Edgcomb, J. H., and Utz, J. P. Fungal endocarditis: Review of the literature and report of three cases. Ann. Intern. Med., 48:242, 1956.
140. Finegold, S. M., Will, D., and Marray, J. F. Aspergillosis: a review and report of 12 cases. Amer. J. Med., 27:463, 1959.
141. Persellin, R. H., Haring, O. M., and Lewis, F. J. Fungal endocarditis following cardiac surgery. Ann. Intern. Med., 54:127, 1961.
142. Zimmerman, L. E. Candida and aspergillus endocarditis. Arch. Path., 50:591, 1950.
143. Kay, J. H., Bernstein, S., Feinstein, D., and Biddle, M. Surgical cure of candida albicans endocarditis with open-heart surgery. New Eng. J. Med., 264:907, 1961.
144. Andriole, V. T., Kravetz, H. M., Roberts, W. C., and Utz, J. P. Candida endocarditis, clinical and pathologic studies. Amer. J. Med., 32:251, 1962.
145. Lillehei, C. W., Shaffer, J. M., Spink, W. W., Bobb, J. R. R., Wargo, J. D., and Visscher, M. B. Role of cardiovascular stress in the pathogenesis of endocarditis and glomerulonephritis: observations including method of experimental production utilizing arteriovenous fistula. Arch. Surg., 63:421, 1951.
146. Oka, M., and Angrist, A. Histochemical studies of thrombotic nonbacterial endocarditis. Lab. Invest., 13:1504, 1964.
147. ———— and Angrist, A. Comparative histochemical studies of nonbacterial and bacterial valvular vegetations. Lab. Invest., 14:48, 1965.
148. ———— Girerd, R. J., Brodie, S., and Angrist, A. Cardiac valve and aortic lesions in Beta-aminopropionitrile (BAPN) fed rats with and without high salt. Amer. J. Path., 48:45, 1966.
149. Zucker, M. B., and Borrelli, J. Platelet clumping produced by connective tissue suspensions and by collagen. Proc. Soc. Exp. Biol. Med., 109:779, 1962.
150. Hovig, T. Aggregation of rabbit blood platelets produced in vitro by saline "extract" of tendons. Thromb. Diath. Haemorrh., 9:248, 1963.
151. ———— Release of a platelet-aggregating substance (adenosine diphosphate) from

rabbit blood platelets induced by saline "extract" of tendons. Thromb. Diath. Haemorrh., 9:264, 1963.

152. Hugues, J., and Lapiere, Ch. M. Nouvelles recherches sur l'accolement des plaquettes aux fibres de collagène. Thromb. Diath. Haemorrh., 11:327, 1964.

153. Glynn, M. F., Movat, H. Z., and Murphy, E. A. Study of platelet adhesiveness and aggregation, with latex particles. J. Lab. Clin. Med., 65:179, 1965.

154. Born, G. V. R. Adenosine triphosphate (ATP) in blood platelet. Biochem. J., 62:32 (abstract) 1956.

155. Born, G. V. R. Aggregation of blood platelets by adenosine diphosphate and its reversal. Nature, 194:927, 1962.

156. ——— and Gross, H. J. The aggregation of blood platelets. J. Physiol., 168:178, 1963.

157. Mitchell, J., and Sharp, A. Platelet clumping in vitro. Brit. J. Haemat., 10:78, 1964.

158. McLean, J. R., Maxwell, R. E., and Hertler, D. Fibrinogen and adenosine diphosphate induced aggregation of platelets. Nature, 202:605, 1964.

159. Oka, M., and Brodie, S. Age sequence of tagged fibroblasts and collagen in the cardiac valves and aorta of rats. Fed. Proc. Part 1, 25:665 (abstract), 1966.

160. Kirk, J. E. Chemistry of the vascular wall of middle sized arteries. *In* The Peripheral Blood Vessels. International Academy of Pathology, Monograph No. 4:47, New York, Williams & Wilkins Co., 1963.

161. ——— Anticoagulant activity of human arterial mucopolysaccharides. Nature, 184:369, 1959.

162. Torii, S., Bashey, R. I., and Nakao, K. Acid mucopolysaccharide composition of human-heart valve. Biochim. Biophys. Acta, 101:285, 1965.

163. Klemperer, P. The concept of collagen diseases. Amer. J. Path., 26:505, 1950.

164. ——— The significance of the intermediate substances of the connective tissue in human disease. Harvey Lectures. series 49, 1953–54. New York, Academic Press Inc., 1955, p. 100.

165. Gersh, I. Ground substance and the plasticity of connective tissues. Harvey Lectures. Series 45, 1949–1950. Springfield, Ill., Charles C Thomas, 1951, p. 211.

166. Ragan, C., Howes, E. L., Plotz, C. M., Meyer, K., Blunt, J. W., and Loftes, R. The effect of ACTH and cortisone on connective tissue. Bull. New York Acad. Med., 26:251, 1950.

167. Layton, L. L. Cortisone inhibition of mucopolysaccharide synthesis in the intact rat. Arch. Biochem., 32:224, 1951.

168. Boström, H., and Odeblad, E. The influence of cortisone upon the sulphate exchange of chondroitin sulphuric acid. Arkiv Kemi, 6:39, 1953.

169. Jacobson, B., and Boström, H. Studies on the biochemistry of heart valves. II. The effect of aging and anti-inflammatory drugs on the synthesis of glucosamine-6-phosphate and phosphoadenosine phosphosulfate by bovine heart valves. Biochim. Biophys. Acta, 83:152, 1964.

170. Selye, H. General adaptation syndrome and the diseases of adaptation. J. Clin. Endocr., 6:117, 1946.

171. ——— Role of somatotrophic hormone in the production of malignant nephrosclerosis, periarteritis nodosa, and hypertensive disease. Brit. Med. J., 1:263, 1951.

172. Geiger, A. J., and Durlacher, S. H. The fate of endocardial vegetations following penicillin treatment of bacterial endocarditis. Amer. J. Path., 23:1023, 1947.

173. Geraci, J. E., and Martin, W J. Antibiotic therapy of bacterial endocarditis: IV. Subacute enterococcal endocarditis, clinical, pathologic and therapeutic consideration of 33 cases. Circulation, 10:173, 1954.

174. ——— The antibiotic therapy of bacterial endocarditis. Med. Clin. North America, 42:1101, 1958.

175. Kaye, D., McCormack, R. C., and Hook, E. W. Bacterial endocarditis. The changing pattern since the introduction of penicillin therapy. *In* Antimicrobial Agents

and Chemotherapy. Finland, M., and Savage, G. M., eds., Ann Arbor, Mich., Braun Brumfield, Inc., 1961, p. 39.

176. Pankey, G. A. Acute bacterial endocarditis at University of Minnesota Hospitals, 1939–1959. Amer. Heart J., 64:583, 1962.

177. Wilson, L. M. Etiology of bacterial endocarditis: before and since introduction of antibiotics. Ann. Int. Med., 58:946, 1963.

178. Eger, W. Verruca endocarditis in cancer patient. Beitr. Path. Anat. Allg. Path., 105:219, 1941.

179. Tiffany, F. B., Stevenson, J. B., and Edwards, J. E. Pancreatic carcinoma and cardiovascular complications. Minnesota Med., 47:1501, 1964.

180. Rohner, R. F., Prior, J. T., and Sipple, J. Mucinous malignancies and terminal endocarditis with embolism: a syndrome. In press. Cancer, 1966.

181. Zeman, F. D., and S. Siegel. Acute bacterial endocarditis in the aged. Amer. Heart J., 29:597, 1945.

182. ——— Subacute bacterial endocarditis in the aged. Amer. Heart J., 29:661, 1945.

183. Lichtman, P., and Master, A. M. Incidence of valvular heart disease in people over fifty and penicillin prophylaxis of bacterial endocarditis. N.Y. J. Med., 49:1693, 1949.

184. Trout, E. F., Carter, J. B., Gumbiner, S. H., and Hench, R. H. Bacterial endocarditis in elderly: Report of 94 autopsied cases. Geriatrics, 4:205, 1949.

185. Anderson, H. J., and Staffurth, J. S. Subacute bacterial endocarditis in the elderly. Lancet, 2:1055, 1955.

186. Wallach, J. B., Glass, M., Lukash, L., and Angrist, A. Bacterial endocarditis in the aged. Ann. Intern. Med., 42:1206, 1955.

187. ——— Glass, M., Lukash, L., and Angrist, A. The distinctive nature of bacterial endocarditis in patients over 50. Geriatrics, 11:35, 1956.

188. Hartman, F. L., and Myers, W. K. Occurrence of bacterial endocarditis in older individuals. Geriatrics, 14:374, 1959.

189. Wedgwood, J. Bacterial endocarditis in old age. Geront. Clinica (Basel), Suppl., 3:11, 1961.

190. Dowling, H. F., Lepper, M., Caldwell, E. R., and Spies, H. W. Staphylococcic endocarditis: analysis of 25 cases treated with antibiotics, together with review of recent literature. Medicine, 31:155, 1952.

191. Fisher, A. M., Wagner, H. N., and Ross, K. S. Staphylococcal endocarditis, some clinical and therapeutic observations on thirty-eight cases. Arch. Intern. Med. (Chicago), 95:427, 1955.

192. Rantz, L. A., and Kirby, W. M. M. Enterococcal infections: An evaluation of the importance of fecal streptococci and related organisms in the causation of human disease. Arch. Intern. Med. (Chicago), 71:516, 1943.

193. Jones, M. Subacute bacterial endocarditis of non-streptococcal etiology. A review of the literature of the thirteen-year period 1936–1948 inclusive. Amer. Heart J., 40:106, 1950.

194. Koenig, M. G., and Kaye, D. Enterococcal endocarditis. Report of nineteen cases with long-term follow-up data. New Eng. J. Med., 264:257, 1961.

195. Cohen, R. A., Geraci, J. E., Dearing, W. H., and Needham, G. M. Salmonellosis: Observations on 94 patients. Mayo Clinic Proceeding, 39:401, 1964.

196. Jawetz, E., and Sonne, M. Penicillin-streptomycin treatment of enterococcal endocarditis: A re-evaluation. New Eng. J. Med., 274:710, 1966.

197. Lawes, F. A. E., Duvie, E. B., Goldsworthy, N. E., and Spies, H. G. Subacute bacterial endocarditis caused by erysipelothrix rhusiopathiae. M. J. Australia, 1:330, 1952.

198. Schiffman, W. L., and Black, A. Acute bacterial endocarditis caused by erysipelothrix rhusiopathiae. New Eng. J. Med., 255:1148, 1956.

199. Keith, T. A., and Lyon, S. D. *Hemophilus aphrophilus* endocarditis. Amer. J. Med., 34:535, 1963.

200. Hirsch, S. R., and Koch, M. L. Herellea (Bacterium anitratum) endocarditis. Report of a case. J.A.M.A., 187:148, 1964.
201. Witorsch, P., and Gorden, P. *Hemophilus aphrophilus* endocarditis. Report of three cases. Ann. Intern. Med., 60:957, 1964.
202. Procter, W. I. Subacute bacterial endocarditis due to erysipelothrix rhusiopathiae. Amer. J. Med., 38:820, 1965.
203. Zimmerman, L. E. Candida and aspergillus endocarditis. Arch. Path., 50:591, 1950.
204. Luke, J. L., Bolande, R. P., and Gross, S. Generalized aspergillosis and aspergillus endocarditis in infancy. Report of a case. Pediatrics, 31:115, 1963.
205. Kirschstein, R. L., and Sidransky, H. Mycotic endocarditis of the tricuspid valve due to *Aspergillus flavus*. Report of a case. Arch. Path., 62:103, 1956.
206. Grist, N. R. Rickettsial endocarditis. Brit. Med. J., 1:1540, June 8, 1963.
207. Derby, B. M., Coolidge, K., and Rogers, D. E. Histoplasma capsulatum endocarditis with major arterial embolism. Arch. Intern. Med. (Chicago), 110:63, 1962.
208. Palmer, R. I., Geraci, J. E., and Thomas, B. J. Histoplasma endocarditis: report on patient treated with amphotericin B, with review of amphotericin B therapy for histoplasmosis. Arch. Intern. Med. (Chicago), 110:359, 1962.
209. Haust, M. D., Wlodek, G. K., and Parker, J. O. Histoplasma endocarditis. Amer. J. Med., 32:460, 1962.
210. Ferguson, I. C., Craik, J. E., and Grist, N. R. Clinical, virological and pathological findings in a fatal case of Q-fever endocarditis. J. Clin. Path., 15:235, 1962.
211. Burch, G. E., and Depasquale, N. P. Viral endocarditis. (Editorial) Amer. Heart J., 67:721, 1964.

Addendum

The incidence of infectious endocarditis in the last decade has increased, as compared to the first 20 years of the postantibiotic era. The change in the spectrum of infectious endocarditis is attributed to an increase of cardiac surgery, the number of narcotic addicts, the appearance of antibiotic-resistant strains of organism, as well as the use of long periods of antibiotic therapy and of chemotherapy for malignant tumors. The increase in Staphylococcal endocarditis on normal heart valves is impressive (Buchbinder and Roberts series,[1] 53 percent of 45 cases of left-sided endocarditis; about 50 percent of Kaye's series [2]).

Recently Buchbinder and Roberts studied 14 habitual alcoholics with infectious endocarditis and found the causative organism was *Diplococcus pneumoniae* in 10 of these patients, though endocarditis caused by *D pneumoniae* all but disappeared soon after the antibiotic era.[3] In heroin addicts, Lessin and Siegel reemphasized the close association of renal disease and infectious endocarditis.[4]

Staphylococcal endocarditis has increased, particularly soon after prosthetic cardiac valve replacement, ie, less than 60 days postoperatively, and in heroin addicts. Kammer and Utz reported a case of Aspergillus endocarditis and reviewed the literature; all 39 Aspergillus endocarditis cases followed cardiac surgery and a characteristic finding was major arterial emboli.[5]

Endocarditis due to group *D. Streptococci* including nonenterococcal *Streptococcus bovis* was reported by Moellering et al.[6] They collected 14 cases of *Streptococcus bovis* and 15 of *Enterococci* from the Massachusetts General Hospital between 1964 and 1973 These patients were older or quite aged. *Streptococcus bovis* was predominant in the female, and no case of enterococcal endocarditis was noted in the childbearing age. Six cases due to *Streptococcus bovis* had a definitive history of dental manipulation, indicating that that old story still applies.

Infectious Endocarditis Related to Prosthetic Cardiac Valve Replacement

Sande et al studied the sustained bacteremia in cardiac surgery patients and found that the group of patients without proven endocarditis had bacteremia in the early postoperative period.[7] Bacteremias were mostly due to intravascular catheters, venous pacemakers, sternal wound infections, and pneumonia with gram-negative bacilli. On the other hand, the group of patients with proven endocarditis were due mostly to gram-positive cocci; *Staphylococci* accounted for two-thirds of cases. Although these strains of organisms are sensitive to the antibiotics used prophylactically, once valvular infection was established, eradication with antibiotics alone was more difficult. A second surgical intervention must be considered. They also suggested that when sustained bacteremia developed later in the postoperative period, gram-positive organisms (*Staphylococcus epidermidis, aureus,* or *diphtheroids*) have to be suspected.

Slaughter et al did retrospective studies on a total of 1,235 patients who had valve replacements from 1960 to 1972, and found bacterial endocarditis in 48 cases, or 3.9 percent.[8] The causative organisms were *Staphylococcus aureus,* 21 percent; *Staphylococcus epidermidis,* 25 percent (*Staphylococcus* 46 percent). *Streptococcus viridans* and *fecalis* had an incidence of 17 percent each, gram-negative bacilli occurred in 10 percent. Dismukes et al analyzed 38 cases of prosthetic valve endocarditis and found that early endocarditis was most commonly caused by *Staphylococci* (7 of 19 patients) and by *Streptococci* in the late stage of endocarditis.[9] They also analyzed the bacteriology of a reported series, revealing *Staphylococci* caused 38 of 65 cases of early endocarditis and 14 of 26 cases in late endocarditis. They also stressed that all patients with prosthetic valves who undergo any kind of manipulation likely to produce a transient bacteremia require adequate prophylaxis during and after the procedure. In prosthetic-valve endocarditis, additional surgical intervention has been stressed in selected patients by Black et al [10] and Okies et al.[11]

Infectious Endocarditis Associated with Drug Addicts

Staphylococci are common causative organisms in heroin addicts. Louria et al found this organism in 16 of 26 cases; [12] Cherubin et al collected 54 cases of infectious endocarditis in addicts and 148 cases in nonaddicts during 1960–67 in New York City [13] The causative organism in addicts was found to be different from that in nonaddicts. For instance, *S aureus* was found in 24 percent of nonaddicts and in 48 percent of addicts; *Candida* species and gram-negative bacilli were found in 10 percent and 24 percent respectively in heroin addicts, and were found in 0 and 4 percent in nonaddicts.

Menda and Gorback saw 23 cases of infectious endocarditis in heroin addicts (Cook County Hospital, Chicago) and found that *Staphylococcus* was the causative organism in 16 of them; solitary tricuspid valve involvement with *Staphylococcus aureus* was found in 11 patients.[14] This data is quite different compared to Cherubin's series, in which solely the tricuspid valve was involved in 7 of 52 cases, while 11 of 52 cases showed the tricuspid involved combined with other valves. Septic pulmonary emboli were common in narcotic addicts with infectious endocarditis. Roberts and Buchbinder studied 12 patients with right-sided infectious endocarditis.[15] Five were alcoholic, four were heroin addicts, two had blood dyscrasias, and one had congenital cardiac disease. In heroin addicts, particularly in chronic cases, the common pulmonary vascular granulomatosis has been stressed by Siegel recently.[16] This pulmonary alteration might be secondary to right-sided infectious endocarditis.

Experimental studies in A-V shunt cases with only a minute bit of vegetation at the attachment at the base demonstrate that it can be picked up only by careful observation of the valve. Very often only a granular or rough surface of the valve represents the site of dislodged fresh nonbacterial thrombotic endocarditis (NBTE). This can be confirmed by histologic section; emboli in the viscera from such sites are often evident. It should be reemphasized that the NBTE which became the site of bacterial contamination is not necessarily obvious on macroscopic examination. In many cases the site of contamination of bacteria is a tiny, flat vegetation consisting of a minute mixture of platelets and fibrin on the edematous surface of the valve. However, once the organisms seed on the surface of the vegetation, they may have a dot-like chalky appearance. The whole vegetation increases rapidly in size and adheres more firmly to the valvular surface. The phenomenon can be seen on studying very early stages of infectious endocarditis in the human and it has been demonstrated experimentally.[21] This is the reason that antibiotic therapy is most effective in the early stages of disease.

Rosen and Armstrong questioned why there was a high frequency of NBTE with adenocarcinoma of lung, while infectious endocarditis was seen more frequently in women with epidermoid carcinoma of the cervix.[22] This may be due to the difficulty in the eradication of the infectious nidus in the latter and the fact that those patients are prone to have a sustained septicemia. NBTE without a sustained bacteremia would not be expected to progress into infectious endocarditis. This also gives a proper explanation for the mode of development of right-sided NBTE to yield bacterial endocarditis by central venous pressure (CVP) catheter.

For cardiac surgery or parenteral feeding, indwelling CVP catheters have been used more frequently, as have intravenous pacemakers recently. These procedures have a potential risk of injury to the tricuspid valve or auricular endocardium, which causes the development of NBTE and right-sided infectious endocarditis when contaminated. Greene and Cummings found that all eight patients who had been treated with a CVP catheter during their final hospitalization had endocardial lesions.[23] Four of the eight patients had NBTE. They also found another four cases with endocarditis of tricuspid valve associated with CVP catheter. Two cases were infected with *Staphylococcus aureus* and two cases had only NBTE. The catheters in the two infected cases were used for parenteral feedings while in the other two cases with NBTE the catheters were used to monitor the CVP.[24] Becker et al also recorded three cases of right-sided endocarditis associated with CVP catheters.[25] In two infected cases the catheter was used for parenteral feeding and the one case with NBTE was used only for monitoring the CVP The incidence of NBTE and infectious endocarditis associated with CVP catheters showed a direct relationship to the duration that the catheter was in place and the chance of contamination. Experimental models based on the above include work by Garrison and Friedman,[26] Durak and Beeson,[27] and Jortner and Angrist.[28]

Endocarditis is an old problem with no real solution until control of blood coagulation and the problem of platelet agglutination are solved. Some light is dawning.

References

1. Buchbinder NA, Roberts WC: Left-sided valvular active infective endocarditis; a study of forty-five necropsy patients. Am J Med 53:20, 1972
2 Kaye D: Changes in the spectrum, diagnosis and management of bacterial and fungal endocarditis. Med Clin North Am 57:941, 1973
3. Buchbinder NA, Roberts WC: Alcoholism: an important but unemphasized factor predisposing to infective endocarditis. Arch Intern Med 132:689, 1973
4. Lessin BE, Siegel L: Endocarditis in drug addicts. JAMA 224:1650, 1973
5. Kammer RB, Utz JP: Aspergillus species endocarditis: the new face of a not so rare disease. Am J Med 56:506, 1974
6. Moellering RC Jr, Watson BK, Kunz LJ: Endocarditis due to group D streptococci: comparison of disease caused by streptococcus bovis with that produced by the enterococci. Am J Med 57:239, 1974
7. Sande MA, Johnson WD, Hook EW, Kaye D: Sustained bacteremia in patients with prosthetic cardiac valves. N Engl J Med 286:1067, 1972
8. Slaughter L, Morris JE, Starr A: Prosthetic valvular endocarditis: 12 year review. Circulation 47:1319, 1973
9. Dismukes WE, Karchmer AW, Buckley MJ, Austen WA, Swartz MN: Prosthetic valve endocarditis, analysis of 38 cases. Circulation 48:365, 1973
10. Black S, O'Rourke RA, Karliner JS: Role of surgery in the treatment of primary infective endocarditis. Am J Med 56:357, 1974
11. Okies JE, Bradshaw MW, Williams TW: Valve replacement in bacterial endocarditis. Chest 63:898, 1973
12 Louria DB, Heusle T, Rose J: The major complication of heroin addiction. Ann Intern Med 67:1, 1967
13. Cherubin CE, Baden M, Kavaler F, Lerner S, Cline W: Infective endocarditis in narcotic addicts. Ann Intern Med 69:1091, 1968
14. Menda KB, Gorback SL: Favorable experience with bacterial endocarditis in heroin addicts. Ann Intern Med 78:25, 1973
15. Roberts WC, Buchbinder NA: Right-sided valvular infective endocarditis: a clinical pathological study of twelve necropsy patients. Am J Med 53 7, 1972
16. Siegel H: Human pulmonary pathology associated with narcotic and other addictive drugs. Hum Pathol 3:55, 1972
17. Oka M, Belenky D, Brodie S, Angrist A: Studies of bacterial susceptibility of heart valves. Lab Invest 19:113 1968
18. Waller BF, Knapp WS Edwards JE: Marantic valvular vegetation. Circulation 48:644, 1973

19. Guinn GA, Ayala A, Liddicoat J: Clinical and therapeutic considerations in nonbacterial thrombotic endocarditis. Chest 64:26, 1973
20. Rosen P, Armstrong D: Nonbacterial thrombotic endocarditis in patients with malignant neoplastic diseases. Am J Med 54:23, 1973
21. Oka M, Angrist A: Histo-enzymatic studies of experimental bacterial endocarditis. J. Pathol Bact 93:637, 1967
22. Rosen P, Armstrong D: Infective endocarditis in patients treated for malignant neoplastic disease: a postmortem study. Am J Clin Pathol 59:241, 1973
23. Greene JF Jr, Cummings KC: Aseptic thrombotic endocardial vegetations: a complication of indwelling pulmonary artery catheters. JAMA 225:1525, 1973
24. Greene JF Jr, Cummings KC: Septic endocarditis and parenteral feeding. JAMA 225:315, 1973
25. Becker AE, Becker MJ, Martin FM, Edwards JE: Bland thrombosis and infections in relation to intracardiac catheter. Circulation 46:200, 1972
26. Garrison PK, Friedman LR: Experimental endocarditis in rabbits. Yale J Biol Med 42:394, 1970
27. Durak DT, Beeson PB: Experimental bacterial endocarditis. 3. Production and progress of the disease in rabbits. Br J Exp Pathol 54:142, 1973
28. Angrist N, Jortner BS: New model improves procedure for NBTE and Bacterial Endocarditis. Comparative Pathology Bulletin 4:1, February 1972

SHOCK

VINCENT J. McGOVERN

The conditions most frequently complicated by shock in general hospital practice are blood loss, myocardial infarction, and infections, particularly infections of a septicemic nature due to gram positive as well as gram negative organisms. Histologically the manifestations of shock are fibrin thrombi in small vessels, hemorrhages, and necrosis of tissues. Although any or all of these features of the shock syndrome may be present in an organ, there are certain patterns which are peculiar to each. Thus, the intestinal lesions are characterized by hemorrhage with fibrin thrombi in small vessels, the heart and liver lesions are chiefly necrotizing, while the lung lesions are dominated by hemorrhages. There is no fixed pattern of organ involvement but certain organs are more vulnerable to hypotensive injury than others, presumably by reason of pre-existent vascular insufficiency.

Fibrin Thrombi

The phenomenon of fibrin deposition in shock has received more attention than either of the other two manifestations.[1-4] Remmele and Harms[4] observed fibrin thrombi in 50 percent of subjects dying within 4 hours of the onset of shock, and in almost all between 24 hours and 48 hours. After 48 hours fibrin thrombi became increasingly difficult to find.

The actual mechanism of fibrin deposition in shock is unknown. It is found in all types of experimental shock[5-10] and is accompanied by alteration in coagulability due to fibrinogen and platelet depletion.[3,7,11-14] Experimentally, the formation of fibrin thrombi can be prevented either by heparin[7-9,15] or by blockade of the α-adrenergic receptor sites,[7,8,16-18] but neither prevents the development of shock though the prevention of fibrin thrombi may prolong life.

The fact that α-adrenergic blockade prevents fibrin deposition, including that arising in the shock produced by continuous catecholamine infusion,[7,8] points to stimulation of the α-adrenergic receptor sites rather than to liberation of thromboplastic substances as the initiating factor in intravascular fibrin deposition. Fibrin thrombi in small vessels such as in the renal glomeruli disappear within a week but those in veins may persist for several weeks depending upon their size.

Hemorrhages

The hemorrhagic lesions of the shock syndrome may be seen in most organs. They are commonest in the suprarenal gland and lungs, but they are most likely to cause death of the patient when they occur in the lungs. Their mechanism of production is probably the escape of blood through damaged vascular endothelium similar to that observed experimentally in the rabbit lung by McKay, Whitaker, and Cruse,[8] augmented in some cases by thrombocytopenia resulting from fibrin thrombus formation.

Necroses

Necrotizing lesions may be associated with fibrin thrombi but in many sites, particularly in the heart, liver, and renal tubules, they occur independently. Experimentally, an increase in plasma levels of catecholamines is found in all kinds of shock.[19-21] Though the rises are usually only temporary, this may well cause the necrotizing lesions through vasoconstriction.

Lesions identical with those of the shock syndrome may occur in the absence of hypotension when the blood supply to an organ has been incompletely or temporarily halted. Anoxia itself does not cause lesions of this type and one must therefore attribute the lesions of shock to the sudden reduction of blood flow.

TABLE 1. Disorders Complicated by Shock with Histologic Manifestations in 100 Consecutive Cases

Bleeding (peptic ulcers, oesophageal varices, ruptured aortic aneurysms)	24
Infections (gram-positive and gram-negative organisms)	19
Myocardial infarction	18
Cardiac operations	8
Miscellaneous cardiac conditions	7
Perforated viscus (peptic ulcers, colitis)	7
Pulmonary embolus	6
Acute pancreatitis	4
Miscellaneous	7
TOTAL	100

The histologic descriptions which follow are based upon experience in more than 13,000 autopsies performed at Royal Prince Alfred Hospital since 1950, reinforced by analysis of the findings in 100 consecutive autopsies in which there were morphologic alterations of organs and tissues due to the shock syndrome. The incidences of the primary disorders are recorded in Table 1 and the sites of organ involvement are recorded in Table 2. These do not include traumatic deaths, autopsies of which, except for donor subjects of organs for transplant, are all performed by the New South Wales State Department of Forensic Pathology.

Heart in Shock

The necrotizing lesions of shock occur in all parts of the heart including the conducting system.

TABLE 2. Sites of Shock Lesions at Autopsy in 100 Cases

Liver	47
Intestine	38
Heart	30
Kidney	
Tubular necrosis	23
Glomerular thrombi	4
Cortical necrosis	1
Suprarenal glands	17
Lung	16
Brain	14
Pancreas	6
Pituitary	2
Skin	2
Urinary bladder	1
Lymph nodes	1

They may take the form of infarction similar to that found in occlusion of a coronary artery, but more commonly there are disseminated focal lesions affecting portions of single fibres or groups of fibres. If death occurs within 24 hours, affected fibres or segments of fibres are found to stain more deeply eosinophilic than adjacent normal fibres, and normal striations within the affected zones can no longer be recognized. Nuclei fade after one day and necrotic cells without nuclei can usually be recognized by the second or third day.

Polymorphonuclear leucocytes make their appearances after about three days and invade the regions with necrotic fibres and also the surrounding zones in which the fibres, though damaged, are probably viable (Figs. 1 and 2). Mononuclear cells consisting of lymphocytes, plasma cells, and Anitschkow cells start

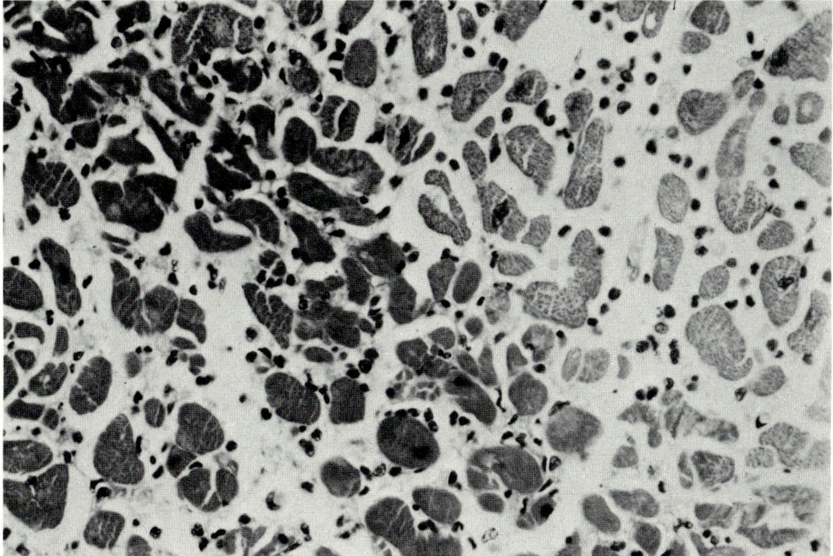

Fig. 1. Heart muscle from a 60-year-old male patient dying 9 days after perforation of duodenal ulcer. The depth of staining varies with the degree of damage to fibres. There are polymorphonuclear leucocytes and a few lymphocytes infiltrating the area. H&E. ×300.

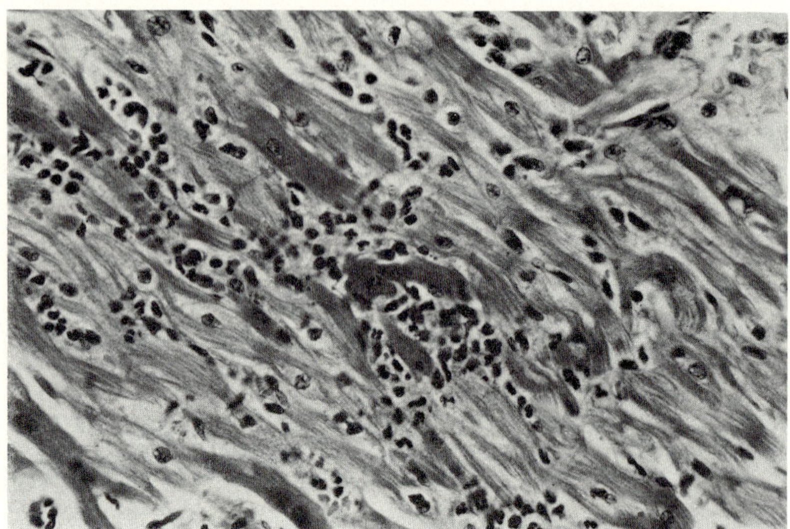

Fig. 2. Necrotic fibre surrounded by leucocytes in random section of left ventricle from a 62-year-old male patient with alcoholic cirrhosis who died 8 days after massive esophageal hemorrhage. H&E. ×320.

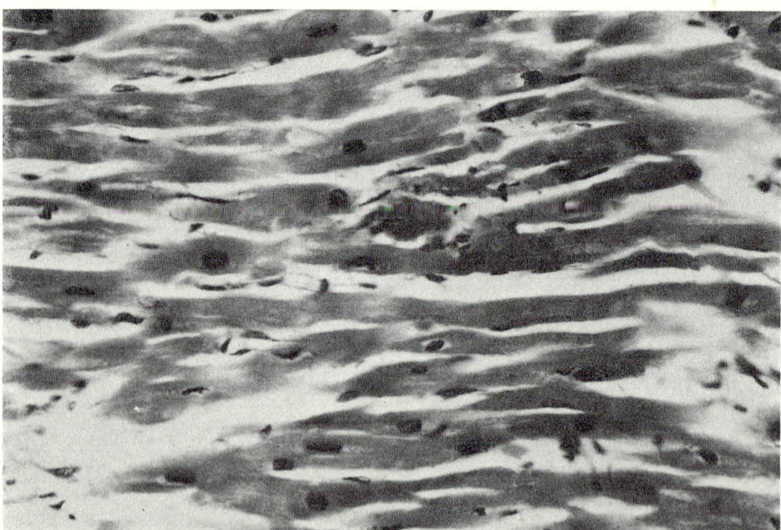

Fig. 3. A focus of necrosis in a random section of left ventricle from a 79-year-old female patient with ischemic disease of the gut. This lesion is about 11 days old. Leucocytes have disappeared from this lesion, though some are still present in other lesions. Necrotic segments of muscle are disintegrating. H&E. ×300.

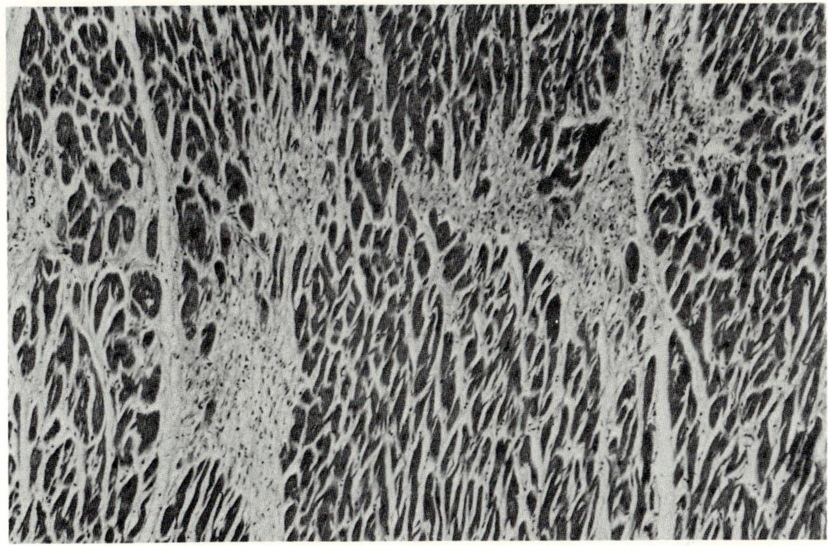

Fig. 4. Random section of heart from a 64-year-old male patient with generalized myopathy who had an attack of profound hypotension exactly 14 days prior to death. It shows foci from which muscle fibres have disappeared leaving only the reticulin framework and a sparse infiltrate of mononuclear cells. H&E. ×60.

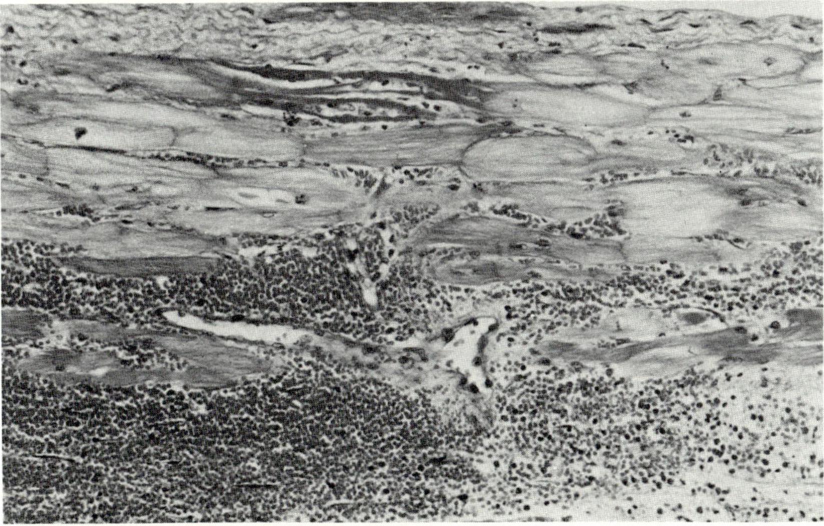

Fig. 5. Hemorrhage into conducting bundle of heart from a 45-year-old female patient who died 2 days after the onset of a coliform septicemia of renal origin. There is also segmental necrosis of a fibre. H&E. ×60.

to replace the polymorphs from about the fifth day. They are never very dense and by the end of two weeks have almost all disappeared. Sometimes the cell reaction consists of mononuclear cells from the beginning.

By the fourteenth day, necrotic muscle fibres in small lesions have disappeared leaving their reticulin framework and a light infiltrate of mononuclear cells amongst which are pigment-containing phagocytes (Figs. 3 and 4). Phagocytosis of necrotic fibres from large areas of necrosis, comparable to those resulting from coronary artery occlusion, take much longer.

Scattered focal lesions of the type described above are frequently found in the vicinity of recent ischemic infarcts of the heart due to coronary artery disease. They are also discoverable in apparently normal portions of heart at a distance from infarcted areas, presumably due to hypotensive episodes between the time of the original infarct and death.

In addition there are two other types of cardiac lesion in shock which are less commonly observed in human material but frequently occur in experimental shock.[18,22,23] The first of these consists of subendocardial hemorrhages with or without muscle fibre necrosis (Fig. 5). The second is a very striking lesion, consisting of transverse tigroid stripes or bands of deeply eosinophilic staining from which the normal fibrillary pattern has disappeared. In some cases the muscle fibre between these bands, particularly in the region of the intercalated discs, is disrupted and fragmented. These lesions have been produced experimentally in dogs with hemorrhagic shock[23] and they have also been observed in a soldier dying from exsanguination.[24] Though they are the least common myocardial lesion in shock in humans[25] they are almost invariably present in the heart of patients dying after open-heart surgery[25, 26] (Fig. 6). As in the experimental animals they are usually subendocardial. Martin et al.[24] postulate that they are due to supercontraction of myocytes at the intercalated discs, and because they were not preventable by hyperbaric oxygen, Ratliff, Hackel, and Mikrat[27] also postulate a mechanical cause. However, they can also be produced by occlusion of a coronary artery in the rat,[20] and one sees them from time to time in the hearts of patients dying suddenly from myocardial ischemia due to coronary artery disease.

Martin and Hackel[23] found that in experimental shock the histochemical reactions at the sites of the tigroid striations or contraction bands differed from those in the necrotizing lesions. They consider that fibres with contraction bands only should be able to recover but the histochemical reactions in the necrotizing lesions resemble those in myocardial infarction and are mainly irreversible.

In the series of 100 consecutive au'opsies at Royal Prince Alfred Hospital, Sydney, in which there were anatomical manifestations of the shock syndrome, cardiac lesions were present in 30 (45 percent) of the 67 noncardiac cases. Seven of these were sufficiently extensive to be classified as infarcts.

As would be expected, most of the cardiac lesions occurred in the elderly, only 7 of the 30 patients being under the age of 50 years. Although coronary atherosclerosis was the main factor predisposing to cardiac injury in shock, severe lesions also occurred in persons without vascular disease. One of these was a boy aged 13 years with leukemia who suffered an episode of shock due to septicemia, which resulted in frank myocardial infarction.

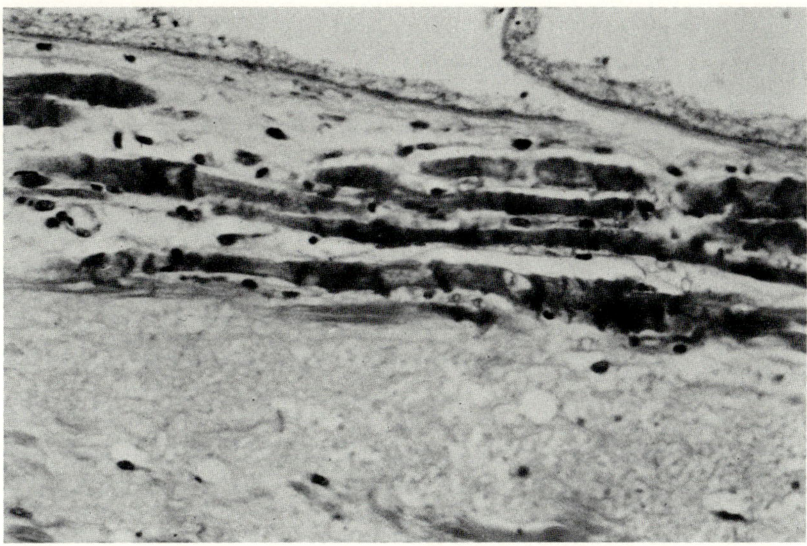

Fig. 6. Tigroid stripes in subendocardial fibres of patient dying 1 day after open-heart surgery. H&E. ×160.

The relationship between the myocardial lesions in shock and the "myocarditis" occurring after head injuries is not clear. Eichbaum[29] described lesions in the heart occurring with head injury which consisted of foci of edema, occasional hemorrhages, and collections of mononuclear cells. Plueckhahn[30] showed similar cardiac lesions in 6 of 15 adolescents dying as a result of head injury. Focal edema and collections of mononuclear cells were present in every instance in which the patient lived more than 6 hours. Plueckhahn and Cameron[31] in a later paper discussed the possibility that such lesions are hypoxic in nature. Agar[32] has shown that patients with head injury may develop arrhythmias accompanied by electrocardiographic tracings of anoxic type. However, until there have been more complete electrocardiographic and hemodynamic studies correlated with histologic appearances, the nature of the "traumatic myocarditis" must remain *sub judice.*

The cardiac lesions of shock are indistinguishable from ischemic lesions in coronary artery insufficiency and stain in a similar manner with the acid fuchsin method.[33]

Lungs in Shock

Patients who survive the acute phases of shock may succumb later to pulmonary complications which are characterized by congestion with hemorrhage into alveoli.[9,10,34] Edema is also present but this much less than one would expect for the degree of congestion, and in a proportion of cases hyaline membranes are present within alveoli. The sequence of events in 30 patients with shock due to soft tissue injury has been described by Blaisdell, Lim, and Stallone.[10] In the first 18 hours there were petechial hemorrhages, microthrombi, scattered foci of congestion and edema, and atelectases of the dependent portions of the lower and middle lobes. From 18 to 72 hours the congestion intensified and hemorrhagic consolidation of entire lobes developed. After 72 hours the cut surface of the lung resembled liver in consistency while microscopically hyaline membranes were found in addition to hemorrhages, and early bronchopneumonia had supervened.

Sixteen percent of the shock autopsies reviewed at Royal Prince Alfred Hospital had hemorrhagic consolidation of the lungs. In seven and probably in an eighth, shock was due to septicemia, in four it followed heart valve replacement, and in four it was due to hemorrhage from ruptured oesophageal varices. Hyaline membranes were present in three of the cardiac cases, and in one of meningococcemia; all of the patients had been treated with 100 percent oxygen.

The presence of microthrombi in the pulmonary vessels has been stressed,[1,10,34,35] but they are seldom recognizable by the time hemorrhages in the lung are well established, i.e., after the third day. Nevertheless, Blaisdell, Lim, and Stallone[10] think that the development of pulmonary hemorrhages depends upon the presence of intravascular thrombi.

In addition to fibrin thrombi there must be vascular factors to account for the congestion and hemorrhages that are so characteristic of the shock lung. On experimental grounds, Cook and Webb[36] came to the conclusion that congestion and hemorrhages are due to venous constriction. On the other hand, Veith et al.[37] concluded that arteriolar vasoconstriction is responsible.

The development of hyaline membranes is a controversial subject. Soloway, Castillo, and Martin[38] believe that oxygen therapy in the shocked patient may produce hyaline membrane changes by a direct toxic action of oxygen on alveolar walls. This is in accord with our experience also.

Apart from lesions directly due to shock, the lung is often indirectly affected by terminal bronchopneumonia and by congestion and edema due to cardiac failure.

Intestine in Shock

For want of a better term, the intestinal lesions found in hypotension have been given the name ischemic enterocolitis.[2,39] There may be involvement of any part of the gut from jejunum to rectum but the site of predilection is the splenic flexure region and descending colon. Even in an affected segment of the intestinal tract the lesions may be focal, appearing initially on the summits of the mucosal ridges.

In acute ischemic enterocolitis the gut lumen often contains blood, the mucosa may be shredded, and there may be ulcers of various shapes, both circumferential and longitudinal (Fig. 7). Histologically, the first lesion is the formation of fibrin thrombi in capillaries and venules of the mucosa and submucosa, almost always accompanied by hemorrhages. Necrosis of the mucosa supervenes and in severe cases extends to the muscularis propria; after a day or two polymorphonuclear leucocytes invade the affected areas (Fig. 8).

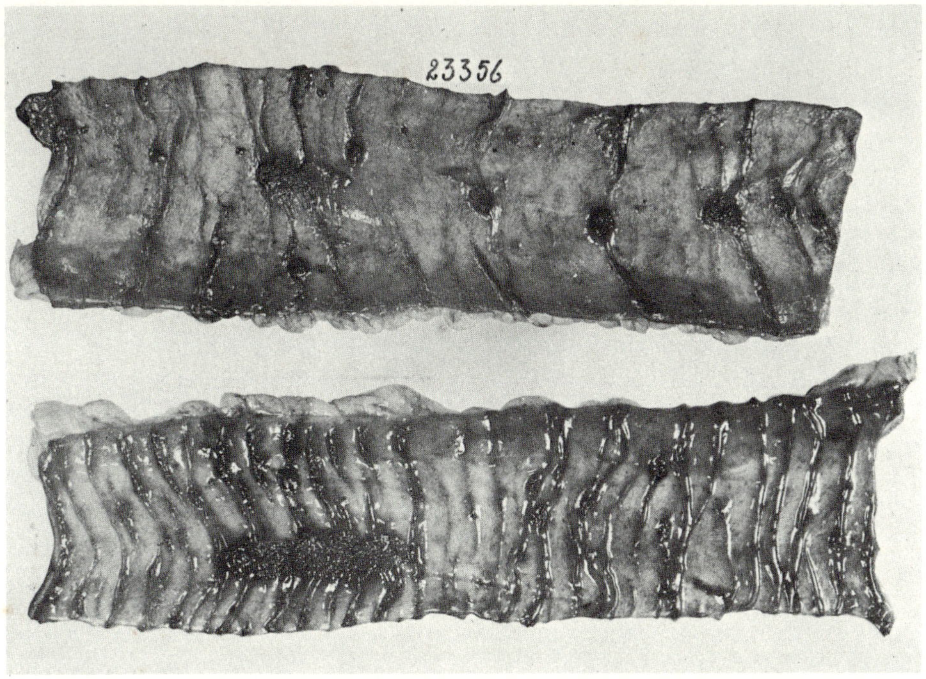

Fig. 7. "Ischemic" enteritis from a 34-year-old male patient with coliform septicemia complicating aplastic anemia.

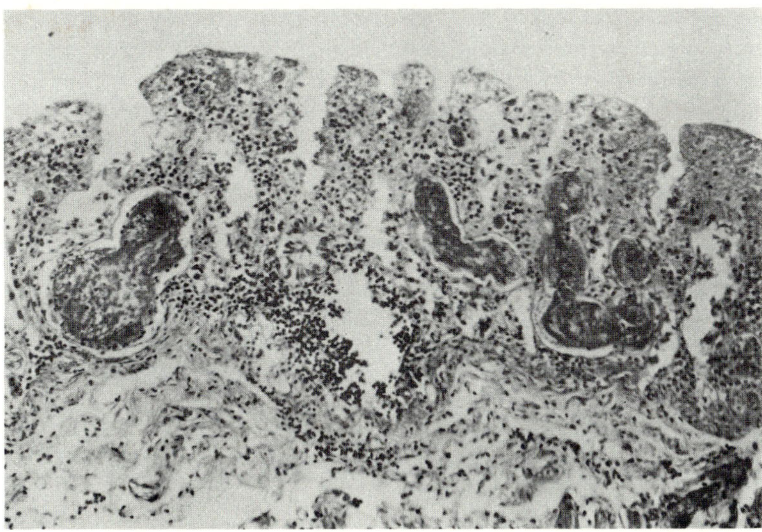

Fig. 8. "Ischemic" colitis from same subject as in Figure 3. Prominent thrombi adjacent to area of ulceration. H&E. ×120.

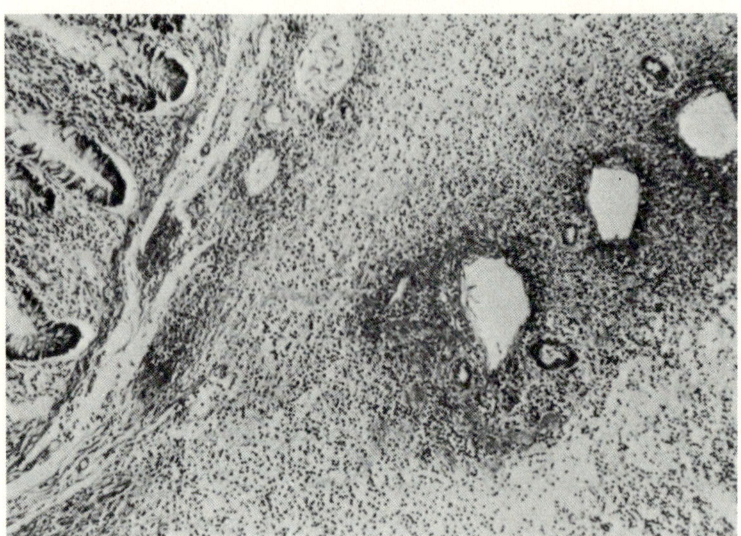

Fig. 9. Colon from a 44-year-old male patient with alcoholic cirrhosis who died 3 days after a massive esophageal hemorrhage. The walls of submucosal venules are impregnated with and surrounded by fibrin. Arterioles are unaffected. There is an extensive infiltrate of polymorphonuclear leucocytes around the affected vessels. H&E. ×100.

Occasionally the vascular lesions of ischemic enterocolitis take the form of edema, hemorrhages, and an angiitis. There may be no fibrin within the lumen of the affected vessels but the wall and adventitia are infiltrated by fibrin and later by polymorphonuclear leucocytes. These lesions are readily differentiated from polyarteritis or sensitivity angiitis by the fact that they occur exclusively in venules and veins; arterioles and arteries are unaffected (Fig. 9).

Benign strictures resulting from ischemic enterocolitis have been well documented by Marston et al.[40] They found that the splenic flexure-descending colon region was the zone most frequently affected. Here the arcade system of the middle colic and left colic arteries is often absent, thereby rendering the affected zone more susceptible to injury by reduction of the blood supply.[39] These lesions may be mistaken for Crohn's disease (granulomatous colitis) but apart from appreciation of the site of predilection, ischemic lesions can be differentiated on histologic grounds.[39] In the first three or four weeks organizing venous thrombi can still be found in the granulation tissue and a helpful feature pointed out by Marston et al.[40] is the presence of hemosiderin-containing phagocytes. Necrosis of the muscularis propria is another very helpful diagnostic feature. Furthermore, strictures of ischemic origin are much more densely cicatricial than strictures due to other causes.

Ischemic enterocolitis, which is so characteristic of the shock syndrome, may occur in the absence of hypotension from partial arterial occlusion due to embolus, thrombosis, volvulus, or incarceration of a loop of intestine in a hernial sac, providing that there is sufficient blood flow through the affected segment of gut to prevent frank infarction.[39] It has also been seen in cardiac failure without hypotension and is attributed to splanchnic vasoconstriction which occurs with the administration of digoxin.[41] Hemorrhagic lesions which were probably of this nature were seen by Szakács and Cannon[42] in patients with phaeochromocytoma. These authors produced similar lesions in dogs with norepinephrine infusions.

Liver in Shock

Zonal necroses of the liver are the most common histologic manifestation of shock encountered at autopsy, but they seldom enter into the clinical assessment of the patient, being overshadowed by the primary disorder or by the circulatory disturbances of shock.

That the necroses are significant is borne out by the fact that from time to time patients who have had an attack of hypotension, from which they have recovered, present with clinical features of liver disease. Biopsies have shown foci of centrilobular cell-fallout which can be dated back to this episode. Recognition of the nature of these foci enables a reassuring prognosis to be given because repopulation with restoration of normal architecture can be expected.

Even quite large necroses may be unrecognized clinically, but they should always be suspected when cirrhotic patients with gastrointestinal bleeding go into liver failure. At Royal Prince Alfred Hospital, 30 percent of cirrhotic patients who have died as a result of bleeding have had liver cell necrosis and in 10 percent it was severe enough to have caused hepatic failure (Fig. 10).

Histologically, zonal necroses occur towards the centres of lobules. They are seldom as symmetrical as the centrilobular degeneration of congestive cardiac failure, and only in severe cases is every lobule involved. After about two days, the affected zones are invaded by polymorphonuclear leucocytes. Remmele and Harms[4] found the hepatic sinusoids to be the most common site for the demon-

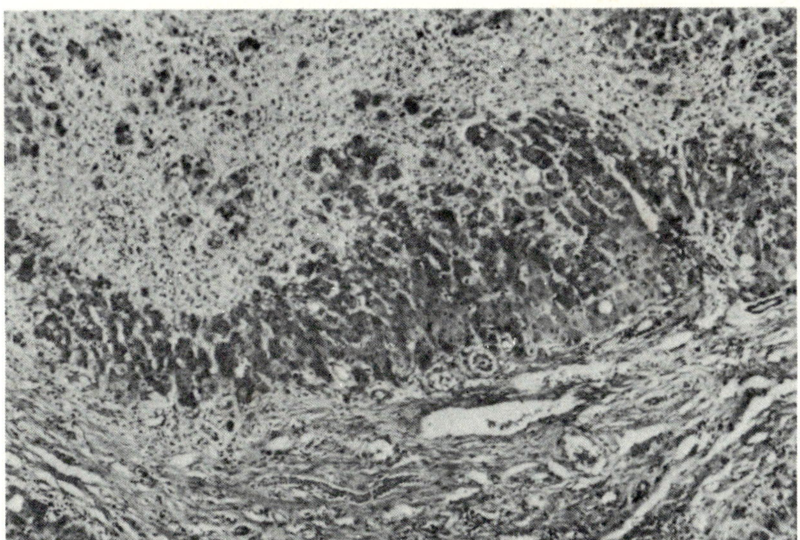

Fig. 10. Cirrhotic liver with extensive necrosis of parenchymal cells from 34-year-old female patient who died of liver failure of about 3 days duration after repeated hemorrhages from esophageal varices. H&E. ×80.

stration of fibrin thrombi in shock but they are seldom seen at this site unless death occurs within three days of the onset of shock.

The mechanism by which hepatic necroses are produced is not clear. Shoemaker, Szanto, and Anderson[43] made direct observations on the transilluminated livers of dogs and rats during hemorrhagic shock and noted that initially there were cellular aggregates in the sinusoids immediately adjacent to the hepatic venules and this was followed by congestion and engorgement. Serial biopsies revealed widening of sinusoids with compression of cell plates followed by necrosis in the centres of lobules.

This sequence of events suggests that the hemodynamic aspects of shock are more important in causing liver necrosis than anoxia and this view is strengthened by the experiments of Ratliff, Hackel, and Mikrat[27] who were not able to prevent hepatic necrosis in experimental shock by hyperbaric oxygen.

Kidney in Shock

Tubular Necrosis

Diminished urine excretion often to the point of anuria is a frequent complication of shock. In a few cases this is due to bilateral cortical necrosis, but the usual histologic change is tubular necrosis of varying extent. Because of this association there is a tendency to use the term "tubular necrosis" for the oliguria (or anuria) of shock. However, as Allen has pointed out, there is no correlation between the severity of the oliguria and the extent of tubular necrosis.[44] The pathogensis of anuria in shock is unknown and there are objections to every theory so far propounded.[45] A shunt mechanism along the lines described by Trueta et al.[46] seems the most likely explanation, accounting for both diminished urine excretion and ischemic necrosis of tubules.

The occurrence of renal tubular necrosis and anuria in the absence of shock has been described in head injury.[47] In these cases it was attributed to vasoconstrictor impulses of cerebral origin. The site of injury was the posterior and orbital regions of the frontal lobes, sites at which hypotensive injury is not uncommon.

A problem confronting the pathologist in a renal transplant team is the recognition of early tubular necrosis in a kidney obtained from a donor who has been shocked. The tubules may appear quite normal in a biopsy taken immediately after the kidney is removed, or during the cold perfusion period, but when a further biopsy is taken a few minutes after the recipient's circulation through the graft has been established, the cytoplasm of some tubular epithelial cells may already show the eosinophilic granulation of early necrosis.

Fibrin Thrombi

Fibrin thrombi occur less commonly in the kidney than tubular necrosis. The glomerular capillaries are the most frequently affected (Fig. 11), and with increasing severity, glomerular arterioles, venules, and even the arcuate veins may have thrombi. But in the absence of cortical necrosis, it is unusual for thrombi to be

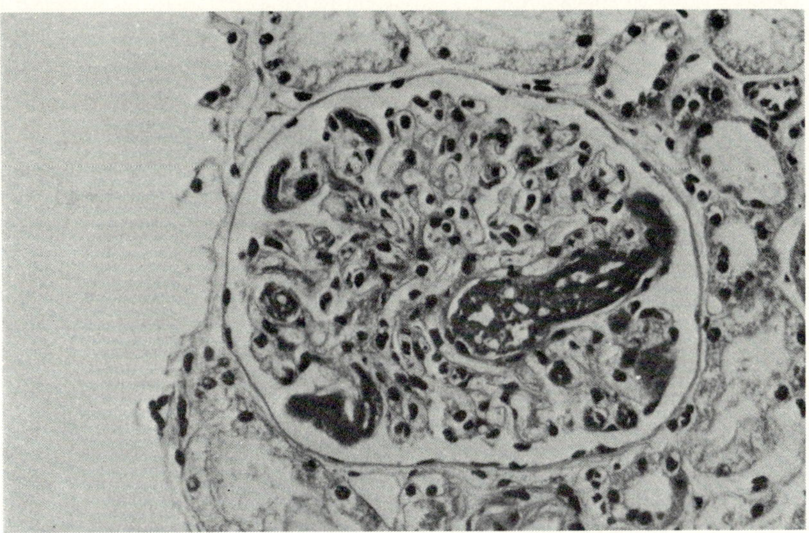

Fig. 11. Fibrin thrombi in glomerulus of 45-year-old male patient who died 24 hours after motor accident. H&E. ×300.

found in vessels other than arterioles, though free fibrin flakes may be seen within the lumen of any vessel. In the absence of cortical necrosis, fibrin thrombi in glomeruli can undergo lysis within a week, even when the biopsy shows almost every glomerulus to be involved. This phenomenon was observed in two recipients of kidney grafts from a donor dying in the shocked state.

Cortical Necrosis

Bilateral cortical necrosis is a very rare condition in which there may be infarct-like necrosis of almost the entire cortex including the columns of Bertini, sparing only a narrow subcapsular zone and the juxtamedullary portion; or there may be discontinuous foci of necrosis resembling a series of infarcts. Histologically it has the main features of the Shwartzman reaction, viz. necrosis, fibrin thrombi, and haemorrhages. The necrosis affects glomeruli, tubules, interstitial tissues, and vessels. The capillary tufts of the necrotic glomeruli are distended by red blood cells and hemorrhages may occur in and around them. Small collections of neutrophil leucocytes are found in necrotic glomerular capillaries and in some small arterioles. Fibrin thrombi are found in glomerular arterioles, veins, and venules. Arteries too, may have fibrin deposits but are seldom occluded. Surviving glomeruli adjacent to the necrotic zone often contain fibrin thrombi but at other times their capillaries are packed with red cells. Bilateral cortical necrosis due to shock is an extremely rare condition and at Royal Prince Alfred Hospital it has been seen once only in the last 13,000 autopsies. This was in a 55-year-old woman with a phaeochromocytoma in whom an episode of shock produced extensive fibrin deposition in the border zones of the brain and an infarct of the heart as well as bilateral renal cortical necrosis.

Because most of the early reports of symmetrical cortical necrosis were from obstetrical cases with abruptio placentae, it was often regarded as an obstetrical complication rather than as a manifestation of the shock syndrome. It is now known to occur in a great variety of conditions which include blood transfusion reactions, burns, gastrointestinal hemorrhage, head injury, and pulmonary infarction, to mention a few. Wells, Margolin, and Gall[48] reviewed the literature up to 1960 and presented 21 further cases of which only three were obstetrical. In 15 of the 18 cases in which the blood pressure was recorded there had been hypotension prior to the advent of anuria.

McKay, Jewett, and Reid[1] were among the first to note the occurrence of renal cortical necrosis in septicemic shock and to point out its resemblance to the Shwartzman reaction. In six patients with *E. coli* infections of the uterus, they found bilateral cortical necrosis of the kidney, in three together with a variety of other histologic manifestations of the shock syndrome including extensive intravascular fibrin deposition. Shock in these cases was attributed to coliform endotoxin. Cortical necrosis has also been recorded in shock due to gram positive organisms[49] and in shock occurring with cholera.[50]

Cortical necrosis identical with that of the shock syndrome has been observed on two occasions at Royal Prince Alfred Hospital in the absence of shock. In each case it occurred in grafted kidneys in which there was thrombosis of renal arteries with incomplete occlusion.

Suprarenal Gland in Shock

As noted by Greendyke,[51] there has in the past been a tendency to interpret suprarenal gland hemorrhage in terms of the disorders with which it has been associated. The best known of these is meningococcemia, in which the hemorrhage used to be regarded as peculiar to the meningococcus rather than as a component of the shock syndrome, which so often complicates septicemias of all types. In the presulfonamide and preantibiotic era, pneumococcal pneumonia was occasionally complicated by suprarenal hemorrhage.

Shock in the suprarenal gland manifests itself by hemorrhages, fibrin thrombi, and necroses.

The hemorrhages may be massive or there may be only congestion with focal extravasation of red blood cells. In the former, fibrin thrombi are always present either in the cortical sinusoids, in the central vein, or both. Smaller hemorrhages are associated with thrombi in about two-thirds of cases. These findings are similar to those of Greendyke[51] who found thrombosis of the central vein, either fresh or old, in more than 75 percent of adrenals with "idiopathic" hemorrhage. We have also observed central vein thrombosis in adrenals without hemorrhage though there was always prominent congestion.

Necroses occur in the cortical portion of the gland and may affect only small groups of cells, but at other times there is necrosis of almost the entire cortex (Fig. 12). Necroses are usually present when there are hemorrhages, but they also occur in the absence of hemorrhage and in half of these, fibrin thrombi are present also.

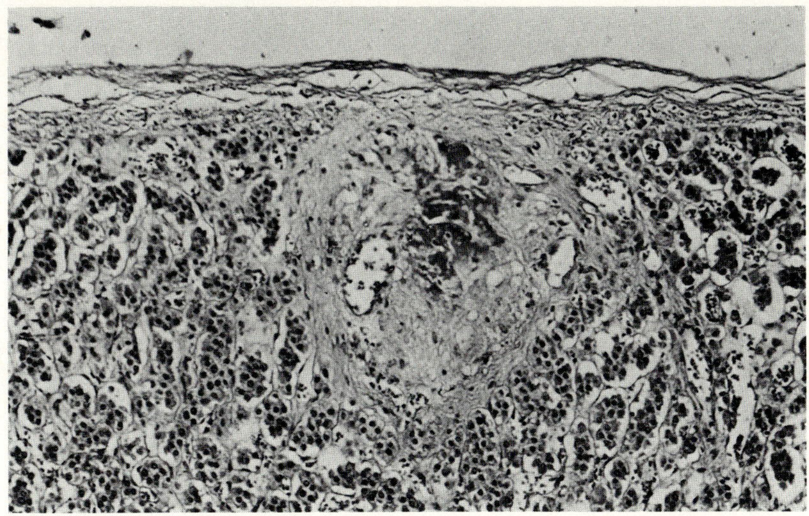

Fig. 12. Healing infarct in suprarenal cortex from same patient as in Figure 4. H&E. ×120.

Fibrin thrombi do not invariably accompany hemorrhages. Although it is likely that thrombi, especially of the central vessels, predispose to hemorrhage either mechanically or through associated thrombocytopenia, there must, in addition, be some vascular component to account for cases in which there are hemorrhages but no thrombi, and also necroses without either thrombi or hemorrhages.

Brain in Shock

The lesions of the brain caused by shock occur most frequently in the sites where the blood supply from the anterior cerebral arteries meets the blood supply from the middle cerebrals, where the middle cerebral blood supply meets that from the posterior cerebrals, and occasionally in the basal ganglia.[52,53]

In any one brain these lesions may be present in any or all of the susceptible sites, but they are found most constantly in the gray matter of the border zones between the anterior and middle cerebral arteries. These lesions are not specific for shock. They occur also when the cerebral circulation has been diminished through vascular disease or reduced cardiac output.[52,53]

In the fresh brain one usually sees a reddened hemorrhagic area in the gray matter, with or without softening. Sometimes it has the appearance of a pure hemorrhage and extends into the white matter (Figs. 13 and 14). Microscopically, the typical feature is that of fibrin thrombi in venules surrounded by a ring of hemorrhage. As in the gut, the vessels may appear necrotic and a light polymorphonuclear leucocytic infiltrate is common (Fig. 15). These lesions are seldom severe enough to cause dangerous elevations of intracranial pressure unless there is ex-

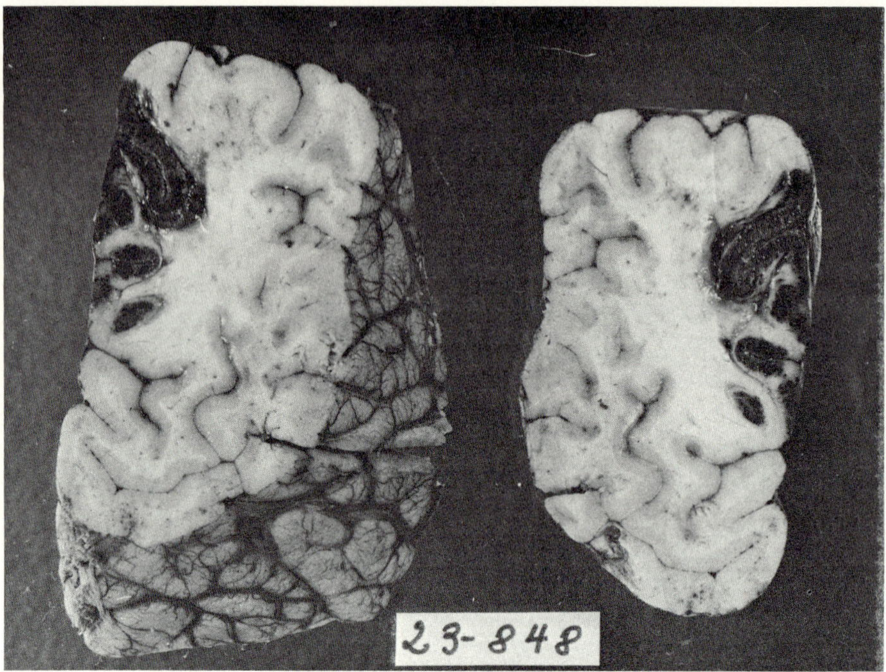

Fig. 13. Brain of 16-year-old male patient who died 20 days after a motor accident, illustrating a typical lesion in the border zone between the middle and posterior cerebral arteries.

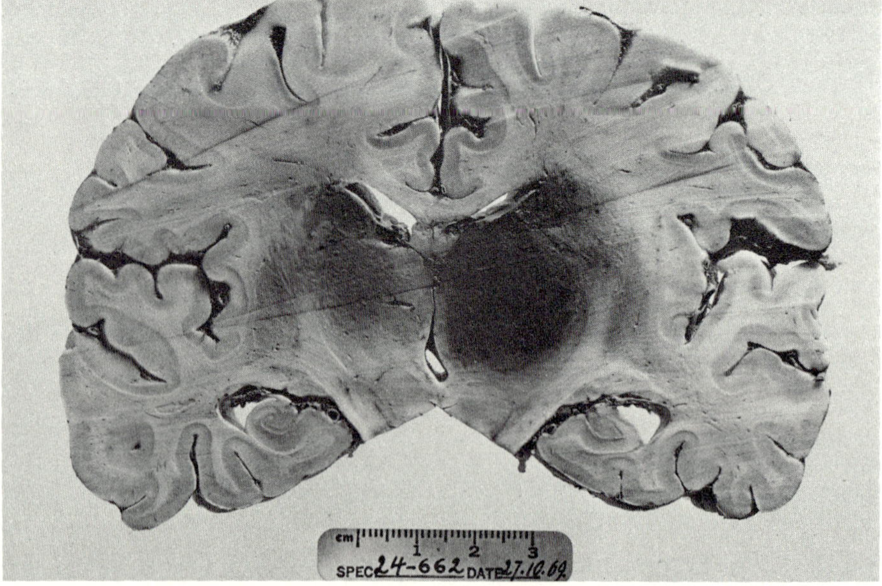

Fig. 14. Brain of a 50-year-old male patient who died 10 days after a pulmonary embolus illustrating basal ganglia lesions.

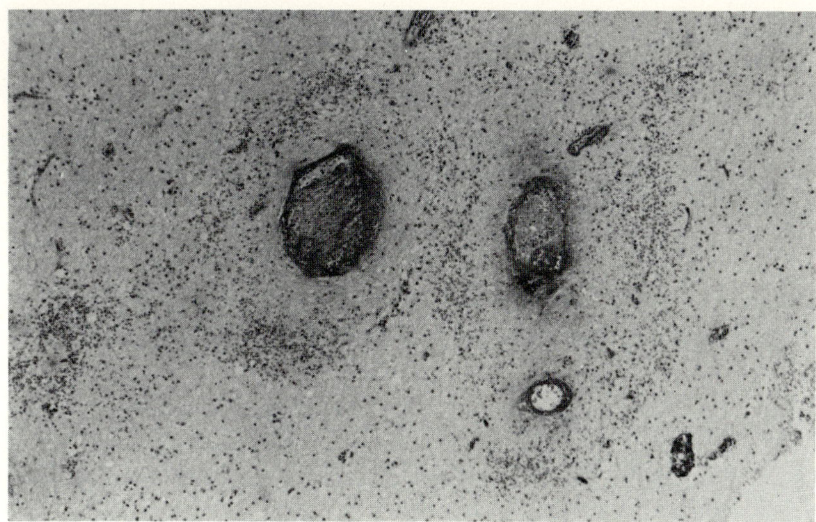

Fig. 15. Fibrin thrombi in vessels surrounded by ring hemorrhages from a less hemorrhagic zone in brain illustrated in Figure 14. H&E. ×48.

tension of thromboses to the superior sagittal and lateral sinuses. In patients with arterial disease, even a brief episode of syncope can cause lesions of this type.

Lesions of the brain identical with those of shock have been described in puerperal women by Martin and Sheehan[54] and by Carroll, Leak, and Lee.[55] In a few case reports, an episode suggestive of shock or hypotension has been recorded but in most, the symptoms are said to have appeared suddenly without warning. Blackwood et al.,[56] in *Greenfield's Neuropathology,* illustrate an example of superior sagittal sinus thrombosis and thrombophlebitis of cortical veins occurring in a puerperal patient with a breast abscess. These lesions are indistinguishable from those found in shock. Until there has been a study with adequate clinical correlation, the etiology and pathogenesis of cortical thrombophlebitis of puerperal women must remain in doubt.

Pancreas in Shock

As well as being a cause of shock, acute necrotizing pancreatitis is one of the complications of shock which can be the direct cause of death. There may be multiple foci of necrosis or there may be massive necrosis. Fibrin thrombi may be associated with some necrotizing lesions extending into normal tissues, but necrotic foci can occur independently of thrombi. Hemorrhages are mainly in lesions with fibrin thrombi.

Acute pancreatitis was encountered in 6 of the 100 autopsies analyzed for the purposes of this review. In each case it was sufficiently extensive to have contributed towards the death of the patient, but in a retrospective study it is not always possible to determine the order of seriousness of the various lesions discovered at autopsy.

Other Organs in Shock

Areas of necrosis in the anterior lobe of the pituitary sometimes associated with fibrin thrombi have been occasionally encountered. The exact incidence cannot be determined as most pituitary glands in Australia are reserved for growth hormone extraction.

Fibrin thrombi have been observed in the skin on two occasions, each time associated with purpura. One was in a patient who died from what was clinically puerperal septicemia and the other was in a patient with meningococcemia.

No organ seems to be immune and fibrin thrombi with hemorrhages and necrosis have been found even in the urinary bladder and lymph nodes.

Summary

The pathology of shock centers upon intravascular fibrin formation, hemorrhages, and necrosis of tissue. These changes can also occur in the absence of hypotension when the blood flow through an organ has been reduced. Anoxia alone without reduction of blood flow cannot produce these effects.

Clinically, intravascular fibrin deposition can be verified by demonstrating a fall in blood platelets. Measurement of the central venous pressure indicates whether the circulatory failure of shock is hypovolemic or due to cardiac damage.[57]

References

1. McKay, D. G., Jewett, J. F., and Reid, D. E. Endotoxin shock and the generalized Shwartzman reaction in pregnancy. Amer. J. Obstet. Gynec., 18:546, 1959.
2. McGovern, V. J., and Goulston S. J. M. Ischemic enterocolitis. Gut, 6:213, 1965.
3. Cafferata, H. T., Robinson, A. J., Aggeler, P. M., and Blaisdell, F. W. Intravascular coagulation in the surgical patient. Its significance and diagnosis. Amer. J. Surg., 118:281, 1969.
4. Remmele, W., and Harms, D. Zur pathologischen Anatomie des Kreislaufschocks beim Menschen. Klin. Wschr., 46:352, 1968.
5. McKay, D. G., Margaretten, W., and Csavossy, I. An electron microscope study of endotoxin shock in rhesus monkeys. Surg. Gynec. Obstet., 125:825, 1967.
6. Goodman, J. R., Lim, R. C. Jr., Blaisdell, F. W., Hall, M. D., and Thomas, A. N. Pulmonary microembolism in experimental shock. An electron microscopic study. Amer. J. Path., 52:391, 1968.
7. Whitaker, A. N., McKay, D. G., and Csavossy, I. Studies of catecholamine shock. I. Disseminated intravascular coagulation. Amer. J. Path., 56:153, 1969.
8. McKay, D. G., Whitaker, A. N., and Cruse, V. Studies of catecholamine shock. II. An experimental model of microangiopathic hemolysis. Amer. J. Path., 56:177, 1969.
9. Stallone, R. J., Herbst, H., Blaisdell, F. W., and Murray, J. F. Pulmonary changes following ischemia of the lower extremities and their treatment. Amer. Rev. Resp. Disease, 100:813, 1969.
10. Blaisdell, F. W., Lim, R. C., and Stallone, R. J. The mechanism of pulmonary damage following traumatic shock. Surg. Gynec. Obstet., 130:15, 1970.

11. Attar, S., Kirby, W. H., Jr., Masaitis, C., Mansberger, A. R., and Cowley, R. A. Coagulation changes in clinical shock. I. Effect of hemorrhagic shock on clotting time in humans. Ann. Surg., 164:34, 1966.

12. ———— Mansberger, A. R., Irani, B., Kirby, W. Jr., Masaitis, C., and Cowley, R. A. Effect of septic shock on clotting time and fibrinogen in humans. Ann. Surg., 164:41, 1966.

13. Corrigan, J. J., Ray, W. L., and May, N. Changes in blood coagulation system associated with septicemia. New Eng. J. Med., 279:851, 1968.

14. Timmons, R. C., Collins, J. A., Heistenkamp, C. A., Mills, D. E., Andren, R., and Phillips, L. L. Coagulation disorders in combat casualties. I. Acute changes after wounding. II. Effects of massive transfusion. III. Post-resuscitative changes. Ann. Surg., 169: 455, 1969.

15. Margaretten, W., McKay, D. G., and Phillips, L. L. The effect of heparin on endotoxin shock in the rat. Amer. J. Path., 51:61, 1967.

16. Lillehei, R. C., and MacLean, L. D. The intestinal factor in irreversible endotoxin shock. Ann. Surg., 148:515, 1958.

17. ———— and MacLean, L. D. The physiological approach to the successful treatment of irreversible endotoxin shock in the experimental animal. Arch. Surg., 78:464, 1959.

18. Brunson, J. G., Kalina, R. E., and Eckman, P. L. Studies on experimental shock. Effects of vasopressor amines and phenothiazin derivatives. Amer. J. Path., 35:1149, 1959.

19. Walker. W. F., Zileli, M. S., Reuther, F. W., Shoemaker, W. C.. Friend. D., and Moore, F. D. Adrenal medullary secretion in hemorrhagic shock. Amer. J. Physiol., 197:773, 1959.

20. Rosenberg, J. C., Lillehei, R. C., Longerbeam, J., and Zimmermann, B. Studies on hemorrhagic and endotoxin shock in relation to vasomotor changes and endogenous circulating epinephrine, norepinephrine and serotonin. Ann. Surg., 54:611, 1961.

21. Spink, W. N., Reddin, J., Zak, S. J., Peterson, M., Starzecki, B., and Seljeskog, E. Correlation of plasma catecholamine levels with hemodynamic changes in endotoxin shock. J. Clin. Invest., 45:78, 1966.

22. Hackel, D. B., and Goodale, W. T. Effects of hemorrhagic shock on the heart and circulation of intact dogs. Circulation, 11:628, 1955.

23. Martin, A. M., Jr., and Hackel, D. B. The myocardium of the dog in hemorrhagic shock. A histochemical study. Lab. Invest., 12:77, 1963.

24. ———— Green, W. I., Simmons, R. L., and Soloway, H. B. Human myocardial zonal lesions. Arch. Path., 87:339, 1969.

25. Reichenback, D. D., and Benditt, E. P. Myofibrillar degeneration. A response of the myocardial cell to injury. Arch. Path., 85:189, 1968.

26. Morales, A. R., Fine, G., and Taber, R. E. Cardiac surgery and myocardial necrosis. Arch. Path., 83:71, 1967.

27. Ratliff, N. B., Hackel, D. B., and Mikrat, E. The effect of hyperbaric oxygen on the myocardial lesions of hemorrhagic shock in dogs. Amer. J. Path., 51:341, 1967.

28. Pacey, N. F. Early changes in experimental myocardial infarction. *In* Reports of Scientific Meetings No. 2 The College of Pathologists of Australia (abstract), 1962, p. 31.

29. Eichbaum, F. W. Myokardveränderungen nach Schädeltraumen. Virchow. Arch. [Path. Anat.], 338:78, 1964.

30. Plueckhahn, V. D. Head injury in the adolescent: pathological factors complicating its early management. Med. J. Aust., 2:1185, 1966.

31. ———— and Cameron, J. M. Traumatic myocarditis or myocarditis in trauma. Med. Sci. Law, 8:177, 1968.

32. Agar, J. M. Head injury in the adolescent: medical complications in the early management. Med. J. Aust., 1182, 1966.

33. Lie, J. T. Detection of early myocardial infarction by the acid fuchsin staining technique. Amer. J. Clin. Path., 50:317, 1968.

34. Collins, J. A. The causes of progressive pulmonary insufficiency in surgical patients. J. Surg. Res., 9:685, 1969.

35. McLaughlin, J. S., Lee-Lacer, R., Attar, S., and Cowley, R. A. Pulmonary dysfunction in shock. Southern Med. J., 62:674, 1969.
36. Cook, W. A., and Webb, W. R. Pulmonary changes in hemorrhagic shock. Surgery, 64:85, 1968.
37. Veith, F. J., Hagstrom, J. W. C., Panossian, A., Nehlsen, S. L., and Wilson, J. W. Pulmonary microcirculatory response. Surgery, 64:95, 1968.
38. Soloway, H. B., Castillo, Y., and Martin, A. M. Adult hyaline membrane disease: Relationship with oxygen therapy. Ann. Surg., 168:937, 1969.
39. McGovern, V. J. The differential diagnosis of colitis. *In* Sommers, S. C., ed. Pathology Annual, 1969. New York, Appleton-Century-Crofts, 1969, p. 127.
40. Marston, A., Pheils, M. T., Thomas, M. L., and Morson, B. C. Ischemic colitis. Gut, 7:1, 1966.
41. Ferrer, M. L., Bradley, S. E., Wheeler, H. O., Enson, Y., Preisig, R., and Harvey, R. M. The effect of digoxin in the splanchnic circulation in ventricular failure. Circulation, 32:524, 1965.
42. Szakács, J. E., and Cannon, A. l-Norepinephrine myocarditis. Amer. J. Clin. Path., 30:425, 1958.
43. Shoemaker, W. C., Szanto, P. B., and Anderson, D. Hepatic hemodynamic and morphologic changes in shock. Arch. Path., 80:76, 1965.
44. Allen, A. C. The Kidney—Medical and Surgical Diseases, 2nd ed. New York, Grune & Stratton Inc., 1962.
45. Heptinstall, R. H. Pathology of the Kidney. Boston, Little, Brown and Company, 1966.
46. Trueta, J., Barclay, A. E., Daniel, P. M., Franklin, K. J., and Prichard, M. M. L. Studies of the Renal Circulation. Springfield, Ill., Charles C Thomas, Publisher, 1947.
47. Steinmetz, P. R., and Kiley, J. E. Renal tubular necrosis following lesions of the brain. Amer. J. Med., 29:268, 1960.
48. Wells, J. D., Margolin E. G., and Gall, E. A. Renal cortical necrosis. Clinical and pathologic features in twenty-one cases. Amer. J. Med., 29:257, 1960.
49. De Navasquez, S. Experimental symmetrical cortical necrosis of the kidneys produced by staphylococcus toxin: A study of the morbid anatomy and associated circulatory and biochemical changes. J. Path. Bact., 46:47, 1938.
50. De, S. N., Sengupta, K. P., and Chand, N. N. Renal changes including total cortical necrosis in cholera. Arch. Path., 57:505, 1954.
51. Greendyke, R. M. Adrenal hemorrhage. Amer. J. Clin. Path., 43:210, 1965.
52. Romanul, F. C. A., and Abramowicz, A. Changes in brain and pial vessels in arterial border zones. A study of 13 cases. Arch. Neurol., 11:40, 1964.
53. Torvik, A., and Jörgensen, L. Thrombotic and embolic occlusions of the carotid arteries in an autopsy series. J. Neurol. Sci., 3:410, 1966.
54. Martin, J. P., and Sheehan, H. L. Primary thrombosis of cerebral veins (following childbirth). Brit. Med. J., 1:349, 1941.
55. Carroll, J. D., Leak, D., and Lee, H. A. Cerebral thrombophlebitis in pregnancy and the puerperium. Quart. J. Med., 35:347, 1966.
56. Blackwood, W., McMenemy, W. H., Meyer, A., Norman, R. M., and Russell, D. S. Greenfield's Neuropathology, 2nd ed. London, Edward Arnold (Publishers) Ltd., 1963, pg. 97.
57. Chalmers, J. P. The management of septicaemia with shock. *In* Modern Medicine of Australia, Vol. 12, No. 15, 1969, pg. 19.

Addendum

The lesions of the shock syndrome seem to be the result of diminished perfusion and consequently are most likely to occur in organs already affected by arterial disease or by imperfect anastomoses. The heart is an important organ in the former category and the likelihood of scattered foci of necrosis in cardiogenic shock, remote from the primary infarct, has been emphasized by Page et al.[1] If the hypotension is sufficiently severe or prolonged, organs which ordinarily have quite adequate circulatory reserves also become affected.

Reduction in the blood flow through single organs, or part of an organ, as in intestinal volvulus or incarcerated hernia, may produce locally the fibrin thrombi, the hemorrhages, and the necroses which characterize the shock syndrome.

Lesions of the shock syndrome due to gram-negative septicemia have a different incidence from those occurring in cardiogenic or hemorrhagic shock. Any of the lesions of shock due to other causes may be found, but the most common and most serious lesions are those occurring in the lung.[2]

In a series of 92 autopsies in which there had been gram-negative septicemia, lesions of the shock syndrome were found in 49, and in 32 of these there were lung hemorrhages. These varied from multiple small foci up to large areas having the consistency of massive infarcts. The sequence of events in septicemic shock was similar to that found in shock from other causes. If the patient lived long enough, pneumonia inevitably supervened, and this was the most common cause of death. Hyaline membranes were found in three of the 32 cases, all of whom had had oxygen therapy. However, hyaline membranes have since been observed in the shock syndrome where oxygen had not been administered.

References

1. Page DL, Caulfield JB, Kastor JA, De Sanctis RW, Sanders CH: Myocardial changes associated with cardiogenic shock. N Engl J Med 285:133, 1971
2. McGovern VJ: The pathophysiology of gram-negative septicemia. Pathology 4:265, 1972

SARCOIDOSIS AND THE HEART

AZORIDES R. MORALES,
SAMUEL LEVY,
JOSEPH DAVIS,
AND GERALD FINE

Sarcoidosis is a granulomatous disease of unknown etiology that may affect almost every organ of the body. Although a variety of agents may produce "sarcoid-like" granulomas, the term sarcoidosis is usually applied to a disease process or syndrome characterized by the presence of noncaseating granulomas of undetermined etiology in involved organs. The possible relationship with tuberculosis has long been debated and the allergic or immunologic nature of the disease attracts many supporters.

Clinical manifestations of sarcoidosis may be purely constitutional (malaise, fever) or referrable to involved organs, but silent forms are as common, sometimes in the presence of extensive disease. Lymph nodes, lungs, liver, spleen, and eyes are the most frequent sites involved. Cardiac involvement is less common but when present may lead to a variety of serious cardiovascular manifestations often terminating in death.

Pathology of Cardiac Sarcoidosis

Gross Pathology

Cardiac enlargement with hypertrophy and ultimately failure of the right ventricle occur in a number of cases as a result of pulmonary sarcoidosis (cor pulmonale). Direct cardiac involvement may produce a gross appearance as variable as the disease itself. Although any cardiac structure may be affected the disease is usually myocardial, manifesting itself as microscopic foci or small, patchy, grey-

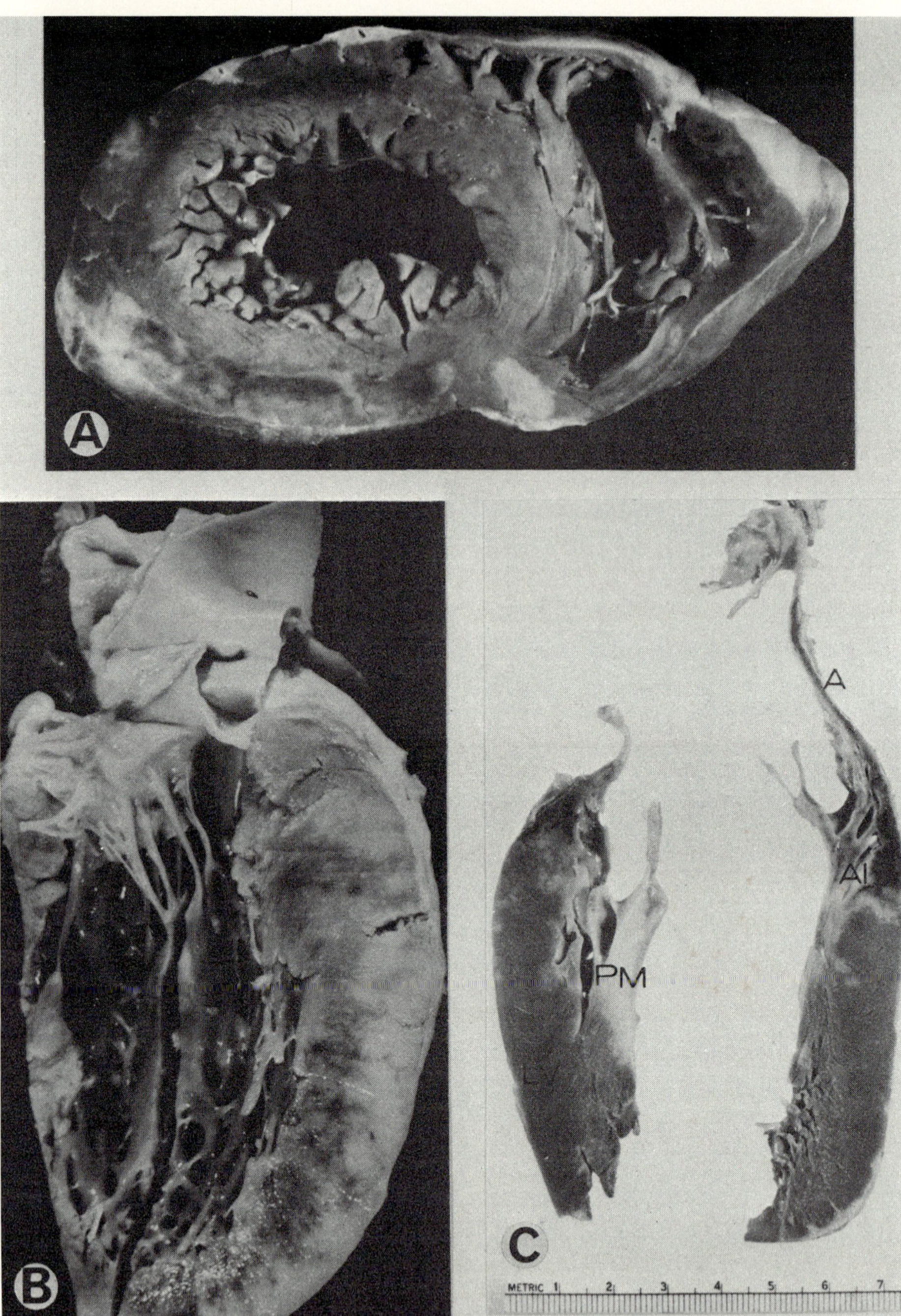

Fig. 1. Gross cardiac changes associated with sarcoidosis. A. Focal but also diffuse, irregular, dark brown, and grey-white areas of myocardial involvement. B. Extensive, diffuse, grey-white mottling reminiscent of a lymphomatous infiltrate. (Courtesy of Dr. Charles Garrett.) C. Left ventricular wall showing focal irregular areas of fibrous tissue replacing the myocardium of the posterior papillary muscle (PM) and left ventricle (LV), and extensive diffuse myocardial replacement resulting in aneurysm formation (A). Active inflammation adjacent to the aneurysm still persists (AI).

white areas diffusely distributed and not unlike scars of myocardial ischemia (Fig. 1A). However, their distribution does not correspond to that of the major coronary arteries. Confluence of cellular areas may resemble the gross appearance of a lymphomatous infiltrate (Fig. 1B) while extensive scar replacement of myocardium may lead to the formation of an aneurysm (Fig. 1C).

Microscopic Pathology

Sarcoid granulomas consist in conglomerates of mononuclear "epithelioid" cells surrounded by a peripheral zone of lymphocytes and a lesser number of plasma cells. Multinucleated giant cells, occasionally with asteroid bodies or calcific concretions, are often present. Special stains fail to demonstrate organisms and characteristically little or no necrosis is associated with the granulomas. Regressive

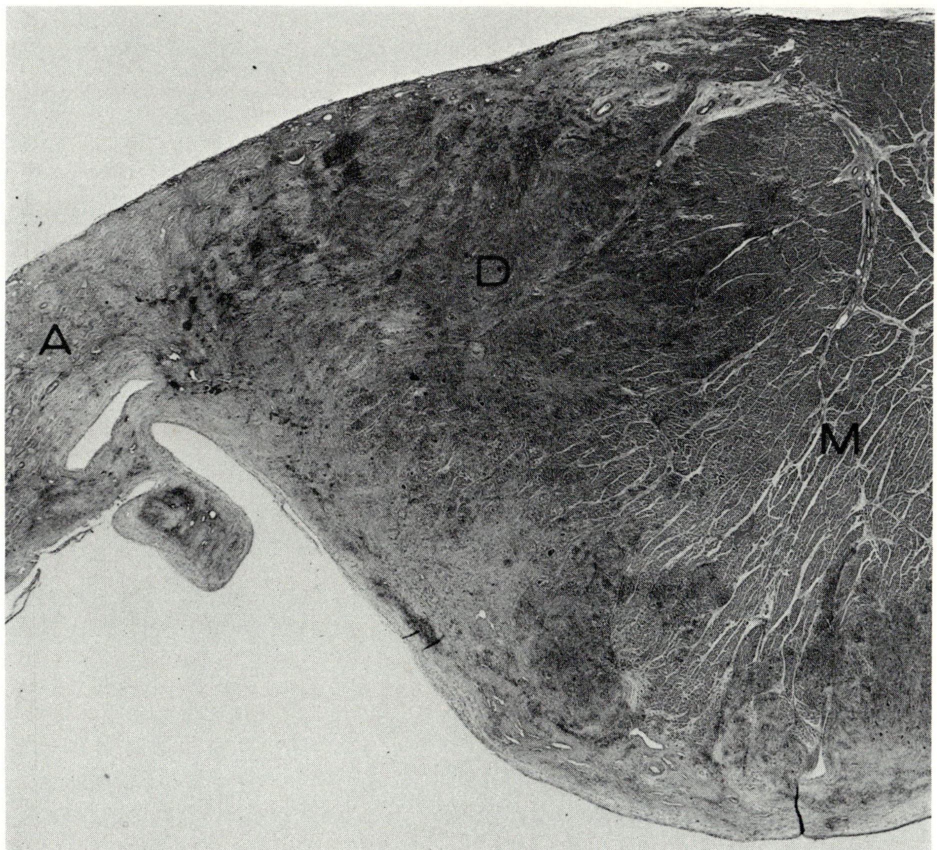

Fig. 2. Same case as Figure 1C. Left ventricular wall showing fibrous replacement of the myocardium in the aneurysm (A), advancing active disease (D), and uninvolved myocardium (M). Hematoxylin and eosin. × 9.

or older lesions are accompanied by a variable number of fibroblasts, inflammatory cell infiltrate, and fibrosis, which may be dense and hyalinized.

Any cardiac structure may be affected but the most constant and characteristic finding is isolated focal or confluent involvement of the interstitial tissue (Figs. 2 and 3) in the form of noncaseating granulomas, lymphocytic infiltration, cellular or hyalinized fibrous tissue, or a combination of the three. Less commonly involved than the interstitial tissue are the pericardium, endocardium, valves, and blood vessels. Valve dysfunction may be secondary to direct involvement or to inflammation of the papillary muscles.[1] Perivascular granulomatous inflammation of the major coronary arteries without involvement of their walls is in contrast to the active inflammatory or reparative process seen in the intramyocardial vessels, which results in disruption of their elastica and intimal proliferation (Fig. 6).

Involvement of the conduction system is of particular significance in view of

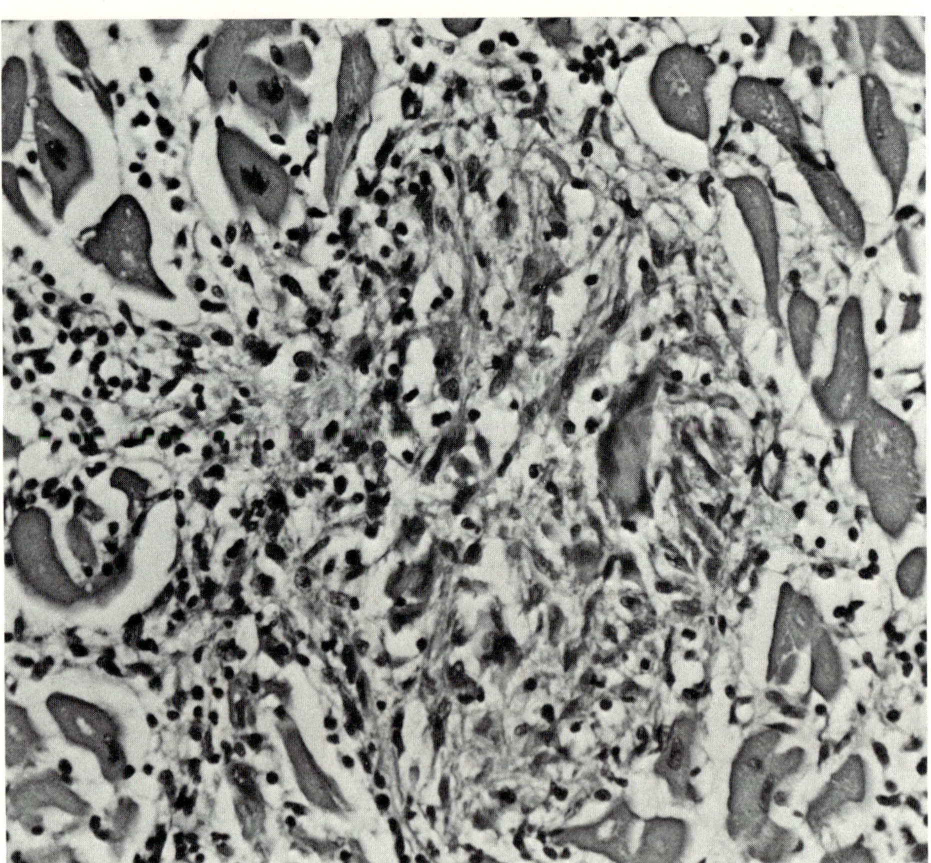

Fig. 3. Magnification of an area of D in Figure 2, illustrating the sarcoid granuloma-epithelioid cells, multinucleated giant cells, and surrounding lymphocytes, which are also present among the fragmented and separated myocardial fibers. Hematoxylin and eosin. × 420.

TABLE 1. Sarcoidosis of the Heart. Summary of Clinical Findings and Pathologic Lesions of the Cardiac Conduction System

Case	Age Race Sex	Clinical Course	ECG Findings	Conduction System					Observations
				SN	*AV*	*His*	*RBB*	*LBB*	
1. RA	32 BF	Recurrent episodes of ventricular tachycardia for four days.	Ventricular tachycardia and ventricular fibrillation	Fibrosis. Lymph. infilt. Artery: fragmentation of elastica and intimal fibrosis	Fibrosis. Lymph. infilt.	Fibrosis. Lymph. infilt.	Fibrosis. Lymph. infilt.	Fibrosis. Lymph. infilt.	
2. JB	41 BM	Three week history of fainting spells. Sudden death	Sinus bradycardia (two weeks prior to death)	Lymph. infilt.	Lymph. infilt.	Fibrosis. Lymph. infilt.	Fibrosis. Lymph. infilt.	Fibrosis. Lymph. infilt.	Ventricular aneurysm
3. BM	46 BF	One week history of "flu" chest pain and dyspnea. Sudden death		Granuloma. Lymph. infilt.	Not available	Granuloma. Lymph. infilt. Scar.	Granuloma. Lymph. infilt.	Granuloma. Lymph. infilt.	
4. KH	67 BF	One week history of congestive heart failure. Died after recurrent episodes of cardiac arrest	RBB and LAH supraventricular arrhythmias. Ventricular fibrillation	Fibrosis. Granuloma. Lymph. infilt.	Normal	Lymph. infilt.	Granuloma. Lymph. infilt.	Normal.	Granuloma in pericardial fat and sarcoid involvement of intramyocardial vessels

B, black; M, male; F, female.

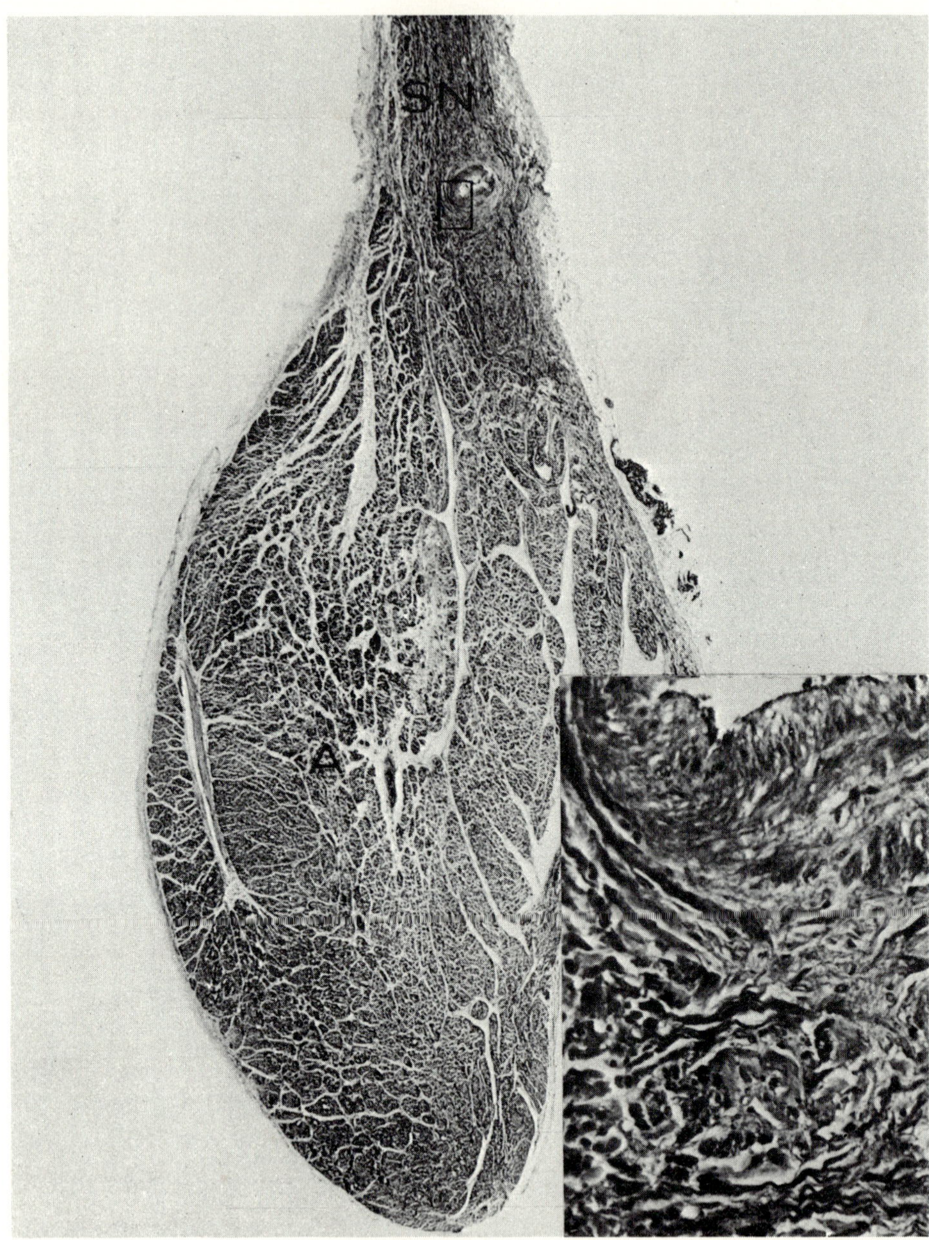

Fig. 4. Normal sinus node (SN) to compare with involved nodes of sarcoidosis (Figs. 5 to 9). The sinus node is located at the junction of the superior vena cava and right atrium (A). Note the central position of the artery within the nodal tissue. Insert: Magnification to illustrate the close relationship of the artery with the surrounding nodal fibers, which are lying in a dense fibrocollagenous framework. Masson trichrome stain. $\times$ 14; insert $\times$ 420.

its association with dysrhythmias and conduction disturbances. Table 1 summarizes the pertinent clinical and pathologic findings in the conduction systems of four patients studied within a one-year period (1971–1972) at Jackson Memorial Hospital in Miami, Florida. Except for case 3 in which no tissue from the atrioventricular node was available for study, the entire conduction system was serially sectioned according to previously reported procedures.[2, 3]

The lesions present in the pathway of conduction system fibers were not unlike those found in the working myocardium, and some or all of the major components of this specialized tissue of the heart (sinus node, atrioventricular node, bundle of His, and bundle branches) were involved by sarcoidosis, although their histology and extent of involvement varied considerably.

In case 1 (Table 1) the sinus node and adjacent myocardium were replaced by dense fibrous tissue (Fig. 5) containing a sparse lymphocytic infiltrate. The sinus node artery, characteristically located in the midst of the nodal substance (Fig. 4), showed marked intimal fibrosis and fragmentation of its elastica (Fig. 6), suggesting healing arteritis. Nerves in the sinus nodal area were also involved by the inflammatory and fibroblastic process (Fig. 7) which extended to the pericardium and endocardium.

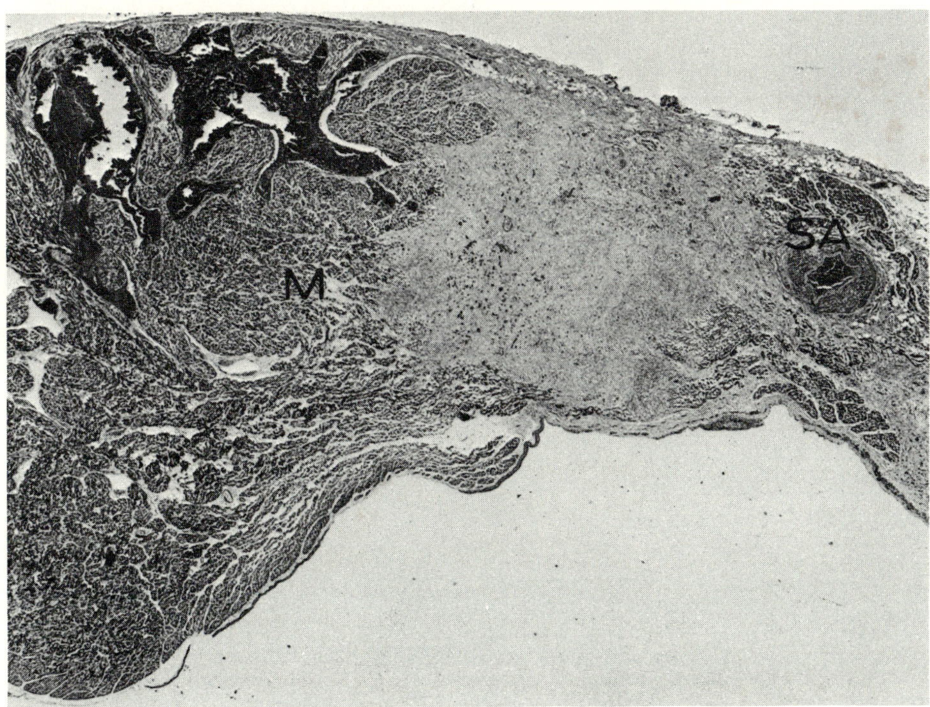

Fig. 5. Sinoatrial node area in Case 1 (Table 1) to illustrate extensive fibrous and inflammatory replacement of fibers of the sinus node and working myocardium (M). SA, sinus node artery. Masson trichrome stain. × 14.

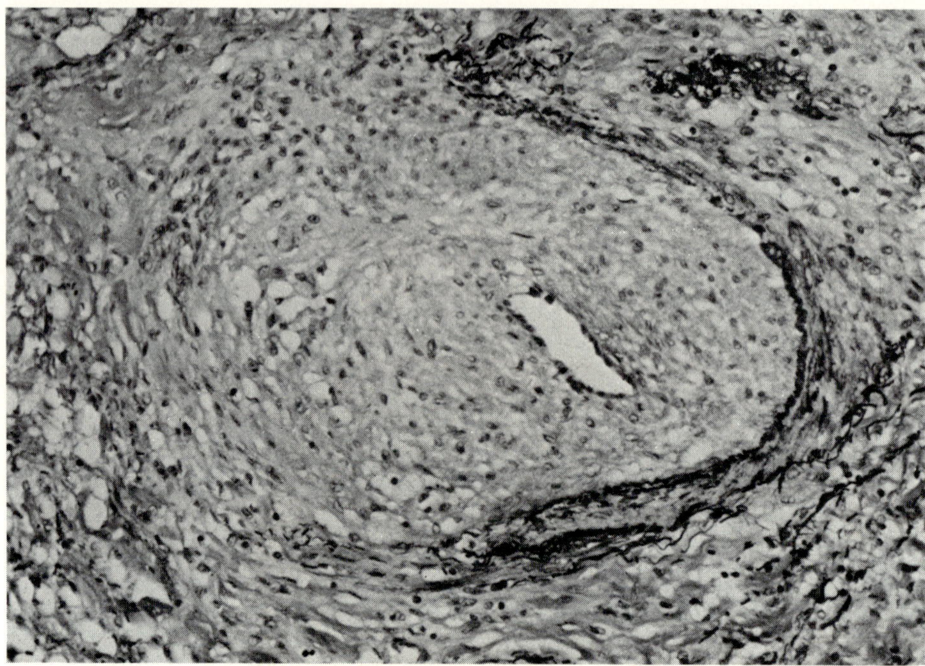

Fig. 6. Alteration of sinus node artery (SA, Fig. 5) by fibroblastic proliferation of intima producing stenosis of the lumen and fragmentation of the internal elastic lamina of the artery. Verhoeff-van Gieson stain. × 210.

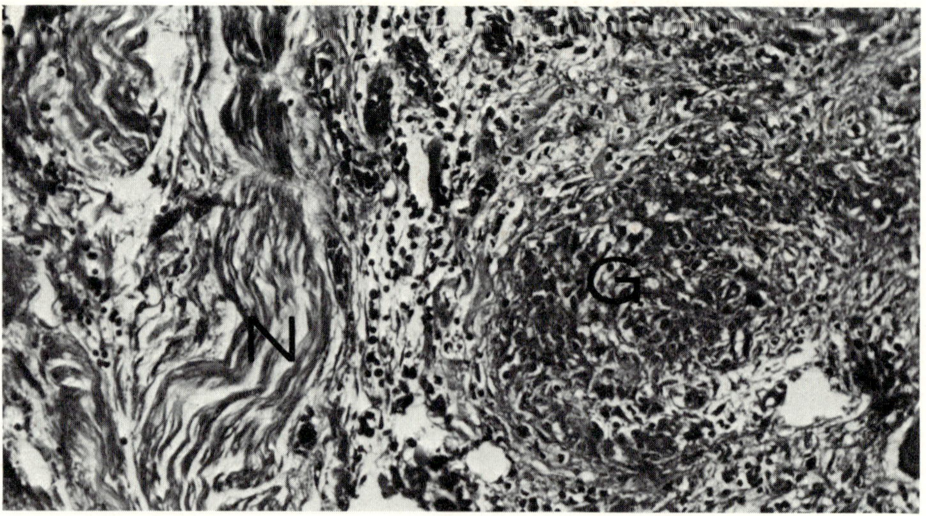

Fig. 7. Sarcoid granuloma (G) with extensive lymphocytic infiltrate adjacent to a nerve (N) in the immediate vicinity of the sinus node. Hematoxylin and eosin. × 210.

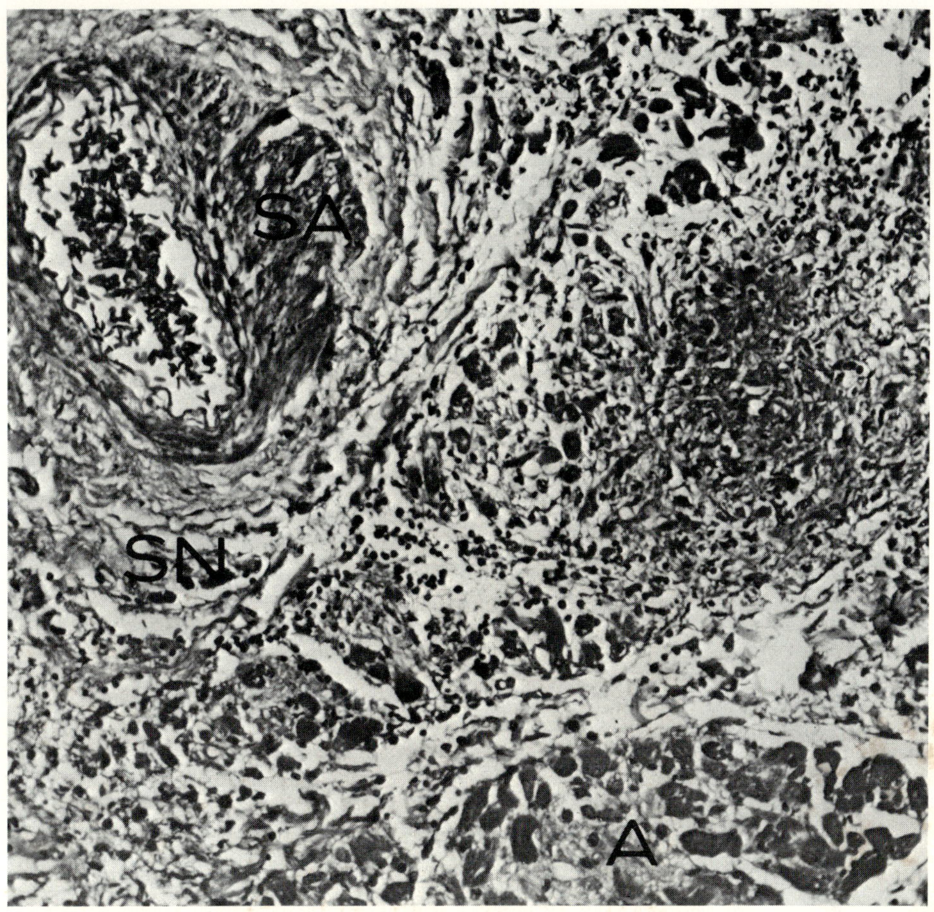

Fig. 8. Sarcoid granuloma in the midst of sinus node tissue adjacent to the sinus node artery (SA). SN, normal nodal fibers; A, right atrial working myocardium. Hematoxylin and eosin. × 210.

In the other cases only portions of the sinus node were partially involved by either granulomas or lymphocytic infiltrate (Fig. 8). In three cases the atrioventricular node (Fig. 9), and its approaches were available for study and showed fibrosis of the most posterior portion of the node in one instance (Fig. 10), diffuse lymphocytic infiltration in another (Fig. 11), and no lesions in case 4 (Table 1). The bundle of His (Fig. 12) was altered in all four cases. Patchy lymphocytic infiltration and fibrosis were evident in two cases and complete replacement in portions of its trajectory by either fibrosis or conglomerate granulomas (Fig. 13) was found in the remaining two cases. Except for case 4 in which no lesions were found in the left bundle branch, portions of both bundle branches were partially replaced in some portions of their trajectories by either granulomas, fibrosis, or lymphocytic infiltrate (Figs. 14 and 15).

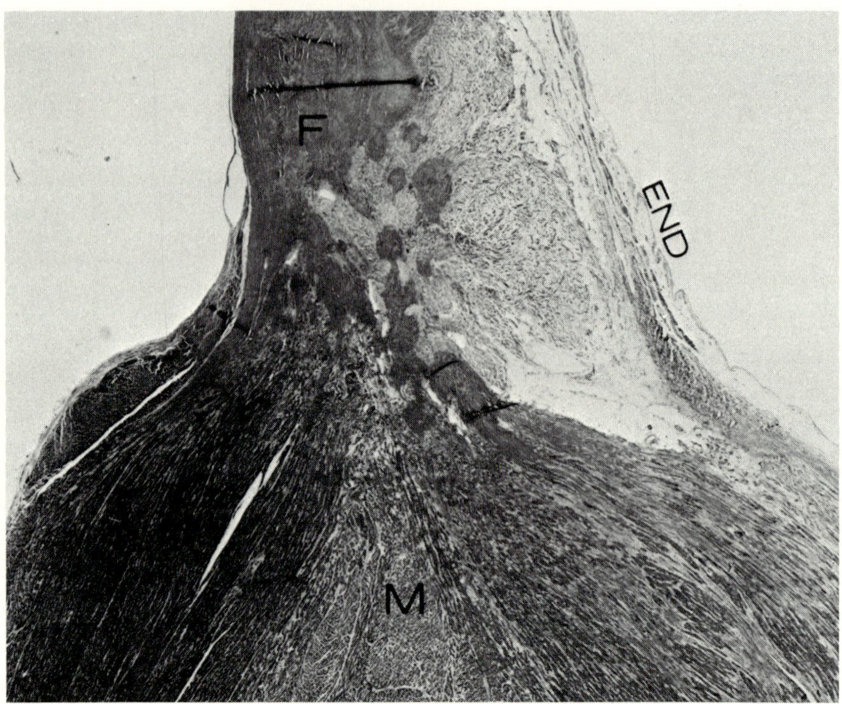

Fig. 9. Normal atrioventricular node for comparison with Figures 10 and 11 of cardiac sarcoidosis. The node with its interweaving fibers lies adjacent to the annulus fibrosus (F), beneath the right atrial endocardium (END). M, ventricular septal myocardium. Masson trichrome stain. × 15.

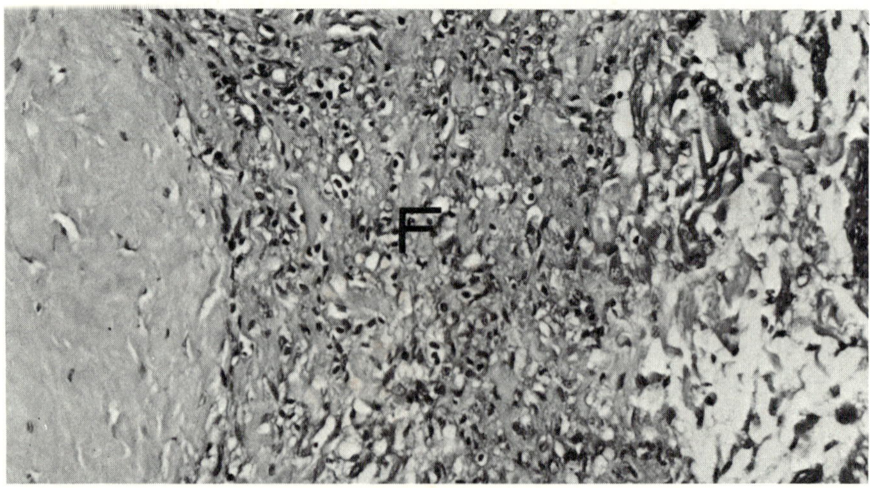

Fig. 10. Fibrous replacement (F) of the most posterior portion of the AV node in a case of sarcoidosis. Hematoxylin and eosin. × 210.

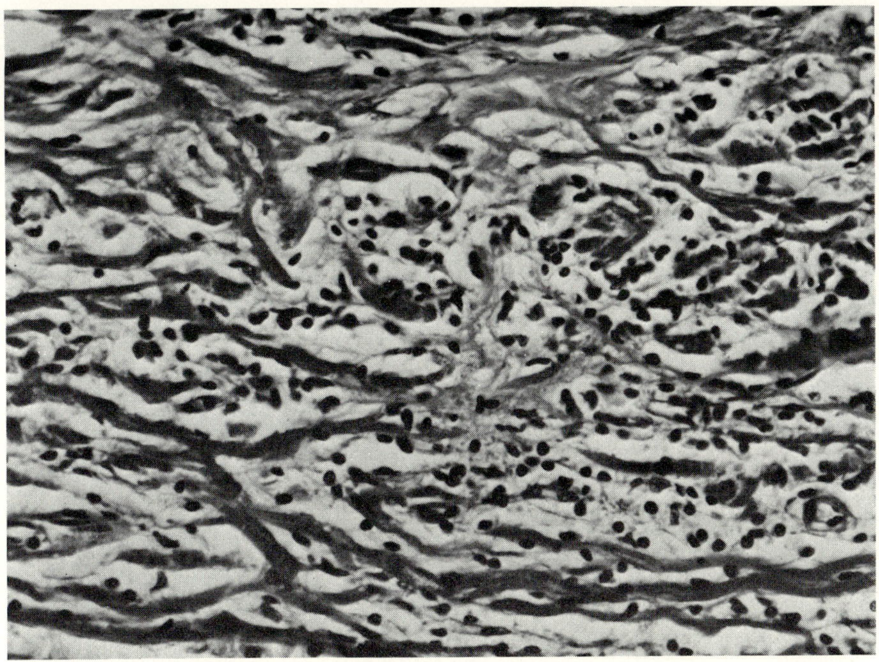

Fig. 11. Atrioventricular node illustrating diffuse interstitial infiltration by lymphocytes. Hematoxylin and eosin. × 420.

Clinical Significance and Pathophysiology of Cardiac Sarcoidosis

Sarcoidosis is not an uncommon disease, affecting mainly women in the third and fourth decades of life. Although autopsy cases from the world literature do not show a racial predominance, in the United States there is a larger incidence in the black population. Cardiac sarcoidosis is part of the systemic disease and no instance of isolated cardiac involvement was found in the literature. Its incidence is difficult to assess and has varied from 0.7 to 20 percent respectively among clinical [1] and autopsy studies.[4] Such a disproportion in incidence may be indicative of the seriousness of cardiac sarcoidosis or the difficulty in detecting antemortem cardiac involvement.

Including the four cases described in the present review, the world literature contains 118 autopsied cases of cardiac sarcoidosis [5] in patients ranging from 18 to 83 years. Men have been affected more frequently than women (57 to 43 percent). Among the 109 cases with racial information, 44 patients were white, 43 black, and 22 Japanese. The almost equal distribution among Caucasoids and Negroids is a reflection of the reports from European countries and does not denote the incidence in the United States, where in some locales sarcoidosis is 11 times more common among blacks than among whites.[6]

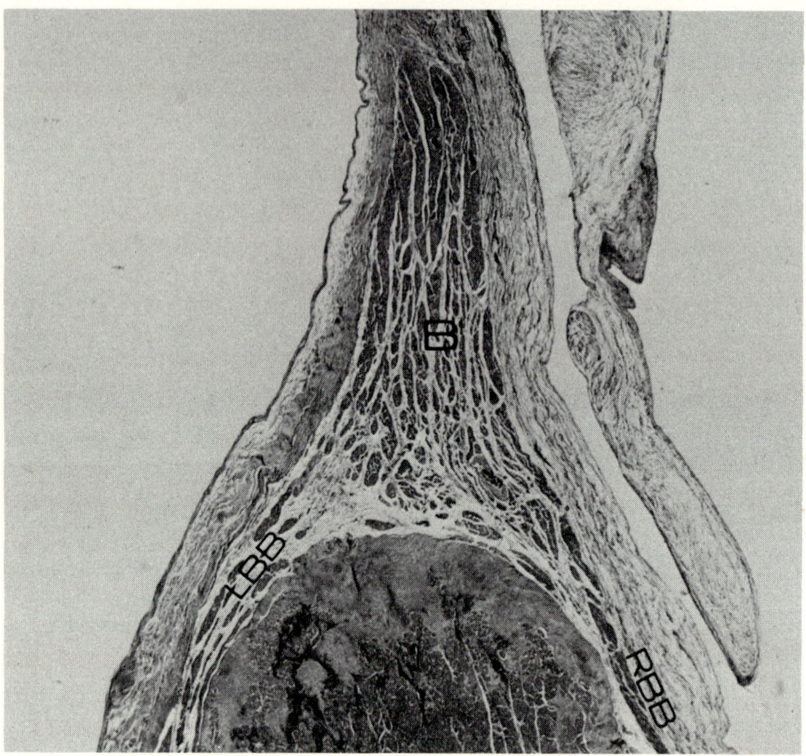

Fig. 12. Normal bundle of His (B) giving off the right (RBB) and left bundle branches (LBB). Hematoxylin and eosin. × 27.

Cardiac sarcoidosis may be manifested by sudden death, conduction disturbances, arrhythmias, aneurysm of the heart, myocardial failure, and electrocardiographic patterns mimicking myocardial infarction. Medical attention may be sought because of dyspnea, palpitations, chest pain, congestive heart failure, or syncope. Sudden death is a constant threat to those afflicted with cardiac sarcoidosis and was observed in 52 (44 percent) of the 118 autopsied cases.[5] Arrhythmia and conduction disturbances were demonstrated in a number of these patients but in 19 cases (16 percent) sudden death was the sole manifestation of the disease.

Arrhythmias and conduction disturbances are by far the most common manifestations of cardiac sarcoidosis. Electrocardiographic findings in 87 autopsied cases[5] showed that 43 patients (50 percent) had some type of cardiac conduction abnormality and 39 patients (42 percent) demonstrated either atrial or ventricular arrhythmias. A pattern similar to myocardial infarction was present in six patients and in only nine cases (10 percent) was the electrocardiogram normal. The single most common conduction disturbance was complete heart block, which was present in 25 of the 87 cases (29 percent). It was persistent in the majority of cases but in three patients it was transient and recurrent. The incidence of arrhythmias and conduction disturbances would even be larger if the cases of sudden death

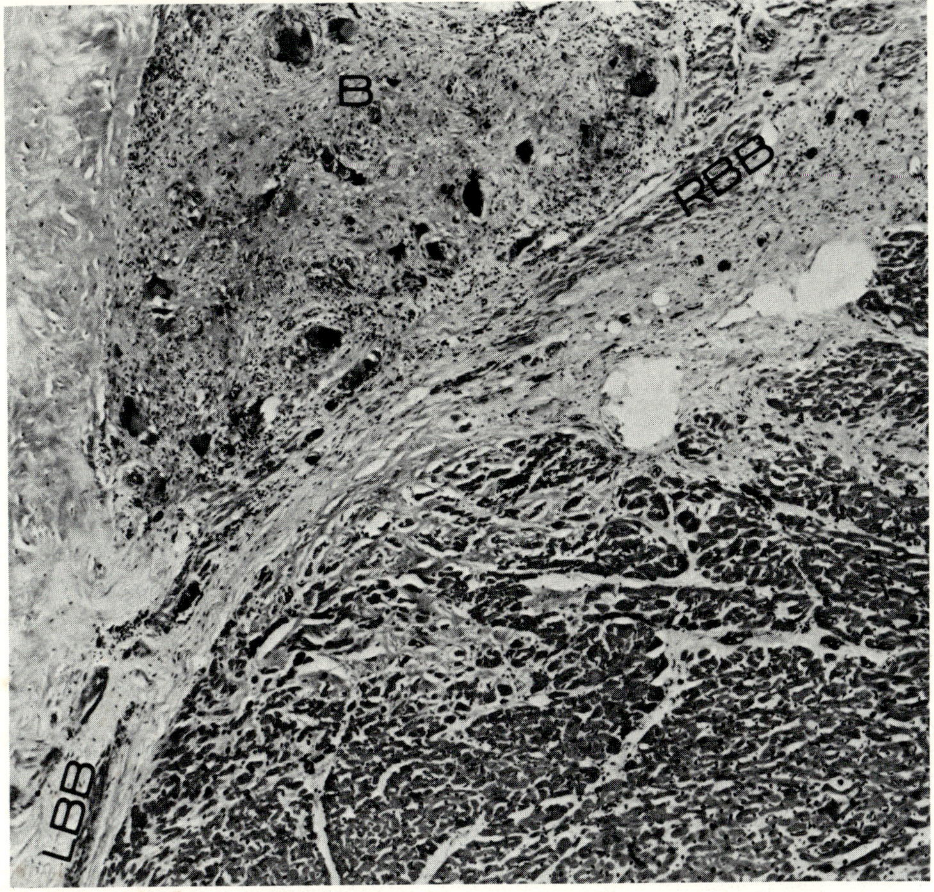

Fig. 13. Sarcoidosis involving the bundle of His at a level similar to the one in Figure 12. The bundle (B) is replaced by a conglomerate of sarcoid granulomas with associated fibrosis. Portions of the left (LBB) and right bundle branches (RBB) are seen adjacent to the granulomas. Hematoxylin and eosin. × 70.

without previous manifestations of the disease were also included, since it is logical to assume that death resulted primarily from involvement of the conduction system.

Despite the frequency of sudden death, arrhythmias, and conduction disturbances associated with cardiac sarcoidosis, detailed histologic study of the conduction system of the heart has not been previously undertaken and only brief reference to the specialized tissue of the heart is present in a limited number of reports (Table 2).[4, 7-14] The sinoatrial node was only mentioned in the studies of Gozo et al [13] and Duvernoy and Garcia,[12] and one cannot evaluate the thoroughness of the examination of the conduction system in the remaining reports in Table 2. The absence of pathologic lesions of this specialized tissue reported by Duvernoy and Garcia in a patient with Stokes-Adams syndrome may be due to inadequate sam-

TABLE 2. Sarcoidosis Involving the Cardiac Conduction System. Reported Cases With Histologic Study of the Specialized Tissue of the Heart

	Age Sex Race	Electrocardiogram	Symptoms Described	Conduction System	Comments
Simkins[7]	50 F?	Complete heart block	Adams-Stokes syndrome, 15 years. Dyspnea, parotitis	Involvement of area of atrioventricular bundle	
Peacock et al[4]	27 FW	Complete heart block	Adams-Stokes syndrome, 6 weeks	Bundle of His replaced by granulomas. AV node negative	
Botti and Young[8]	32 FW	Complete heart block	Adams-Stokes syndrome, 6 months. Signs of aortic stenosis	AV node and bundle destroyed by granulomatous inflammation	Myocardial sarcoidosis confined to AV node, bundle, and a solitary epicardial granuloma. Gross and histologic evidence of rheumatic valvulitis
Porter[9]	19 MW	Complete heart block	Adams-Stokes syndrome. Bilateral uveitis	Bundle of His replaced by fibrous tissue with giant cells	
Phinney[10]	51 FW	Complete heart block	Adams-Stokes syndrome, 3 weeks	Bundle of His replaced by granuloma	Myocardial disease grossly and microscopically, confined to the upper portion of the ventricular septum
Smith[11]	54 FW	Complete heart block alternating with paroxysmal ventricular tachycardia	Dyspnea, chest pain	Ventricular septum including area of AV node involved by sarcoidosis	IVS from base of the heart to apex replaced by the disease. An additional focal involvement in left atrium. No evidence of disease in other areas of the heart.
Duvernoy and Garcia[12]	30 FB	Premature ventricular contractions. Ventricular tachycardia	Dyspnea. Transient Adams-Stokes episodes	No involvement of the sinus node or conduction system	
Gozo et al[13]	27 FB	2 degree AV block, Wenckeback type	Congestive heart failure, pericardial effusion	Areas of sinus and AV nodes extensively involved. No nodal architecture was identified	Hemorrhagic pericardial effusion. Diffuse infiltration of atrial and ventricular walls by sarcoidosis
Ghosh et al[14]	50 F?	Atrial premature contractions	Iridocyclites, progressive dyspnea	Hyaline scars in the atrioventricular node	

W, white; B, black; M, male; F, female

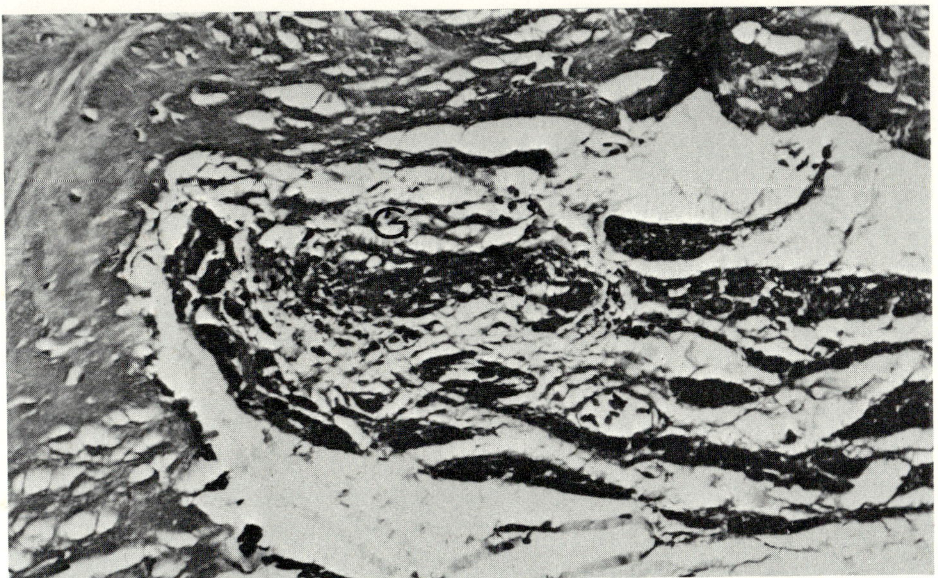

Fig. 14. Sarcoid granuloma (G) at the origin of the right bundle branch. Hematoxylin and eosin. $\times$ 210.

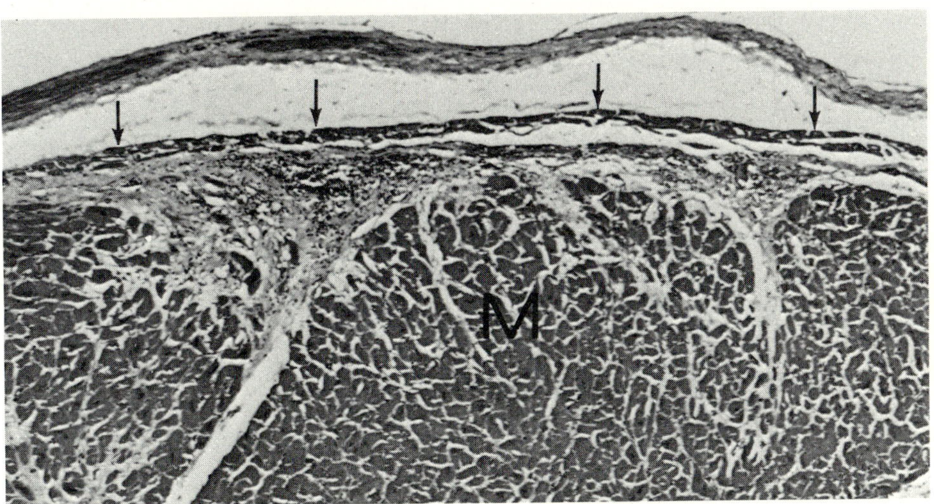

Fig. 15. A number of sarcoid granulomas along the course of a left fascicle (arrows). M, working septal myocardium. Hematoxylin and eosin. $\times$ 70.

pling of conduction tissue. The importance of a systematic and complete sampling of the conduction system whenever this study is undertaken has been repeatedly emphasized since casual sections may lead to serious misinterpretations.

The high incidence of arrhythmias and conduction disturbances and concomitant involvement of the conduction system in sarcoidosis (Tables 1 and 2) indicate a relationship between the two resulting from (1) discontinuity of the conduction system fibers caused by scar tissue, or (2) interference with electrical impulses by lymphocytic or granulomatous foci. Stokes-Adams attacks may result from complete heart block secondary to lesions of the AV node, bundle of His, or the bundle branches.[15] Sarcoidosis may affect any portion of the conduction system; however, the bundle of His in its course through the annulus fibrosus has a maximum diameter of 4 mm [16] and seems to be a particularly vulnerable area, thus accounting for the frequency of complete heart block and sudden death associated with sarcoidosis.

The role of sinus node involvement in the genesis of the syncopal attacks cannot be overlooked.[17, 18] Atrial arrhythmias may result from lesions of the nodal artery, nodal muscle, atrial myocardium, or nerves, which are particularly abundant in the vicinity of and within the sinus node. In addition to the inflammatory and reparative lesions involving nodal and working myocardial fibers, the changes in the nodal artery in sarcoidosis must be considered. The unique anatomic relationship between the sinus node and its nutrient artery has led some investigators to suggest that motion of this vessel may play a role in cardiac pacemaking, either by facilitating transport of extracellular fluid to the surface of nodal fibers or by transmission of motion to the fibers.[19] Intimal proliferation, fragmentation of elastica, and stenosis of the vessel lumen as observed in case 1 (Table 1) may lead to a derangement of the anatomicophysiologic association between the artery and nodal fibers. Sinus node artery changes have also been implicated in causing atrial arrhythmias in Marfan's syndrome,[20] systemic lupus erythematosus,[21] polyarteritis nodosa,[22] and thrombotic thrombocytopenic purpura.[23]

The frequently encountered cardiac failure associated with sarcoidosis results from one or a combination of factors—right ventricular failure secondary to extensive pulmonary disease with fibrosis (cor pulmonale), myocardial replacement by inflammatory or scar tissue, or conduction system abnormalities and arrhythmias with their resulting hemodynamic alterations.

Conclusion

The malignant nature of cardiac sarcoidosis appears to be greatly influenced by the frequent involvement of the conduction system of the heart by disease similar to that in the working myocardium. Anatomic alterations in the conduction system can be correlated well with the functional abnormalities of this system—electrocardiographic findings, arrhythmias, heart block, and attacks of syncope—providing that more than random histologic sections of the entire conduction system are examined. In view of the extent and nonregressive nature of the cardiac lesions, permanent artificial pacing of the heart may be the best solution in patients with conduction system dysfunction due to cardiac sarcoidosis.

References

1. Scadding JG (ed): Sarcoidosis. London, Eyre and Spottiswoode, 1967, pp 291–305
2. James TN: Anatomy of the human sinus node. Anat Rec 141:109, 1961
3. James TN: Morphology of the human atrioventricular node, with remarks pertinent to its electrophysiology. Amer Heart J 62:756, 1961
4. Peacock RA, Lippschutz EJ, Lukas A: Myocardial sarcoidosis. Circulation 16:67, 1957
5. Levy S, Morales AR, Sommer LS, Pemparkul S: Sarcoid heart disease. In preparation.
6. Mayock RL, Bertrand P, Morrison CE, Scott JH: Manifestations of sarcoidosis. Analysis of 145 patients, with a review of 9 series selected from the literature. Amer J Med 35:67, 1963
7. Simkins S: Boeck's sarcoid with complete heart block mimicking carotid sinus syncope. Report of a case. JAMA 146:794, 1951
8. Botti RE, Young FE: Myocardial sarcoid, complete heart block and aortic stenosis. Ann Intern Med 51:811, 1959
9. Porter GH: Sarcoid heart disease. New Eng J Med 263:1350, 1960
10. Phinney AO Jr: Sarcoid of the myocardial septum with complete heart block. Report of two cases. Amer Heart J 62:270, 1961
11. Smith WP: Primary sarcoid heart disease. Report of a case. J Fla Med Ass 51:625, 1964
12. Duvernoy WFC, Garcia R: Sarcoidosis of the heart presenting with ventricular tachycardia and atrioventricular block. Amer J Cardiol 28:348, 1971
13. Gozo EG, Cosnow I, Cohen HC, Okun L: The heart in sarcoidosis. Chest 40:4:379, 1971
14. Ghosh P, Fleming HA, Gresham GA, Stovin PG: Myocardial sarcoidosis. Brit Heart J 34:769, 1972
15. Lev M: The conduction system. In Gould SE (ed): Pathology of the Heart, 3rd ed. Springfield, Ill, Thomas, 1968, pp 180–220
16. Truex RC, Smythe MO: Recent observations on the human cardiac conduction system with special considerations of the atrioventricular node and bundle. In: Taccardi B and Marchetti G (eds) Electrophysiology of the Heart. Proceedings of the meeting held on October 11–13, 1963, at the Instituto di Cardiologia Sperimentale dei Servizi Scientifici Simes, Milan, Italy. Pergamon Press, 1964, pp 177–198
17. Kaplan BM, Langendorf R, Lev M, Pick A: Tachycardiabradycardia syndrome (so-called "sick sinus syndrome"). Pathology, mechanisms and treatment. Amer J Cardiol 31:497, 1973
18. Rasmussen K: Chronic sinoatrial heart block. Amer Heart J 81:38, 1971
19. James TN, Sherf L, Fine G, Morales AR: Comparative ultrastructure of the sinus node in man and dog. Circulation 34:139, 1966
20. James TN, Frame B, Schatz IJ: Pathology of cardiac conduction system in Marfan's syndrome. Arch Intern Med 114:339, 1964
21. James TN, Rupe CE, Monto RW: Pathology of the cardiac conduction system in systemic lupus erythematosus. Ann Intern Med 63:402, 1965
22. James TN, Birk RE: Pathology of the cardiac conduction system in polyarteritis nodosa. Arch Intern Med 117:561, 1966
23. James TN, Monto RW: Pathology of the cardiac conduction system in thrombotic thrombocytopenic purpura. Ann Intern Med 65:37, 1966

LESIONS OF THE CONDUCTION SYSTEM AND THEIR FUNCTIONAL SIGNIFICANCE*

MAURICE LEV AND
SAROJA BHARATI

The pathology of the conduction system mirrors the pathology of the myocardium. However, this pathology is modified by the location of the various components of the conduction system. It is therefore necessary to discuss the anatomy briefly before considering the pathology.

Anatomy of the Conduction System

In a broad sense the conduction system encompasses the entire heart. In a narrow sense, the conduction system consists of the sinoatrial (SA) node, the atrial pathways, the atrioventricular (AV) node, the AV bundle, the right and left bundle branches, the peripheral Purkinje nets, and the terminal Purkinje cells.

SA Node

The SA node [1-3] is a sizeable structure lying in the region of the sulcus terminalis between the superior vena cava and the right atrial appendage (Fig. 1). It is related to the epicardium, Bachmann's bundle, the posterior (terminal) crest, and the musculature of the atrial appendage. Histologically (Fig. 2) it consists of fusiform cells, whose transverse diameters are smaller than those of the remainder of the atrium. These cells are arranged in a serpentine manner with a tendency toward longitudinality along the path of the linea terminalis. Their cytoplasm stains more lightly with eosin or picric acid than that of the ordinary atrial cells. Their nuclei

* Aided by Grant HL-07605-11 from the National Institutes of Health, National Heart and Lung Institute, Bethesda, Md, and by a Grant-in-Aid from the American Heart Association.

 Maurice Lev and Saroja Bharati

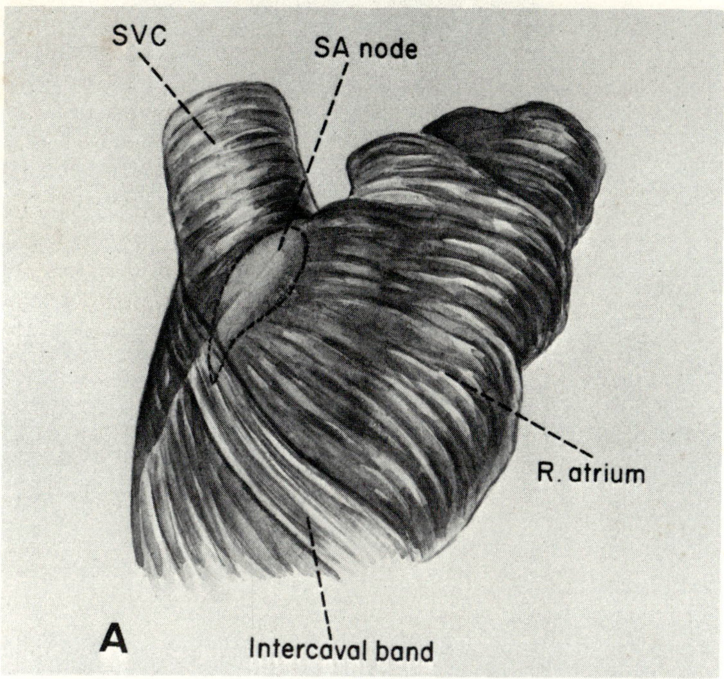

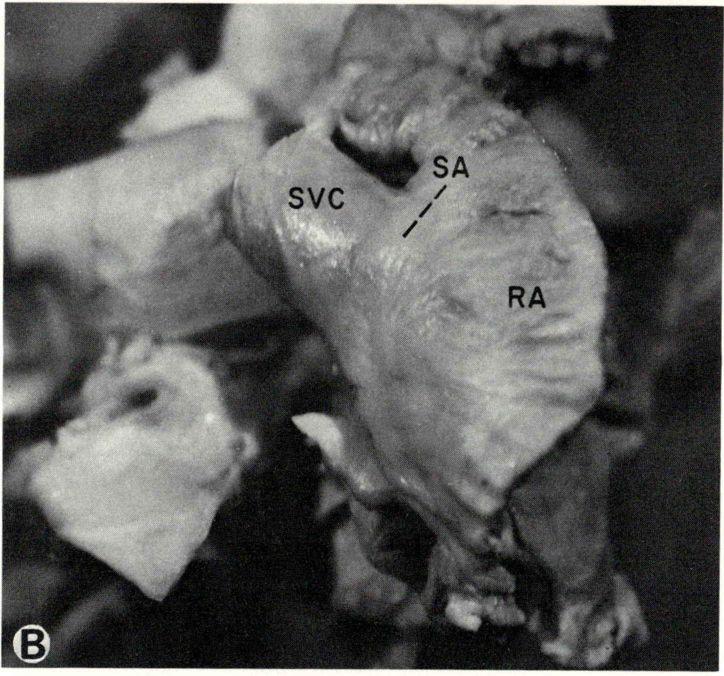

Fig. 1. Gross anatomy of SA node. A. Diagrammatic sketch. (From Lev. In Gould (ed): Pathology of the Heart, 1968. Courtesy of Charles C Thomas, Publishers.) B. SA node region in an infant. SVC, superior vena cava; RA, right atrium; SA, SA node. (From Lev, Watne: Arch Path 57:168, 1954)

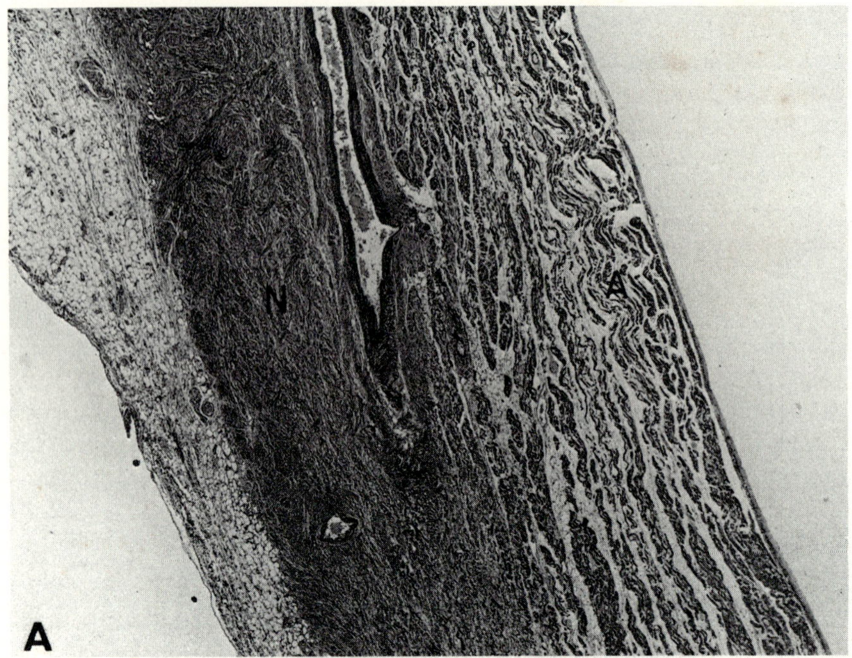

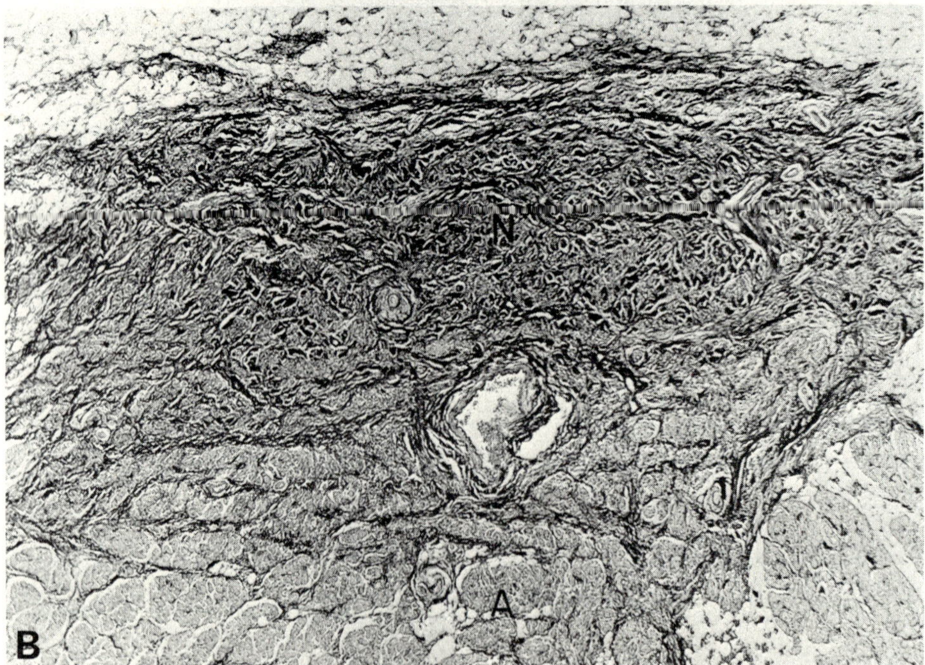

Fig. 2. Histology of SA node. A. Longitudinal section. Hematoxylin-eosin stain. × 16. B. Transverse section. Weigert-van Gieson stain. × 43. N, SA node; A, atrial musculature. (From Lev, Watne: Arch Path 57:168, 1954)

are slightly smaller in diameter than those of the atrial myocardium. The cells are striated after birth, but show no intercalated discs at the light level. The SA node contains a large amount of elastic and collagenous tissue, much more than is present in the ordinary atrial musculature. The node connects with the surrounding atrium by means of ordinary atrial cells.

With advancing age the SA node grows more slowly than the atrial myocardium. The amount of collagenous fibers increases until about the age of 40, and scarcely at all thereafter; the amount of elastic tissue increases until about the age of 50 to 60. After the age of 40 apparently some muscle fibers are lost and fat cells surround the node and partly infiltrate it.

Three preferential pathways, the upper, middle, and lower, connect the SA to the AV node.[4-7] The upper starts at the head of the node at its junction with Bachmann's bundle, and proceeds along the upper part of the atrial septum and curves downward to the AV node. The middle pathway skirts around the posterior part of the atrium and enters the atrial septum lying along the limbus fossae ovalis. This joins the upper pathway to reach the AV node. The inferior pathway travels along the crista terminalis to the lower part of the atrial septum, proceeds to the coronary sinus region, and joins the AV node. These three pathways consist of ordinary atrial muscle at the light level. They are not tracts separated by connective tissue sheaths from the remainder of the atria but wide masses of muscle making up the entire atrial septum.

AV Node, AV Bundle (Bundle of His), and Bundle Branches

The AV node is a sizeable structure, lying in the inferodistal portion of the atrial septum between the mouth of the coronary sinus and the medial leaflet of the tricuspid valve (Fig. 3). It lies somewhat below or is related medially to the right side of the central fibrous body, but occasionally it lies more distally, adjacent to the right side of the left ventricular-right atrial component of the pars membranacea.[8] Histologically it consists of a plexiform arrangement of striated cells which have a smaller diameter than atrial cells, but are larger than SA nodal cells (Fig. 4). Their cytoplasm stains more lightly with eosin or picric acid and their nuclei are oval. Intercalated discs are present at the light level. The AV node also contains increased elastic and collagenous fibers compared to the atrial or ventricular musculature, but much less than does the SA node.[3, 9]

As the AV node dips into the central fibrous body (or sometimes the atrioventricular portion of the pars membranacea) it becomes more compact, and is now the penetrating portion of the AV bundle or bundle of His (Fig. 3). The latter travels in the central fibrous body and lower confines of the pars membranacea. In the former position it is related to the posterior commissure of the mitral valve. At the level of the middle or distal portion of the posterior aortic cusp, the bundle of His gives off fine fasciculi of the main left bundle branch (Fig. 3). As it does so it becomes the branching portion of the AV bundle. This reaches the region of the commissure between the posterior and right aortic cusp, where the bifurcation or pseudobifurcation is reached. At this point the right bundle branch is given off, together with the remaining portion of the main left bundle branch.

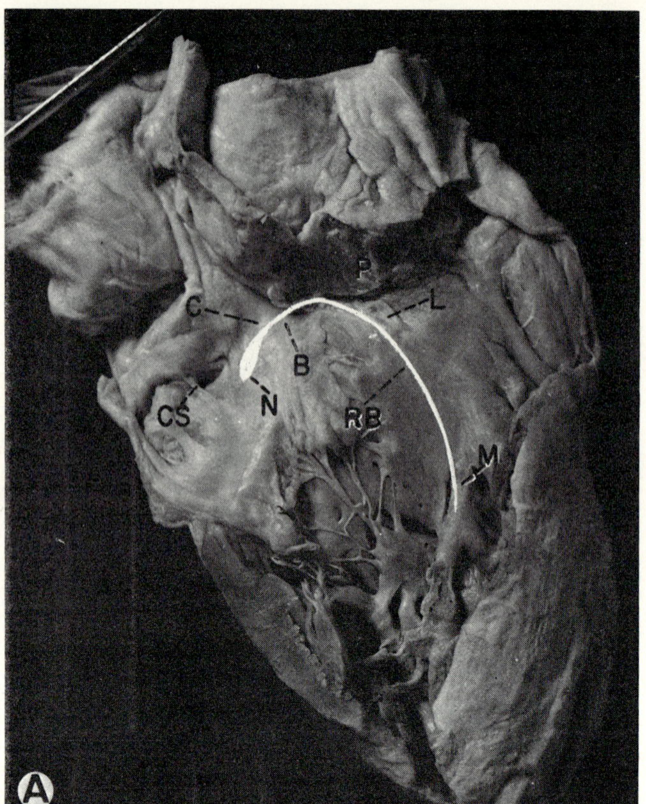

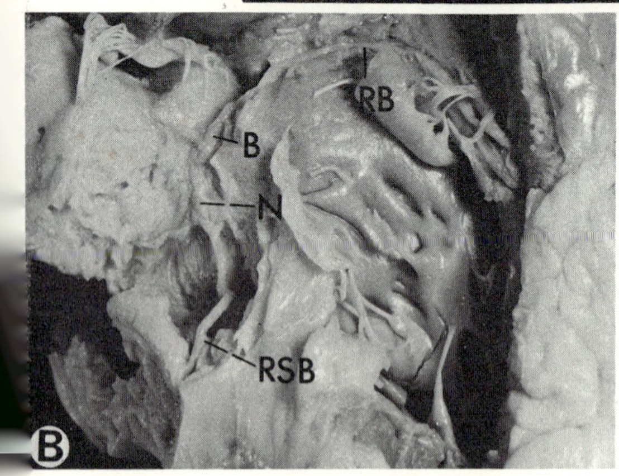

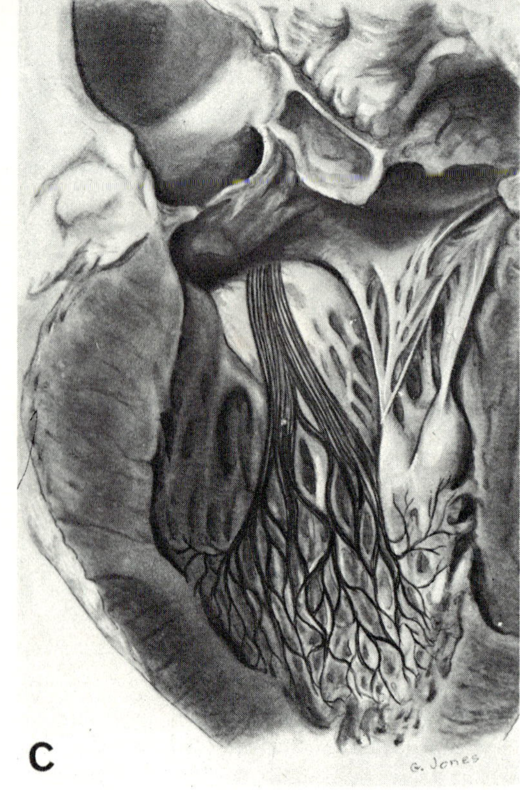

Fig. 3. A. Diagrammatic sketch of AV node, bundle, and right bundle branch. B. Actual dissection of AV node, bundle, and right bundle branch. (From Widran, Lev: Circulation 4:863, 1951) C. Diagrammatic sketch of left bundle branch stained with Lugol's solution. (After Uhley and Rivkin [10]) White line in "A" denotes course of AV node, bundle, and right bundle branch. CS, coronary sinus; C, central fibrous body; P, parietal band; L, muscle of Lancisi; M, moderator band; LM, main left bundle; AR, anterior radiation or fasciculi; PR, posterior radiation or fasciculi; RSB, ramus septi fibrosi; N, AV node; B, AV bundle; RB, right bundle branch.

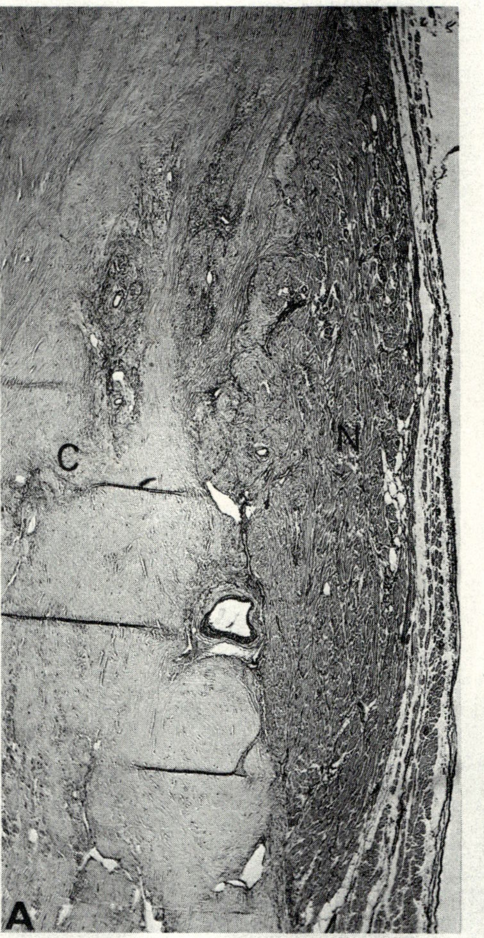

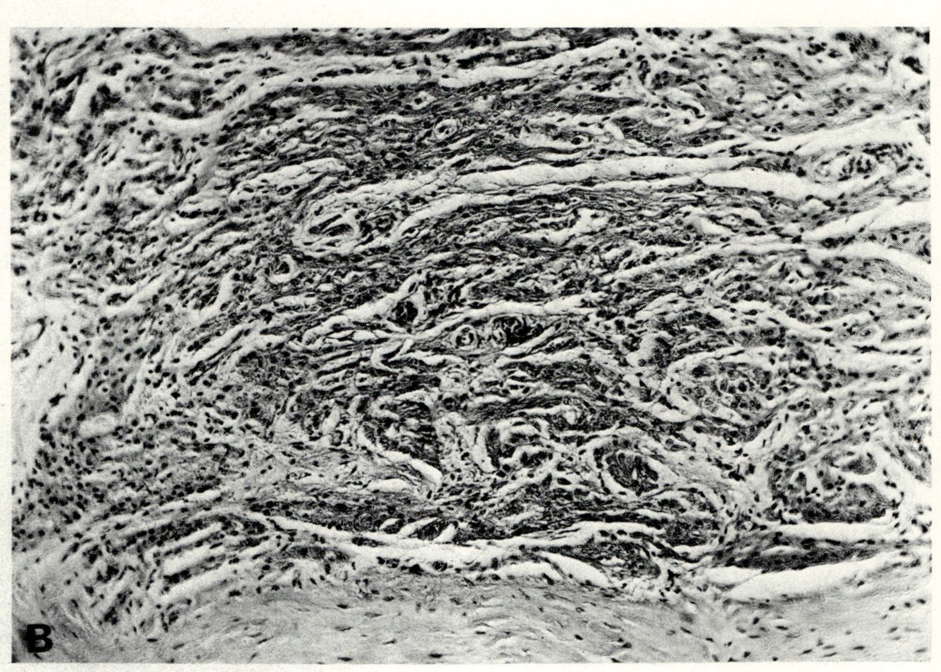

Fig. 4. Histology of AV node in adult. A. Weigert-van Gieson stain. × 35. B. Hematoxylin-eosin stain. × 77. C, central fibrous body; N, node. (From Erickson, Lev: J Geront 7:1, 1952)

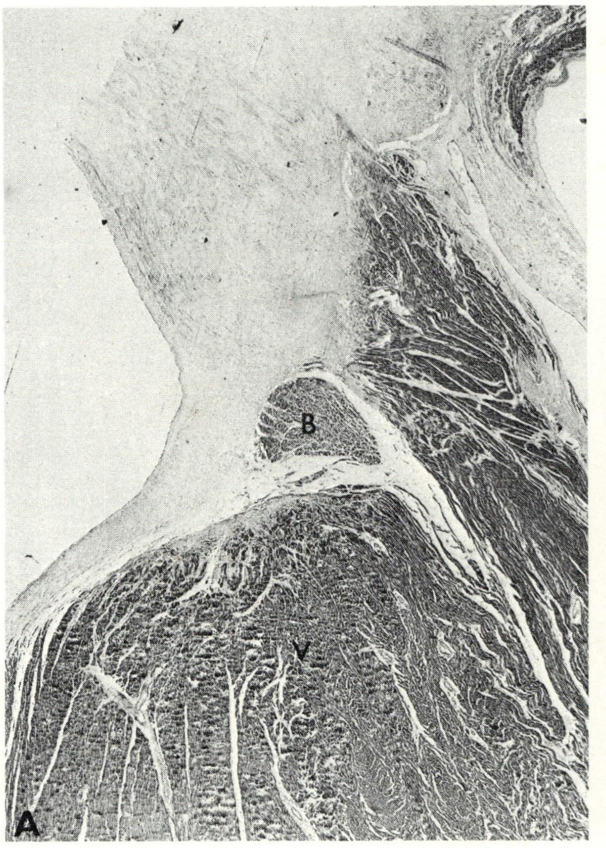

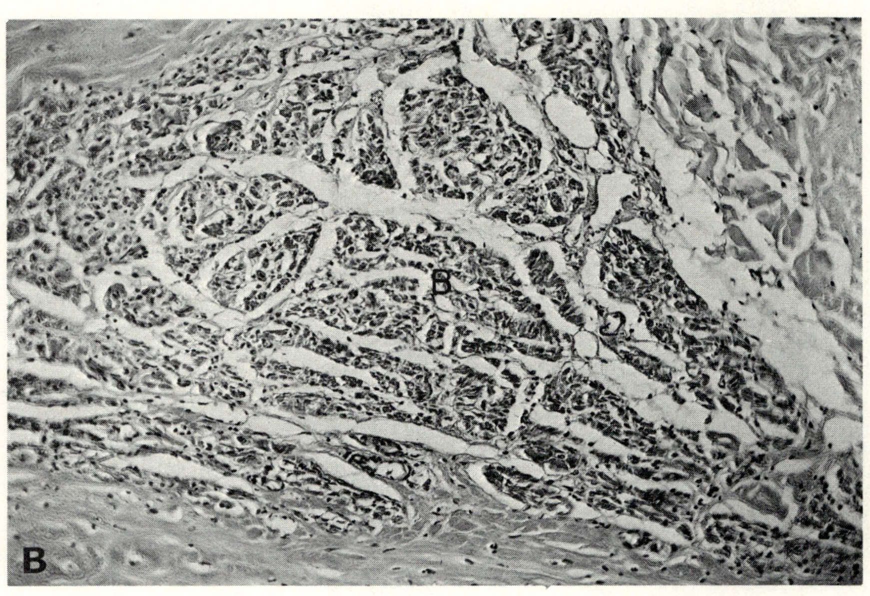

Fig. 5. Histology of AV bundle in adult. A. Hematoxylin-eosin stain. × 14. B. Hematoxylin-eosin stain. × 125. B, AV bundle; V, ventricular myocardium. (From Erickson, Lev: J Geront 7:1, 1952)

Thus it is clear that the penetrating portion of the AV bundle is related to the mitral annulus, the central fibrous body, and part of the interventricular portion of the pars membranacea, while the branching portion is related to the pars membranacea, the summit of the ventricular septum, and indirectly to the base of the aortic valve.

Both portions of the bundle of His have a similar histologic structure. Their cells are arranged in a longitudinal fashion with some bridges between the fasciculi. The diameter of these cells is less than that of the cells of the ventricular myocardium. Their cytoplasm stains more lightly with eosin or picric acid. They are distinctly striated and they have intercalated discs (Fig. 5).

The right bundle branch proceeds from the pseudobifurcation along the lower part of the septal band about 1 mm below the muscle of Lancisi to the moderator band (Fig. 3). It is divided into three parts. The first part is usually subendocardial but may be intramyocardial. The second part is intramyocardial but lies in the right side of the ventricular septum. The third part is again subendocardial.

Histologically (Fig. 6) the cells of the first part of the right bundle branch are the same size as cells of the branching portion of the AV bundle. The cells of the second part are about the same size as those of the ventricular myocardium. The cells of the third part are larger than components of ventricular myocardium and are Purkinje cells. The cytoplasm of all of these cells stains lighter than that of the ventricular myocardium; they are striated and contain intercalated discs. There is a distinct increase in elastic fibers as compared to the ventricular myocardium.

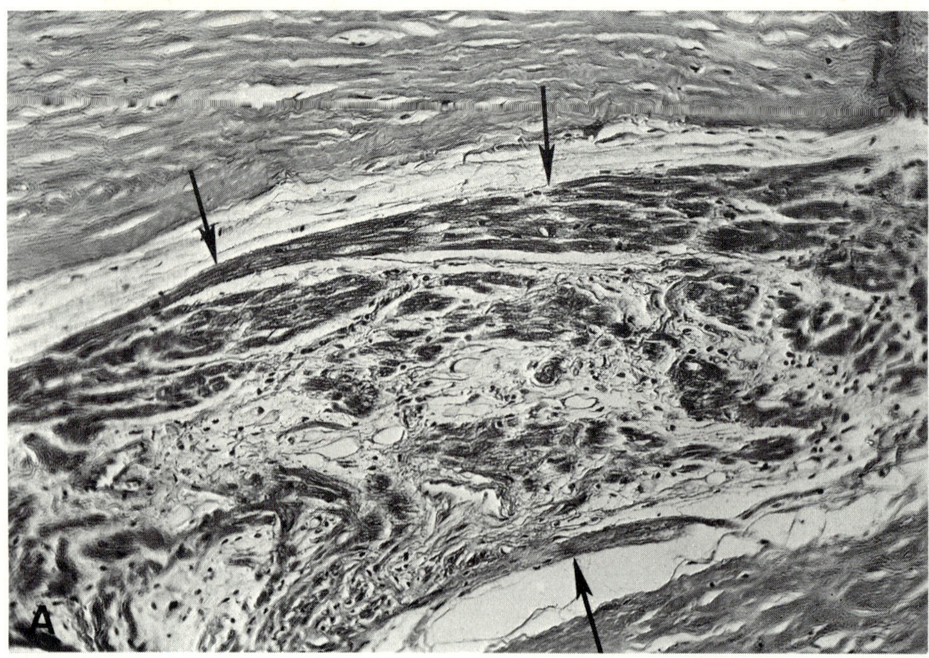

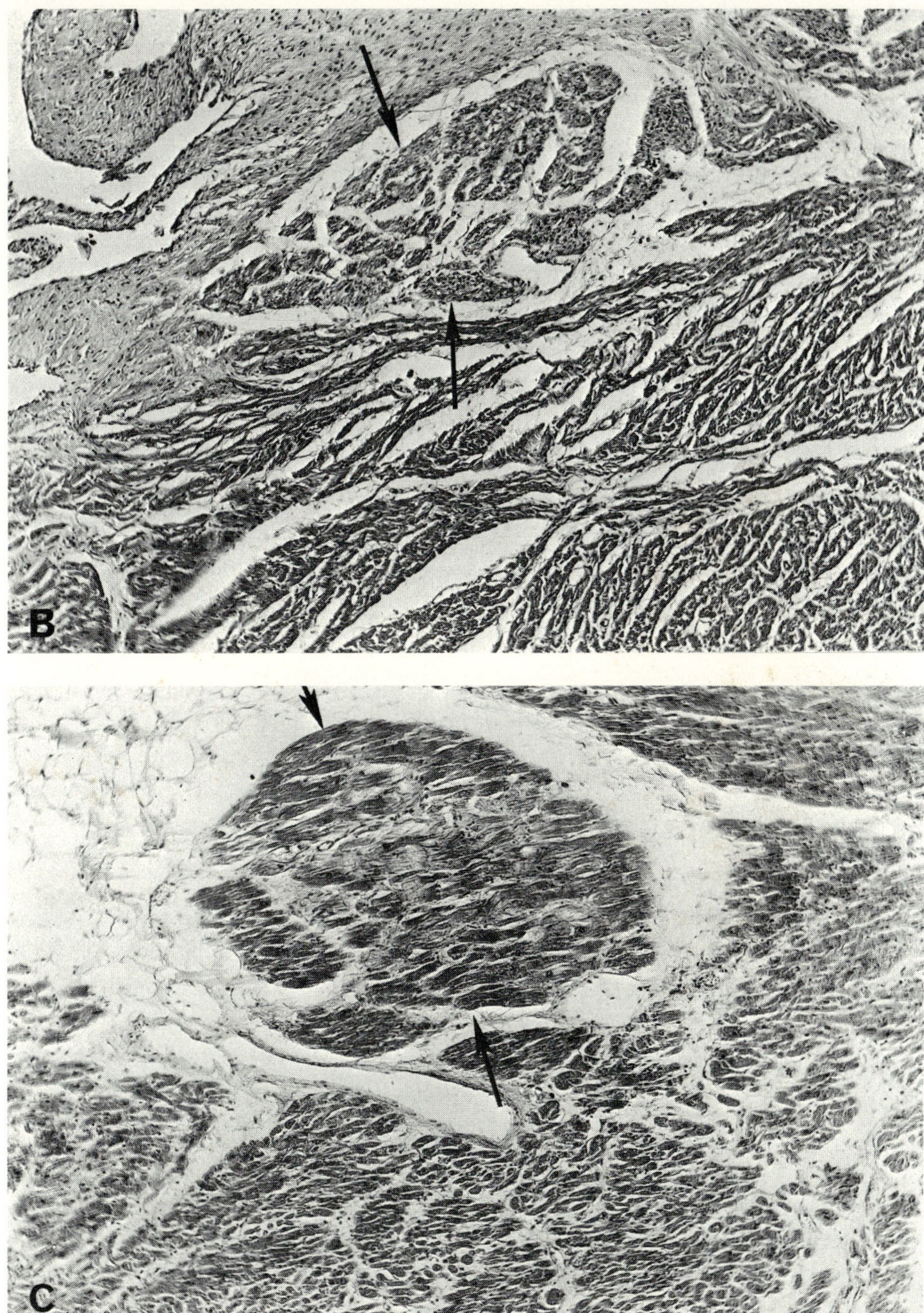

Fig. 6. Histology of right bundle branch. Hematoxylin-eosin stain. A. At origin from bundle in adult. × 137. B. First portion in new born × 76. C. Second portion in old age. × 152. Arrows point to right bundle branch. (From Erickson, Lev: J Geront 7:1, 1952)

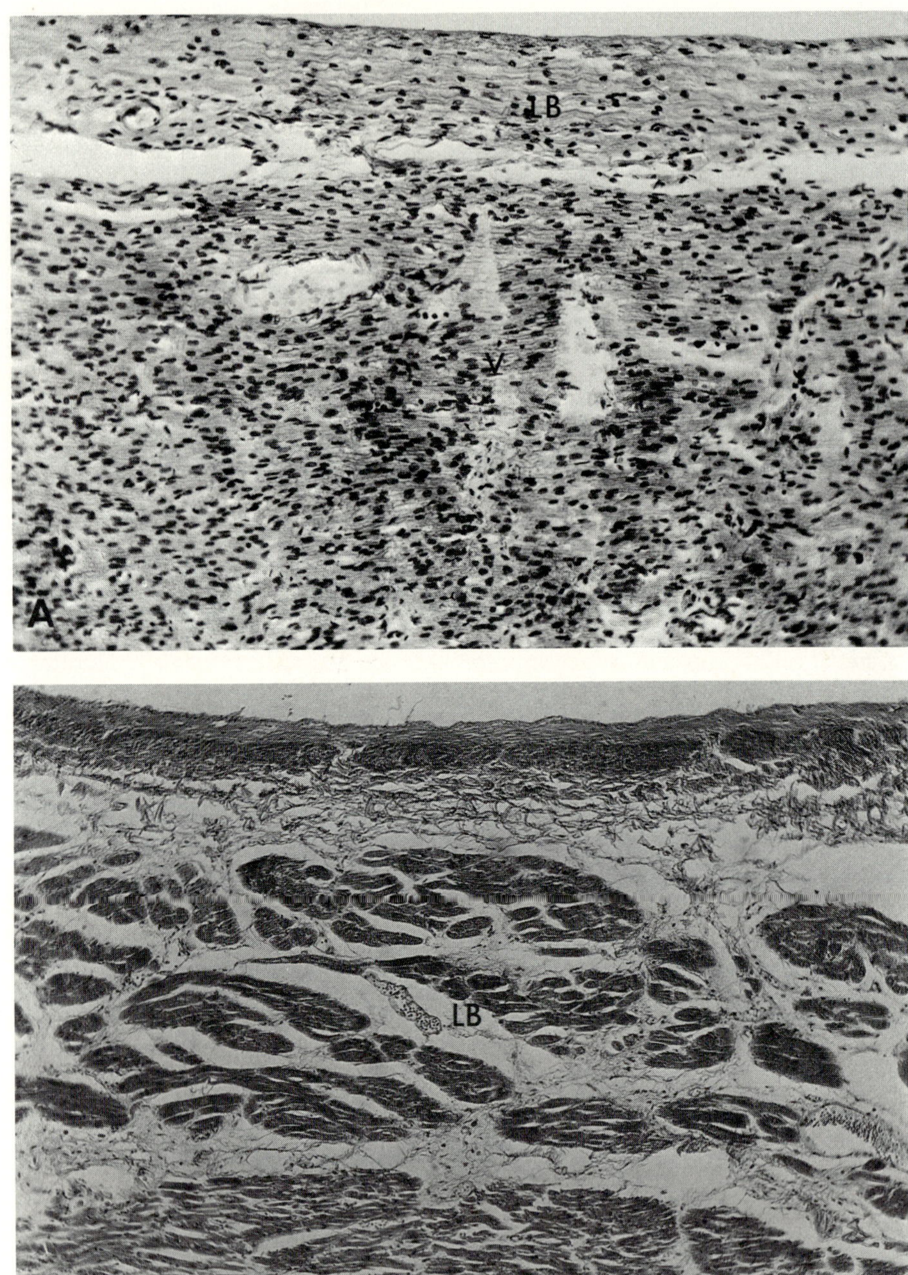

Fig. 7. Histology of left bundle branch. Hematoxylin-eosin stain. A. In newborn. $\times$ 152. B. In adult. $\times$ 76. The darker color of Purkinje cells is due to photography. Actually they stain lighter than the myocardium as in "A." LB, left bundle branch; V, ventricular myocardium. (From Erickson, Lev: J Geront 7:1, 1952)

The main left bundle,[10] as stated above, begins to be given off in fine sub-endocardial fasciculi before the right bundle branch is reached (Fig. 3). At the pseudobifurcation the remaining fibers of the main left bundle are given off with the right bundle branch. Thus the main left bundle branch is as much as 1 cm in width in its origin. It continues down for 1 to 3 cm and bifurcates into two radiations, the anterior and posterior, going to the anterior and posterior group of papillary muscles, respectively. The anterior is smaller in diameter than the posterior radiation. After some distance these radiations give off branches which swing medially ending in a plexiform arrangement of Purkinje nets in the apical region. The remainder of the anterior and posterior radiations likewise end in Purkinje cells at the bases of the papillary muscles.

Histologically (Fig. 7) the cells of the left bundle branch as they leave the bundle rapidly become Purkinje cells. The Purkinje cell is a large cell with pale clear cytoplasm and with round or oval nuclei; some cells contain more than one nucleus. In this paper only the large cells of the left bundle branch and the periphery of the right bundle branch are called Purkinje cells. The left bundle branch and its Purkinje network contain more elastic tissue than the ventricular myocardium.

There is a space surrounded by mesothelial cells about the AV bundle (Fig. 5) and the bundle branches. The nature of this space is today unknown. Similar mesothelial cells with small spaces are present in the AV node (Fig. 4).

With advancing age the AV node, bundle, and bundle branches grow less than the remainder of the heart. There is a greater increase in elastic and connective tissue than in the atrial and ventricular myocardium and an infiltration of fat in the AV node, bundle, and in the first portion of the right bundle branch.[9]

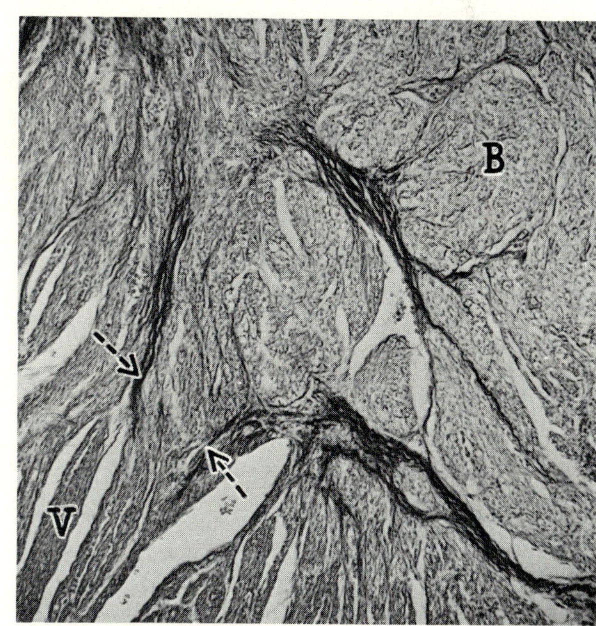

Fig. 8. Fibers of Mahaim from bundle to ventricular septum in 6-month fetus. Weigert-van Gieson stain. × 100. B, bundle; V, ventricular septum. Arrows point to Mahaim fibers.

Bundles of Kent

The bundles of Kent [11, 12] are fasciculi of ordinary atrial fibers connecting the free walls of the right atrium and right ventricle or the left atrium and left ventricle. They are present normally up to the age of 6 months, but have not been found later.

Fibers of Mahaim

There are muscle connections between the end of the AV node and the ventricular septum, the penetrating portion of the AV bundle and the ventricular septum, and the beginning of the left bundle branch and the ventricular septum, known as the Fibers of Mahaim (Fig. 8).[5, 11, 13] They may be present in all age groups.

A Method of Studying the Conduction System

Opening the Fresh Heart

The first cut is made from the inferior vena cava into the right atrial appendage, thus sparing the SA node. The second cut is made along the acute margin of the heart to the apex, making sure not to injure the anterolateral papillary muscle. The third cut is made in the anterior wall of the right ventricle anterior to the tricuspid leaflets and medial to the moderator band and the anterolateral papillary muscle, through the pulmonary orifice into the pulmonary trunk, thus sparing the periphery of the right bundle branch. The fourth cut is made across the base of the left atrium from the left pulmonary veins to the right. The fifth cut is made along the obtuse margin of the heart between the anterior and posterior groups of papillary muscles to the apex. The sixth cut is made along the junction of the anterior and septal walls of the left ventricle (paraseptally) into the aorta (Fig. 9).[14, 15]

The heart is then fixed in 4 percent formaldehyde (10 percent formalin) with cotton packed in all chambers and crevices, and with heart suspended in a large container. Whenever possible the formaldehyde is changed in 48 hours. Fixation is complete in about a week.

Microscopic Examination of the Conduction System

In our view, the purpose of studying the conduction system is to accumulate data which can be used for electrocardiographic and His bundle recording correlation. Therefore, in any type of electrophysiologic abnormality the whole heart should be studied.[14, 15]

To cut the heart into proper blocks for histologic sections, we use the following method (Fig. 10). After fixation, the heart is washed for 4 to 8 hours. The aorta is cut short above the sinuses of Valsalva. The cut made originally from the

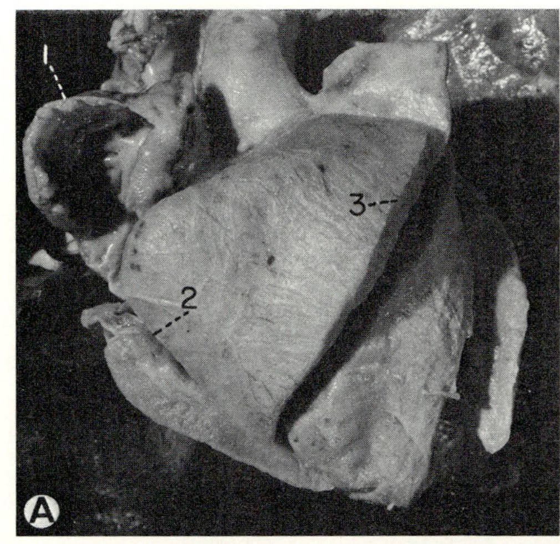

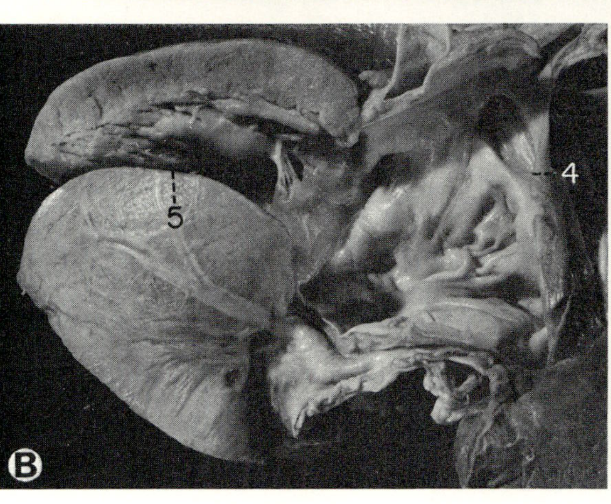

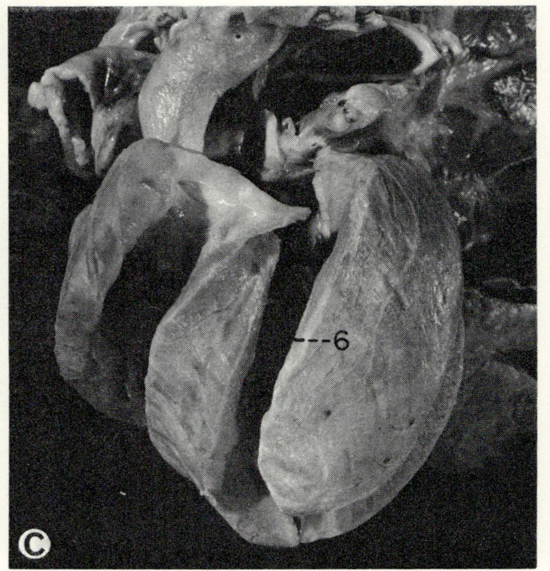

Fig. 9. Method of opening a heart. A. Right side. B. Left side. C. Paraseptal cut on left side. Numbers 1 to 6 indicate the cuts described in text.

inferior vena cava into the right atrial appendage is now extended over the roof of the atrium for 0.5 to 1 cm (Fig. 10A, cut 1). Another cut is made along the proximal side of the sulcus terminalis where the anterior wall of the atrium meets the atrial septum into the superior vena cava (Fig. 10B, cut 2). A transverse cut is made from cut 1 into the superior vena cava (Fig. 10A, cut 3). This gives the block containing the SA node and its approaches.

To obtain the superior and middle preferential atrial pathways and the blood supply to the SA node, cuts are made paraseptally into the roofs of the right and left atrium to their distal terminations, care being taken not to cut into the aorta (Fig. 10A, cuts 4 and 5). Cuts are then made into the opposite sides of the roofs of the atria to the AV groves (Fig. 10A, cuts 6 and 7) and transverse cuts at the AV groove free both roofs of the atria (Fig. 10A, cuts 8 and 9). One of these blocks so fashioned contains the SA nodal artery, dependent upon whether the artery arises from the main right or left circumflex. If these blocks are too long to place into a rotary microtome, they are cut in half. The atrial septum and its

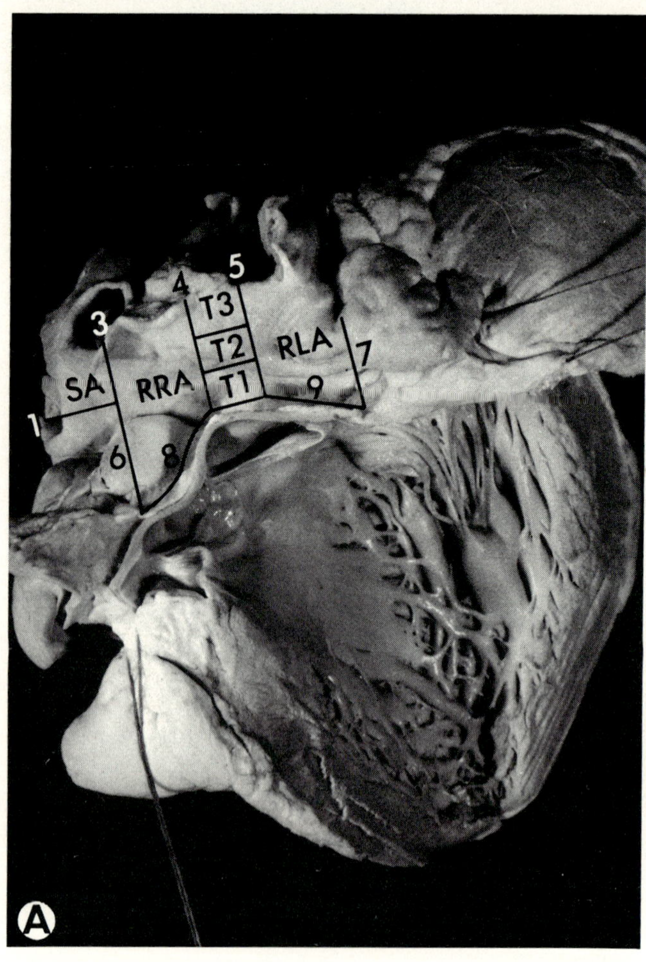

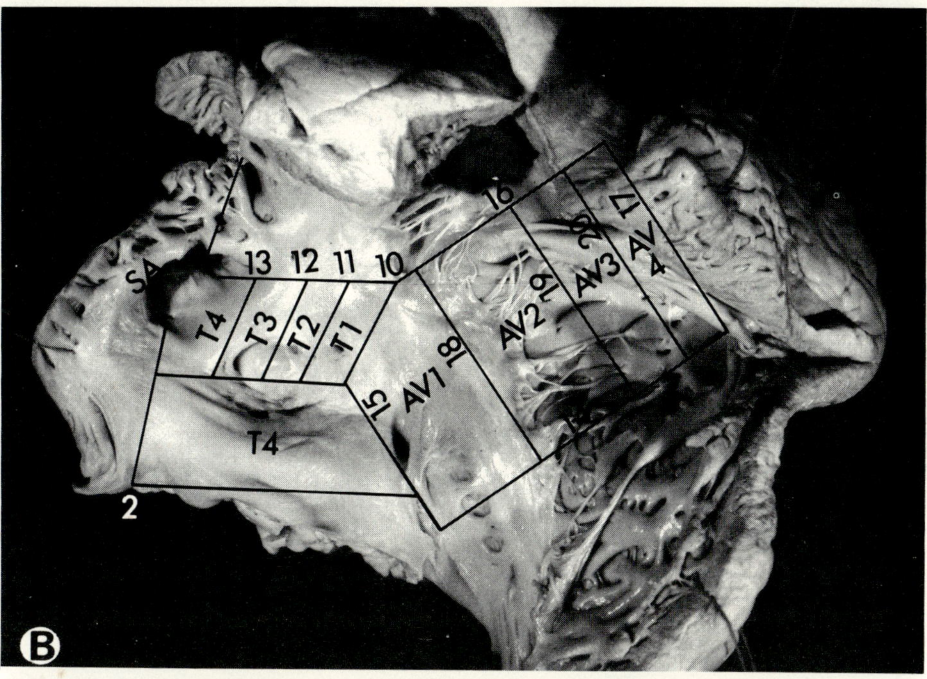

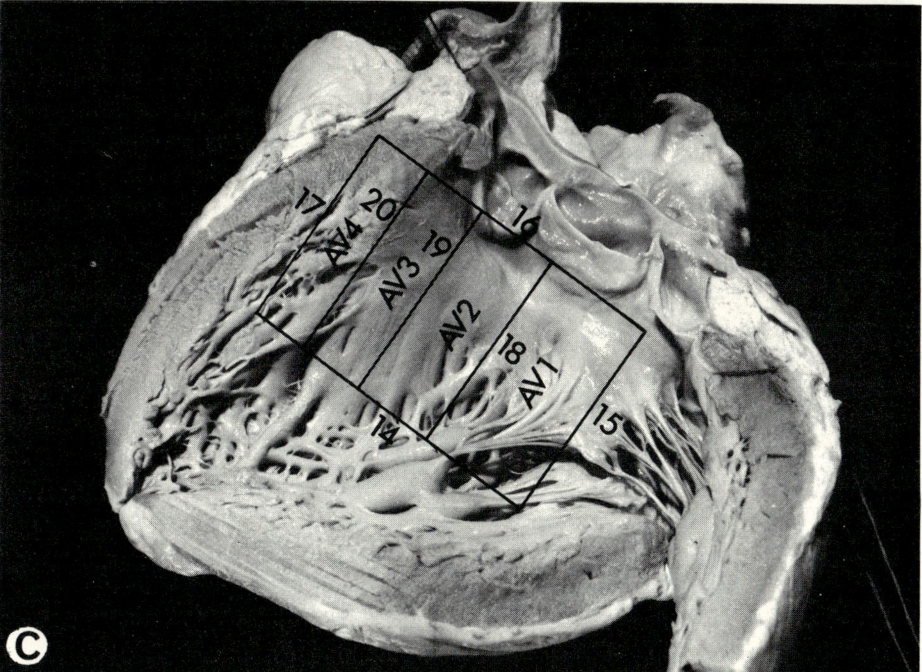

Fig. 10. Method of cutting heart for conduction system studies. Numbers indicate cuts and the labels indicate blocks. T_1 to T_4, atrial tracts; RRA, roof right atrium; RLA, roof left atrium; SA, SA node; AV_1 to AV_4, blocks containing AV node and approaches, AV bundle, and bundle branches.

accompanying piece of atrial roof are now free to be cut into blocks to obtain the superior and middle atrial pathways. Cuts are made consecutively from distally to proximally in a manner slanting proximally so as not to injure the approaches to the AV node (Fig. 10B, cuts 10, 11, 12, and 13). These cuts pass through the area of the fossa ovalis and the limbus. The number of blocks made depends upon the size of the atrial septum. No block can be larger than two inches in greatest dimension.

The inferior walls of the atria and ventricles are now separated from the septum by paraseptal cuts. The anterior wall of the right ventricle is separated from the septum by a cut through the parietal band and the pulmonary trunk. The more apical part of the anterior wall is added later. A cut is made through the aortic-mitral annulus into the aorta thus separating the anterior wall of the left ventricle. Thus a portion of the atrial septum and all of the ventricular septum now remain.

We study the AV node, bundle, and bundle branches in an oblique fashion. This is because these structures describe an arc. Hence horizontal or longitudinal sectioning short-changes part of the conduction system, unless complete serial sections are done. To achieve this oblique sectioning, a cut is made in the region of the anterior papillary muscle passing through a line ending proximally just below the crux (Fig. 10B, cut 14). A second cut is now made through the coronary sinus at right angles to the first cut (Fig. 10B, cut 15). A third cut is now made through the base of the aorta in the lower part of the pockets of the sinuses of Valsalva at right angles to the second cut (Fig. 10B, cut 16). The fourth cut is made just distal to the anterolateral papillary muscle meeting the first and third cut (Fig. 10B, cut 17). Thus a rectangular block is obtained which houses the approaches to the AV node, the AV node, the AV bundle, and the bundle branches up to the level of the moderator band. This includes the complete right bundle branch, the main left bundle branch, and the anterior and posterior radiations and some of their more peripheral branches.

This block is now divided into portions which can be suitably embedded as follows. A cut is made in the block in the region of the pars membranacea, parallel to cut 15 (Fig. 10B, cut 18). This produces a block containing the approaches to the AV node, the AV node, and the penetrating portion of the bundle. Another cut is now made in the original block through the muscle of Lancisi parallel to cut 18 (Fig. 10B, cut 19). This separates out the branching portion of the bundle and the beginning of the main bundle branches and the posterior peripheral portion of the left bundle branch. If the block so fashioned is too thick it may be divided into two parts. The remainder of the original block is divided into portions by parallel cuts. These contain the remainder of the right bundle branch and the anterior more peripheral portion of the left bundle branch.

If the electrocardiographic diagnosis is left anterior or posterior hemiblock then the method of Davies [16] is used instead of the above method. In this method the AV node, bundle, and the beginning of the bundle branches are cut from the posterior wall upward, while the remainder of the bundle branches are cut horizontally at right angles to the other blocks.

The inferior interatrial pathway is contained in the remaining atrial septal fragment. The walls of the ventricles and atria and the remainder of the atrial septum are now cut into small blocks and properly labelled, leaving fragments of atrium and ventricle in the event special stains become necessary.

Blocks containing the SA node, and the AV node, their approaches, and the penetrating portion of AV bundle, are serially sectioned and every tenth section is retained. The blocks containing the branching bundle and the beginning of the bundle branches are serially sectioned and every fifth section is retained. The blocks containing the remainder of the bundle branches are serially sectioned and every tenth section is retained. The blocks containing the atrial tracts are serially sectioned and every 40th section is retained. Two sections are taken from each of the remainder of the blocks.

In the SA node and the branching bundle and beginning of the bundle branches successive sections are stained with hematoxylin-eosin, Weigert-van Gieson, and Gomori trichrome. In the other sections alternate slides are treated with hematoxylin-eosin and Weigert-van Gieson stain.

It may be necessary to completely serial section some conduction systems in some cases of congenital heart block in infants. In a case where a diagnosis of Wolff-Parkinson-White syndrome is made, complete serial sections must be cut throughout the conduction system and both AV grooves and the adjacent atria and ventricles.

General Pathology of the Conduction System

The conduction system may be involved in any pathologic process which involves the myocardium itself. Thus the basic processes of congenital malformation, inflammation, degeneration, necrosis, and neoplasia may affect the conduction system. In addition, there may be a tendency toward an increase in spaces in the AV bundle and the bundle branches. These processes are manifest in congenital heart disease, coronary heart disease, hypertensive heart disease, rheumatic heart disease, syphilitic heart disease, myocarditis, collagen disease, and other rarer disease entities and states. In addition, because of the location of the AV node, bundle, and bundle branches, they may be involved in "sclerosis of the left side of the cardiac skeleton."

Congenital Heart Disease

In congenital heart disease,[3, 17-23] the conduction system may display malposition, discontinuity, aberrancy of development, or the presence of accessory bundles.

MALPOSITION.   In atrial septal defect of the fossa ovalis type the conduction system is normal, except where the defect is large, extending far forward. Here the AV node may be displaced posteriorly. In common AV orifice (Fig. 11)[24] and persistent ostium primum, the AV node is displaced posteriorly. The AV bundle lies on the inferior (posterior) rim of the defect and gives off the left bundle branch more posteriorly than normally. The right bundle branch lies on the distal wall of the combined defect and, in the region of the muscle of Lancisi, proceeds in its usual manner. In ventricular septal defect (Fig. 12)[25-32] the position of the conduction system is related to the position of the defect. Where the defect is at

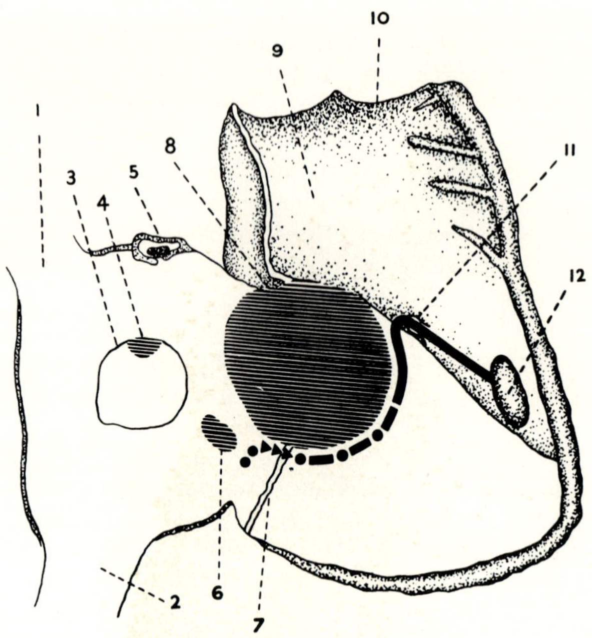

Fig. 11. Diagram of the course of the AV node, bundle, and right bundle branch in common AV orifice. Right atrial and right ventricular view. . . AV node; ▲, penetrating portion of AV bundle; .—.—, branching portion of AV bundle; ———; right bundle branch. 1, Superior vena cava; 2, inferior vena cava; 3, limbus; 4, patent foramen ovale; 5, cut edge of atrial appendage; 6, entry of coronary sinus; 7, base of tricuspid valve; 8, combined atrial and ventricular septal defect; 9, conus; 10, base of pulmonary valve; 11, muscle of Lancisi; 12, cut edge of moderator band. (From Lev: Arch Path 65:174, 1958)

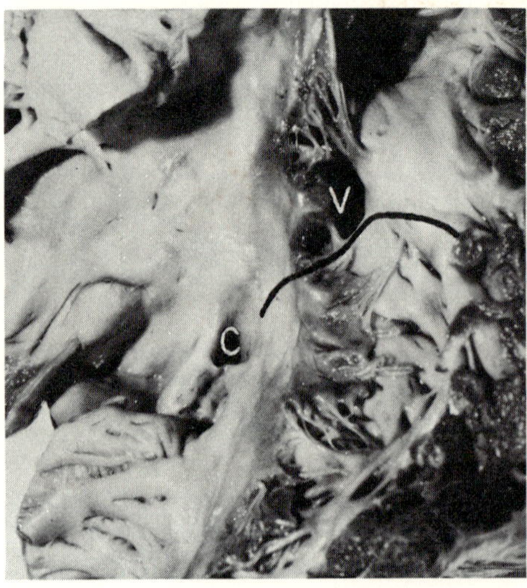

Fig. 12. Course of conduction system in one type of ventricular septal defect. C, coronary sinus opening; V, ventricular septal defect. (From Lev: Arch Path 70:529, 1960)

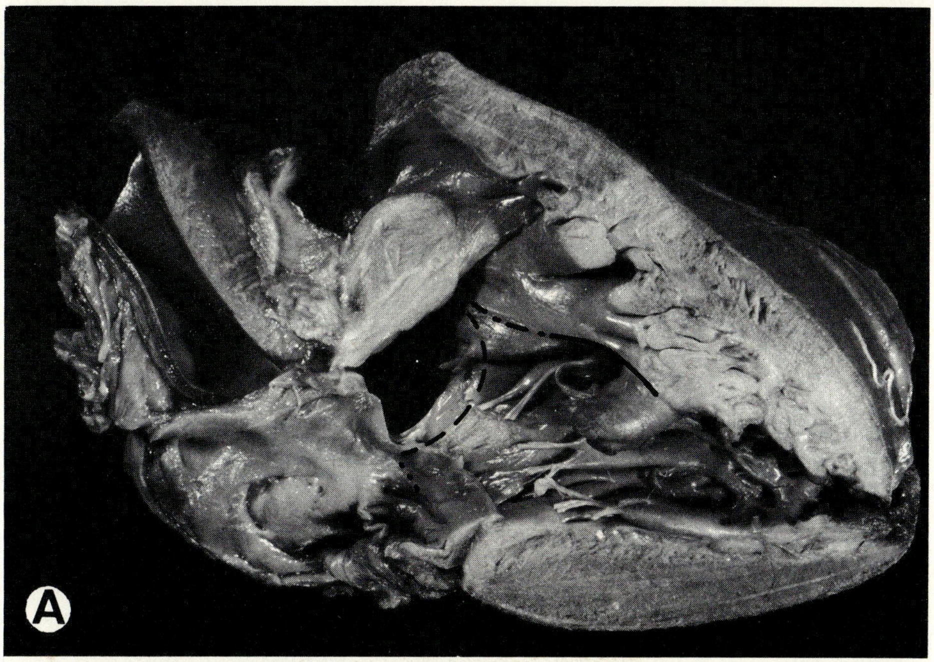

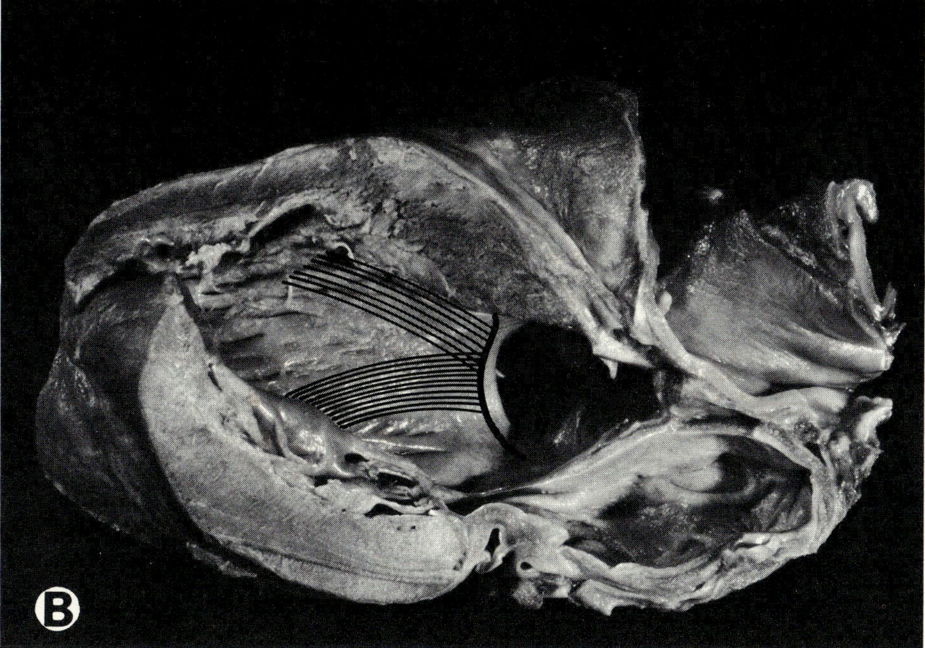

Fig. 13. Diagrammatic sketch of the course of the AV node, bundle, and bundle branches in tetralogy of Fallot. A. Right ventricular septal view. B. Left ventricular septal view. (From Lev: Arch Path 67: 572, 1959)

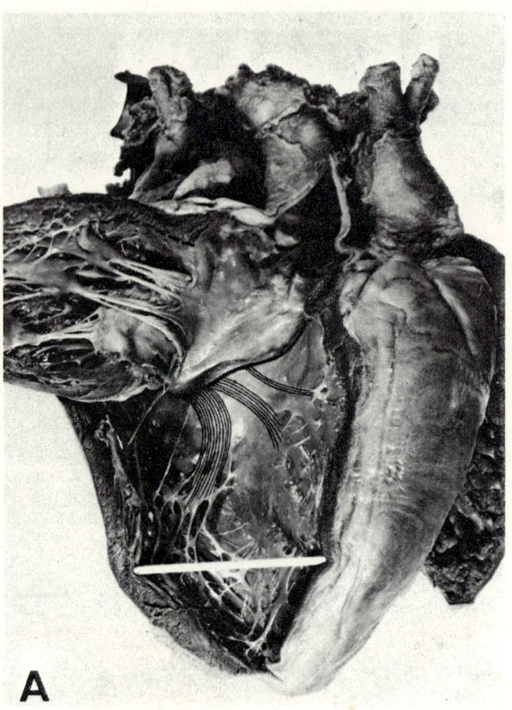

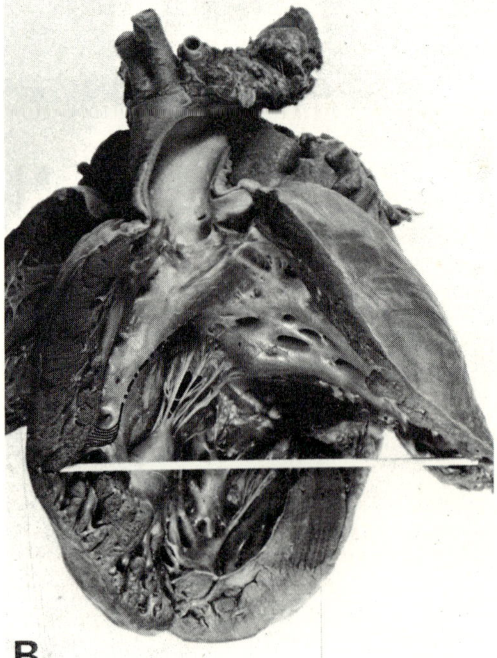

Fig. 14. The course of the conduction system in mixed levocardia with ventricular inversion (corrected transposition). A. Left ventricular view. B. Right ventricular view. (From Lev, Licata, May: Circulation 28:232, 1963)

the base, if it is related to the pars membranacea, the AV node is normal. The AV bundle lies on the inferior (posterior) rim of the defect, usually shifted slightly to the left side of the rim. The bundle branches are normal. If there is a common AV canal type of ventricular septal defect, then the AV node, bundle, and bundle branches are as in common AV canal. If the ventricular septal defect is in the conus, unrelated to the pars membranacea, then the AV bundle is unrelated to the defect. Likewise, if the defect is posterior, unrelated to the pars membranacea, the AV bundle is unrelated to the defect. If the defect is in the more apical region, the conduction system is normal except occasionally for deviation of either the right or left bundle branch fibers around the defect.

In single ventricle,[32] the AV bundle lies on a muscle bundle present on the posterior wall of the main ventricular chamber between the mitral and tricuspid orifices. In tetralogy of Fallot (Fig. 13) [31, 33, 34] the AV node is normal, unless there is a left superior vena cava entering the coronary sinus, when it is displaced either to the right or superiorly. The AV bundle lies distinctly to the left side of the inferior (posterior) rim of the defect. The position of the right bundle branch depends on the architecture of the septal band. In mixed levocardia with ventricular inversion (corrected transposition) [35] the bundle branches are inverted, and in some cases the AV node and bundle are also inverted (Fig. 14). All these deviations have no functional component, unless they are accompanied by discontinuity of structures.

DISCONTINUITY.   There may be lack of connection between the atrial musculature and the AV node (Fig. 15).[36] This may be accompanied by partial or complete absence of the AV node. Fat tissue and vascular channels take the place of atrial muscle in these circumstances. Or there may be discontinuity in the penetrating or branching portion of the bundle of His (Fig. 16),[37] the gaps in the structure being occupied either by connective tissue or clear spaces. Occasionally the pathology lies in the bundle branches, with lack of formation, being complete or incomplete in the right or left bundle branch. The results of these discontinuities or lacks of formation may be partial or complete AV block, or right or left bundle branch block electrocardiographically.

ABERRANCY OF FORMATION.   Occasionally the conduction system is abnormally formed.[38] Thus in one case the AV node ended blindly and an accessory AV node situated anteriorly formed a bundle of His which went off into the bundle branches. The bundle of His showed fibrosis and hemorrhage and there was complete AV block. This may be seen in corrected transposition, and single ventricle.

Congenital AV block due to any of the above mechanisms may be found unassociated or associated with other congenital malformations. It has been described in patent foramen primum,[39] atrial septal defect of the fossa ovalis type,[40] inversion of the atria or ventricles,[41] cor biatriatum triloculare,[42] large ventricular septal defect,[43] absence of the atrial septum,[44] idiopathic hypertrophy with fibroelastosis,[36] aneurysm of the pars membranacea,[45-47] hypoplasia of the aortic tract complex,[48, 49] tetralogy of Fallot,[50] bicuspid aortic valve,[51] complete transposition with single ventricle and with pulmonary atresia,[52] complete transposition with tricuspid stenosis or atresia,[53-55] fetal coarctation,[36] patent ductus arteriosus with double aortic arch,[56] pulmonary atresia with intact ventricular septum,[57] isolated

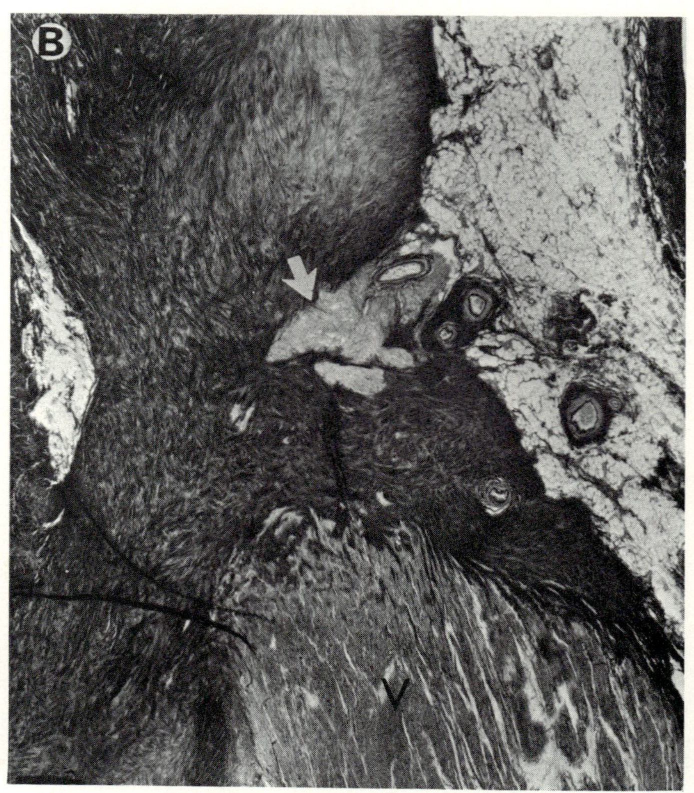

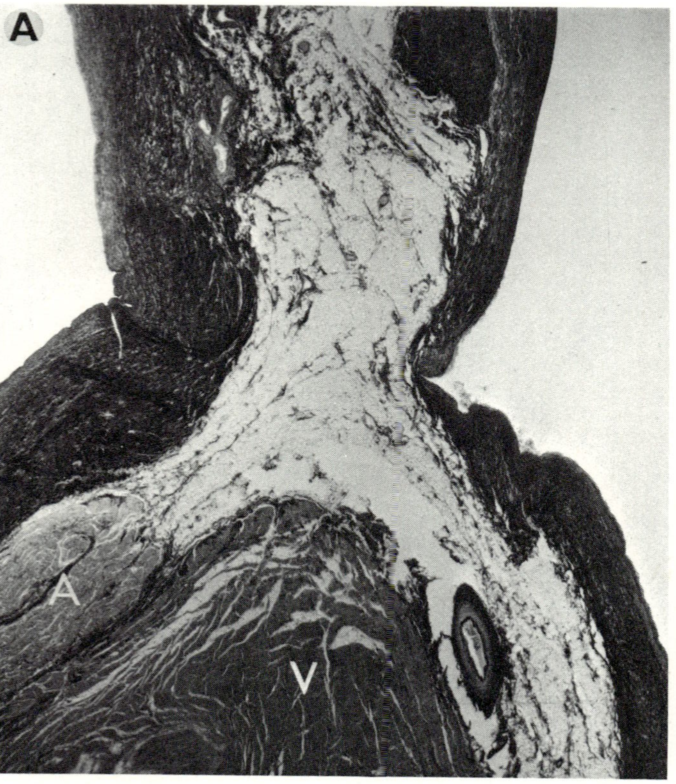

Fig. 15. Lack of connection between the atria and the AV node with congenital complete AV block. A. Approaches to the AV node showing dearth of muscle. Weigert-van Gieson stain. × 10. B. Fragment of AV node or bundle lying in central fibrous body. Weigert-van Gieson stain. × 20, **A,** left atrial muscle; V, ventricular muscle. Arrow points to AV node. (From Lev et al: Amer J Cardiol 27:481, 1971)

tricuspid insufficiency,[58] aneurysm of an aortic sinus of Valsalva,[45] muscular sub-aortic stenosis,[59] Marfan's disease,[60-62] and congenital absence of the left pericar-dium.[63] In cases of persistent ostium primum there may be absence of the left [64] or right [30] bundle branch; in cases of common AV orifice there may be absence of the left bundle branch.[32] In one case of isolated ventricular septal defect the right bundle branch was absent; in another the left bundle branch was abnormal, re-sembling a right bundle branch.[65] In Ebstein's disease disconnection between the right bundle branch and the AV bundle has been described,[32] as well as encase-ment of the right bundle branch in fibrous tissue; [66] in other cases of this disease, high connections of the right bundle branch with the ventricular septum have been reported.[32, 67] In a case of complete transposition no connection between the right

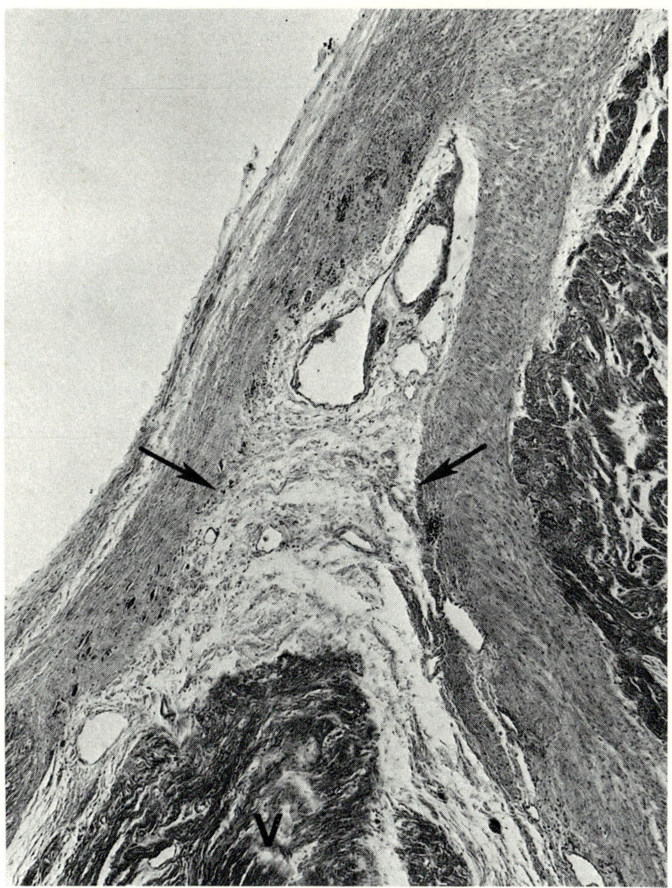

Fig. 16. Interruption of penetrating portion of AV bundle with congenital complete AV block. Hematoxylin-eosin stain. × 38. V, ventricular muscle. Arrows point to region of penetrating portion of bundle. (From Lev, Cuadros, Paul: Circulation 43:703, 1971)

bundle branch and the ventricle was found,[27] and in a case of cor biloculare no bundle branches were present.[32] In otherwise normal hearts the right bundle branch may be absent.[68,69] In subaortic stenosis the left bundle branch may be encased in fibrous tissue and interrupted.[70]

Cases of atrial septal defect and ventricular septal defect may be associated with acquired AV block. This is probably due to hemodynamic stress on the AV bundle.[40]

ACCESSORY COMMUNICATIONS.   Bundles of Kent may be found in the right or left AV rim and be related to Wolff-Parkinson-White syndrome (Fig. 17).[67, 71-74] Likewise, a tract between the atrial septum and the bundle of His may bypass the AV node. This may be associated with Mahaim fibers to produce the Wolff-Parkinson-White syndrome (Fig. 18).[75] Fibers of Mahaim may be more developed than usual and be related to the formation of the widened QRS with a Δ wave.[76]

SURGICAL INJURY TO THE CONDUCTION SYSTEM.   In any type of open heart surgery the SA node may be injured due to the atriotomy.[77] In closure of a ventricular septal defect (VSD) or repair of tetralogy and common AV canal and calcific aortic stenosis, the AV bundle may be injured (Fig. 19) proximal to the branching point of the left bundle branch to produce AV block. Repair of a VSD in corrected transposition very often results in block, probably due to injury of the AV bundle during its long course. The block in these conditions may be evanes-

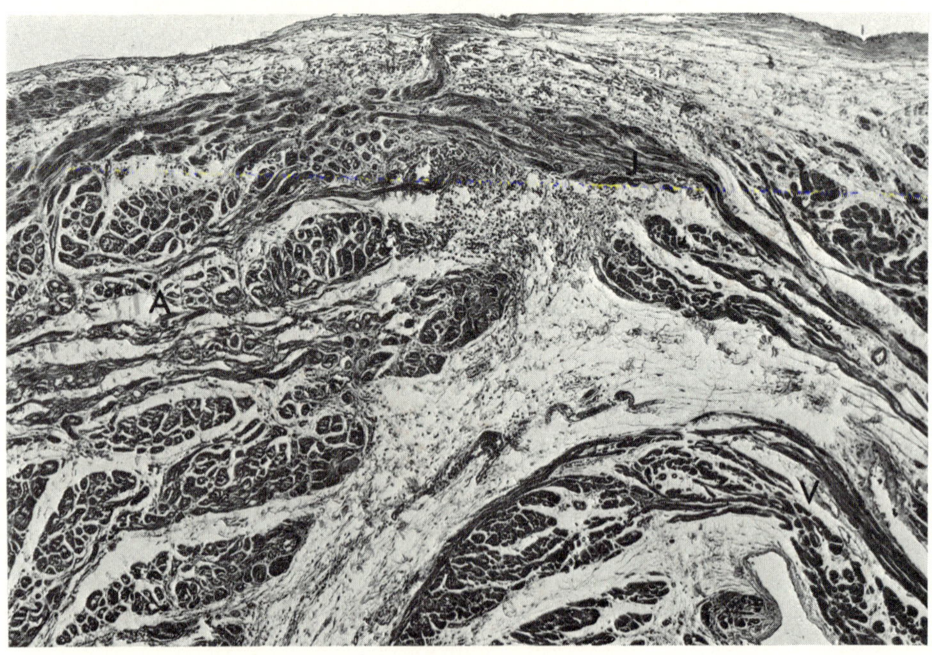

Fig. 17. Bundle of Kent in WPW. Hematoxylin-eosin stain. $\times$ 80. A, atrial musculature; V, ventricular musculature; J, junctional muscular tissue. (From Lev et al: Circulation 24:41, 1961)

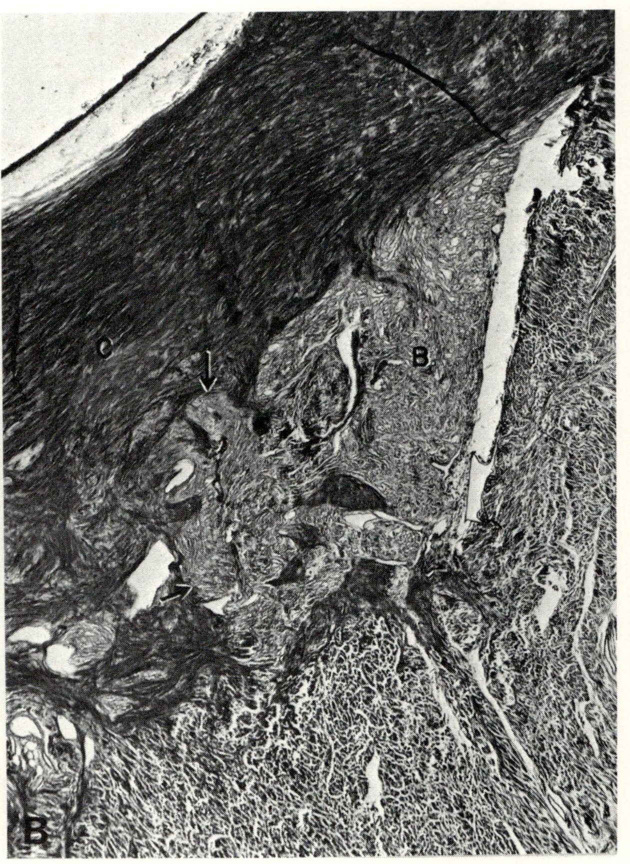
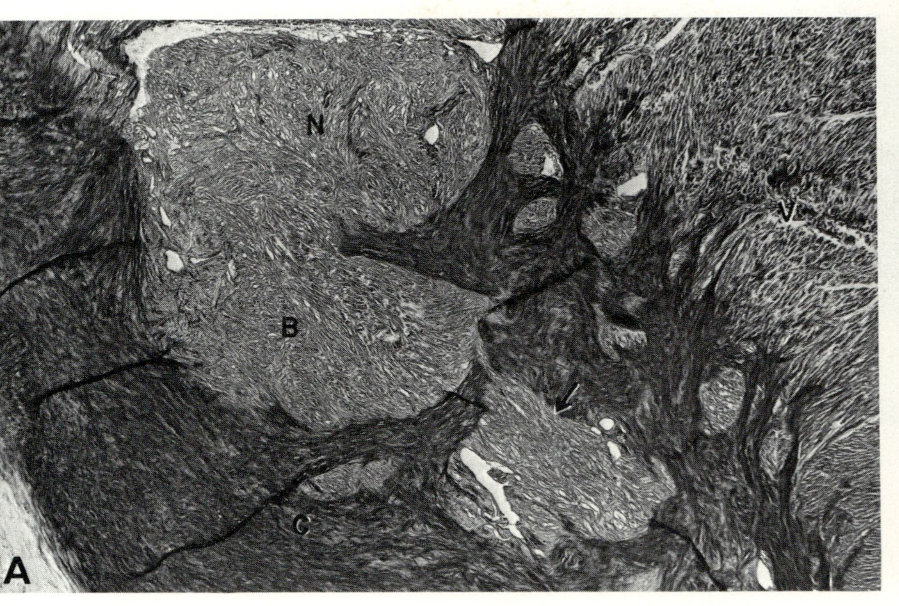

Fig. 18. Case of WPW, showing AV nodal bypass and fibers of Mahaim. A. Section through the junctional area between the AV node and bundle showing termination of bypass tract in AV bundle. Weigert-van Gieson stain. ×17. N, AV node; B, AV bundle; V, ventricular musculature; C, central fibrous body. Arrow points to the bypass tract. (From Lev et al: Circulation 34:718, 1966) B. Section through the penetrating portion of AV bundle showing copious Mahaim fibers. Weigert-van Gieson stain. × 18. C, central fibrous body; B, AV bundle; V, ventricular muscle. Arrows point to Mahaim fibers.

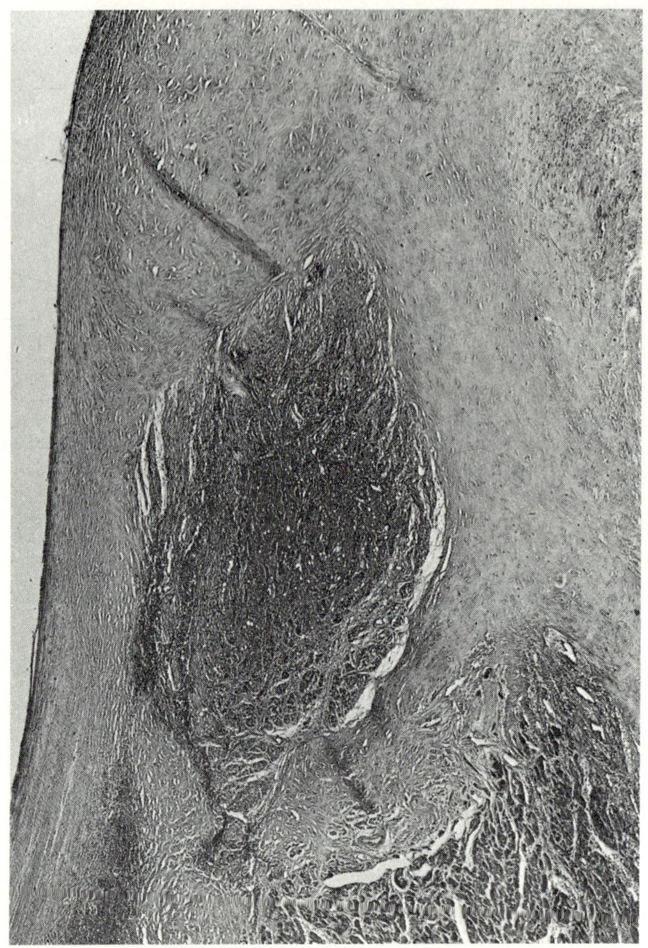

Fig. 19. Replacement of penetrating portion of AV bundle by hemorrhage related to surgery. Hematoxylin-eosin stain. × 30. (From Lev et al: Amer J Cardiol 14:464, 1964)

cent as hemorrhage clears up, or it may be permanent. Block may appear long after the operation, presumably due to fibrosis of the AV bundle related to the previous repair.

The question of the cause for the frequent occurrence of right bundle branch block in repair of VSD and tetralogy has not been answered. According to some it is due to the ventriculotomy.[78] According to others some cases are due to injury to the right bundle branch.[77]

In the Mustard procedure, the SA node and/or the atrial pathways between the SA and AV nodes may be disturbed, producing atrial arrhythmias.[79,80] In operative intervention on the aortic valve or subaortic region, the left bundle branch may be injured producing left bundle branch block.[45,81-84]

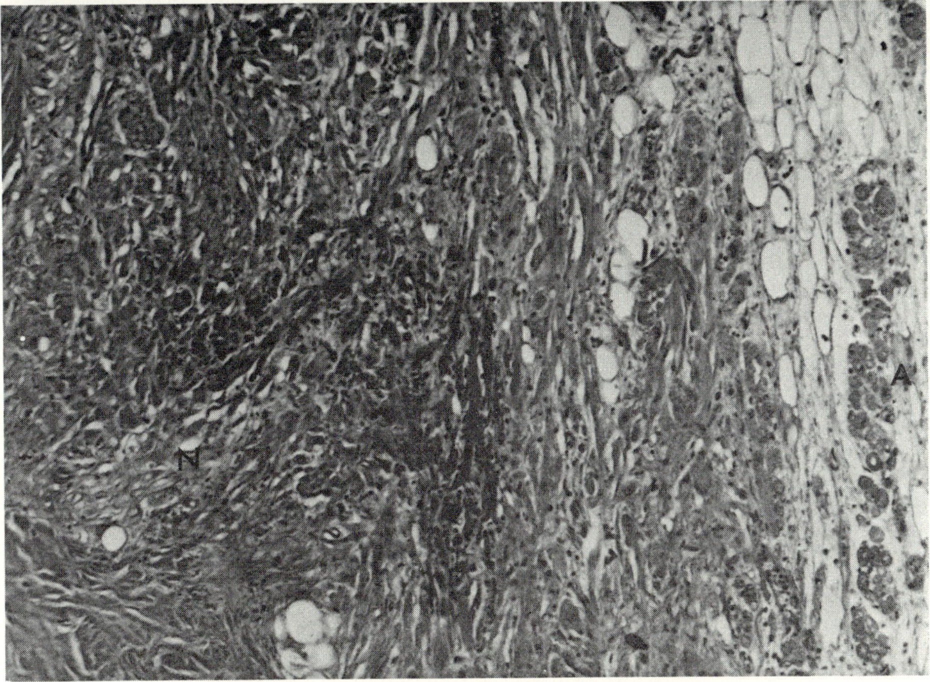

Fig. 20. Focal necrosis of AV node and recent infarct of the approaches in acute postero-septal infraction. Hematoxylin-eosin stain. × 115. A, approaches; N, AV node. (From Lev, Kinare, Pick: Circulation 42:409, 1970)

Coronary Heart Disease

Lesions may be present in the conduction system in acute myocardial infarction.[85-88] In cases in which the infarct is in the posterior wall, there may be infarction of the periphery of the SA node, infarction of the approaches to the AV node, and focal necrosis of the AV node (Fig. 20), bundle, and bundle branches. In some cases the bundle branches are severely involved, and in others there is no involvement of the conduction system at all. The above changes may be associated with atrioventricular block, which is usually evanescent if the patient recovers. Where the acute infarct is in the anteroseptal wall, infarction of the branching portion of the AV bundle and bundle branches is maximal (Fig. 21) with lesser involvement of the conduction system more proximally. This likewise may be associated with atrioventricular block which may also be evanescent if the patient recovers, but the mortality here is higher than in posterior infarction. Such pathologic change in anteroseptal infarction may involve both bundle branches, with more involvement of one than the other to produce temporary right or left bundle branch block. These electrocardiographic changes may however proceed into complete AV block.

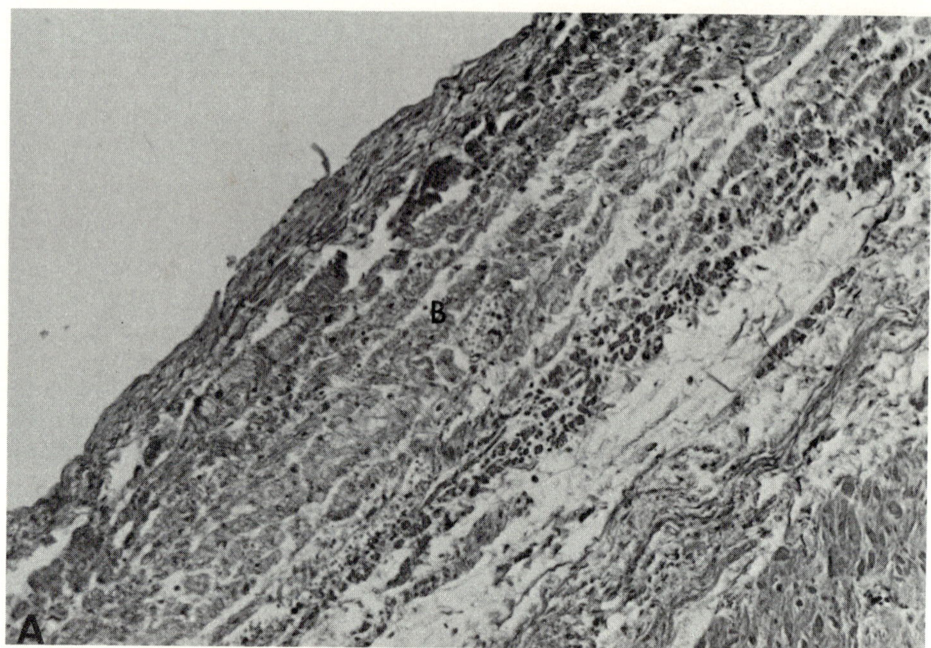

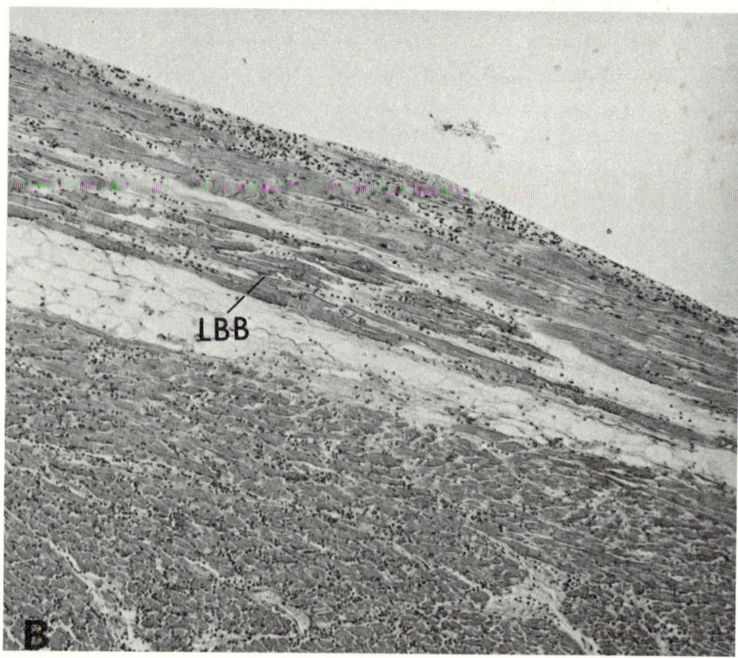

Fig. 21. Necrosis of branching bundle and left bundle branch in anteroseptal infarction. Hematoxylin-eosin stain. $\times$ 115. A. Branching bundle. B. Left bundle branch. B, AV bundle; LBB, left bundle branch. (From Lev, Kinare, Pick: Circulation 42:409, 1970)

In chronic coronary insufficiency with or without infarction, involvement of various parts of the conduction system may occur.[87, 89, 90] Thus, fibroelastosis of the SA node, the atria, and the AV node may manifest electrocardiographic changes. There may be fibrosis of the AV node and bundle of His to produce AV block. However, it is more common in chronic coronary disease to have fibroelastosis of the beginning of the left main bundle branch and of the second portion of the right bundle branch under these circumstances (Fig. 22). The fibrosis of the left main bundle is probably mechanical and that of the right bundle branch ischemic in origin. Chronic complete AV block or right or left bundle branch block may thus ensue.

The site of occlusion of the coronary arteries is not as important as the site of infarction in the production of lesions in the conduction system. Also, the pathology in the main coronary arteries may be exacerbated by arteriolosclerosis. In an occasional case arteriolosclerosis may be present alone.

Hypertensive Heart Disease

In addition to the associated coronary disease dealt with above, the effects of hypertension are both mechanical and due to arteriolosclerosis. The mechanical effect is the injury to the beginning of the left bundle branch due to stress and strain upon the fibrous skeleton of the heart. Arteriolosclerosis of the heart is often seen in hypertensives with conduction disturbances. Thus the SA, AV node, bundle, and bundle branches may be involved in arteriolosclerosis (Fig. 23).[91] This may be associated with SA block, atrial standstill, complete AV block, or right or left bundle branch block.

Rheumatic Heart Disease

In the acute phase of rheumatic heart disease there may be specific or nonspecific fibrositis, and arteriolitis of the conduction system. This may be associated with prolongation of the PR time, and rarely is responsible for complete AV block. Upon healing, all these changes disappear. A rare case of chronic AV block may be due to the fibrosis of various parts of the conduction system related to healed rheumatic fever.[90]

Where mitral stenosis and insufficiency or aortic stenosis and insufficiency ensue as sequelae of rheumatic fever, there may be an extension of the fibrotic process to the AV node, bundle, and bundle branches. This may be associated with right or left bundle branch block.[92]

Syphilitic Heart Disease

In the early part of the century, involvement of the conduction system by gummatous myocarditis was very common,[92] with the frequent production of AV block. Today it is rare.[47, 93, 94]

Maurice Lev and Saroja Bharati

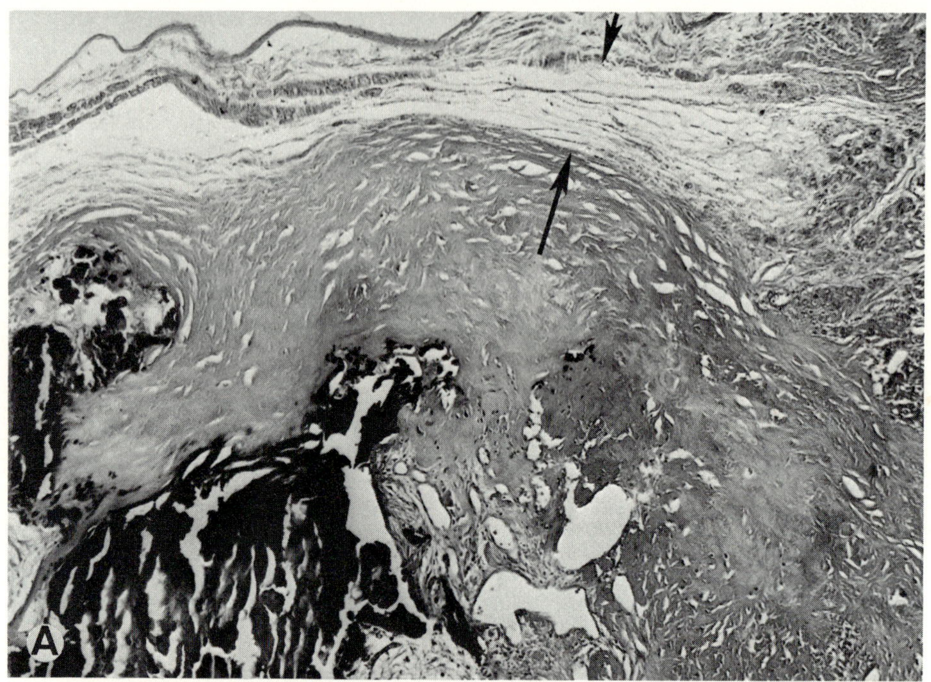

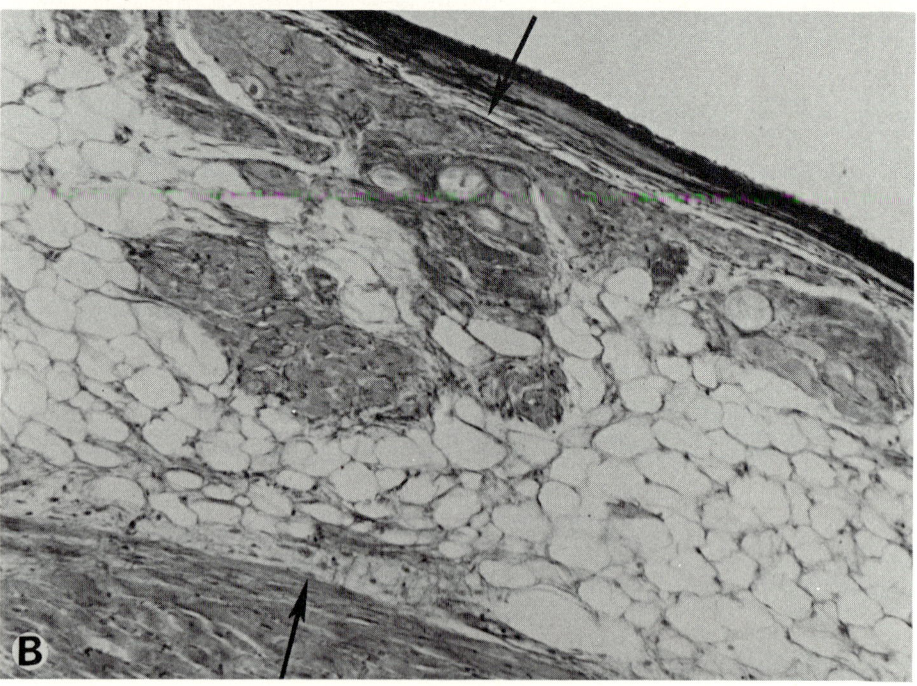

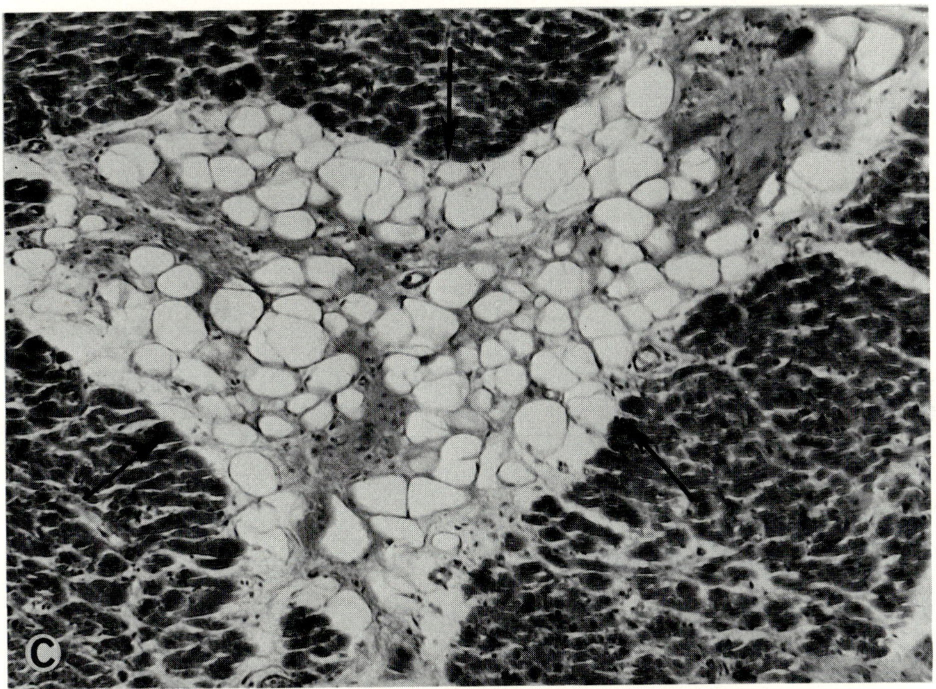

Fig. 22. Involvement of bundle branches in chronic coronary disease with chronic AV block. A. Beginning of LBB compressed by calcific mass. Hematoxylin-eosin stain. × 69. B. LBB more distally showing fatty infiltration and replacement. Weigert-van Gieson stain. × 115. C. RBB, second portion showing replacement by fibrous and fatty tissue. Hematoxylin-eosin stain. × 115. Arrows point to right and left bundle branches in various views. (From Lev, Kinare, Pick: Circulation 42:409, 1970)

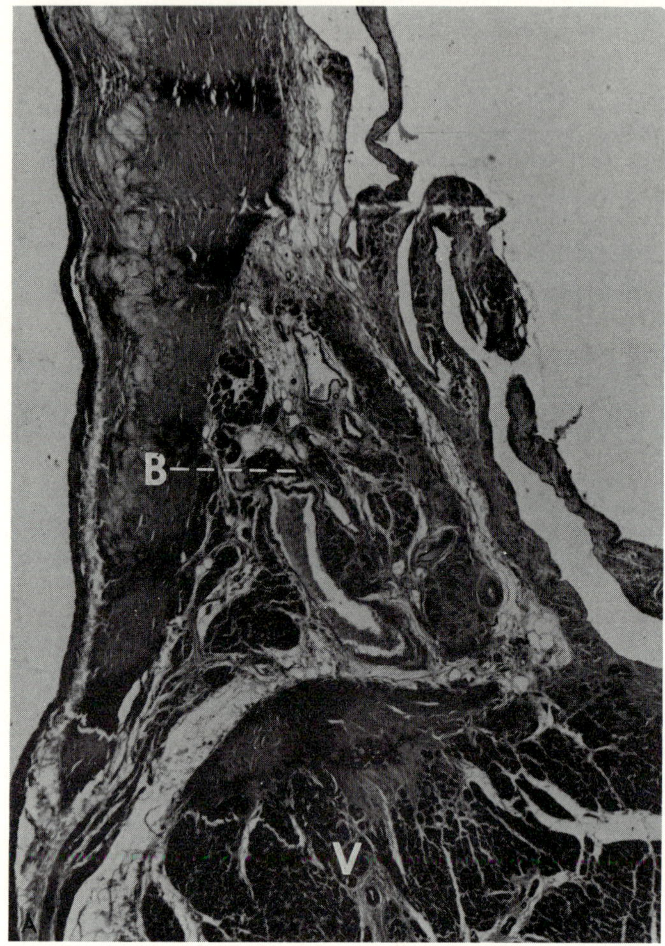

Fig. 23. Arteriolosclerotic involvement of the AV bundle with fibrosis. Hematoxylin-eosin stain. × 34. B, AV bundle; V, ventricular muscle. (From Lev, Kinare, Pick: Circulation 42:409, 1970)

Acute Inflammatory Disease of the Heart

Acute, nonspecific myocarditis associated with almost any disease may involve the conduction system (Fig. 24). The involvement is minimal in the SA node, but progressively more severe distally so that the bundle branches are maximally involved. However, any part of the conduction system may be selectively involved. There may be marked involvement of the myocardium with minimal involvement of the conduction system or vice-versa; these changes may produce temporary AV block. If the patient gets well this usually disappears. It is very

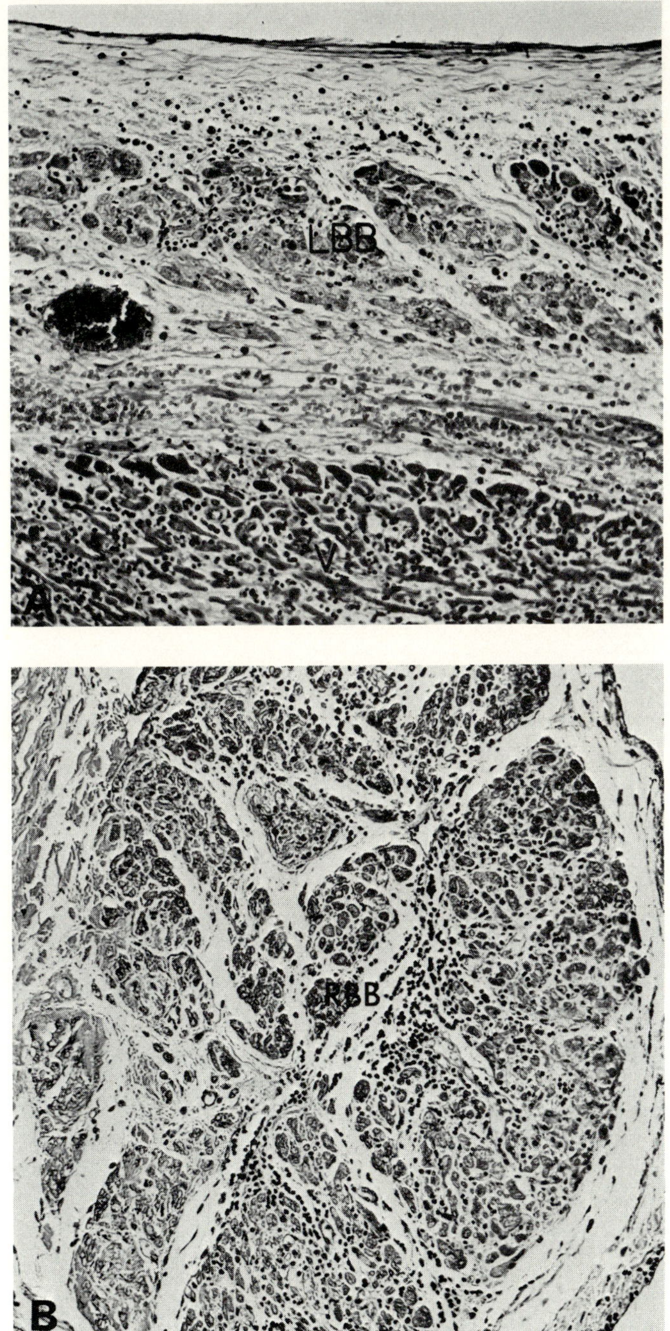

Fig. 24. Acute myocarditis involving the bundle branches. Hematoxylin-eosin stain. $\times$ 120. A. LBB. B. RBB. V, ventricular muscle.

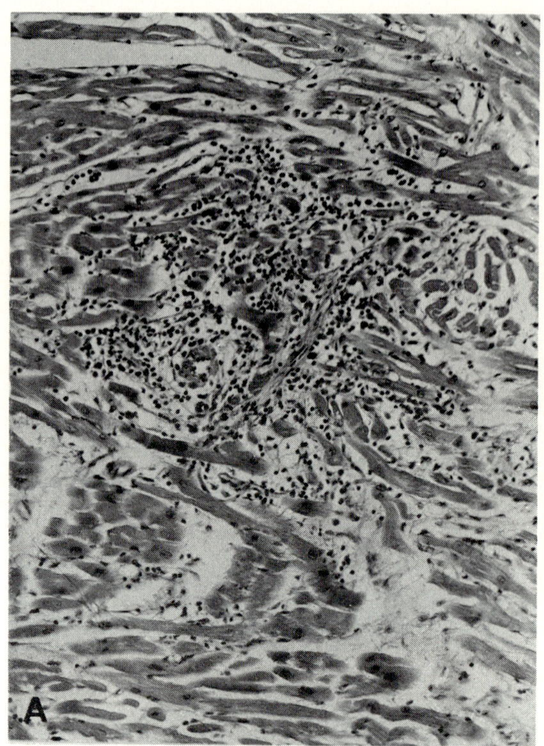

Fig. 25. Smoldering myocarditis with involvement of the conduction system and AV block. A. Myocarditis. Hematoxylin-eosin stain. × 125. B. Left bundle branch. Weigert-van Gieson stain. × 20. C. Right bundle branch. Hematoxylin-eosin stain. × 68. LBB, left bundle branch. Arrows point to right bundle branch. F, fibrosis. (From Harris, Siew, Lev: Amer J Cardiol 24:880, 1969)

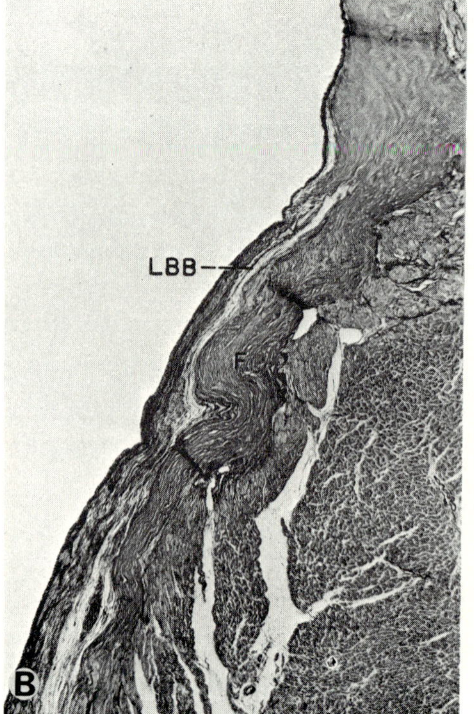

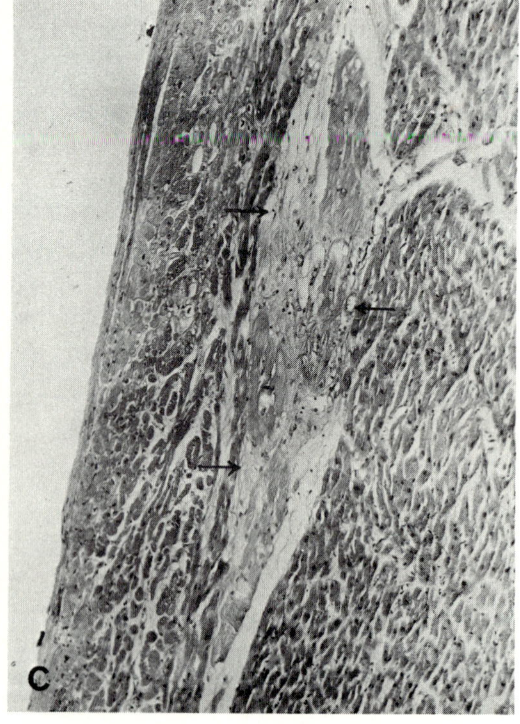

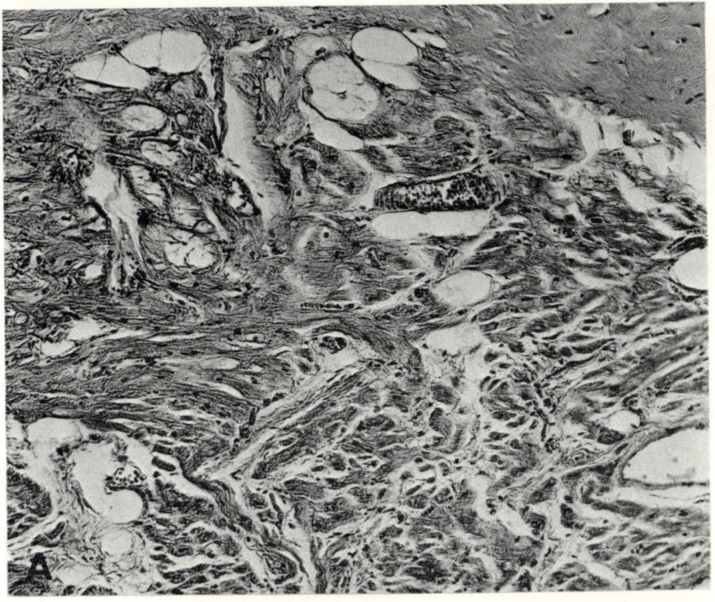

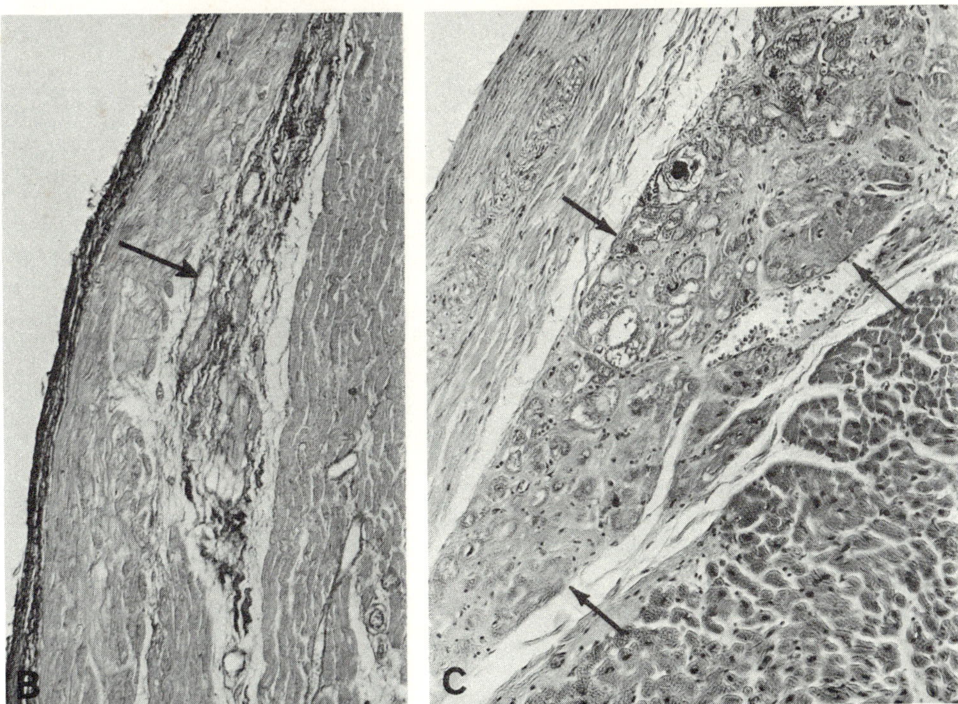

Fig. 26. Involvement of the conduction system in scleroderma with complete AV block. A. Penetrating portion of AV bundle, showing marked vacuolar degeneration of bundle cells. Hematoxylin-eosin stain. × 110. B. Right bundle branch showing fibroelastic replacement of part of bundle with degeneration of remaining cells. Weigert-van Gieson stain. × 41. C. Left bundle branch showing fibroelastic replacement of part of bundle with degeneration of remaining cells. Hematoxylin-eosin stain. × 115. (From Lev et al: Amer Heart J 72:13, 1966)

rare to find a previous or smoldering myocarditis implicated in the production of chronic conduction disturbance (Fig. 25).[95]

Complete AV block has been reported in diphtheria,[96-109] scarlet fever, [110, 111] mumps,[112, 113] German measles,[114] influenza,[104] typhoid fever,[104] pneumonia,[115] measles,[116] typhus fever,[104] malaria,[117] amebic hepatitis,[118] tuberculosis,[119, 120] varicella,[121] sarcoidosis,[122-124] whooping cough,[125] toxoplasmosis,[126] African trypanosomiasis,[127] Chagas disease,[127] and Keshan's disease.[128] Endocarditis may spread from the aortic valve to the AV bundle to produce AV block.[129-131] Likewise, acute pericarditis may involve the SA node to produce conduction disturbances.

Collagen Disease

In lupus erythematosus disseminatus,[132-136] generalized arteritis,[137] dermatomyositis,[136, 138] and scleroderma (Fig. 26),[136, 139-141] the conduction system may be involved in the basic process. This may produce complete AV block, or other conduction disturbances.

Rheumatoid Arthritis and Ankylosing Spondylitis

In rheumatoid arthritis, the diffuse myocarditis with granuloma may involve the AV bundle and bundle branches, either in the active or healed state, to produce

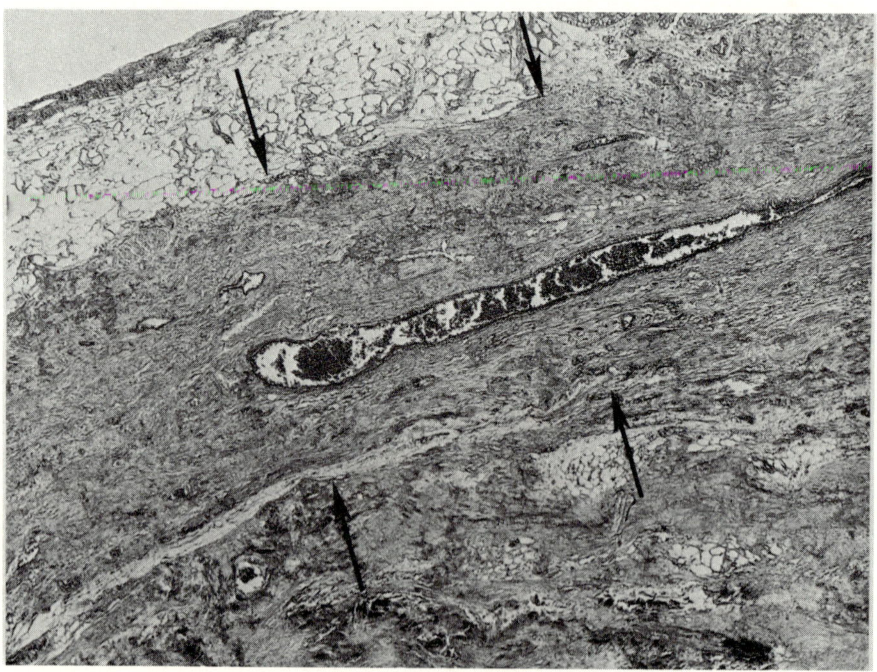

Fig. 27. Amyloid infiltration of SA node. Hematoxylin-eosin stain. $\times$ 32. Arrows point to node.

AV block. In ankylosing spondylitis, there is a spread of the aortitis to the aortic annulus, the pars membranacea, and hence to the AV node and bundle to produce AV block.[142-149]

Amyloid Disease

In the older age group, primary amyloidosis [150-152] is common and amyloid infiltration may involve the SA node, the atria, and the bundle branches (Fig. 27). The AV node and AV bundle are less commonly involved. This may manifest itself as complete AV block, or as other electrocardiographic abnormalities.

Fatty Infiltration

In older age groups fatty infiltration (Fig. 28) is seen frequently about and in the SA node, at the approaches to the AV node, within the bundle of His, and

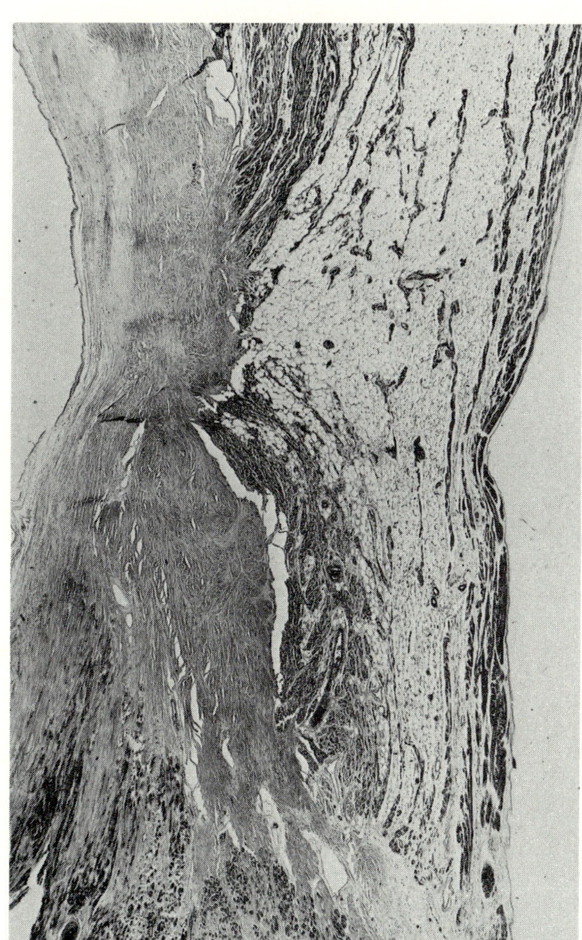

Fig. 28. Fatty infiltration and separation of AV node. Hematoxylin-eosin stain.   × 15. (From Lev, Widran, Erickson: Arch Path 52:73, 1951)

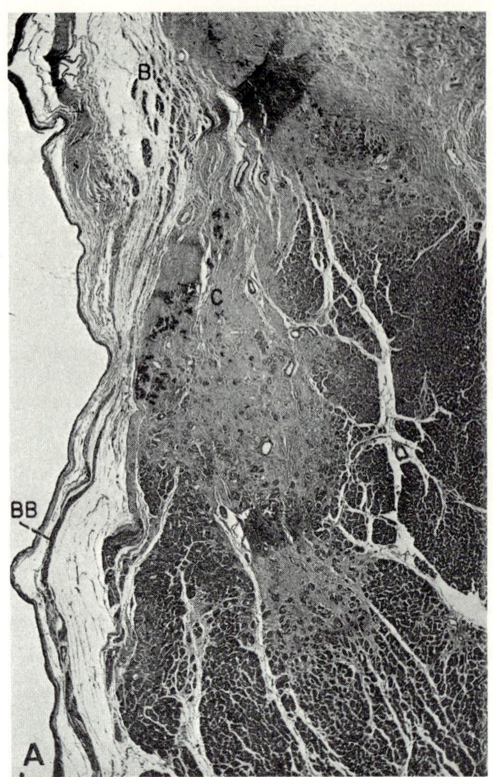

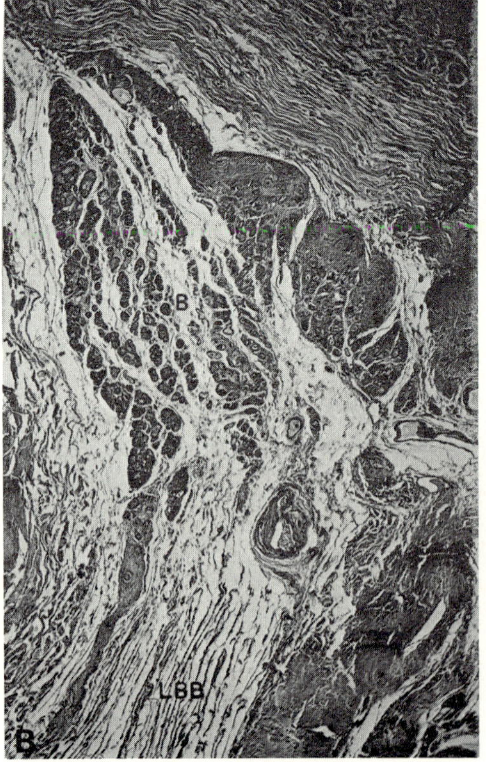

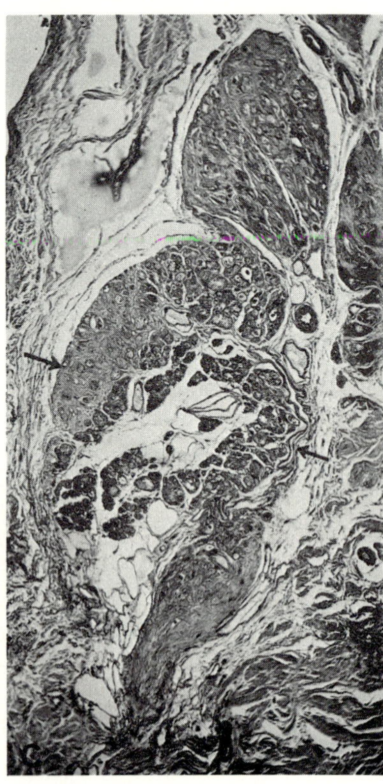

Fig. 29. The AV bundle and bundle branches in a case of sclerosis of the left side of the cardiac skeleton with complete AV block. Note the destruction of AV bundle in "A" and "B" and fibrosis and necrosis of right bundle branch in "C." Hematoxylin-eosin stain. A, × 27; B, × 89; C, × 89. B, AV bundle; BB and LBB, left bundle branch; C, fibrocalcareous lesion. (From Lev: Prog Cardiovasc Dis 6:317, 1964)

in the bundle branches beyond that which is found in ordinary aging. The functional significance of this is not clear. It is often associated with electrocardiographic abnormality, but even marked involvement may not show any conduction effects. Where the fatty tissue takes the place of conductive tissue, as is often seen in the left bundle branch, it is usually of functional importance. A rare case of AV block may be due to separation of the AV node by fatty tissue in an older person.

Sclerosis of the Left Side of the Cardiac Skeleton

Beginning about the age of 40, the summit of the ventricular septum, the mitral annulus, the pars membranacea, the aortic annulus, and sinuses of Valsalva show degenerative changes. These consist in fibrosis, and hyalinization with or without calcification. We have called this degenerative process "sclerosis of the left side of the cardiac skeleton" (Fig. 29).[22] We consider this a process of stress and strain in a high pressure system. These changes may involve by pressure the AV node, bundle, and bundle branches. A favorite spot for such involvement is the bifurcation and the beginning of the right and left bundle branches. The left bundle branch may also be separated from the main bundle while the second part of the right bundle branch is replaced by a fibroelastic process, the cause of which is unknown. These changes may produce complete AV block or left bundle branch block.

Tumors

Primary or secondary tumors of the heart [153-159] may invade the conduction system. Such invasion has been described in myeloma, Hodgkin's disease, carcinoma, and sarcoma. One of the primary tumors of the heart which merits attention is the mesothelioma of the AV node (Fig. 30). This consists of cyst-like formations with intracapillary projections and collections of flat or polygonal cells with no evidence of anaplasia. They involve the distal part of the atrial septum replacing the AV node. The process usually stops at the AV bundle. This produces partial progressing to complete AV block.

Other Disease Processes and Lesions Affecting the Conduction System

In hemochromatosis,[160-162] pigment may be deposited in the conduction system to produce AV block. Hyperthyroidism,[104,163] myxedema,[164] Paget's disease,[165] gout,[166] cor pulmonale,[89] lead poisoning,[167] hypocalcemia,[168] hyperkalemia,[169] thrombotic thrombocytopenic purpura,[170] transfusion sclerosis,[90] external ophthalmoplegia,[171] generalized lentigo,[172] progressive ophthalmoplegia with retinitis pigmentosa,[173] polymyositis,[174] dystrophia myotonica,[175-177] progressive muscular dystrophy,[178] limb girdle dystrophy,[179] and peroneal muscular atrophy [180] may all involve the conduction system and may produce AV block. Uremia [181] may be associated with changes in the conduction system. Trauma may also produce lesions of the SA and AV node and bundle.[182-185]

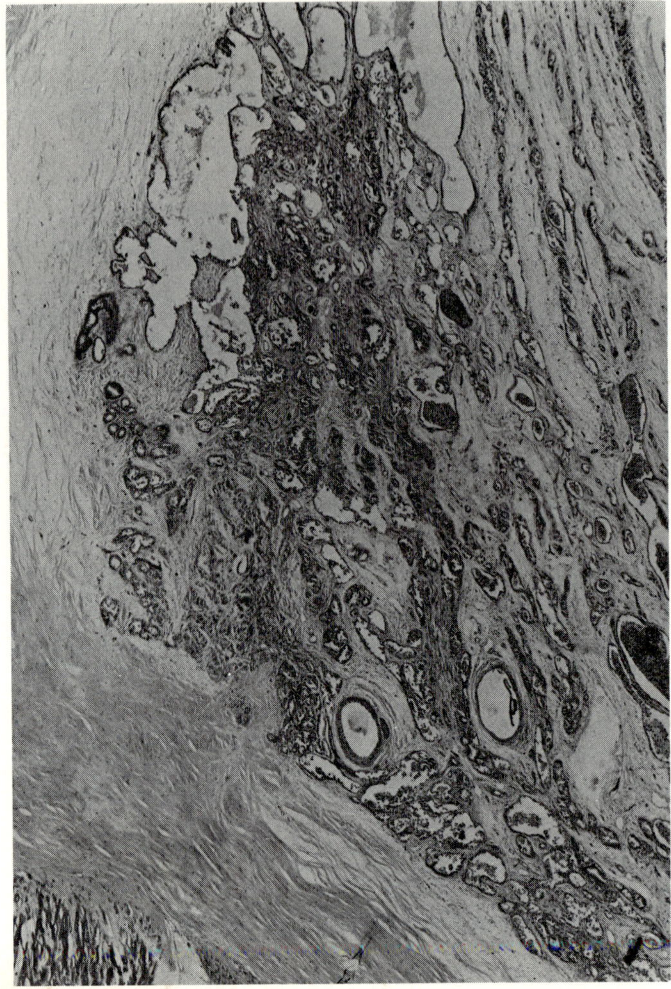

Fig. 30. Mesothelioma of AV node. Hematoxylin-eosin stain. $\times$ 15.

Correlation of Lesions of the Conduction System with Electrocardiography and His Bundle Recordings

It is now clear that chronic acquired AV block is in most cases associated with lesions of the branching bundle and of both bundle branches.[186, 188, 190] It is caused in most cases by sclerosis of the left side of the cardiac skeleton (in some cases exacerbated by coronary disease) or it is idiopathic. In this so-called primary block, either the beginning of the left bundle branch and the second portion of the right bundle branch are involved, or the branching bundle and the beginning of the left bundle branch show lesions, or the beginning of the left bundle branch and the periphery of both bundle branches are involved. A lesser number of cases are due to chronic coronary insufficiency caused by either athero- or arteriolosclerosis, aortic disease, cardiomyopathy, previous myocarditis, or other diseases.

The pattern of incomplete right bundle branch block is in most cases not associated with lesions of the right bundle branch. It is probably related to right ventricular hypertrophy. This is seen especially in congenital heart disease, mitral, or pulmonary disease. The pattern of permanent complete right bundle branch block is usually associated with lesions of the right bundle branch (Fig. 31). This is found especially in coronary disease, hypertensive, and aortic disease, but sometimes in congenital, mitral, and pulmonary disease. The pattern of permanent complete left

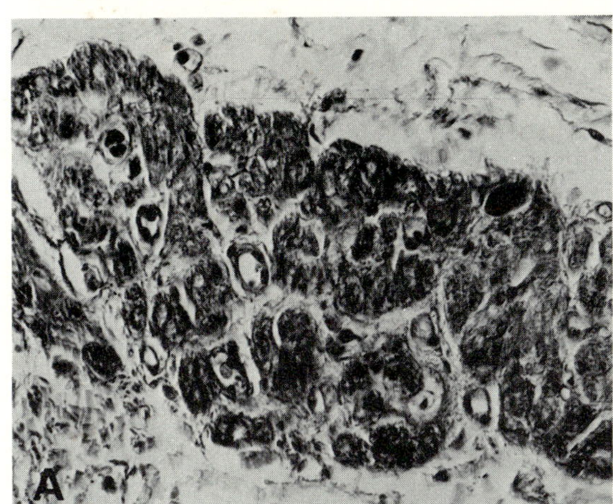

Fig. 31. Right bundle branch lesions in right bundle branch block. A. Acute necrosis. Hematoxylin-eosin stain. × 230. (From Lev, Unger: Arch Path 60:502, 1955) B. Fibroelastosis. Weigert-van Gieson stain. × 61. Arrows point to right bundle branch. (From Lev et al: Amer Heart J 61:593, 1961)

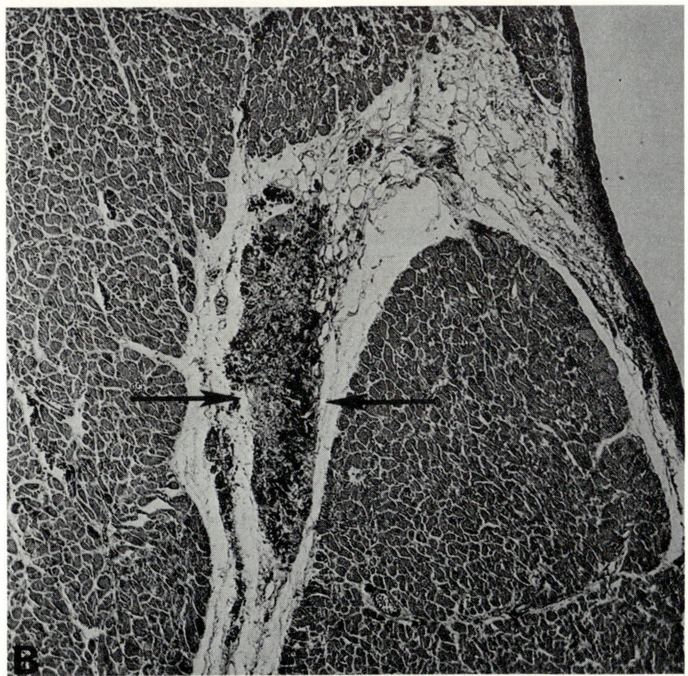

bundle branch block is usually associated with lesions of the left bundle branch. This is seen in aortic, coronary, or hypertensive heart disease. The pattern of incomplete left bundle branch block is also usually associated with lesions of the left bundle branch (Fig. 32). This again occurs in aortic, coronary, or hypertensive heart disease. The pattern of bilateral bundle branch block is usually associated with lesions of both bundle branches.[186-189, 191-193]

From the standpoint of His bundle recordings,[91, 194] only tentative statements can be made at present, since not enough correlative work has been done in this field. P-A prolongation is usually associated with sinus node and/or atrial pathology. However, a normal P-A time does not exclude pathologic changes in these structures. Prolonged A-H time is usually associated with pathologic change in the

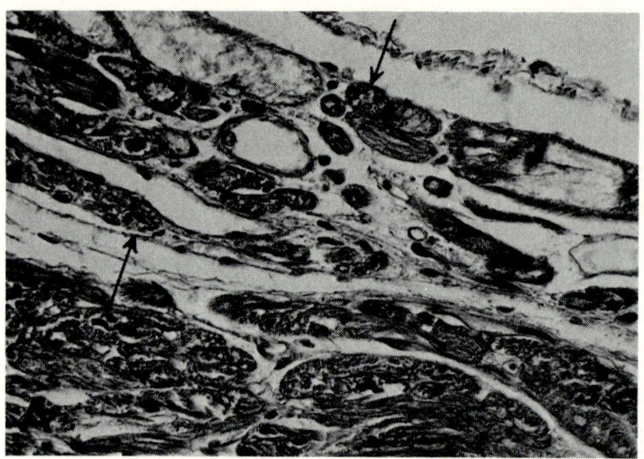

Fig. 32. Left bundle lesions in left bundle branch block. A. Acute necrosis. (From Lev, Unger; Arch Path 60:502, 1955) Hematoxylin-eosin stain. × 115. B. Fibroelastosis with space replacement. Arrows point to left bundle branch. B, AV bundle. Weigert-van Gieson stain. × 6.

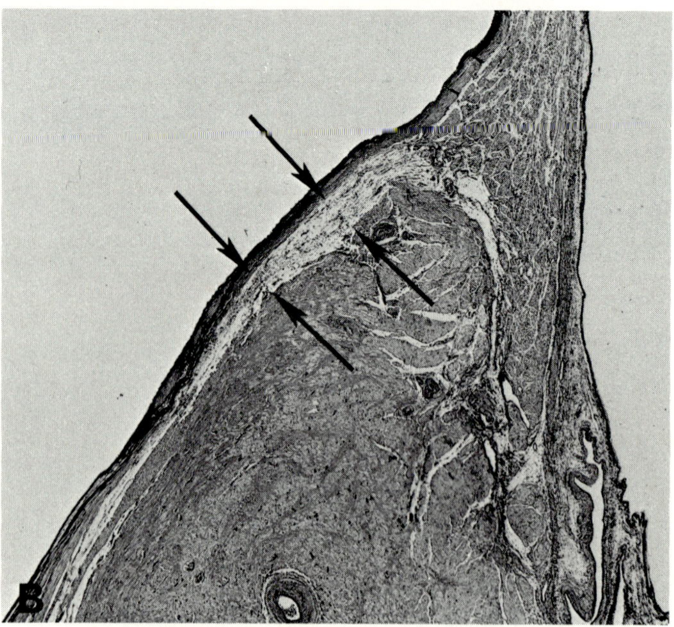

AV node and its approaches. Prolonged H time is associated with lesions in the AV bundle. Split His potentials are likewise associated with a lesion in the bundle of His. Prolonged H-V time is usually associated with bundle branch disease. Unilateral bundle branch block with prolonged H-V time is usually associated with lesions in both bundle branches.

Acknowledgments

We are indebted to Mr. Milorad Ralevich for his technical assistance and to Florence Kotal for her assistance in the preparation of this paper.

References

1. Lev M, Watne AL: Method for routine histopathologic study of the sinoatrial node. Arch Path 57:168, 1954
2. Lev M: Aging changes in the human S-A node. J Gerontol 9:1, 1954
3. Lev M: The conduction system In Gould SE (ed): Pathology of the Heart, 3rd ed. Springfield, Ill, Thomas, 1968, p 180
4. James TN: The connecting pathways between the sinus node and A-V node and between the right and the left atrium in the human heart. Amer Heart J, 66:498, 1963
5. Truex RC, Smythe MQ: Recent observations on the human cardiac conduction system, with special considerations of the atrioventricular node and bundle. In Taccardi B and Marchetti G (eds) Electrophysiology of the Heart. New York, Pergamon Press, 1964
6. Merideth J, Titus JL: The anatomic atrial connections between sinus and A-V node. Circulation 37:566, 1968
7. Spach MS, Lieberman M, Scott JG, et al: Excitation sequences of the atrial septum and the AV node in isolated hearts of the dog and rabbit. Cir Res 29:156, 1971
8. Widran J, Lev M: The dissection of the human AV node, bundle and branches. Circulation 4:863, 1951
9. Erickson EE, and Lev, M. Aging changes in the human atrioventricular node, bundle and bundle branches. J Gerontol 7:1, 1952
10. Uhley HN, Rivkin LM: Visualization of the left branch of the human atrioventricular bundle. Circulation 20:419, 1959
11. Lev M, Lerner R: The theory of Kent. A histologic study of the normal atrioventricular communications of the human heart. Circulation 12:176, 1955
12. Truex RC, Bishof JK, Hoffman EL: Accessory atrioventricular muscle bundles of the developing human heart. Anat Rec 131:45, 1958
13. Mahaim I, Winston MR: Recherches d'anatomie comparée et de pathologie expérimentale sur les connexions hautes du faisceau de His-Tawara. Cardiologia 5:189, 1941
14. Lev M, McMillan JB: A semiquantitative histopathologic method for the study of the entire heart for clinical and electrocardiographic correlations. Amer Heart J 58:140, 1959
15. Lev M, Rowlatt UF, Rimoldi HJA: Pathologic methods for study of congenitally malformed heart. Methods for electrocardiographic and physiologic correlation. Arch Path 72:493, 1961
16. Davies MJ: Pathology of Conducting Tissue of the Heart. New York, Appleton, 1971
17. Lev M: The pathology of atrioventricular block. Cardiovasc Clin 4:159, 1972

18. Lev M: The pathogenesis of congenital atrioventricular block. Prog Cardiovasc Dis 15:145, 1972

19. Lev M: The conduction system in congenital heart disease. Amer J Cardiol 21:619, 1968

20. Lev M: The anatomic basis for disturbances in conduction and cardiac arrhythmias Prog Cardiovasc Dis 2:360, 1960

21. Lev M: The pathology of complete atrioventricular block. Prog Cardiovasc Dis 6:317, 1964

22. Lev M: The normal anatomy of the conduction system in man and its pathology in atrioventricular block. Ann NY Acad Sci 111:817, 1964

23. Lev M: Anatomic basis for atrioventricular block. Amer J Med 37:742, 1964

24. Lev M: The architecture of the conduction system in congenital heart disease. I. Common atrioventricular orifice. Arch Path 65:174, 1958

25. Lev M: The architecture of the conduction system in congenital heart disease. III. Ventricular septal defect. Arch Path 70:529, 1960

26. Reemtsma K, Copenhaver WM: Anatomic studies of the cardiac conduction system in congenital malformations of the heart. Circulation 17:271, 1958

27. Truex RC, Bishof, JK: Conduction system in human hearts with interventricular septal defects. J Thorac Surg 35:421, 1958

28. Urumova E: Der Verlauf des Reizleitungssystems bei Ventrikelseptum-defekt. Arch Kreislaufforsch 31:1, 1959–1960

29. Richter M: Die Topographie des Ventrikel-Septum Defekts und seine Beziehung zum Reizleitungssystem. Thoraxchirurgie 7:456, 1960

30. Rossi L: Studio istologico sulla patogenesi del blocco A-V in 19 casi e osservazioni sul sistema A-V in 5 cuori con malformazioni congenite. Minerva Cardioangiol 12:329, 1964

31. Titus JL, Daugherty GW, Edwards JE: Anatomy of the atrioventricular conduction system in ventricular septal defect. Circulation 28:72, 1963

32. Visiolo O, Baragan J, Lenègre J: Les voies de la conduction intracardiaque dans les cardiopathies par anomalie congénitale du septum. Arch Mal Coeur 55:1024, 1962

33. Lev M: The architecture of the conduction system in congenital heart disease. II. Tetralogy of Fallot. Arch Path 67:572, 1959

34. Hasegawa T: Studies on the conduction system in congenital malformations of the heart, especially of tetralogy of Fallot. Jap Heart J 2:377, 1961

35. Lev M, Licata RH, May RC: The conduction system in mixed levocardia with ventricular inversion (corrected transposition). Circulation 28:232, 1963

36. Lev M, Silverman J, Fitzmaurice F.M, et al: Lack of connection between the atria and the more peripheral conduction system in congenital atrioventricular block. Amer J Cardiol 27:481, 1971

37. Lev M, Cuadros H, Paul MH: Interruption of the atrioventricular bundle with congenital atrioventricular block. Circulation 43:703, 1971

38. Lev M, Fielding RT, Zaeske D: Mixed levocardia with ventricular inversion (corrected transposition) with complete atrioventricular block. A histopathologic study of the conduction system. Amer J Cardiol 12:875, 1963

39. Wallgren A, Winblad S: Congenital heart block. Acta Paediatr 20:175, 1938

40. Lev M, Paul MH, Cassels DE: Complete atrioventricular block associated with atrial septal defect of the fossa ovalis (secundum) type. A histopathologic study of the conduction system. Amer J Cardiol 19:266, 1967

41. Yater WM: Congenital heart block. Review of the literature; report of a case with incomplete heterotaxy; the electrocardiogram in dextrocardia. Amer J Dis Child 38:112, 1929

42. Linder E, Landtman B, Tuuteri L, Hjelt L: Congenital complete heart block. II. Histology of the conduction system. Ann Paediatr Fenniae 11:11, 1965

43. Huntingford PJ: The aetiology and significance of congenital heart block. (The report of a case studied by serial section of the heart.) J Obstet Gynaecol Brit Comm 67:259, 1960

44. Yater WM, Leaman WG, Cornell VH: Congenital heart block. Report of the third case of complete heart block studied by serial sections through the conduction system. JAMA 102:1660, 1934

45. Hudson REB: Surgical pathology of the conduction system of the heart. Brit Heart J 29:646, 1967

46. Cohn AE, Lewis T: Auricular fibrillation and complete heart-block. A description of a case of Adams-Stokes syndrome, including the postmortem examination. Heart 4:15, 1912–1913

47. Harris A, Davies M, Redwood D, Leatham A, Siddons H: Aetiology of chronic heart block. A clinico-pathological correlation in 65 cases. Brit Heart J 31:206, 1969

48. Donoso, E, Braunwald, E, Jick S, Grishman A: Congenital heart block. Amer J Med 20:869, 1956

49. Bernard R, Gérard R, Gras A: Les hypoplasies congénitales de l'aorte. (A propos d'une observation avec bloc auriculo-ventriculaire associé chez un nourrisson de 18 mois.) Arch Fr Pédiatr 17:921, 1960

50. Bernreiter M, O'Connell F: Congenital heart block. Report of a case. JAMA 150:792, 1952

51. Clark RJ, Firminger HI: Coarctation of the aorta associated with Adams-Stokes syndrome, complete heart block and bicuspid calcareous aortic valve. New Eng J Med 24:710, 1949

52. Wilson JG, Grant RT: A case of congenital malformation of the heart in an infant associated with partial heart block. Heart 12:295, 1925–1926

53. Dickson RW, Jones JP: Congenital heart block in an infant with associated multiple congenital cardiac malformations. Amer J Dis Child 75:81, 1948

54. Aitchison JD, Duthie RJ, Young JS: Palpable venous pulsations in a case of transposition of both arterial trunks and complete heart block. Brit Heart J 17:63, 1955

55. Wyss S, Töndury G: Zum kongenitalen totalen Atrioventrikular-Block. Z Kreislaufforsch 52:478, 1963

56. Jennings GH: Two contrasted cases of complete heart block observed over many years. Brit Heart J 33:50, 1971

57. Hoekenga MT: Complete heart block in an infant associated with multiple congenital cardiac malformations. Amer J Dis Child 69:231, 1945

58. Belobradek Z, Herout V, Jurkovic V: Isolated tricuspid insufficiency combined with Adams-Stokes syndrome. Acta Cardiol (Brux) 14:486, 1959

59. Gilgenkrantz JM, Cherrier F, Petitier H, et al: Cardiomyopathie observative du ventricule gauche avec bloc auriculo-ventriculaire complet. Considérations therapeutiques. Arch Mal Coeur 61:439, 1968

60. Bawa YS, Gupta PD, Goel BG: Complete heart block in Marfan's syndrome. Brit Heart J 26:148, 1964

61. Moretti GF, Staeffen J, Bertrand E, Broustet A: Bloc auriculo-ventriculaire complet dans le syndrome de Marfan. Presse Méd 72:605, 1964

62. Chopra KL, Krishnan S, Joseph PP: Intermittent bundle branch block and complete heart block in Marfan's syndrome. Indian Heart J 22:53, 1970

63. Varriale P, Rossi P, Grace WJ: Congenital absence of the left pericardium and complete heart block. Chest 52:405, 1967

64. Morison A: The auriculo-ventricular node in a malformed heart, with remarks on its nature, connexions and distribution. J Anat Physiol 47:459, 1913

65. Lev M, Licata RH, Arcilla R: A congenitally abnormal left bundle branch. Arch Path 76:182, 1963

66. Yater WM, Shapiro MJ: Congenital displacement of the tricuspid valve (Ebstein's disease). Review and report of a case with electrocardiographic abnormalities and detailed histologic study of the conduction system. Ann Intern Med 11:1043, 1937

67. Lev M, Gibson S, Miller RA: Ebstein's disease with Wolff-Parkinson-White syndrome. Amer Heart J 49:724, 1955

68. Coakley JB: Congenital absence of the right branch of the bundle of His. Brit Heart J 13:148, 1951

69. Botti G, Visioli O: Assenza congenita della branca destra del fascio di His con blocco di branca omologo. G Clin Med 38:271, 1957

70. Lenègre J, Deglaude L, Hazim A: Étude clinique, électrique et anatomique d'un cas de bloc de branche. Arch Mal Coeur 38:154, 1945

71. Lev M, Kennamer R, Prinzmetal M, deMesquita QH: A histopathologic study of the atrioventricular communications in two hearts with Wolff-Parkinson-White syndrome. Circulation 24:41, 1961

72. Lev M, Sodi-Pallares D, Friedland C: A histopathologic study of the atrioventricular communications in a case of WPW with incomplete left bundle branch block. Amer Heart J 66:399, 1963

73. Truex RC, Bishof JK, Downing DF: Accessory atrioventricular muscle fibers. II. Cardiac conduction system in a human specimen with Wolff-Parkinson-White syndrome. Anat Rec 137:417, 1960

74. Rosenberg HS, Klima T, McNamara DG, Leachman RD: Atrioventricular communication in the Wolff-Parkinson-White syndrome. Amer J Clin Path 56:79, 1971

75. Lev M, Leffler WB, Langendorf R, Pick A: The anatomic findings in a case of ventricular pre-excitation (WPW) terminating in complete atrioventricular block. Circulation 34:718, 1966

76. Miller RA, Mehta AB, Coronel A, Lev M: Congenital atrioventricular block with multiple ectopic pacemakers. Electrocardiographic and conduction system correlation. Amer J Cardiol 30:554, 1972

77. Lev M, Fell EH, Arcilla R, Weinberg MH: Surgical injury to the conduction system in ventricular septal defect. Amer J Cardiol 14:464, 1964

78. Gelband H, Waldo AL, Kaiser GA, et al: Etiology of right bundle-branch block in patients undergoing total correction of tetralogy of Fallot. Circulation 44:1022, 1971

79. El-Said G, Rosenberg HS, Mullins CE, et al: Dysrhythmias after Mustard's operation for transposition of the great arteries. Amer J Cardiol 30:526, 1972

80. Isaacson R, Titus JL, Merideth J, Feldt RH, and McGoon DC: Apparent interruption of atrial conduction pathways after surgical repair of transposition of great arteries. Amer J Cardiol 30:533, 1972

81. Sayed HM: Complete heart block following open heart surgery. J Cardiovasc Surg 6:426, 1965

82. Hurwitz RA, Riemenschneider PA, Moss AJ: Chronic postoperative heart block in children. Amer J Cardiol 21:185, 1968

83. Smith TW, McFarland JC, Buckley MJ, Austen WG: Late recovery of conduction following surgically induced atrioventricular block. Ann Thorac Surg 9:372, 1970

84. Averill KH, Vogel JHK, Pryor R, Blount SG Jr: Complete heart block following intracardiac surgery. Reversion to normal sinus rhythm after twenty-five months. Amer J Cardiol 14:556, 1964

85. Blondeau M, Rizzon P, Lenègre J: Les troubles de la conduction auriculo-ventriculaire dans l'infarctus myocardique recent. II. Étude anatomique. Arch Mal Coeur 54:1104, 1961

86. James TN: Arrhythmias and conduction disturbances in acute myocardial infarction. Amer Heart J 64:416, 1962

87. Lev M, Kinare SG, Pick A: The pathogenesis of atrioventricular block in coronary disease. Circulation 42:409, 1970

88. Harper JR, Harley A, Hackel DB, Estes EH Jr: Coronary artery disease and major conduction disturbances. A pathologic study designed to correlate vascular and conduction system abnormalities with electrocardiogram. Amer Heart J 77:411, 1969

89. Lenègre J: Les blocs auriculo-ventriculaires complets chronique. Étude des causes et des lésions à propos de 37 cas. Mal Cardiovasc 3:311, 1962

90. Davies MJ: A histological study of the conduction system in complete heart block. Pathol 94:351, 1967

91. Rosen KM, Rahimtoola SM, Gunnar RM, Lev M: Site of heart block as defined by His bundle recording. Pathologic correlations in three cases. Circulation 45:965, 1972

92. Mahaim I: Les Maladies Organiques du Faisceau de His-Tawara. Paris, Masson, 1931

93. Braunstein AL, Bass JB, Thomas S: Gummatous myocarditis and aneurysm of the left ventricle, with nodal tachycardia, and, subsequently bundle branch block. Report of a case. Amer Heart J 19:613, 1940

94. Ramamoorthy K, Sahiar KH, Golwalla AF: Complete atrioventricular heart block due to gumma of the interventricular septum. Amer J Cardiol 10:879, 1962

95. Harris R, Siew S, Lev M: Smoldering myocarditis with intermittent complete A-V block and Stokes-Adams Syndrome. A histopathological and electrocardiographic study of "Trisfascicular" bundle branch block. Amer J Cardiol 24:880, 1969

96. Fleming GB, Kennedy AM: A case of complete heart block in diphtheria, with an account of post-mortem findings. Heart 2:77, 1910–1911

97. Marvin HM: The effect of diphtheria on the cardiovascular system. I. The heart in faucial diphtheria. Amer J Dis Child 29:433, 1925

98. Stecher RM: Electrocardiographic changes in diphtheria. I. Complete auriculo-ventricular dissociation. Amer Heart J 4:545, 1929

99. Neubauer C: Heart block in diphtheria. Brit J Child Dis 40:93, 1943

100. Butler S, Levine SA: Diphtheria as a cause of the late heart-block. Amer Heart J 5:592, 1930

101. Kocher RA: Fatal myocarditis with complete heart block from diphtheria. Calif Med 66:27, 1947

102. Massey FC, Walker WJ: Complete atrioventricular block in diphtheritic myocarditis. Report of a case with serial electrocardiographic tracings. Arch Intern Med 81:9, 1948

103. Engle MA: Recovery from complete heart block in diphtheria. Pediatrics 3:222, 1949

104. Wright JC, Hejtmancik MR, Herrmann GR, Shields AH: A clinical study of complete heart block. Amer Heart J 52:369, 1956

105. Visioli O, Botti G: Contributo allo studio anatomo-clinico delle dissociazioni atrio-ventricolari: Dissociazioni A-V completa ad alta frequenza atriale e ventricolare da emorragia interruttiva del tronco commune. Riv Anat Patol Oncol 12:665, 1957

106. Hoel J: Reappearance of complete heart block years after diphtheritic myocardial disease. Acta Med Scand 160:237, 1958

107. Claman HN: Progressive myocardial damage following recovery from diphtheria. A case showing development of complete heart block. Amer J Cardiol 9:790, 1962

108. James TN, Reynolds EW Jr: Pathology of the cardiac conduction system in a case of diphtheria associated with atrial arrhythmias and heart block. Circulation 28:263, 1963

109. Morales AR, Vichitbandha P, Chandruang P, Evans H, Bourgeois CH: Pathological features of cardiac conduction disturbances in diphtheric myocarditis. Arch Path 91:1, 1971

110. Bernstein M: Auriculoventricular dissociation following scarlet fever. Report of a case. Amer Heart J 16:582, 1938

111. Paul WD, Rhomberg C, Cole J: Transitory A-V block occurring during scarlet fever. Amer Heart J 31:138, 1946

112. Rosenberg DH: Electrocardiographic changes in epidemic parotitis (mumps). Proc Soc Exp Biol Med 58:9, 1945

113. Thompson WM Jr, Noland TR: Atrioventricular dissociation associated with Adams-Stokes syndrome presumably due to mumps myocarditis. J Pediatr 68: 601, 1966

114. Logue RB, Hanson JF: Complete heart block in German measles. Amer Heart J 30:205, 1945

115. Swift EV, Smith HL: Complete heart block associated with pneumonia and peritonitis. Review of the literature and report of a case in which a lesion was demonstrated histologically. JAMA 109:2038, 1937

116. Clark NS: Complete heart block in children. Report of three cases possibly attributable to measles. Arch Dis Child 23:156, 1948

117. Kanatsoulis A: Les troubles du faisceau de His d'origine palustre. Arch Mal Coeur 51:250, 1958

118. Rawkins MD, Konstam GLS: Complete heart block associated with amoebic hepatitis. Normal rhythm restored with emetine. Lancet 2:152, 1949

119. Menon TB, Rao CKP: Tuberculosis of the myocardium causing complete heart block. Amer J Pathol 21:1193, 1945

120. Kinare SG, Deshmukh MM: Complete atrioventricular block due to myocardial tuberculosis. Report of a case. Arch Path 88:684, 1969

121. Morales AR, Adelman S, Fine G: Varicella myocarditis. A case of sudden death. Arch Path 91:29, 1971

122. Botti RE, Young FE: Myocardial sarcoid, complete heart block and aortic stenosis. Ann Intern Med 51:811, 1959

123. Phinney AO, Jr: Sarcoid of the myocardial septum with complete heart block. Report of two cases. Amer Heart J 62:270, 1961

124. Johansen A: Isolated myocarditis versus myocardial sarcoidosis. Acta Pathol Microbiol Scand 67:15, 1966

125. Johansson BW: Adams-Stokes syndrome. A review and follow-up study of forty-two cases. Amer J Cardiol 8:76, 1961

126. Shee JC: Stokes-Adams attacks due to toxoplasma myocarditis. Brit Heart J 26:151, 1964

127. Bertrand E, Sentilhes L, Baudin L, Barabe P, Aye H: Troubles de conduction cardiaque dans la trypanosomiase humaine Africaine a trypanosoma Gambiense. Bull Soc Pathol Exot 61:613, 1968

128. Lu YJ, Wang KL: Pathologic changes of the conduction system of the heart in 43 cases of Keshan disease. China's Med (Peking) 83:430, 1964

129. Lenègre J, Himbert J: Les troubles de la conduction intracardique dans les endocardites à hémocultures négatives. Bull Soc Med Hop Paris 113:279, 1962

130. Meshel JC, Wachtel HL, Graham J: Bacterial endocarditis presenting as heart block. Amer J Med 48:254, 1970

131. Wang K, Gobel F, Gleason DF, Edwards JE: Complete heart block complicating bacterial endocarditis. Circulation 46:939, 1972

132. James TN, Rupe CE, Monto RW: Pathology of the cardiac conduction system in systemic lupus erythematosus. Ann Intern Med 63:402, 1965

133. Moffitt GR Jr: Complete atrioventricular dissociation with Stokes-Adams attacks due to disseminated lupus erythematosus. Report of a case. Ann Intern Med 63:508, 1965

134. Becker JH: Systemic lupus erythematosus causing heart block. Wis Med J 64:396, 1965

135. Hull D, Binns BAO, Joyce D: Congenital heart block and widespread fibrosis due to maternal lupus erythematosus. Arch Dis Child 41:688, 1966

136. Motté G, Papritz J, Slama R: Les blocs auriculo-ventriculaires complets dans les collagénoses. (A propos de 5 observations personnelles.) Ann Cardiol Angeiol (Paris) 17:313, 1968

137. James TN, Birk RE: Pathology of the cardiac conduction system in polyarteritis nodosa. Arch Intern Med 117:561, 1966

138. Siquier F, Binet JP, Godeau P, Levy R, Hamida B: Dermatomyosite compliquée de bloc auriculo-ventriculaire complet avec syndrome d'Adams-Stokes. Implantátum d'un stimulateur interne. Bull Soc Med Hop Paris 113:1126, 1962

139. Lev M, Landowne M, Matchar JC, and Wagner JA: Systemic scleroderma with complete heart block, report of a case with comprehensive study of the conduction system. Amer Heart J 72:13, 1966

140. Raynaud R, Benatre A, Brochier M, Morand P, Raynaud P: Coeur sclérodermique et bloc auriculo-ventriculaire complet. Arch Mal Coeur 60:1865, 1967

141. Barr IM, Abramov A, Dreyfuss F, Yahini JH, Neufeld HN: Progressive heart block in a case of scleroderma. Isr J Med Sci 6:373, 1970

142. Gowans JDC: Complete heart block with Stokes-Adams syndrome due to rheumatoid heart disease. Report of a case with autopsy findings. New Eng J Med 262:1012, 1960

143. Sobin LH, Hagstrom JWC: Lesions of cardiac conduction tissue in rheumatoid aortitis. JAMA 180:1, 1962

144. Julkunen H, Luomanmäki K: Complete heart block in rheumatoid (ankylosing) spondylitis. Acta Med Scand 176:401, 1964

145. Hoffman FG, Leight L: Complete atrioventricular block associated with rheumatoid disease. Amer J Cardiol 16:585, 1965

146. Julkunen H: Atrioventricular conduction defect in ankylosing spondylitis. Geriatrics 21:129, 1966

147. Weed CL, Kulander BB, Mazzarella JA, Decker JL: Heart block in ankylosing spondylitis. Arch Intern Med 117:800, 1966

148. Liu SM, Alexander CS: Complete heart block and aortic insufficiency in rheumatoid spondylitis. Amer J Cardiol 23:888, 1969

149. Harris M: Rheumatoid heart disease with complete heart block. J Clin Pathol 23:623, 1970

150. Brownstein MH: Cardiac amyloidosis and complete heart block. NY State J Med 66:397, 1966

151. De Maros S, Polzella A: Studio istologico del sistema specifico di conduzione nella amiloidosi cardiaca. Boll Soc Ital Cardiol 12:13, 1967

152. Tricot R, Valère P, Guérot C, Castillo A, Vissuzaine C: Bloc trifasciculaire au cours d'une amylose cardiac primitive. Arch Mal Coeur 63:1278, 1970

153. Mahaim I: Les Tumeurs et les Polypes du Coeur. Paris, Masson, 1945

154. Kellaway G, Gardner DL: Metastatic reticulum cell sarcoma of the heart causing complete heart block. Scott Med J 4:575, 1959

155. Arduini U, Botti G, Visioli O: Etude anatomo-clinique d'un cas de syndrome de Morgagni-Adams-Stokes. Acta Cardiol (Brux) 14:255, 1959

156. Goggio AF, Harkness JT, Palmer WS: Stokes-Adams syndrome in Hodgkin's granuloma. JAMA 176:687, 1961

157. Buckberg GD, Fowler NO: Complete atrioventricular block due to cardiac metastasis of bronchogenic carcinoma. Circulation 24:657, 1961

158. Lenègre J, Moreau P, Iris L: Deux cas de bloc auriculo-ventriculaire complet par sarcome primitif du coeur. Arch Mal Coeur 56:361, 1963

159. Lafargue RT, Hand AM, Lev M: Mesothelioma (coelothelioma) of the atrioventricular node. Chest 59:571, 1971

160. Schellhammer PF, Engle MA, Hagstrom JWC: Histochemical studies of the myocardium and conduction system in acquired iron-storage disease. Circulation 35:631, 1967

161. Aronow WS, Meister L, Kent JR: Atrioventricular block in familial hemochromatosis treated by permanent synchronous pacemaker. Arch Intern Med 123:433, 1969

162. Slama R, Motté G, Coumel P, Passa P, Perrault M: A-V heart block and hemochromatosis. Presse Méd 79:747, 1971

163. Stern MP, Jacobs RL, Duncan GW: Complete heart block complicating hyperthyroidism. JAMA 212:2117, 1970

164. Lee JK, Lewis JA: Myxoedema with complete A-V block and Adams-Stokes disease abolished with thyroid medication. Brit Heart J 24:253, 1962

165. King M, Huang J, Glassman E: Paget's disease with cardiac calcification and complete heart block. Amer J Med 46:302, 1969

166. Virtanen KSI, Halonen PI: Total heart block as a complication of gout. Cardiologia 54:359, 1969

167. Myerson RM, Eisenhauer JH: Atrioventricular conduction defects in lead poisoning. Amer J Cardiol 11:409, 1963

168. Griffin JH: Neonatal hypocalcemia and complete heart block. Amer J Dis Child 110:672, 1965

169. Fisch C, Greenspan K, Edmands RE: Complete atrioventricular block due to potassium. Circ Res 19:373, 1966

170. James TN, Monto RW: Pathology of the cardiac conduction system in thrombotic thrombocytopenic purpura. Ann Intern Med 65:37, 1966

171. Ross A, Lipschultz D, Austin J, Smith J Jr: External ophthalmoplegia and complete heart block. New Eng J Med 280:313, 1969

172. Smith RF, Pulicicchio LU, Holmes AV: Generalized lentigo. Electrocardiographic abnormalities, conduction disorders, and arrhythmias in three cases. Amer J Cardiol 25:501, 1970

173. Shastri SD, Tulgan H, Budnitz J, Colker JL: Progressive ophthalmoplegia, retinitis pigmentosa, and complete heart block. NY State J Med 71:587, 1971

174. Schaumburg HH, Nielsen SL, Yurchak PM: Heart block in polymyositis. New Eng J Med 284:480, 1971

175. Soffer A: Delayed conduction in dystrophica myotonia. Chest 40:594, 1961

176. Bulloch RT, Davis JL, Hara M: Dystrophia myotonica with heart block. A light and electron microscopic study. Arch Path 84:130, 1967

177. Bache RJ, Sarosi GA: Myotonia atrophica. Arch Intern Med 121:369, 1968

178. James TN: Observations on the cardiovascular involvement including cardiac conduction system in progressive muscular dystrophy. Amer Heart J 63:48, 1962

179. Champion P: Limb girdle dystrophy and heart block. Proc R Soc Med 62:733, 1969

180. Littler WA: Heart block and peroneal muscular atrophy. Q J Med 39:431, 1970

181. Kettner M: Akute haemolytische Anaemie (Lederer) mit Uraemie und Herzblock. Z Kinderheilkd 65:1, 1947

182. Bharati S, Chervony A, Gruhn J, Rosen KM, Lev M: Atrial arrhythmias related to trauma to sinoatrial node. Chest 61:331, 1972

183. Armand P, Padritge R, Morel M, Bereni J, Camelin A: Syndrome d'Adams-Stokes par bloc A-V consécutif à une plaie thoracique par balle. Arch Mal Coeur 51:1187, 1958

184. Paulin C, Rubin IL: Complete heart block with perforated interventricular septum following contusion of the chest. Amer Heart J 52:940, 1956

185. Sims BA, Geddes JS: Traumatic heart block. Brit Heart J 31:140, 1969

186. Rossi L: Histopathologic Features of Cardiac Arrhythmias. Milano, Casa Edifrice Ambrosiana, 1969

187. Lenègre J: Contribution a l'Étude des Blocs de Branche Comportant Notamment les Confrontations Électriques et Histologiques. Paris, Ballière, 1958, p 341

188. Mahaim I: Les Maladies Organiques du Faisceau de His-Tawara. Paris, Masson, 1931, p 595

189. Lev M: Complete left bundle branch block. A physiologic-pathologic correlation. Report of a case. Amer Heart J 61:149, 1961

190. Lev M, Unger PN: The pathology of the conduction system in acquired heart disease. Severe atrioventricular block. Arch Path 60:502, 1955

191. Lev M, Unger PN, Lesser ME, Pick A: Pathology of the conduction system in acquired heart disease. Complete right bundle branch block. Amer Heart J 61:593, 1961

192. Lev M: The pathology of bundle branch block. Heart Bulletin 16:107, 1967

193. Unger PN, Greenblatt M, Lev M: The anatomic basis of the electrocardiographic abnormality in incomplete left bundle branch block. Amer Heart J 76:486, 1968

194. Rosen KM, Rahimtoola SH, Gunnar RM, Lev M: Transient and persistent atrial standstill with His bundle lesions, electrophysiologic and pathologic correlations. Circulation 44:220, 1971

THE HISTOGENESIS OF CARDIAC MYXOMAS:
Relation to Other Proliferative Diseases of Subendothelial Vasoform Reserve Cells *

ARTHUR A. STEIN
JACQUELINE MAURO
LLOYD THIBODEAU
RALPH ALLEY

During the past few years four primary intracavitary myxomas of the heart have been diagnosed and removed surgically. The clinical course of these patients will be reported later.[1] The gross pathologic tumor findings are summarized in Table 1. Microscopically, the tumor presented a loose vascular myxomatous pattern

Table 1.   Four Primary Intracardiac Myxomas

IDENTITY	AGE	SEX	LOCATION	WEIGHT IN GRAMS	GROSS APPEARANCE
J.S.	44 yr	M	left atrium	41.3	yellow white, mucoid cystic
R.B.	52 yr	F	bilateral atrium	87.0, rt 15.2, lt	yellow-white, focally hemorrhagic, spongy
K.L.	17 yr	F	left atrium	50.0	hemorrhagic, focally cystic, grey, mucoid
L.D.	3 mo	M	right atrium	12.0	lobulated, grey white, myxomatous

* This study was supported primarily by Morphology for Biologic Research, Inc., Albany, N. Y.

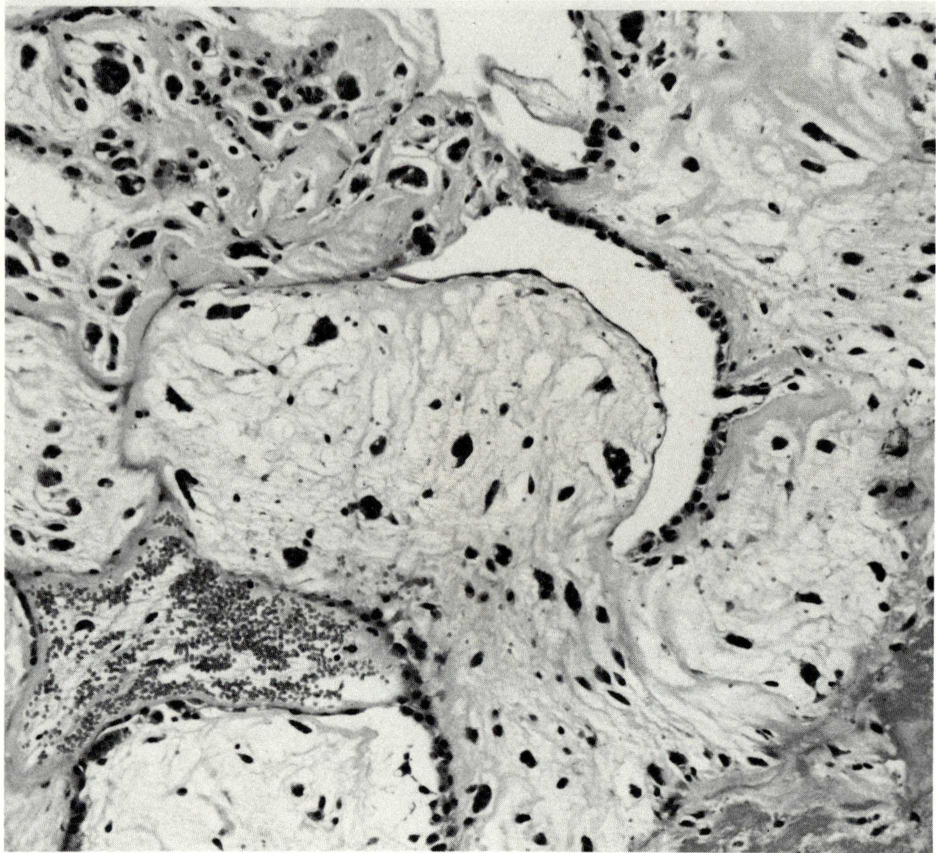

Fig. 1.   Cardiac myxoma. Nests of tumor cells are found singly or in clusters in abundant myxoid stroma. H&E. X150.

with foci of fibrosis, calcification and hemorrhage. The tumor cells were spindle shaped with oval vesicular nuclei and moderate amounts of cytoplasm. Commonly, these cells, singly or in clumps, lay in pools of mucoid stroma (Fig. 1).

This report will present the electron microscopic findings, which indicate that myxomas are benign tumors of subendothelial vasoformative reserve cells. These findings will also be correlated with other proliferative diseases of the subendothelial vasoformative reserve cell.

Materials and Methods

Immediately upon elective surgical excision of three of the intracardiac myxomatous tumors, portions were obtained from the surface and from the base of each tumor. The tissues were fixed in 4 percent glutaraldehyde. Later the material was postfixed in osmium tetroxide, dehydrated in graded alcohols, embedded in Epon, and cut on a Porter-Blum microtome. Sections were stained with 1 percent uranyl acetate, followed by Karnovsky's method[2] or by lead citrate.[3] Sections were examined and photographed under a Zeiss EM-9A electron microscope.

Results

Although several types of cells were seen within the tumor, the dominant type was a relatively mature smooth muscle cell. Sections from these tumors in multiple locations repeatedly demonstrated a large branched smooth muscle cell in which the nucleus appeared to occupy approximately 50 percent of the total volume. The cytoplasm was electron dense, limited by a basement membrane and contained myofilaments, fusiform bodies, and many micropinocytotic vesicles (Figs. 2, 3, 4). Few strands of granular endoplasmic reticulum and a few mitochondria also were present. There were other cells whose morphology suggested a smooth muscle histogenesis, but they appeared less mature. These cells were characterized by variable numbers of the above characteristic internal organelles, an increased amount of rough endoplasmic reticulum, and increased numbers of mitochondria.

Another group of cells, believed to be fibrocytes (Fig. 5) were characterized by abundant granular endoplasmic reticulum with saccular and tubular outlines, increased numbers of oval mitochondria, and prominent Golgi apparatuses.

A third group of cells, believed to be endothelial (Figs. 6, 7, 8), were characterized by a partial basement membrane, microvilli, numerous pinocytotic vesicles, clusters of fine fibrils including rod-shaped bodies,[4] and varying numbers of lipid droplets.

In many micrographs, clear definition and classification of individual cells could not be made. Small numbers of primitive cells had so few internal organelles that they could not be classified. In other cells, there were cytoplasmic organelles which indicated lines of differentiation other than the dominant pattern within the cell. These immature or abortive structural characteristics support the multipotentiality of the reserve cell. However, it was clear that we were documenting at least three lines of differentiation that included smooth muscle cells, fibrocytes, and endothelial cells. Each of these was associated with its characteristic location or end product. The muscle cells were related to electron microscopically acellular stroma associated with mucopolysaccharides; the fibrocytes were associated with collagen or elastic fibrils; the endothelial cells were associated with lipid accumulation, necrosis, and the linings of small vessels that contained red blood cells.

Discussion

Matsuyama and Ooneda[5] have discussed the histogenesis of primary myxoma of the heart based on electron microscopic examination. They noted a preponderance of electron-dense spindle cells with surrounding basement membranes and central oval large nuclei. Abundant rough endoplasmic reticulum and filamentous elements, in addition to other common organelles, were present in the sarcoplasm. The matrix contained a small amount of collagen, elastic fibers, and diffusely distributed fine electron-dense granules. We have observed the same tumor cells electron microscopically.

In 9 of 11 autopsies on infants under four months of age, islands of myxomatous or myxofibromatous tissue were found in the endocardium near the foramen ovalis with the use of light microscopy.

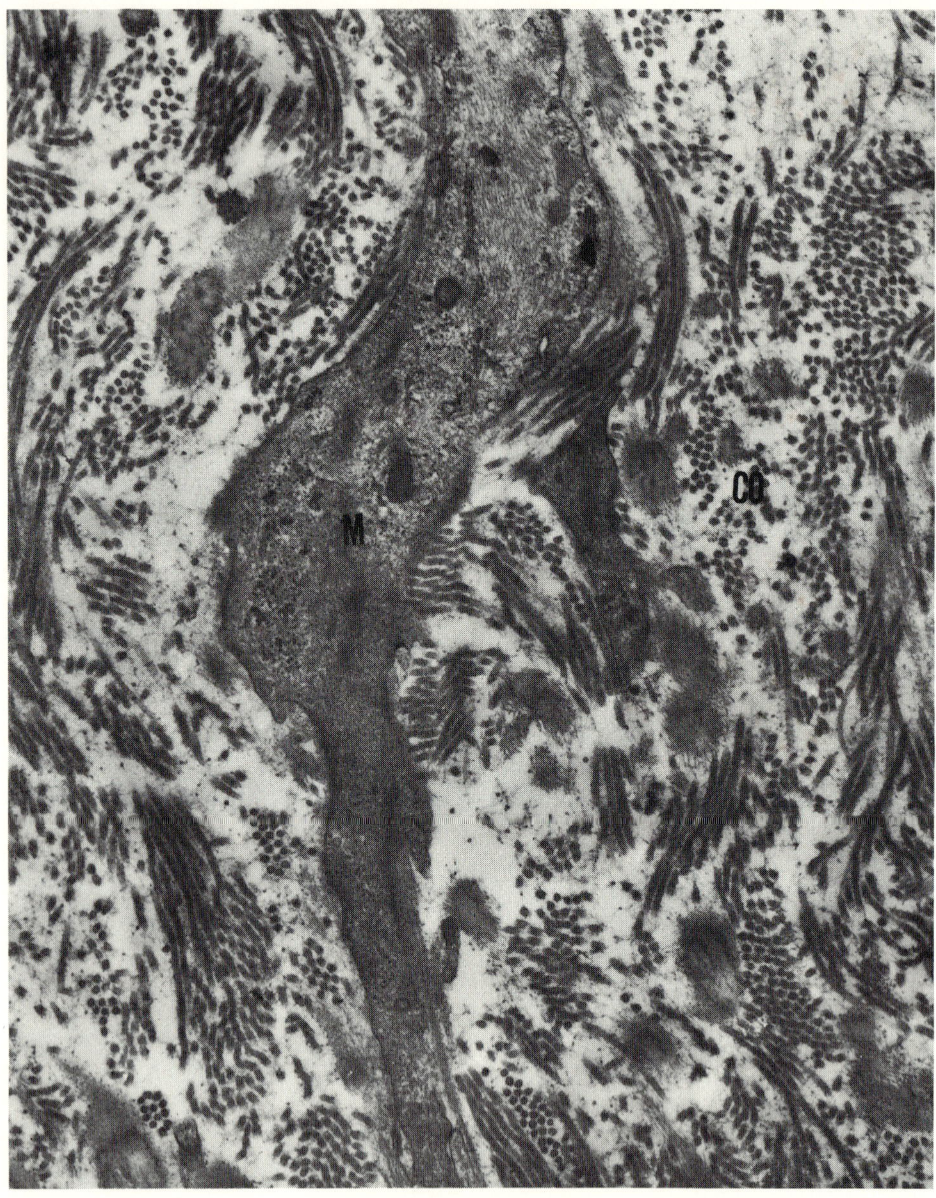

Fig. 2.   Cardiac myxoma. A mature smooth muscle cell is surrounded by collagen fibrils in mucopolysaccharide-rich stroma. M = smooth muscle cell; CO = collagen. X28,000.

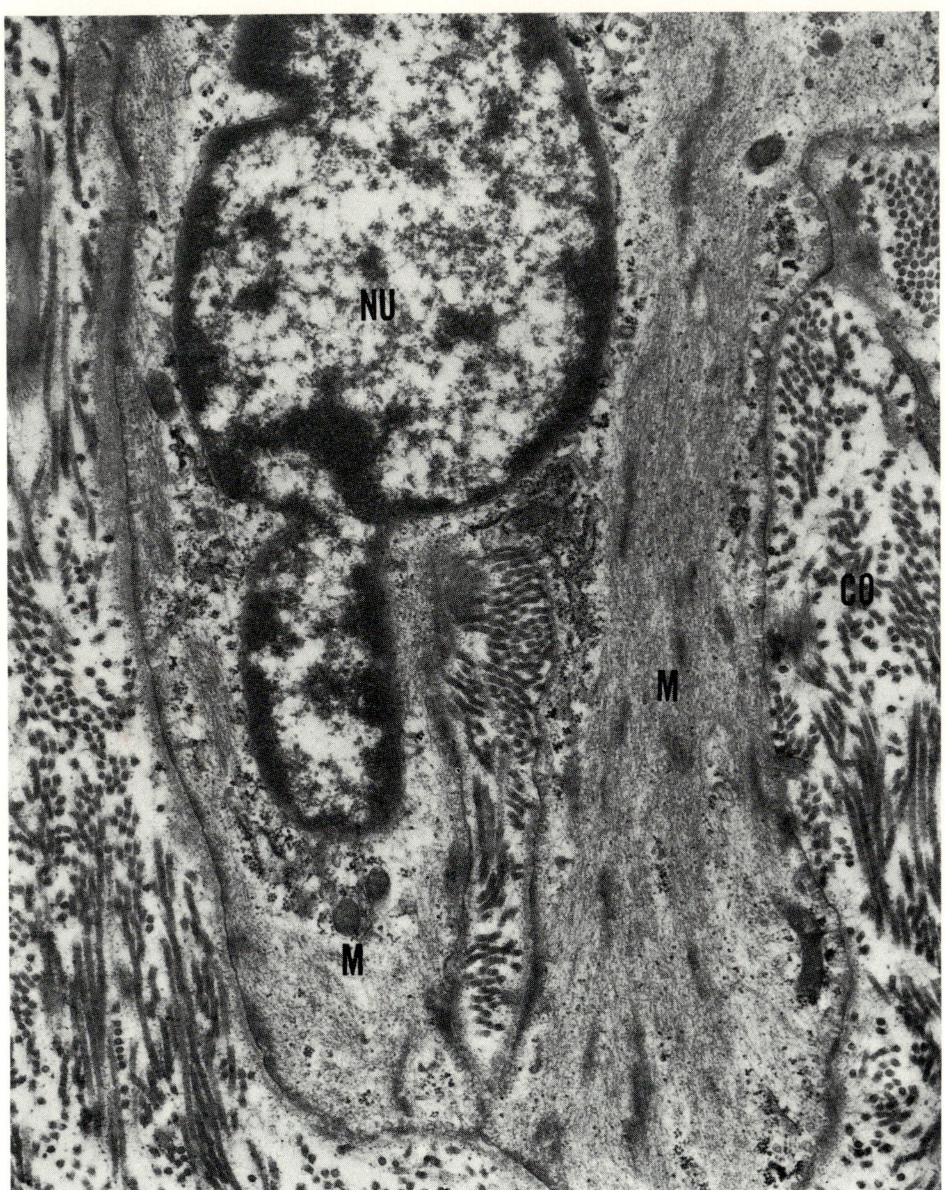

Fig. 3. Cardiac myxoma. NU = nucleus. X28,000.

                                    Stein, Mauro, Thibodeau, and Alley

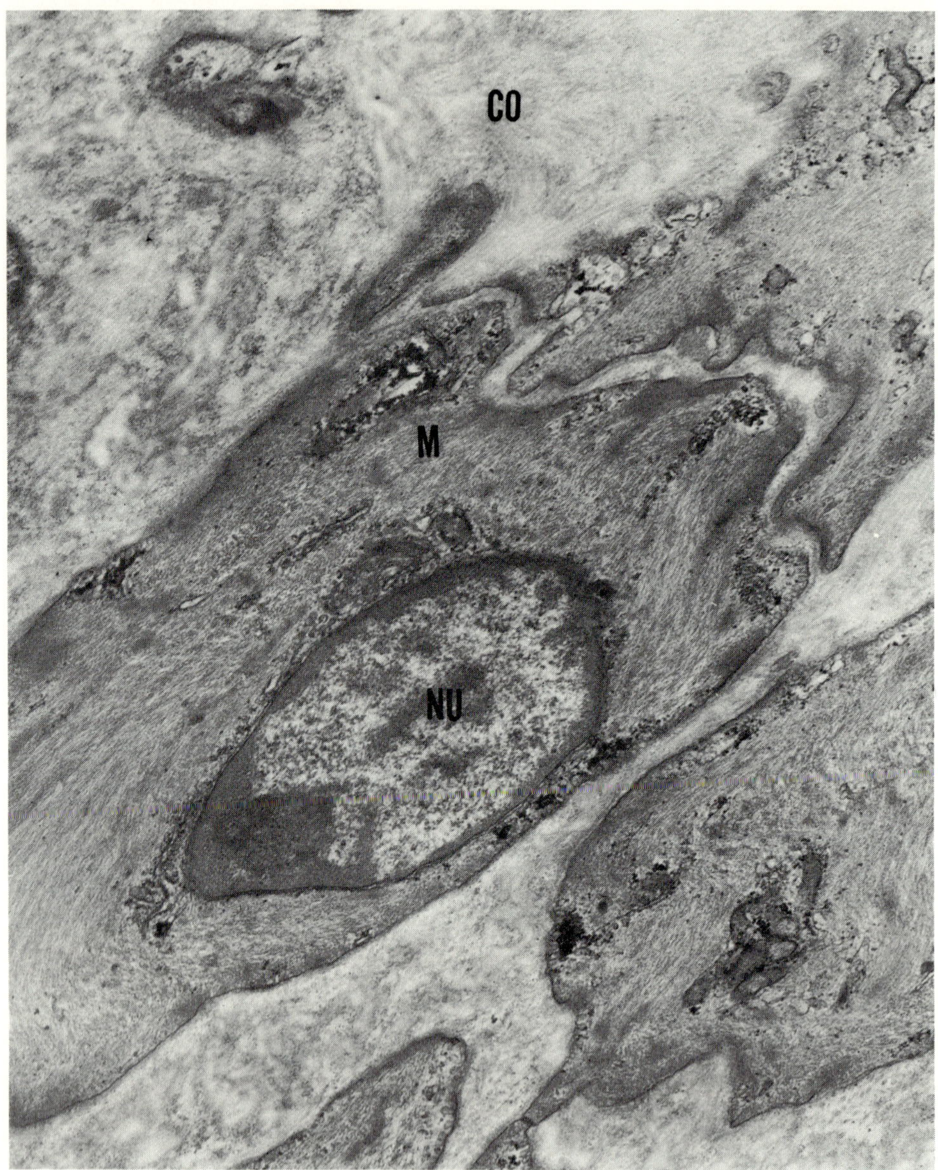

Fig. 4.   Cardiac myxoma. The characteristic internal organelles, including myofilaments, fusiform bodies, and micropinocytic vesicles, are demonstrated. X28,000.

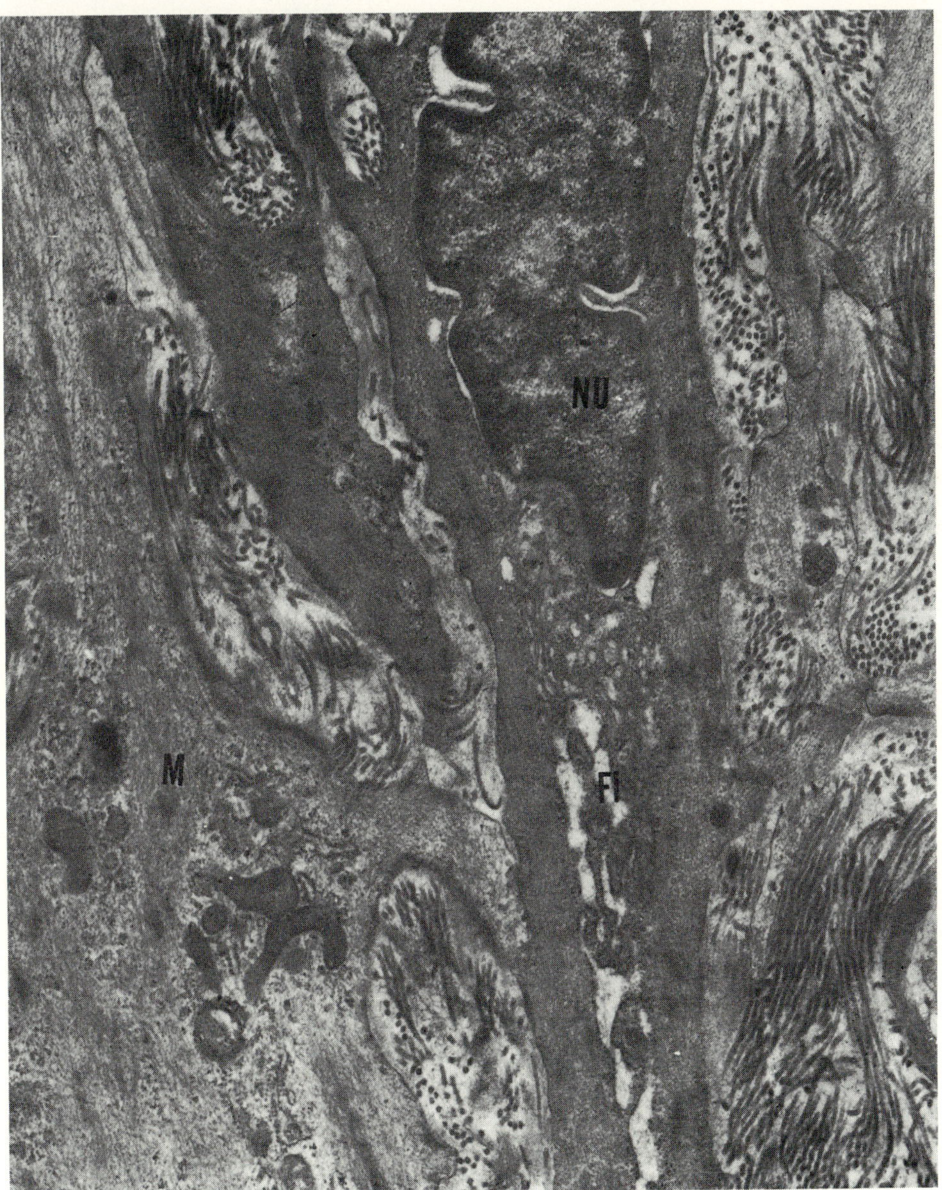

Fig. 5.   Cardiac myxoma. The central elongate cell has the structural characteristics of a fibrocyte embedded in collagen. Nearby a portion of a smooth muscle cell is seen. FI = fibrocyte. X28,000.

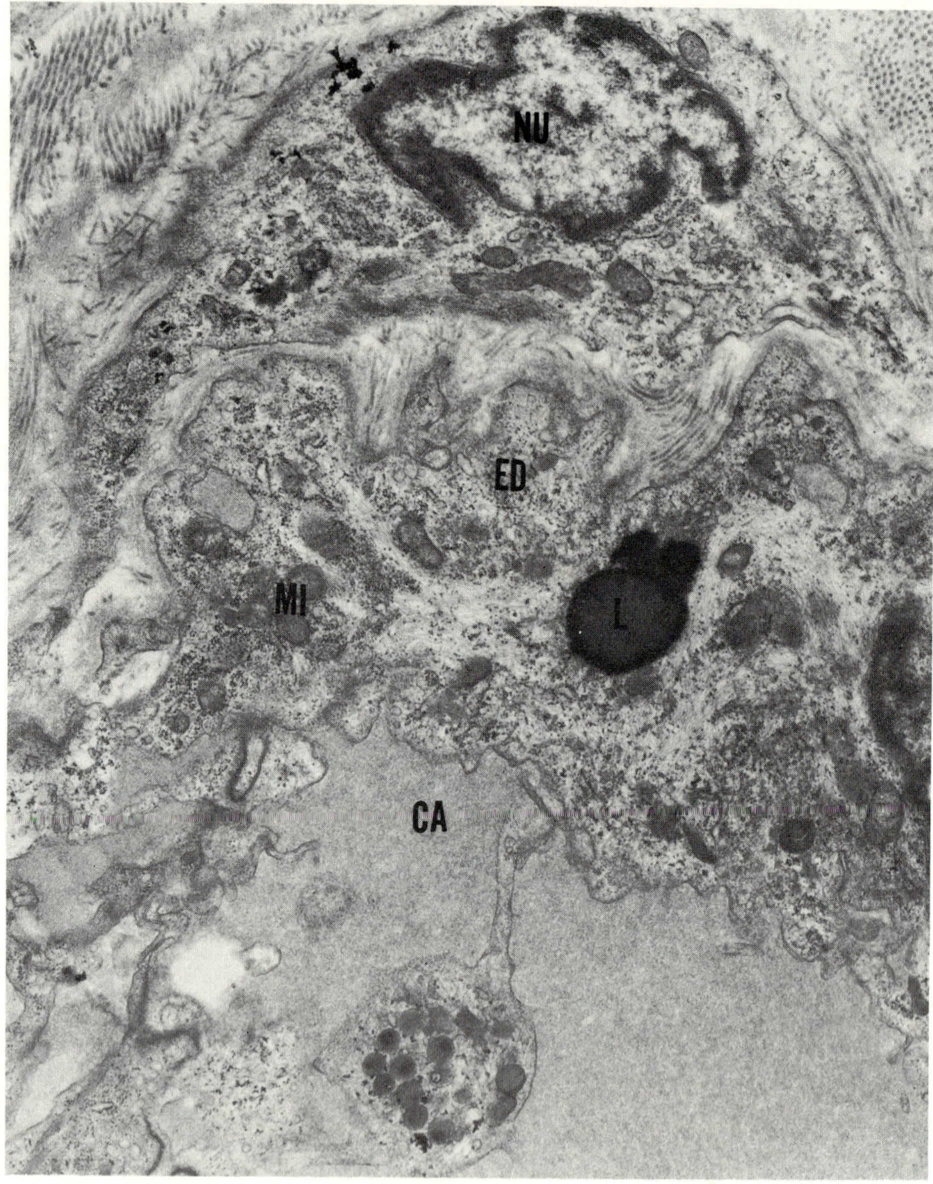

Fig. 6. Cardiac myxoma. ED = endothelial cell; MI = mitochondria; CA = capillary lumen; L = lipid. X28,000.

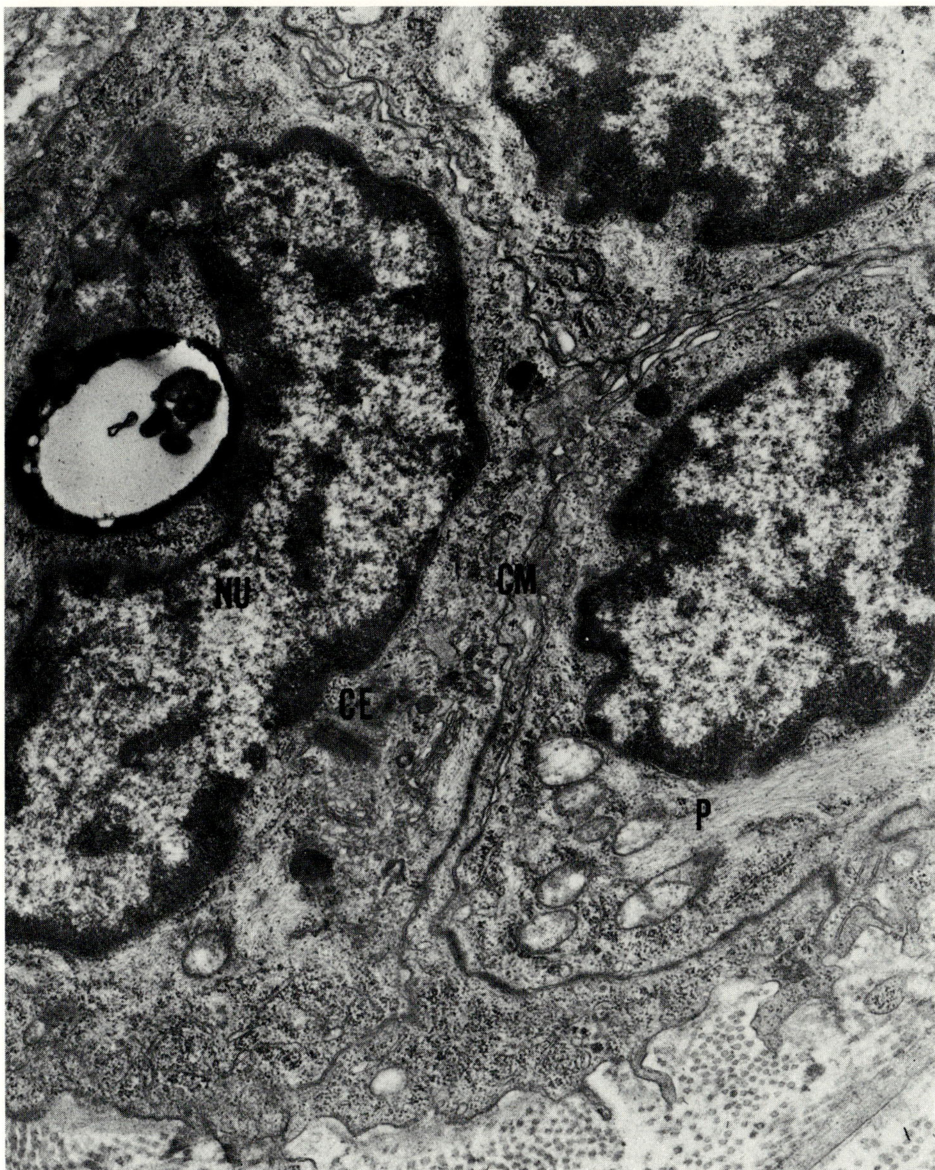

Fig. 7.   Cardiac myxoma. An endothelial cell lining a capillary is seen. In the sarcoplasm there are large lipid droplets. CE = centriole; P = primitive cell; CM = cell membrane. X28,000.

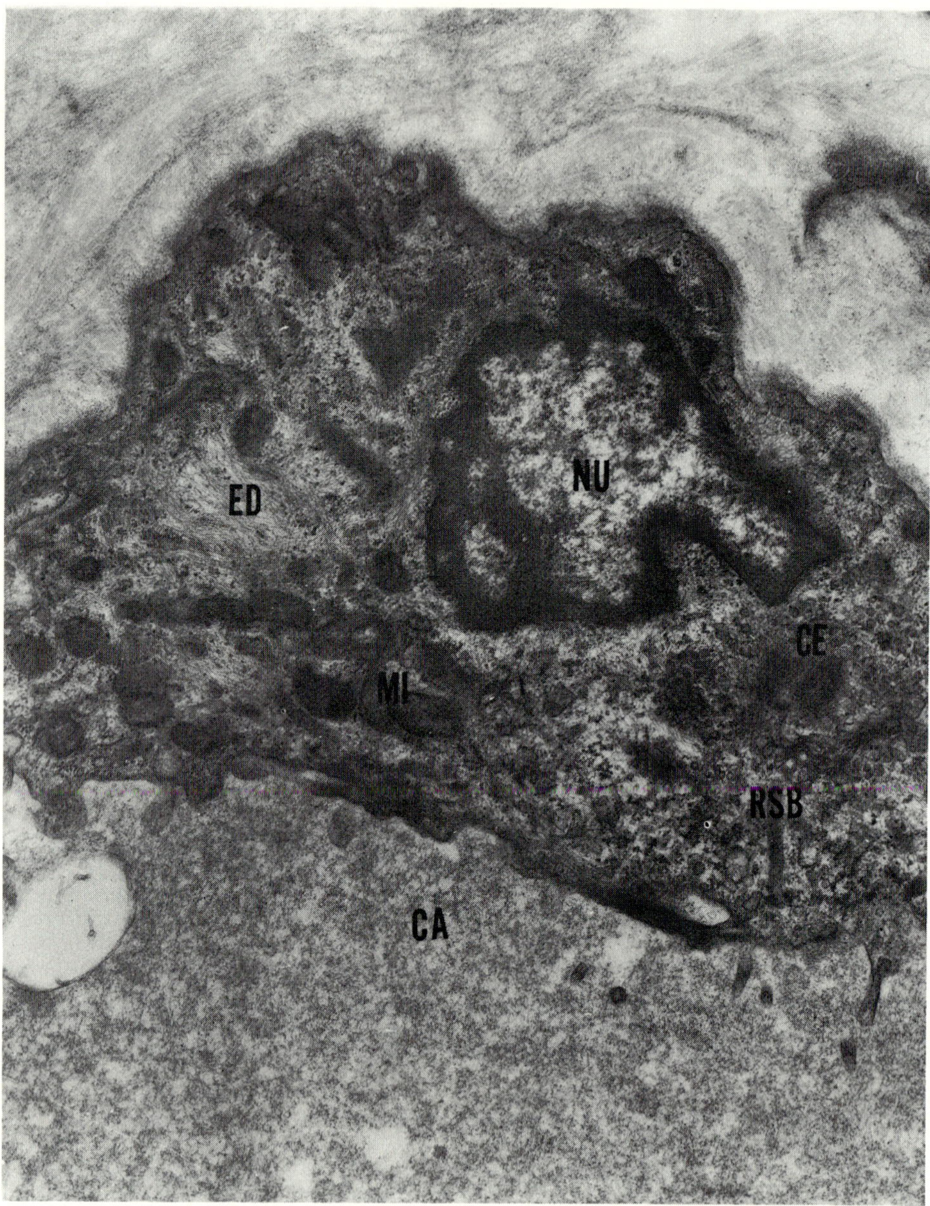

Fig. 8.   Cardiac myxoma. More details of internal organelles of endothelial cells including pinocytic vesicles and rod-shaped bodies. RSB = rod-shaped bodies. X28,000.

Matsuyama and Ooneda[5] concluded that the myxoma was derived from residual islands of embryonal undifferentiated residual tissue in the endocardium, believed to be closely related to embryonal botryoid rhabdomyosarcoma. However, we believe that myxomas represent a benign tumor of the ubiquitous subendothelial vasoformative reserve cell. The residual islands of myxomatous tissue in the endocardium near the fossa ovalis may represent foci of vasoformative reserve cell hyperplasia related to intrauterine flow patterns through the foramen ovale.

Relation to Other Prospective Diseases of the Subendothelial Vasoformative Reserve Cell

To further the concept, we reviewed other vascular lesions characterized electron microscopically by proliferation of these subendothelial reserve cells. In the proliferative phase of the intimal atherosclerotic lesion, the predominant cell electron microscopically is the smooth muscle cell. It has been described in experimental atherosclerosis in the rat,[6, 7] rabbit,[8, 9] dog,[10] and monkey.[11, 12] The smooth muscle cells in the human intimal proliferative lesion have been described by Geer et al.,[13, 15] Haust et al.,[14] and Scott et al.[16]

Electron microscopic studies of the proliferative lesions induced by diet in the rhesus monkey indicated several morphologic type of cells which have been interpreted as being interrelated histogenetically.[11] Clearly evident were mature smooth muscle cells with surrounding basement membrane and electron dense sarcoplasm in which marginal pinocytic vesicles and myofilaments were readily demonstrated. In less mature cells, there were still abundant myofilaments, the hallmark of the smooth muscle cell. Also noted were large lipid-laden cells whose histogenesis could not be definitely related to the smooth muscle cell or to macrophages. In addition, fibroblast-like cells and primitive cells were described. This group of cells closely resembled the cell types seen electron microscopically in the myxomas of the heart.

We collected tissue in the operating room from the thickened whitish endocardium overlying hypertrophied infundibular muscle beneath the pulmonary stenosis of two children with tetralogy of Fallot. Electron microscopic study of this thickened endocardium again demonstrated abundant proliferation of subendothelial cells including numerous smooth muscle cells and fibrocytes (Figs. 9, 10, 11, 12, 13).

We studied a thickened aortic cusp from a 52-year-old patient with rheumatic aortic stenosis. Again, different cells, including smooth muscle cells and fibrocytes, were found within abundant collagen electron microscopically. We also obtained portions of congenitally abnormal stenosed pulmonary valve leaflet from a child with tetralogy of Fallot (Fig. 14). Again, there was abundant proliferative response with different cells, including smooth muscle cells.

Comments on Comparative Histogenesis

Sabin[17, 18] has described embryogenesis of blood vessel walls from the area vasculosa of the yolk sac in chicks. She concluded that angioblasts differentiated from mesenchyme and produced blood vessels, primitive plasma, and red blood cells. Within angioblastic cell masses, the formation of vessels was initiated by marked cytoplasmic vacuolization, death, and liquefaction of central cells, with resultant

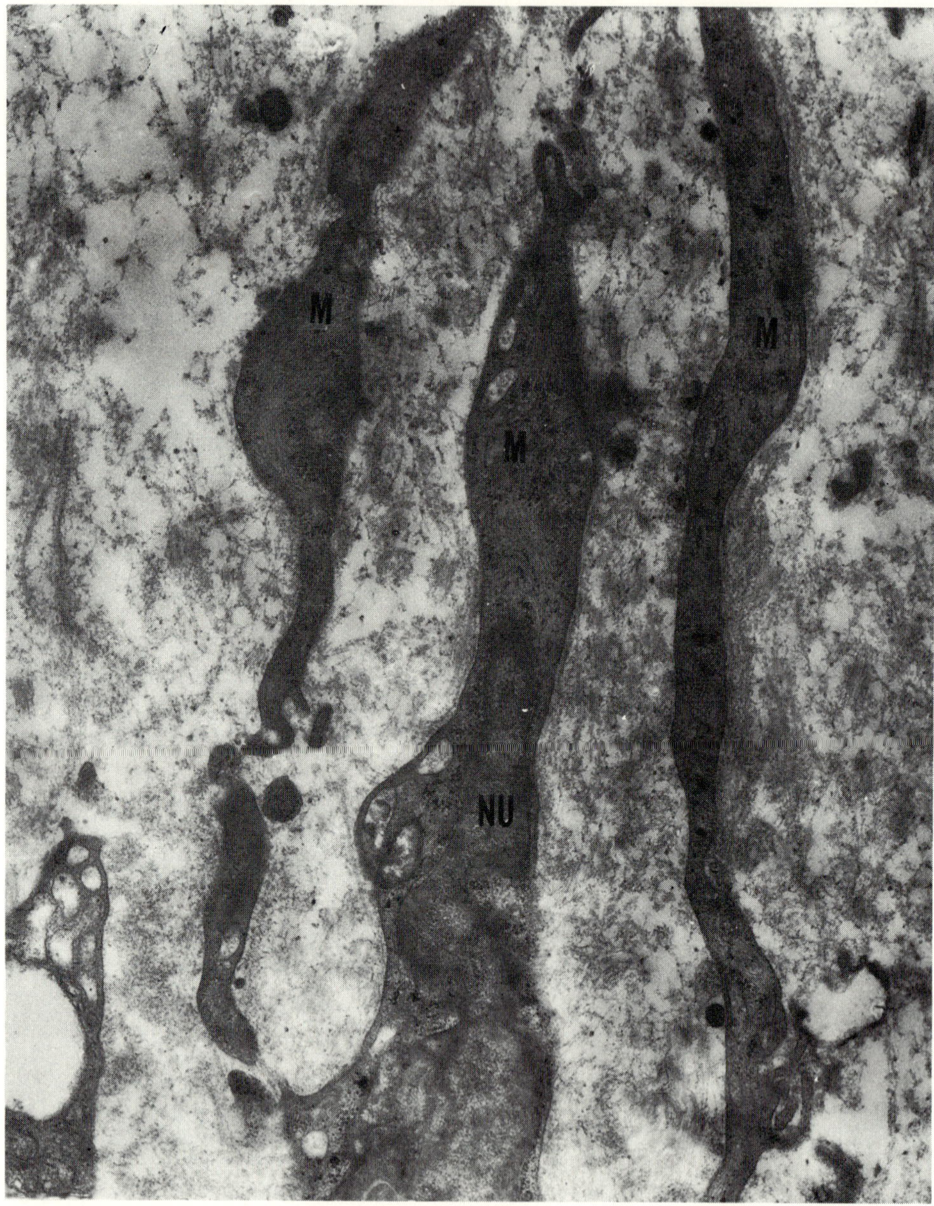

Fig. 9.   Thickened endocardium over hypertrophied infundibular muscle, from tetralogy of Fallot. X28,000.

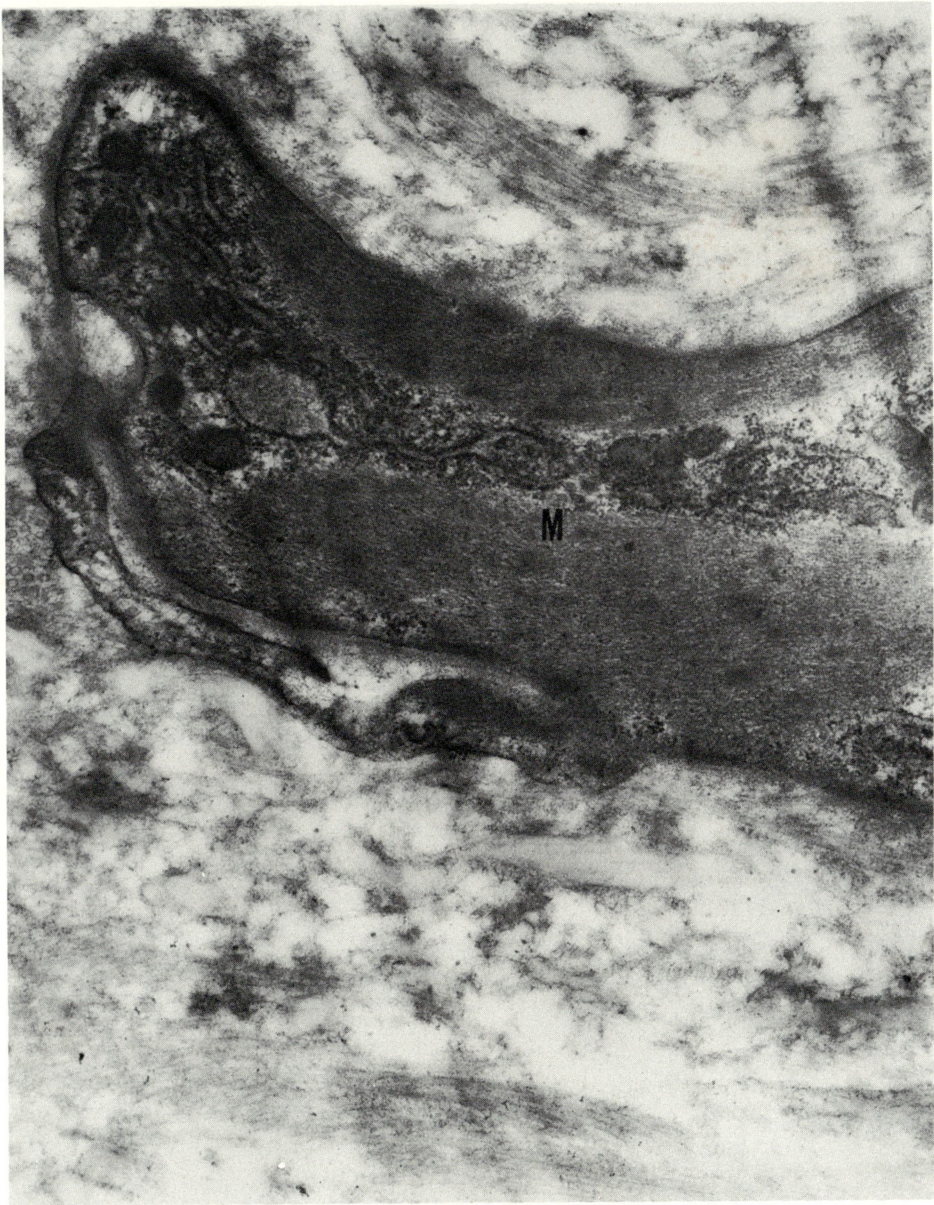

Fig. 10.   Thickened endocardium over hypertrophied infundibular muscle from tetralogy of Fallot. Smooth muscle cells are surrounded by collagen fibrils in mucopolysaccharide-rich stroma. X40,000.

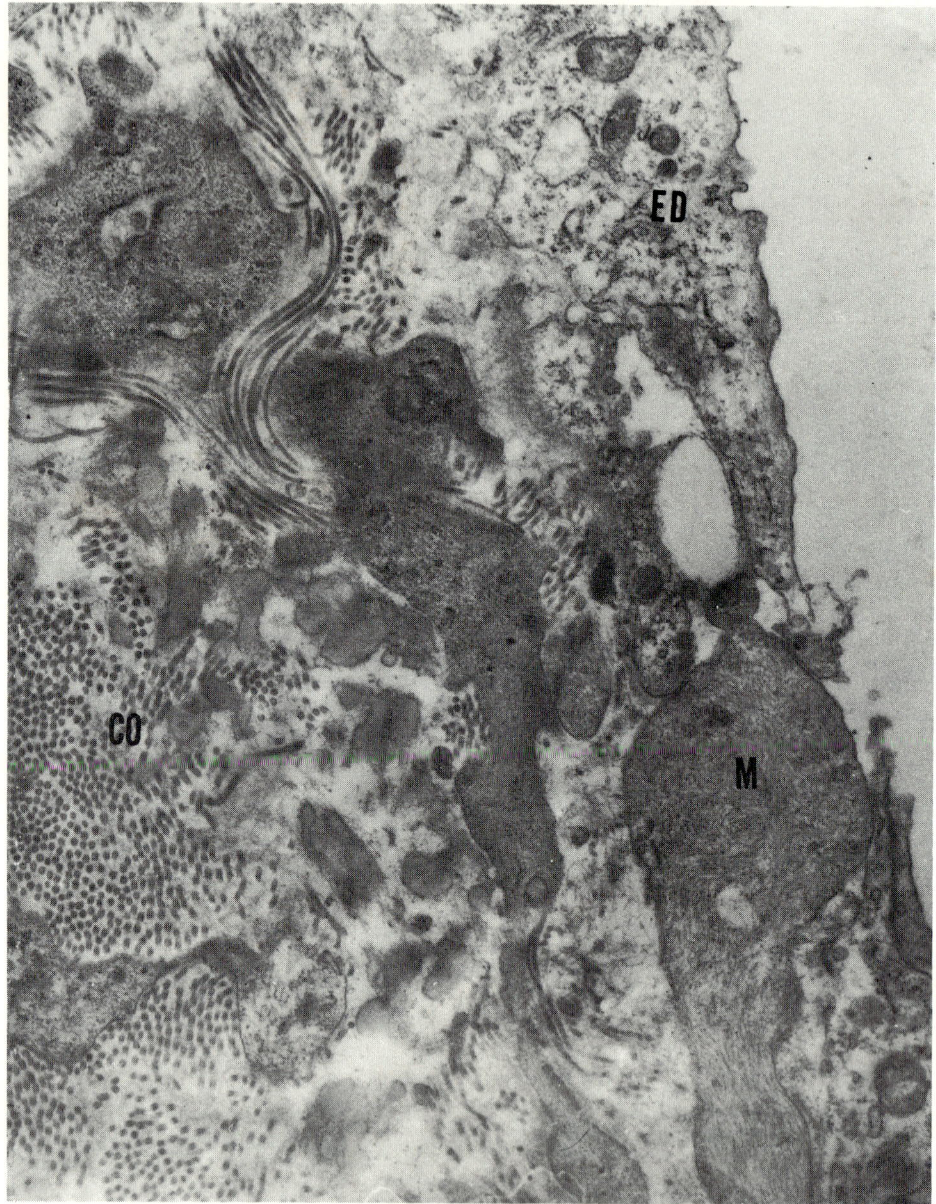

Fig. 11.   Thickened endocardium over hypertrophied infundibular muscle from tetralogy of Fallot. X28,000.

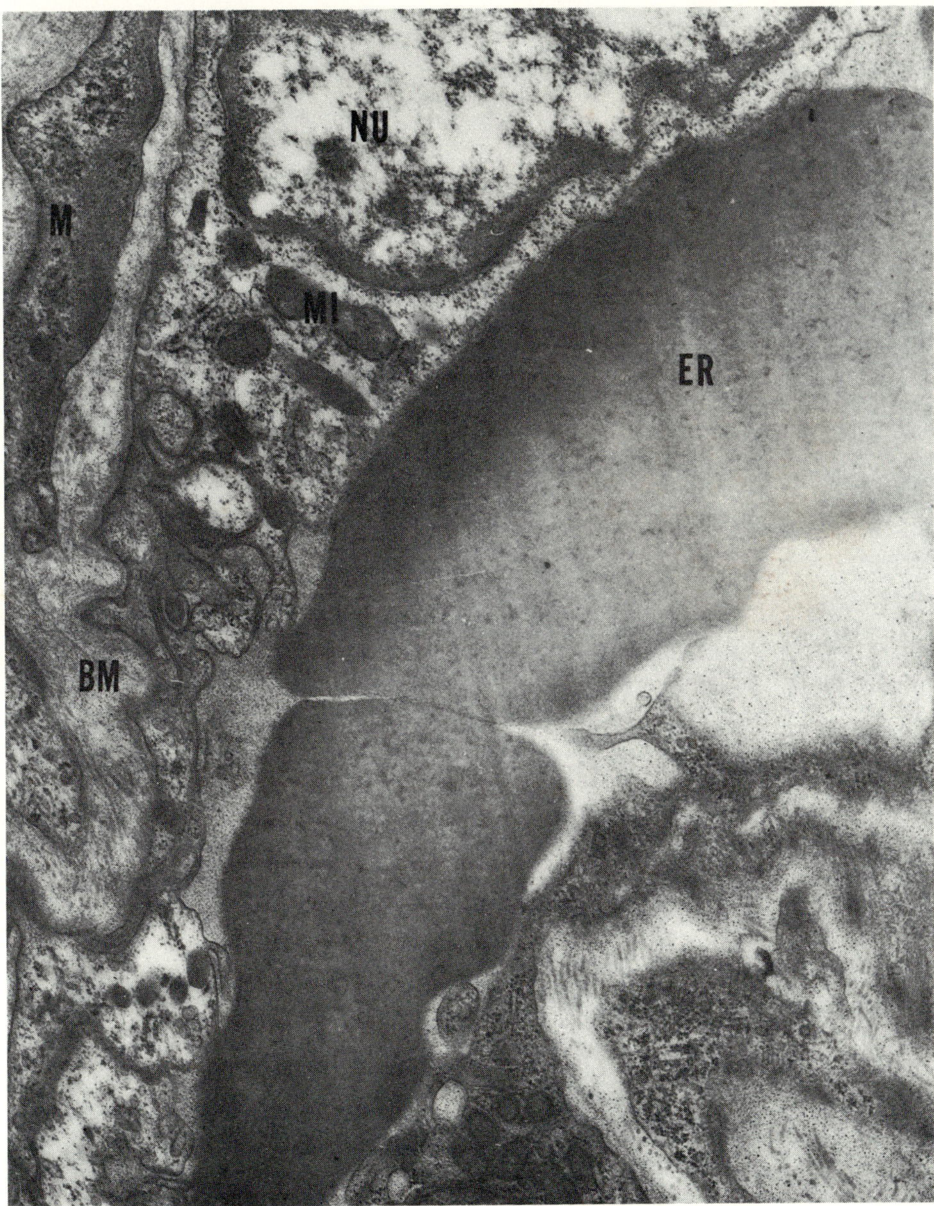

Fig. 12.   Thickened endocardium over hypertrophied infundibular muscle from tetralogy of Fallot. ER = erythrocyte, X28,000.

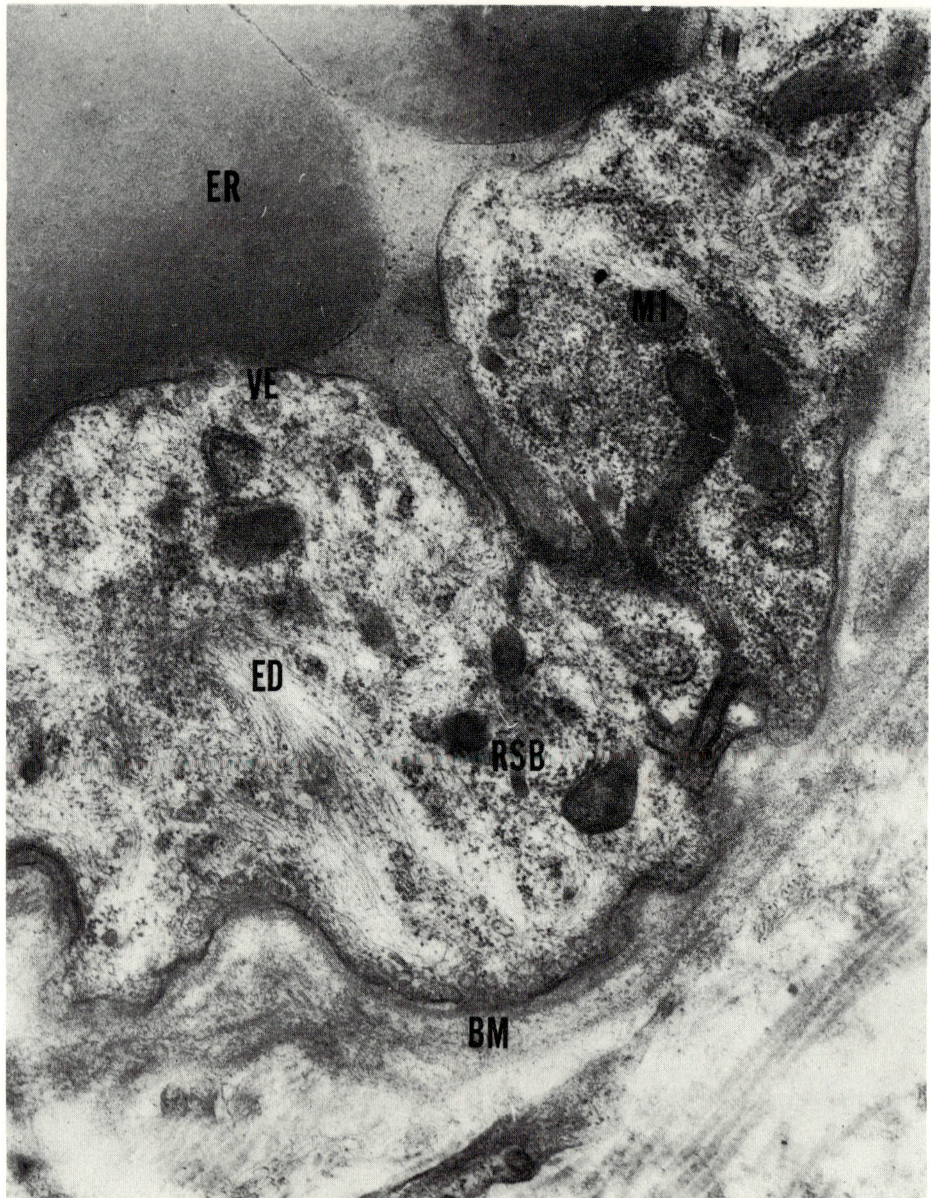

Fig. 13.   Thickened endocardium over hypertrophied infundibular muscle from tetralogy of Fallot. Endothelial cell differentiation can be seen. Foci of varying degrees of maturation are present. BM = basement membrane; VE = pinocytic vesicles. X40,000.

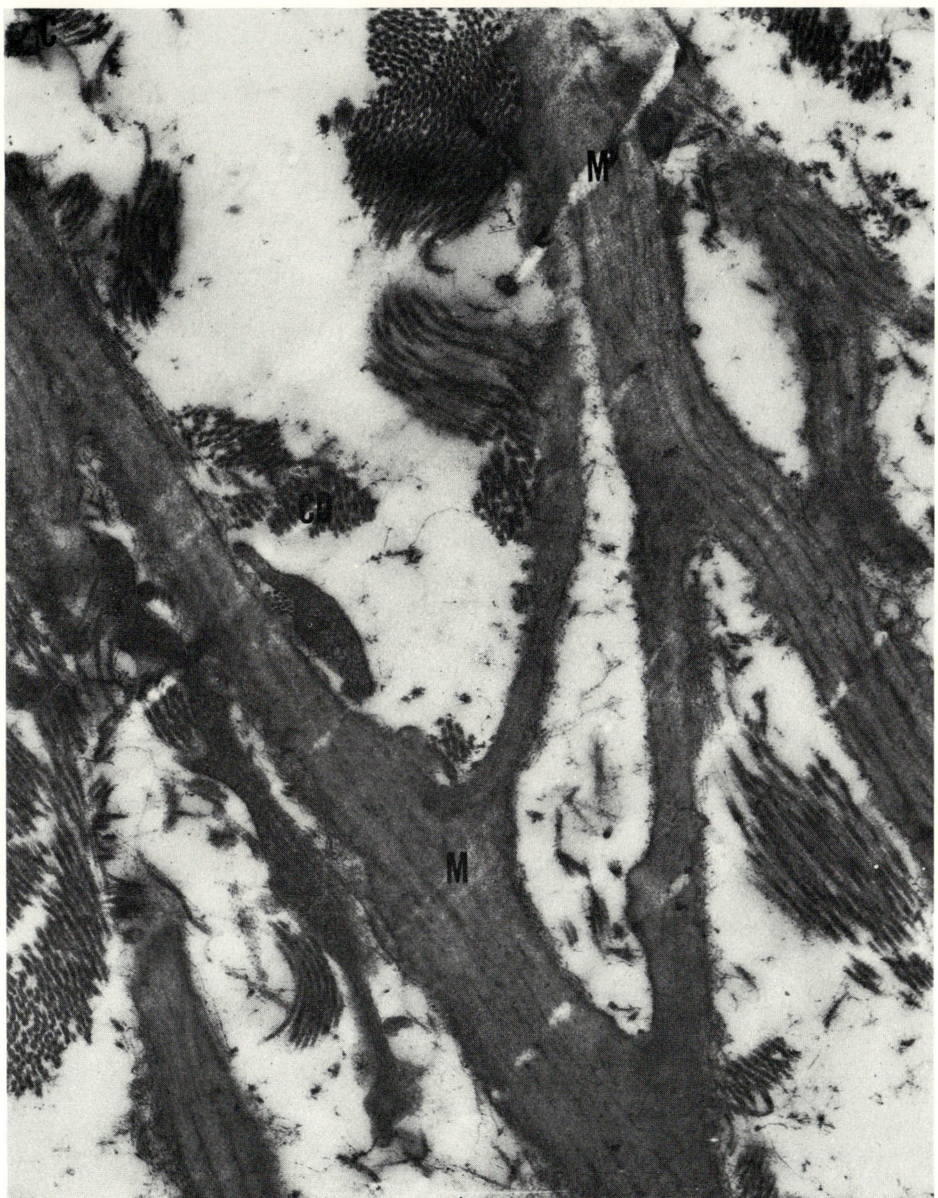

Fig. 14.   Thickened congenitally abnormal stenotic pulmonary valve in tetralogy of Fallot. Branching smooth muscle cells are found in abundant mucopolysaccharide stroma. X28,000.

production of primitive plasma. The future lining cells of the vascular channels also developed large eccentric cytoplasmic vacuoles and liquefied until only a rim of granular cytoplasm surrounded an elongated nucleus. Primitive red blood cells were formed from angioblasts and endothelial cells, but this differentiation did not occur before the formation of primitive plasma.

Utilizing these observations, the histogenetic origin of multiple gross variants of hemangioblastoma of the brain have been considered.[19]

Comments on Kinetics of Cell Replacement

In many hollow organs such as the bronchus, cervix, urinary bladder, esophagus, and others, the lining cell is continuously replaced by a sublining multipotent reserve cell. In these different situations, we recognize the concept of reserve cell hyperplasia. In some locations, the foci of reserve cell hyperplasia may persist for years without apparent differentiation or maturation. However, they may undergo spontaneous regression or may show different lines of differentiation with varying degrees of maturation. On the other hand, functional stimulation of the reserve cells with or without cellular hyperplasia may produce a local increase in secretory products.

Generally, at the light microscope level, we recognize differentiation through morphologic structural characteristics and intra- or extra-cellular elements identified by specific or nonspecific histochemical techniques.

There is a multipotent vasoformative reserve cell in the subendothelial layer of vascular channels. This cell appears to be a normal reserve cell required for continuous replacement of the overlying endothelial cells. Numerous studies indicate that, in the early proliferative vasoformative reserve cell intimal response to injury, the subendothelial smooth cells are characterized by the production of mucopolysaccharides.[20, 21, 22] In other areas, or later, there may appear focal deposits of lipid, focal necrosis, and strands of collagen and elastic fibrils. These products, readily demonstrated by light microscopy, are manifestations of different lines of differentiation in the proliferative vasoformative reserve cell response. The interrelation of these variants is schematically represented in Table 2.

Table 2.   Lines of Differentiation of Vasoformative Reserve Cells

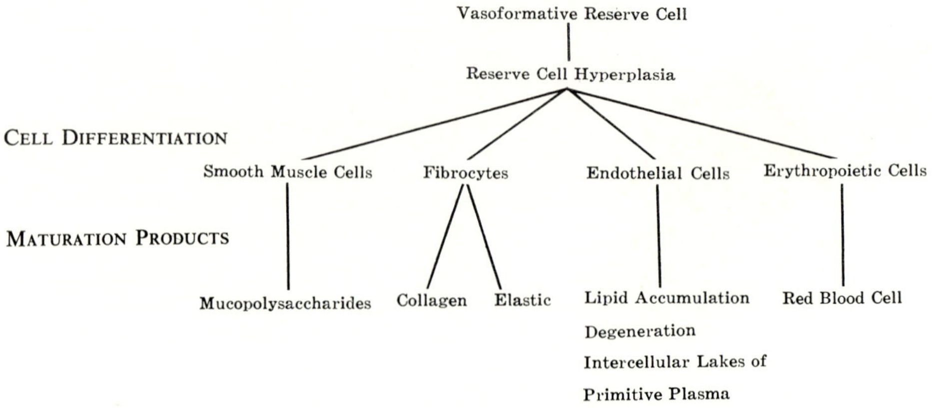

Vasoformative Reserve Cell
|
Reserve Cell Hyperplasia

CELL DIFFERENTIATION

Smooth Muscle Cells   Fibrocytes   Endothelial Cells   Erythropoietic Cells

MATURATION PRODUCTS

Mucopolysaccharides   Collagen   Elastic   Lipid Accumulation   Red Blood Cell

Degeneration

Intercellular Lakes of

Primitive Plasma

Complications in Vascular Sclerosis

The local complications of proliferative vasoformative disease are most commonly related to mixed maturation towards primitive vessel formation. The accumulation of cytoplasmic lipid, cell necrosis, and development of intercellular lakes of fluid can facilitate local hemorrhage and calcification. The development of a subintimal mass produced either by proliferative disease or excessive (mucopolysaccharide) secretory activity can result in direct or indirect injury and loss of the overlying endothelial cell or disturbance in its replacement, with resultant mural thrombus formation.

Structural Variations in Vascular Sclerosis

Morphologic patterns of vascular sclerosis in clinical material vary with age, sex, location, and anatomy and microcirculation of the vessel. By ultrastructural study, smooth muscle cells have also been demonstrated in the media of arteries.[16] Review of surgical specimens would suggest that vasoformative reserve cells are present in the adventitia. Perhaps the variation of vasoformative reserve cell proliferation with different lines and degrees of maturation and cellular metabolic activity can correlate with the various anatomic patterns. Morphologic responses are obviously final common pathways for many chemical and physical incitants whose immediate delivery is primarily dependent upon local physiologic mechanisms.

Molecular Pharmacology

This concept of vasoformative proliferative disease allows a molecular approach to mechanisms in cell stimulation and to proliferation, differentiation, and metabolic activity. Possibly, the chemotherapeutic search can utilize short-term experimental models such as the chick embryo, tissue culture, or even the induction by standardized physical techniques[23] of vasoformative cell proliferations in small experimental animals. We must seek compounds to inhibit proliferation or metabolic activity or to direct the maturation of vasoformative proliferative disease rather than compounds to treat the complications of this disease. This concept may prove of equal basic interest in studies on the mechanism of induction of vascular support in neoplasia.

References

1. Jain, A.C. Personal communication.
2. Karnovsky, M.J. Simple methods for "staining with lead" at high pH in electron microscopy. J. Biophys. Biochem. Cytol., 11:729, 1961.
3. Reynolds, L.S. The use of lead cytole at high pH as an electron-opaque stain in electron microscopy. J. Cell Biol., 17:208, 1963.
4. Weibel, E.R., and Palade, G.F. New cytoplasmic components in arterial endothelia. J. Cell Biol., 23:101, 1964.
5. Matsuyama, K., and Ooneda, G. Histogenesis of primary myxoma of the heart: A case report. Gann, 58:435, 1967.
6. Thomas, W.A., Jones, R., Scott, R.F., Morrison, E., Goodale, F., and Imai, H. Production of early atherosclerotic lesions in rats characterized by proliferation of "modified smooth muscle cells." Exp. Molec. Path. (Supp. 1), 2:40, 1963.

7. Scott, R.F., Morrison, E.S., Thomas, W.A., Jones, R., and Nam, S.C. Short-term feeding of unsaturated versus saturated fat in the production of atherosclerosis in the rat. Exp. Molec. Path., 3:421, 1964.

8. Imai, Lee, K.T., Pastori, S., Panlilio, E., Florentin, R., and Thomas, W.A. Atherosclerosis in rabbits: Architectural and subcellular alterations of smooth muscle cells of aorta in response to hyperlipemia. Exp. Molec. Path., 5:273, 1966.

9. Parker, F., and Odland, G.F. A correlative histochemical, biochemical and electron microscopic study of experimental atherosclerosis in the rabbit aorta with special reference to the myo-intimal cell. Amer. J. Path., 48:197, 1966.

10. Westlake, G., Grundy, S.M., and O'Neal, R.M. The effect of an atherogenic diet on pre-existing aortic intimal thickenings in old dogs. Exp. Molec. Path. (Suppl. 1), 2:1, 1963.

11. Scott, R.F., Jones, R., Daoud, A.S., Zumbo, O., Coulston, F.. and Thomas, W.A. Experimental atherosclerosis in rhesus monkeys. Cellular elements of proliferative lesions and possible role of cytoplasmic degeneration in pathogenesis as studied by electron microscopy. Exp. Molec. Path. 7:34, 1967.

12. Wissler, R.W., Getz, G.S., Vesselinovitch, D., Frazier, L.E., and Hughes, R.W. Acute severe atherosclerosis in rhesus monkeys. Fed. Proc., 25:597, 1966 (Abstract).

13. Geer, J.C., McGill, Henry C., and Strong, J.P. The fine structure of human atherosclerotic lesions. Amer. J. Path., 38:263, 1961.

14. Haust, M.D., Balis, J.U., and More, R.H. Electron microscopic study of intimal lipid accumulations in human aorta and their pathogenesis. Circulation, 26:656, 1962.

15. Geer, J.C. Fine structure of human aortic intimal thickening and fatty streaks. Lab. Invest., 14:1764, 1965.

16. Scott, R.F., Florentin, R.A., Daoud, A.S., Morrison, E.S., Jones, R.M., and Hutt, M.S.R. Coronary arteries of children and young adults. A comparison of lipids and anatomic features in New Yorkers and East Africans. Exp. Molec. Path., 5:12, 1966.

17. Sabin, F.R. Preliminary note on the differentiation of angioblasts and the method by which they produce blood vessels, blood plasma and red blood cells as seen in the living chick. Anat. Rec., 13:199, 1917.

18. ——— Studies on the origin of blood vessels and of red blood corpuscles as seen in the living blastoderm of chicks during the second day of incubation. Contrib. Embryol. Carney Institute (No. 272), 9:213, 1920.

19. Stein, A., Schilp, A.O., and Whitfield, R.D. Histogenesis of hemangioblastoma of the brain. J. Neurosurg., 17:751, 1960.

20. Bunting, C.H., and Bunting, H. Acid mucopolysaccharides of the aorta. Arch. Path., 55:257, 1953.

21. Taylor, J.E. Role of mucopolysaccharides in the pathogenesis of intimal fibrosis and arteriosclerosis of the human aorta. Amer. J. Path., 29:871, 1953.

22. Braunstein, H. Histochemical study of the adult aorta. Arch. Path., 69:29, 1960.

23. Glagor, S., Rowley, D.A., and Wolinsky, H. Pulsating tubes induce tissue growth. J.A.M.A., 205:29, 1968.

Addendum

Cardiac Myxoma

Since 1969 cardiac myxomas have been studied electronmicroscopically by several investigators.[1-4] Most of these studies identified a mixture of cells similar to those previously described. The authors concluded that the lesion was probably a neoplasm and of subendothelial vasoformative reserve cell origin.[2–4] A study on the monoclonal nature of this tumor, similar to the Benditt and Benditt publication on atherosclerotic plaques,[5] would lend further support to its neoplastic histogenesis.

Also, there have been several clinical reports on cardiac myxomas. These cases usually demonstrated unusual complications, unusual histories, or the value of newer diagnostic techniques. The complications included infection, calcification, recurrence embolization, and variations in size and locations.[6–10] Some articles stressed the problems of diagnosis by cardiac catheterization and the value of phonocardiograms,[11] apex cardiograms,[12] and other techniques. Krause et al made the first report of intracardiac myxomas in siblings.[13]

Relation to Other Proliferative Diseases of Subendothelial Vasoformative Reserve Cell

A number of challenging mechanisms which may play a role in the pathogenesis of the arteriosclerotic plaque have been presented recently.

Focal proliferative subintimal vasoformative cellular response is a final common pathway for a number of discrete or interacting incitants. The induction of this cellulo-proliferative response may be mediated by one or more genetic, metabolic, and/or hormonal intrinsic individual factors; as well as by extrinsic environmental chemicals, physical agents, or viruses. One or more of these factors may act at different points locally or systemically in a complex chain of positive or negative feedback controlling molecular events in cell division.

Cellular differentiation and maturation are the means of resolution of the vasoformative celluloproliferative response The type of resolution will dictate the risk of local anatomic complications. Within the plaque. apparent biochemical defects may be related to the irregular and incomplete maturation of the vaso- formative cells.

The genetic aspects of risk usually have been assessed by clinical epidemiologic methods. However, recent studies provide more direct evidence.

In benign uterine smooth muscle tumors, glucose-6-phosphate dehydrogenase exists as a pair of X-linked cellular isoenzymes. One of the two X-chromosome-linked isoenzymes is randomly inactivated early in embryonic development. The analysis of the isoenzymes may be used as an index of monoclonal growths. Benditt and Benditt reported that multiple samples taken from four female patients showed that the fibrous caps of plaques were composed of cells that produced predominantly one enzyme type consistent with monoclonal cell proliferation.[5] This study appears to lend support to the concept of proliferation of a single cell source. the vasoformative reserve cell.

Recent studies concerned with the binding of cholesterol to the surface membrane of human fibroblasts indicate that there are significant individual genetic differences.[14] The development of high-risk atherosclerotic rabbits and pigeon strains as experimental models is a further application of genetic selection.[15, 16]

The role of immunologic mechanisms in the development of atherosclerosis has been recently reawakened and reviewed.[17, 18, 20] Davies reported that a higher proportion of heart attack patients than controls had antibodies in their blood to milk protein and egg white.[19]

The role of a viral agent in induction or interaction with other incitants in the development of a plaque is again considered.[21]

Florentin et al and Lee et al have shown that aqueous extracts of aortic tissues injected intraperitoneally in swine drastically reduce the rate of smooth muscle cell entry into mitosis.[22, 23] It was suggested that this extract may contain a chalone, which plays a role in natural cell growth mechanisms. Simard et al recently reported that, using a rabbit hepatic chalone, mitosis of liver cells could be blocked during interphase or at metaphase in partially hepatectomized rats.[24] This hepatic chalone appeared to be organ specific but not species specific

Apoptosis is a cell death mechanism, which has been long appreciated but recently reexamined.[25, 26] In tissue the dropout of cells is normal in stimulated foci and can be demonstrated by light and electronmicroscopy but is difficult to quantitate. The factors which trigger or inhibit the rate of apoptosis are not clear. However, focal necrosis is a frequent hazard of cellular proliferation in a plaque.

Hille has been studying the mechanisms which turn on protein synthesis in the first stages of embryonic development in the sea urchin egg.[27] There is a protein inhibitor which has been isolated from the ribosomes of unfertilized eggs. Following fertilization this inhibitor of protein synthesis disappears and is followed by an increase in the rate of incorporation of amino acids into protein until the egg reaches embryo stage. There may be mechanisms of control of cell proliferation which are age or differentiation dependent in the totipotent vasoformative reserve cell.

Mizejewski and Allen have shown that antibodies made against α fetoprotein (AFP) can suppress AFP secretory hepatic tumors in mice.[28] These studies suggest that immature proliferating cells such as proliferating totipotent vasoformative reserve cells may have surface embryo antigens which can induce host antibodies for the internal target humoral immunotherapeutic control of proliferation (a form of cell surveillance mechanism).

The effects of numerous chemicals in the development or resolution of experimental plaques continue to be reported.

Modern living places mongrel man in a multifactorial milieu and the result of the total body burden countered by all levels of host adaptation will dictate the topography of risk and disease.

References

1. Jones-Williams W, Jenkins D, Erasmus D: The ultrastructure of cardiac myxoma. Thorax 25:756, 1970
2. Glasser SP, Bedynek JL, Hall RS, et al: Left atrial myxoma. Am J Med 50:113, 1971
3. Silverberg SG, Kay S: Ultrastructure of a cardiac myxoma. Am J Clin Pathol 54:650, 1970
4. Kelley M, Bhagwat AG: Ultrastructural features of a recurrent endothelial myxoma of the left atrium. Arch Pathol 93:219–226, 1972

5. Benditt EP, Benditt JM: Evidence for a monoclonal origin of human atherosclerotic plaques. Proc Natl Acad Sci USA 70:1753, 1900

6. Maranhao V, Gooch AS, Yang SS, Goldberg H: Regrowth of left atrial myxoma. Chest 63:98, 1973

7. Case records of the Massachusetts General Hospital. Weekly clinicopathological exercises. Case 37-1972. N Engl J Med 287:555, 1972

8. Goldschlager A, Popper R, Goldschlager N, Gerbode F, Prozan G: Right atrial myxoma with right to left shunt and polycythemia presenting as congenital heart disease. Am J Cardiol 30:82 1972

9. Pindyck F, Peirce EC 2nd, Baron MG, Lukban SB: Embolization of left atrial myxoma after transseptal cardiac catheterization. Am J Cardiol 30:569, 1972

10. Resection of regrowth of a left atrial myxoma complicated by complete heart block three years following its primary resection. J Cardiovasc Surg (Torino) 14:338, 1973

11. Becker LC, Conti CR: Left atrial myxoma—evidence of tumor movement by apex-cardiogram Chest 60:280, 1971

12. Craige E, Algary WP: Left atrial myxoma. Diagnosis with the help of the phono-cardiogram and apexcardiogram. Arch Intern Med 129:470, 1972

13. Krause S, Adler LN, Reddy PS, MacGovern GJ: Intracardiac myxoma in siblings. Chest 60:404, 1971

14. Brown MS, Goldstein JL: Familial hypercholesteremia: defective binding of lipo-proteins to cultured fibroblasts associated with impaired regulation of 3-hydroxy-3 methylglutaryl co-enzyme A-reductase activity. Proc Natl Acad Sci USA 71:788, 1974

15. Wagner WD, Clarkson TB, Feldner MA, Prichard RW: The development of pigeon strains with selected atherosclerosis characteristics. Exp Mol Pathol 19:304, 1973

16. Adams WC, Gaman EM, Feigenbaum AS: Breed differences in the responses of rabbits to atherogenic diets. Atherosclerosis 16:405, 1972

17. Minick CR, Murphy GE: Experimental induction of atheroarteriosclerosis by the synergy of allergic injury to arteries and lipid-rich diet. II. Effect of repeatedly injected foreign protein in rabbits fed a lipid-rich, cholesterol-poor diet. Am J Pathol 73:265, 1973

18. Lamberson HV Jr, Fritz KE: Immunological enhancement of atherogenesis in rabbits. Arch Pathol 98:9, 1974

19. Davies DF, Johnson AP, Rees BWG, Elwood PC: Food additives and myocardial infarction. Lancet 1:1012, 1974

20. Poston RN, Davies DF: Immunity and inflammation in the pathogenesis of atherosclerosis. A review. Atherosclerosis 19:353, 1974

21. Hayes KC, Westmoreland NP, Faherty TP: An aortitis in the squirrel monkey and its effect on atherosclerosis. Exp Mol Pathol 17:334, 1972

22. Florentin R, et al: Population dynamics of arterial smooth muscle cells. Arch Pathol 95:317, 1973

23. Lee KT, et al: Genesis of atherosclerosis in swine fed high fat cholesterol diets. Med Clin North Am 58:281, 1974

24. Simard A, Corneille L, Deschamps Y, Verly WG: Inhibition of cell proliferation in the livers of hepatectomized rats by a rabbit hepatic chalone. Proc Natl Acad Sci USA 71:1763, 1974

25. Kerr JFR, Wyllie AH, Currie AR: A basic biological phenomenon with wide ranging implications in tissue kinetics. Br J Cancer 26:239, 1972

26. Wyllie AH, Kerr JFR, Currie AR: Cell death in the normal neonatal rat adrenal cortex. J Pathol 3:255, 1972

27. Hille MB: Inhibitor of protein synthesis isolated from ribosomes of unfertilized eggs and embryos of sea urchins. Nature 249:556, 1974

28. Mizejewski GJ, Allen RP: Immunotherapeutic suppression in transplantable solid tumors. Nature 250:50, 1974

RECENT ADVANCES IN THE UNDERSTANDING OF THE PATHOGENESIS AND THE REVERSAL OF ATHEROSCLEROSIS

R. W. WISSLER

D. VESSELINOVITCH

The pathogenesis of atherosclerosis in man and experimental animals, long a subject of varying viewpoints and conflicting evidence, is now approaching the point where essential agreement can be anticipated. Two monographs[1, 2] and a number of scientific papers have appeared in 1967 and 1968 which have increased substantially the understanding of the complex pathogenesis of this disease. Furthermore, observations of reversal of this disease process, long a neglected subject, have now been made in man and to a lesser extent in experimental animals, aided substantially by in vivo coronary arteriography.

Geographic Pathology and Epidemiology

One of the most comprehensive and useful studies of the geographic pathology of atherosclerosis which is pertinent to pathogenesis and reversal has just been published in monograph form.[1] This study involves quantitation and clinical-pathologic correlation of atherosclerosis of the aorta, coronary arteries, and cerebral arteries in a standard autopsy sample collected during a five-year period from each of 14 countries and involving data from more than 23,207 sets of aortas and coronary arteries from patients, aged 10 to 69 years.[3] Cerebral arteries were collected from 1,547 autopsies on patients in the same age group from five countries.[4] These cases represent 25 geographic and ethnic population groups. Attention is concentrated in much of the study on the "raised" atherosclerotic lesions which are directly responsible for narrowing the coronary arteries and for setting the stage for the other events which lead to the ischemic and thromboembolic complications of atherosclerosis.[5]

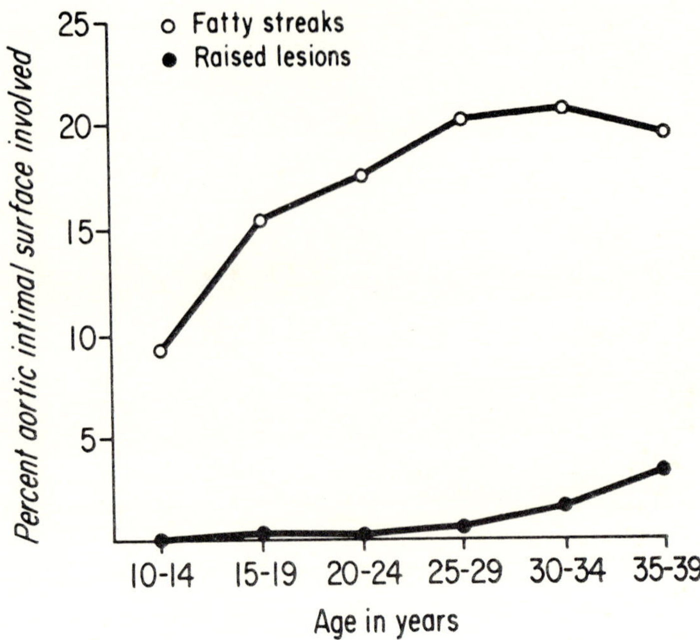

Fig. 1.   Percent of aortic intimal surface involved with fatty streaks and raised lesions in males from Santiago, Chile. (From McGill. *Lab. Invest.*, 18:560, 1968. Courtesy of The Williams & Wilkins Co.)

Factors Affecting Progression

The study revealed that quantitatively similar *aortic* fatty streaks appear to develop during the first two decades in all of the populations regardless of economic state, diet, race, or other recognizable factors. Furthermore, there was little correlation between aortic fatty streaks in young people and aortic raised lesions in older people (Fig. 1).[6] This led the author to conclude that there must be conditions or factors other than lipid deposition that critically influence the development of raised fatty lesions with a fibrous cap in aortas of middle-aged to elderly subjects.

On the other hand, coronary fatty streaks increased continuously during the same period of life, and the accelerated development of fatty streaks correlated well with the accelerated development of raised coronary lesions (Fig. 2). McGill concluded that coronary fatty streaks, unlike aortic fatty streaks, are influenced by environmental or ethnic factors which are likely to control their progression into advanced lesions.

Atherogenesis and Intercurrent Disease

Although the results of this study confirmed the long observed direct association of the severity of atherosclerosis with hypertension and diabetes mellitus,[7] it did not confirm the inverse relationship of atherosclerosis with other diseases such as tuberculosis, cirrhosis of the liver, cancer of the stomach, and other forms of malignant neoplasia.[8]

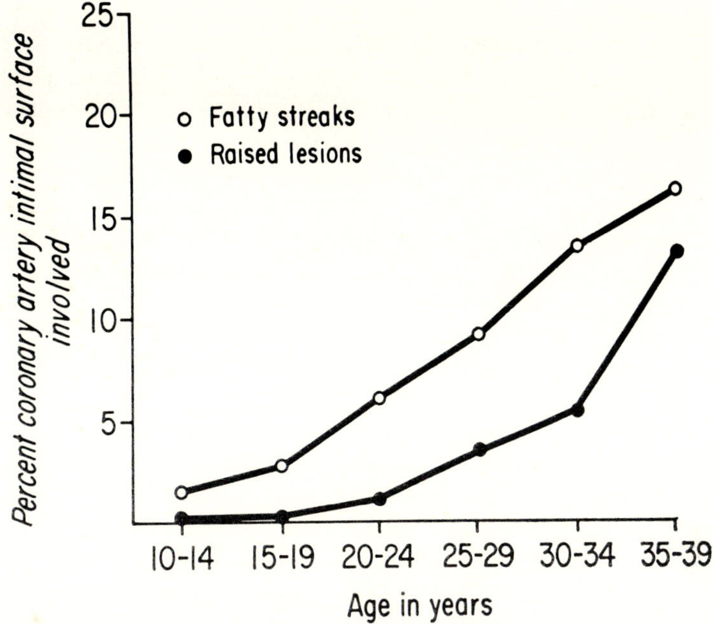

Fig. 2.   Percent of intimal surface involved with fatty streaks and raised lesions in Negro males from New Orleans. (From McGill. *Lab. Invest.*, 18:560, 1968. Courtesy of The Williams & Wilkins Co.)

A borderline suggestive association of cancer of the lung with increased severity of atherosclerosis was revealed in this study. No correlation was found between body weight, body height or trunk length, and severity of atherosclerosis.[9] The authors concluded that if obesity by itself is a risk factor in coronary artery disease, then it would seem to act by a mechanism other than by aggravating mural atherogenesis.

Correlation of Severity of Atherosclerosis with Mortality

The severity of atherosclerosis and its correlation with environmental agents revealed a change in the severity of the disease in the populations several years before morbidity and mortality statistics from coronary heart disease reveal any such association.

An especially important contribution of the study was the finding that with few exceptions the ranking of autopsy groups according to the severity of raised atherosclerotic plaques correlated closely with the ranking of the same population by mortality from coronary heart disease.[10] Furthermore, the ranking was similar among the various autopsy groups regardless of sex, arteries evaluated, or the decade being considered.[11] These observations strongly support the prevailing view that environmental factors exert predominant control over the pathogenesis of this disease and that the severity of the disease in the artery wall is closely correlated with the incidence of clinical manifestations.

Reversal of Lesions?

This study also contributed tantalizing facts regarding reversal of atherosclerotic lesions, since in some of the populations aortic fatty lesions tended to diminish in extent over those seen in earlier decades.[6] This observation could, of course, be a reflection of changing social and economic patterns of living rather than true reversal of lesions. Since the autopsies were performed in a relatively small span of years, one could assume that the younger representatives of the postmortem populations had been exposed more heavily early in life to changing mores which cause acceleration of the atherosclerotic process, such as the consumption of richer diets, decreasing exercise, increasing use of cigarettes, etc.

Histogenesis and Progression

In one of the most challenging parts of the study, the histologic characteristics of the atherosclerotic lesions were determined from a standard site in the left anterior descending coronary artery of 315 males between 10 and 39 years of age from seven different populations.[12] These seven location-race groups were ranked according to the mean extent of atherosclerotic lesions in the coronary artery and aorta as a measure of the tendency of each group to develop atherosclerosis. It was found that the amount of deposited intimal lipid and the degree of cellular infiltration and of intimal proliferation all helped to predict the disposition toward the development of severe raised atherosclerotic plaques with fibrous caps later in life. As will be summarized in the following section of this paper, a similar conclusion can be made from the study of experimentally induced lesions in animals such as Rhesus monkeys[13] and swine.[14] In general, the essential features of the histogenesis of progressive atherosclerosis in the artery wall were proliferation or immigration of medial cells into the intima and evidence of injury or "irritation" of the artery as indicated by signs of cell damage and/or inflammation.

Report of First International Symposium

Signs of reaction of the arterial wall to injury, particularly when certain food fats are fed to experimental animals, were reported in a second monograph on atherosclerosis published within the last few months. This monograph entitled *Recent Advances in Atherosclerosis* contains the complete proceedings, including the discussions, of the First International Symposium on Atherosclerosis held in Athens in June of 1966.[2] Although publication was delayed, it is the only recently available volume which presents a comprehensive review of recent progress in the study of this disease. It, too, reflects substantial progress in the understanding of the pathogenesis of this disease.

Epidemiology and Atherosclerosis Control

Two of the epidemiologic studies which are reported in the first section of this monograph have important implications in terms of pathogenesis, prevention, and reversal of atherosclerosis. J. J. Groen[15] of Israel reported recent studies indicating that members of the Bedouin population as well as Jewish portworkers and Arab villagers with serum cholesterol levels below 150 mg percent demonstrated a virtual absence of myocardial infarction or coronary heart disease; whereas patients with serum cholesterol in the 200 to 300 mg percent range demonstrated a substantial attack rate from this disease. Groen and his co-workers further interpreted some of the very low attack rates, particularly those in the Bedouin and in the Jewish portworkers, as reflecting the protective effects of habitual vigorous physical exercise combined with diets conducive to low serum lipid levels.[16] They emphasized the predominance of cereals in these diets.

In a most stimulating report, Dr. Jeremiah Stamler[17] presented early results of his long-term study of "high risk" male participants in the Coronary Prevention Evaluation Program of the Board of Health of the City of Chicago which is supported by the Chicago Heart Association and the National Heart Institute. The 6-year mortality rate of the 82 very high-risk participants, who were included in the study and who had followed the multiple recommendations designed to reduce their risk factors, was approximately one-tenth of that of a control group composed of dropouts from the program who had had similar but no more severe risk factor abnormalities. The two death rate figures available at the time of this report were 21.7 per thousand for the treated group and 228.7 for the dropout group (Table 1).

Table 1. Six Year Mortality Rates from Coronary Heart Disease in Very High Risk Participants in the Coronary Prevention Evaluation Program*

GROUP	NUMBER OF MEN	NUMBER OF DEATHS	DEATH RATE	S.E.
All	117	6	108.9	45.3
Non-drop-outs	82	1	21.7	19.8
Drop-outs	35	5	228.7	90.0

* From Stamler, et al. *Progr. Biochem. Pharmacol.,* 4:30, 1968. Courtesy of S. Karger, Basel.

Of the 35 dropouts, five died, all of coronary heart disease. These results must be considered as preliminary, but they are encouraging and certainly demonstrate the ability to maintain free-living, high-risk, middle-aged men in a coronary disease prevention program designed to counteract multiple risk factors on a long-term basis.

Control of Cholesterol Synthesis

In the section on lipid metabolism of intact animals, two contributions—one by C. Bruce Taylor's group of Chicago[18] and one by Professor Börgstrom of Lund which was quoted by Ahrens in his presentation[19]—indicate that two of the long-held opinions regarding the lack of danger in consuming large amounts of dietary cholesterol are probably incorrect. Dr. Taylor reported a virtual absence of depression of hepatic cholesterol synthesis when large amounts of dietary cholesterol are given to man. Dr. Börgstrom's report suggested that there is no effective ceiling for cholesterol absorption in man. He reported that with intakes varying from 150 mg to 2 g of dietary cholesterol per day the same percent of the daily intake was absorbed. This means that at least 600 mg per day can be absorbed from dietary sources. Each of these reports have important implications in terms of pathogenesis, prevention, and the reversal of atherosclerosis in man.

Lipoprotein Deposition in the Artery

Many of the intact artery and tissue culture studies reported in this volume[2] helped reinforce the emerging view that intact lipoproteins, particularly the low-density varieties, make their way into the artery wall[20, 21] and into the pre-existing medial (smooth muscle) mesenchymal cells where a number of important biochemical events take place. These include splitting off the protein moiety of the lipoprotein,[22] further synthesis or at least a change in the fatty acids of the cholesterol ester molecules,[23] and stimulation of synthesis of phospholipid by these arterial wall cells.[23, 24, 25] Furthermore, increasing evidence indicates that the cells of the artery wall, far from being inert and static, have a remarkable capacity for proliferation in response to various kinds of stimuli.[26, 27, 28] This appears to be true of the subintimal smooth muscle cells, the endothelial cells, and the stellate cells of the actual atheromatous lesions. In contrast, endothelial and smooth muscle cells located away from the plaque are rarely labelled by tritiated thymidine and probably divide relatively rarely. Of particular interest was the report by Hollander, Kramsch, and Inoue,[29] whose more recent work will be reviewed later in this report. They have obtained substantial evidence that extractable low-density lipoproteins but not high-density lipoproteins accumulate in the human and experimental atherosclerotic plaque (Table 2).[30] Much of the accumulated cholesterol is deposited

Table 2. Extractable Lipoprotein Content of the Human Aortic Intima with Atherosclerosis*

| | | Low-density fractions | | High-density fractions |
| | $d < 1.063$ | % | | d 1.063– 1.210 |
Content	mg/g.d.t.	$d < 1.019$	d 1.019–1.063	mg/g.d.t.
Lipoprotein content	101	44%	56%	8.6
Total lipid	91	40%	47%	4.3
Total protein	10	4%	9%	4.3

* From Hollander. *Exp. Molec. Path.,* 7:248, 1967. Courtesy of Academic Press, Inc.

intracellularly and still retains its linkage to low-density lipoproteins. The reduced cholesterol specific activity in the plaque, together with radioautographic findings, suggest that there is an impaired transport of arterial cholesterol in the plaques. This metabolic deficiency may play an important role in the accumulation of cholesterol in the arterial intima (Table 3).

Anoxia and Other Factors in Pathogenesis of Atherosclerosis

Studies reported by Abel Robertson[22] indicate that reduced oxygen availability at the cellular level may play an important part in accelerating human atherogenesis

 275

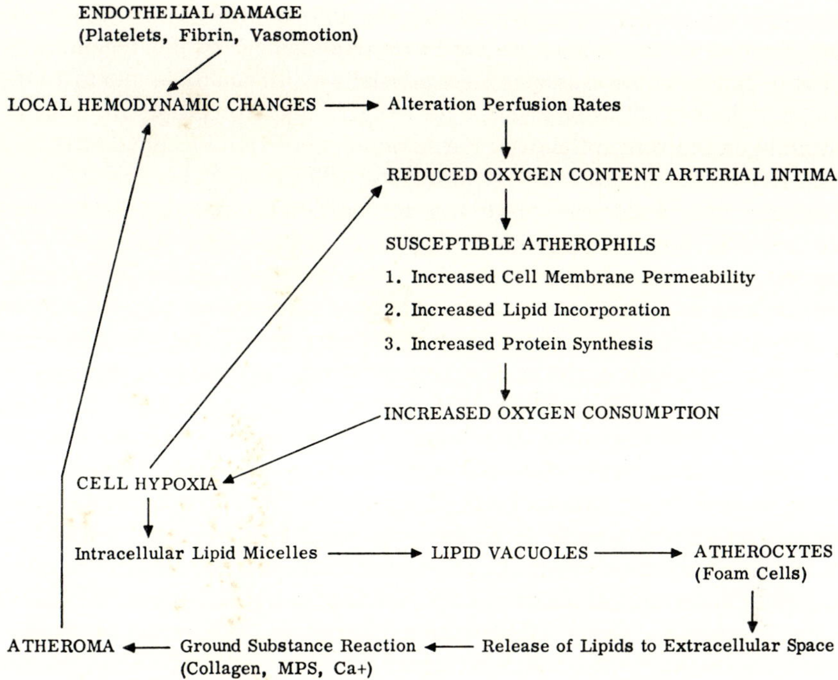

Fig. 3. Reduced oxygen availability at the cellular level and its part in accelerating human atherogenesis by initiating a chain-reaction of self-sustaining metabolic abnormalities. (Lazzarini-Robertson. *Progr. Biochem. Pharmacol.*, 4:305, 1968. Courtesy of S. Karger, Basel.)

by initiating a chain reaction of sustained metabolic abnormalities (Fig. 3). He concludes that many of the theories of pathogenesis of atherosclerosis may be explained by a common denominator of reduced oxygen transport.

There appears to be emerging evidence that enzyme activity in the intact smooth muscle cell is important in determining the overall metabolic activity in the artery wall. The smooth muscle cell appears to be vulnerable to anoxia, and its metabolic activity declines rapidly after various injuries. In fact, Adams et al.[31] have reported that respiratory function is decreased in the senescent aorta. This is correlated with depression of lipolytic and triglyceride degrading enzyme activity.

Table 3. Subcellular Distribution of Intravenously Administered ^{3}H Cholesterol in Aortic Intima of Man Suggests Accumulation in the Arterial Intima*

	Uninvolved Intima			Atherosclerotic Plaque		
Fraction	CHOLESTEROL MG/G.D.T.	^{3}H-CHOLESTEROL CPM/G.D.T.	CHOLESTEROL SP. ACTIVITY	CHOLESTEROL MG/G.D.T.	^{3}H-CHOLESTEROL CPM/G.D.T.	CHOLESTEROL SP. ACTIVITY
Nuclear debris	15.6	8946	573	71.3	7653	107
Mitochondria	2.4	574	239	7.6	1436	189
Microsome	1.5	416	277	13.8	1894	137
Supernatant	3.7	1686	455	50.4	4328	86

A.C. ♀, 34.

* From Hollander, et al. *Progr. Biochem. Pharmacol.*, 4:270, 1968. Courtesy of S. Karger, Basel.

Progressive intimal thickening also impairs the diffusion of oxygen into the inner and middle parts of the media, leading to hypoxic damage of this region.[32]

The thickness of the avascular inner arterial wall in man (0.84 mm to 1.00 mm) borders on a limiting diffusion distance for oxygen. Therefore, this part of the artery is constantly on the verge of anoxia. Furthermore, cholesterol feeding alters respiratory kinetics of the arterial cell. It lowers the efficiency of phosphorylation and depresses the mitochondrion's machinery for fatty acid synthesis. Anaerobic glycolysis then makes the largest contribution to this cell's energy requirement due to inadequate supply of oxygen and deficient "Pasteur effect" in the artery wall.[33]

When middle arterial zones are poorly supplied with oxygen, the activity of many enzymes decline, but lactate dehydrogenase rises.[34] This is compatible with the view that the hypoxic middle layers of the artery wall utilize partial glycolysis for their energy needs. This is also true in the atherosclerotic lesion according to the results of lactate dehydrogenase isoenzyme studies by Lojda and Fric.[35] In a recent article, Zemplenyi[36] explains the relationship between enzymatic disturbances and some events of genesis in atherosclerosis as follows: In arteries susceptible to atherosclerosis, the activity of Krebs cycle enzymes decreases, respiration and oxidative phosphorylation are impaired, so that there is a decreased production of energy rich phosphate bonds and reduced vascular synthetic activity. The result of the above biochemical abnormalities might be expected to be reduced protein and phospholipid synthesis which in turn could result in decreased solubilization of hydrophobic lipids (especially cholesterol) and the decreased removal of "sclerogenic" lipids from the arterial wall. Therefore, Zemplenyi reasons, it appears that the defensive mechanism in the arterial medial cells of the artery wall is reduced, resulting in an unfavorable balance between lipid transportation from plasma and the artery's metabolism.

Other new and informative data which may have a bearing on the pathogenesis of atherosclerosis in man and which were presented for the first time at the Athens Symposium are reported by Beaumont[37] who studied patients who have produced antibodies to their own low-density (beta) lipoproteins. The report by K. W. Walton[38] implicated and also demonstrated connection of the low-density lipoproteins to the pathogenesis of human atherosclerosis both in the male and in the female. Furman, et al.,[39] taking into consideration the importance of the serum lipids, particularly their physical state, in atherogenesis, indicated that androgen-induced reduction in apoliprotein A synthesis (a-lipoproteins) will result in diminution of serum lipoprotein stability and will thus augment atherogenesis.

Effects of Drugs on Reversal of Atherosclerosis

New data on the effects of some of the most promising therapeutic agents were recorded for the first time. Among these was the report by Lars Karlson[40] of Stockholm who reviewed the most recent advances in the understanding of the blood lipid lowering effects of nicotinic acid. It now appears that it lowers lipoprotein concentration by inhibiting the usual free fatty acid supply to the liver from adipose stores, thus resulting in a decrease of lipoprotein synthesis in the liver, which in turn results in decreasing concentrations of lipoproteins in the blood. Gould and

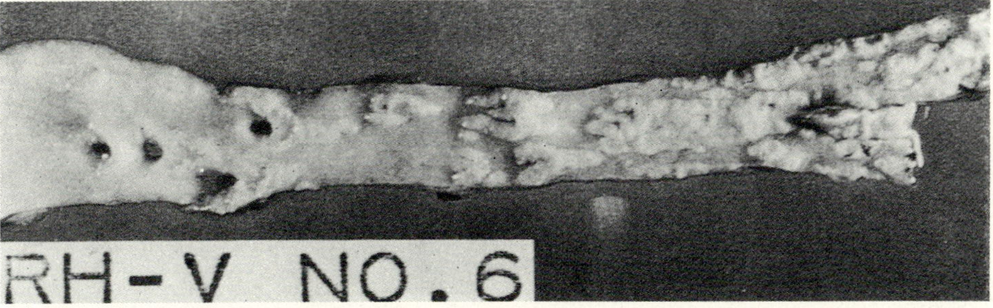

Fig. 4.   Severe atherosclerotic lesion in the abdominal aorta of the Rhesus monkey fed a mixture of butterfat and coconut oil. (From Wissler. *Progr. Biochem. Pharmacol.*, 4:378, 1968. Courtesy of S. Karger, Basel.)

Swyryd[41] presented extensive evidence indicating that CPIB (Atromid S) inhibits cholesterol synthesis in the liver at a very early biochemical stage in the conversion of acetate to mevolonate, with no resulting accumulation of any identifiable intermediate in the cholesterol biosynthesis chain. They concluded that the CPIB acts in a manner similar to exogenous cholesterol in inhibiting cholesterol synthesis and thus should be considered as having a physiologic mechanism of action.

Experimental Atherogenesis

Among the reports most pertinent to an understanding of the pathogenesis of atherosclerosis were those which dealt with the development of this disease in primates and nonprimates, both experimentally manipulated and studied in the normal situation. The accelerated development of severe, far advanced atherosclerosis in the Rhesus monkey by pure dietary means involving the use of a mixture of butterfat and coconut oil was documented (Figs. 4, 5).[28] In addition, the importance of certain food fats such as coconut oil and peanut oil in the stimulation

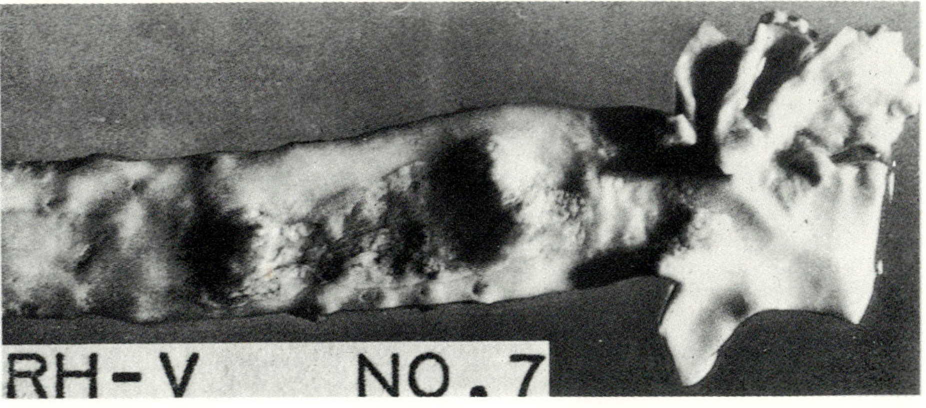

Fig. 5.   Severe atherosclerotic lesion in the thoracic aorta of a Rhesus monkey fed a mixture of butterfat and coconut oil. (From Wissler. *Progr. Biochem. Pharmacol.*, 4:378, 1968. Courtesy of S. Karger, Basel.)

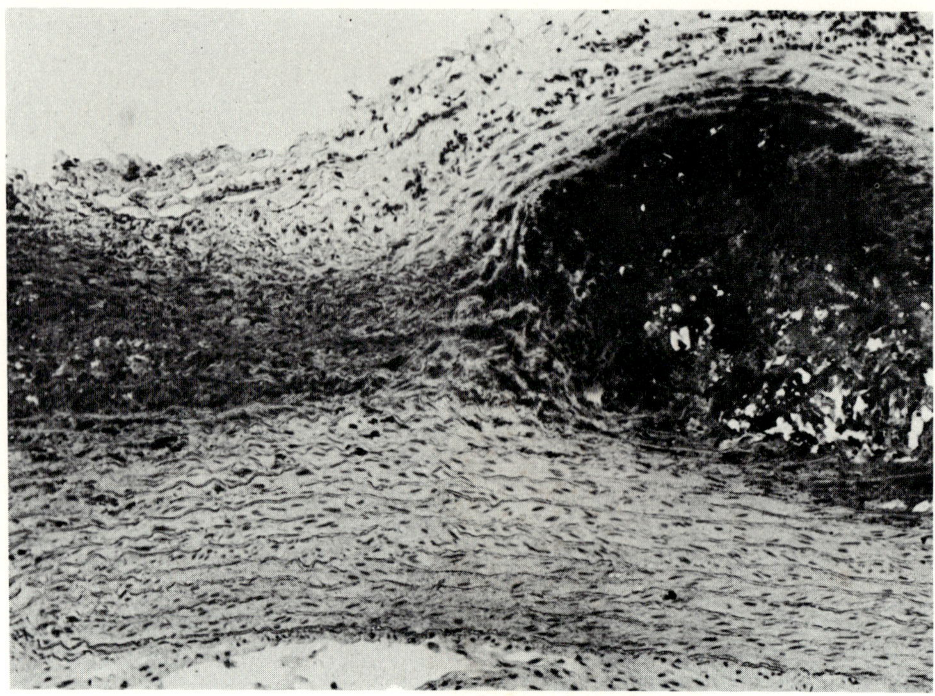

Fig. 6.   Photomicrograph of a severe atherosclerotic lesion produced by a diet containing butterfat and coconut oil in the aorta of a Rhesus monkey. Oil Red 0. X 100. (From Wissler. *Progr. Biochem. Pharmacol.*, 4:378, 1968. Courtesy of S. Karger, Basel.)

of arterial medial cells proliferation was reported in several species. These included studies in the squirrel monkey, rabbit, and dog.[42, 43, 44] The ensuing discussion suggested that myristic acid or perhaps lauric acid may be particularly potent in producing this substantial arterial cell reaction. This phenomenon is of considerable practical importance since some populations, notably Scandinavians, are recorded to consume very large amounts of coconut oil. Furthermore, the experimental disease produced by rather simple manipulation of the monkey so closely resembles the complicated and far advanced lesions in man (Figs. 6, 7) that this model may present a promising approach to further studies of methods to additional documentation of the important factors influencing pathogenesis, prevention, and reversal of atherosclerosis.

Platelets, Fibrin and Atherogenesis

There were numerous reports in this monograph which indicates the growing recognition of the substantial role played by platelets and fibrin in the development of the atherosclerotic lesion in man and experimental animals. Although the precise mechanisms are not yet clear, it is becoming more and more evident that platelets or platelet products not only enter the arterial wall, but they may have an important role in unlocking the arterial endothelium so that larger quantities of low-density lipoproteins can be deposited in focal areas. Of particular interest were the results

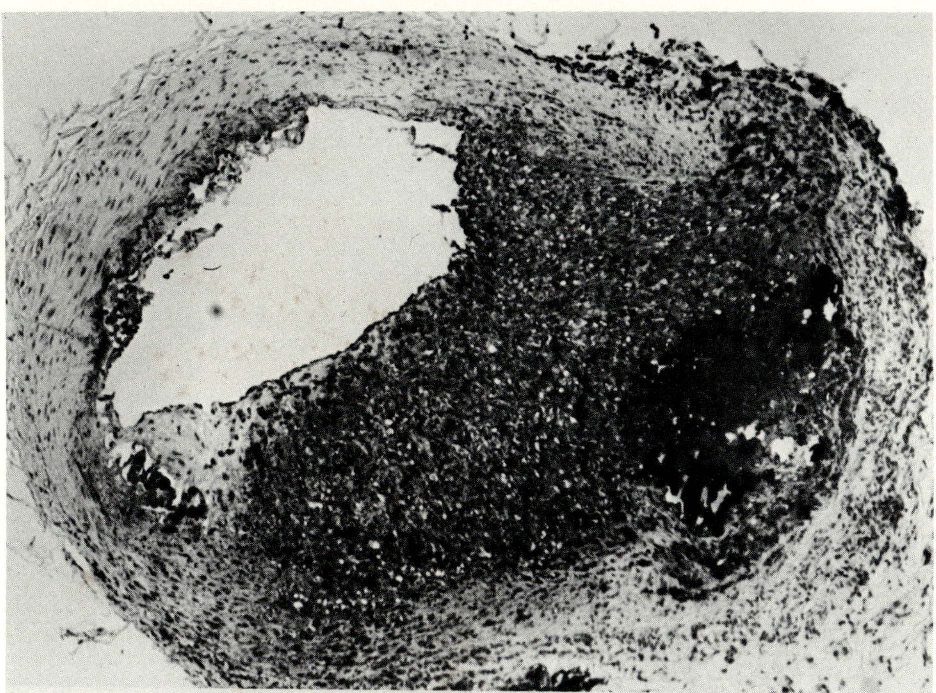

Fig. 7   Photomicrograph of a severe atherosclerotic lesion in the cross section of a major coronary artery of a Rhesus monkey fed a mixture of butterfat and coconut oil. Oil Red 0. X 100. (From Wissler. *Prog. Biochem. Pharmacol.*, 4:378, 1968. Courtesy of S. Karger, Basel.)

summarized by Frazier Mustard[45] which indicate that adenosine diphosphate causes platelet aggregation and appears to be a final common pathway for many stimuli which induce platelet aggregation. He suggests that surfaces such as collagen and particulate matter such as antigen-antibody complexes, viruses and bacteria all induce platelet aggregation (Fig. 8). Further, the interaction of platelets with these stimuli can be inhibited by several "anti-inflammatory" compounds. The electron-microscopic and immunohistochemical studies of "fatty streaks" of the human aorta by M. Daria Haust[46] also implicate fibrin in the early atherosclerotic lesion in man and further support the concept that several blood elements as well as the smooth muscle cell are involved in the development and progression of the fatty lesion.

In general, these studies further emphasize the combined roles of lipoprotein and fibrin (with or without platelet products) in the development of atherosclerosis in man. They also indicate the importance of further studies of the interactions among these substances if we are to understand completely the early pathogenesis of this important disease.

Arterial Localization and Metabolism of Lipid

The importance of lipoprotein inhibition in the development of atherosclerosis has been given a further impetus from the recent work on the composition of the

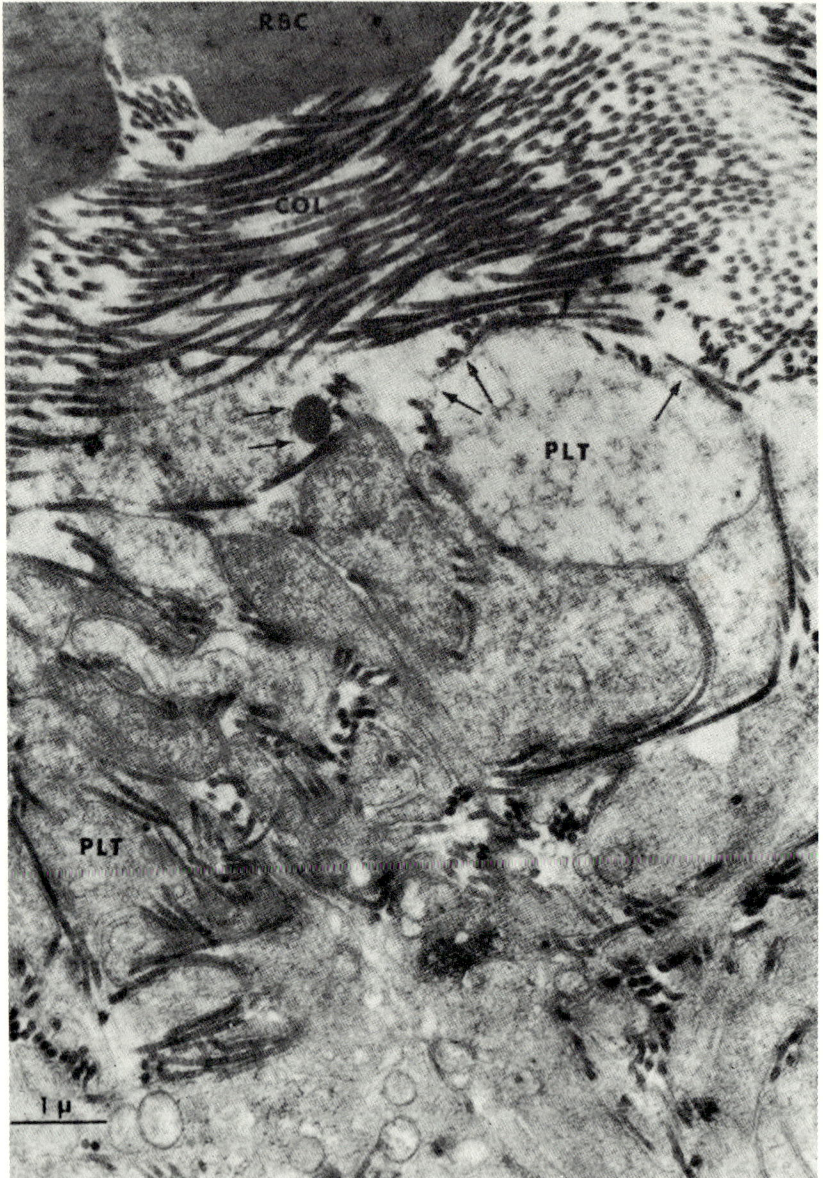

Fig. 8.   Electronmicrograph of the platelets in contact with collagen on an injured vessel wall. X14,500. (From Mustard, et al. *Progr. Biochem. Pharmacol.*, 4:508, 1968. Courtesy of S. Karger, Basel.)

atherosclerotic plaque as compared to normal intima.[30] Hollander[29] and his co-workers have found that the plaque area in both man and dog is much more likely to take up labelled cholesterol than is the normal-looking area (Table 3). Furthermore, they report that the concentration of low-density lipoproteins is about four times as high in atherosclerotic plaques as compared to normal intima, while high density lipoprotein content is comparable in diseased and normal intima. By means of other calculations, it is apparent that low-density to high-density lipoprotein ratios are about 14 to 1 in diseased intima and about 2.5 to 1 in "normal" intima.[30] In contrast, nonprotein bound cholesterol is not readily transportable or metabolizable by the artery; in addition, it is capable of producing substantial inflammation. Studies on the subcellular distribution of intravenously administered tritium-labelled cholesterol in dog and monkey indicated that the uptake is greatest in the microsomal fraction with decreasing amounts in "nuclear debris," mitochondria, and in supernatant fluid.

More recent studies by Hollander[47] indicate the ^{131}I-labelled low-density lipoprotein are also taken up by both the aortic intima and media of the dog. In the intima, much of this appears in the nuclear debris fraction and in the supernatant fluid which may contain some of the "plasma membrane." In the aortic media, the largest proportion of the label appears in the supernatant fluid and lesser quantities are associated with the microsomes, mitochondria, and with the "nuclear debris." Similar results are obtained with samples of femoral artery.

Of equal interest is the fact that over 80 percent of ^{14}C-labelled acetate was incorporated with both the lipid and protein components of the low-density lipoprotein fractions when intimal segments are incubated for eight hours. About three times more ^{14}C acetate was converted into the protein associated with the low-density fraction than in the proteins bound with the high-density fractions. Additional incubation studies with ^{14}C leucine revealed a similar distribution of radioactive protein moieties. In general, the results of these studies by Hollander and his collaborators suggest that lipid and protein components of the low-density lipoprotein fractions are being incorporated into and kept by the artery wall to a much greater extent than those of the high-density fraction.[30, 47, 48]

The studies of Hollander and co-workers also help to increase the evidence that the medial mesenchymal cell of the artery is of critical importance in trapping low-density lipoproteins. In fact, the accumulation of these lipid moieties appears to be of paramount importance in the development of the typical atherosclerotic lesion in man.[48] The importance of localization of low-density lipoprotein in this cell has also been recently supported by new evidence which indicates that the cells in which low-density lipoprotein (and lipid droplets) can be identified by immunohistochemical means are also the same cells which contain myosin.[49, 50] Furthermore, there is increasing evidence that most, if not all, of the cells which proliferate in a number of types of experimentally induced atherosclerosis are modified, lipid-containing, and smooth muscle-containing cells when studied by electronmicroscopy.[51, 52, 53, 54] This concept of a single cell type which responds to injury by means of proliferation and migration, and in some instances by altered synthesis of collagen, elastin, and ground substance, offers an unitarian (Fig. 9) hypothesis for the understanding of the pathogenesis of atherosclerosis.[54, 55] Assuming that this medial cell is more easily injured by accumulating lipid or lipid products than is a histocyte or a fibroblast, this helps one to understand the severe necrosis that is observed in human and non-human primate atherosclerosis, as compared to a relative absence of necrosis in the typical acute foam-cell lesions which have been studied as a part

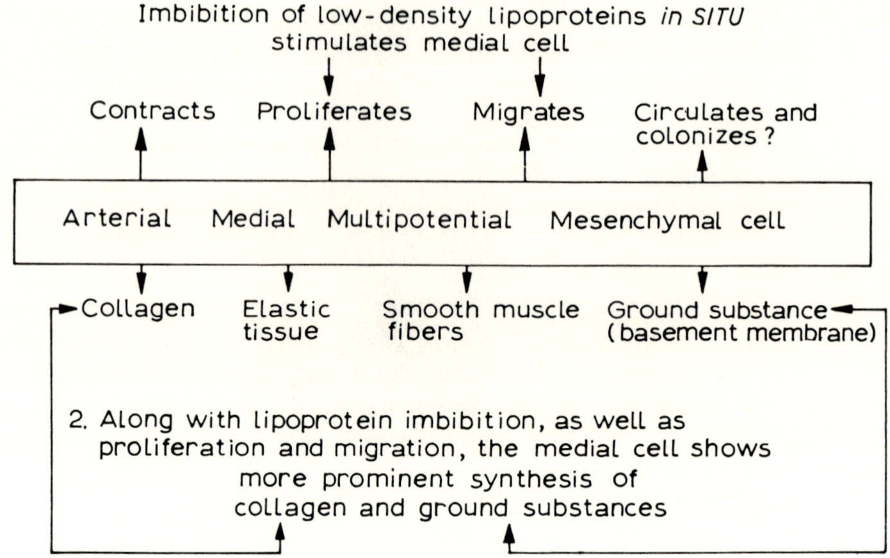

Fig. 9.   Unitarian cellular hypothesis for atherogenesis. (From Wissler. *J. Atheroscler. Res.*, 8:201, 1968. Courtesy of Elsevier Publishing Co., Amsterdam.)

of cholesterol induced generalized xanthomatosis in rabbits and fowl, and to a lesser extent in the cholate-thiouracil-treated, cholesterol-fed rat.[56]

Recently, the major questions which need to be answered about the reaction of the medial cell to this disease have been listed.[49] These include further study of the factors which control the entrance of a number of serum constituents into the arterial medial cell, the factors which stimulate the proliferation and migration of this cell type, identification of the constituents of lipoprotein molecules which are injurious to this cell especially when certain food fats are fed, and the constituents of the lipoprotein molecules which are difficult or impossible for the cells to metabolize. Furthermore, it appears that the mechanisms which can divert the cell from elastin formation to a more abundant collagen or acid mucopolysaccharide formation should be identified.

Thomas and his co-workers[56] have recently reported studies of the pre-proliferative phase of the atherosclerosis in swine fed cholesterol in combination with peanut oil and butter. Observations were made on the abdominal aorta before proliferative lesions became evident. They observed that an increased rate of DNA synthesis in both the intima and media began three days after the experimental dietary regimen was started. At the same time, they observed ultrastructural changes in small clusters of cells in the intima and inner media suggestive of cell damage or even death. Although they did not imply that this pre-proliferative phase always develops into proliferative lesions, it is highly probable that progression by cell multiplication occurs in many cases (Figs. 10, 11).

Imai and Thomas[51] examined and described middle cerebral arteries of young swine fed either a stock or an "atherogenic" diet for 160 days. They observed a transitional state of lesions in the artery between the proliferative and atheromatous

I PRE-PROLIFERATIVE PHASE

> *1 IMBIBITION OF CHOLESTEROL - RICH FLUID INTO EXTRACELLULAR AND INTRACELLULAR COMPARTMENTS OF ARTERIAL WALL.*
>
> *2 DAMAGE AND OCCASIONAL DEATH OF SCATTERED ENDOTHELIAL AND S.M. CELLS USUALLY IN SMALL CLUSTERS IN INNER WALL*
>
> *3 FOCI OF FORMED AND NON-FORMED ELEMENTS OF BLOOD INTO INTIMAL EXTRACELLULAR COMPARTMENT*
>
> *4 INCREASED TURNOVER RATE OF ENDOTHELIAL AND S.M. CELLS TO REPLACE DAMAGED CELLS AND/OR AS A RESULT OF DIRECT STIMULATION*

II PROLIFERATIVE PHASE

> *1 FOCAL PROLIFERATION OF S.M. CELLS TO EXCEED REPLACEMENT NEEDS PRODUCING SMALL MASSES IN INTIMA AND INNER MEDIA*
>
> *2 CYCLE OF DAMAGE AND EXCESSIVE PROLIFERATION PROCEEDS AT VARIABLE PACE IN THE ABOVE MASSES*

III ATHEROMATOUS PHASE

> *1 LARGER FOCI OF DEAD CELLS APPEAR (NECROSIS) RESULTING IN BEGINNING OF ATHEROMA*
>
> *2 THESE FOCI INCREASE IN NUMBER AND COALESCE MAKING LARGER MASSES OF NECROTIC DEBRIS*
>
> *3 IN AREAS OF NECROSIS, CHOLESTEROL (IMBIBED AND RELEASED) PRECIPITATES AND CRYSTALIZES AS DO OTHER SUBSTANCES SUCH AS CALCIUM.*

Fig. 10.   Postulated pathogenesis of atherosclerosis in cholesterol fed swine. Cellular and non-cellular events in the three phases. (From Thomas, et al. *Arch. Path.*, 86:621, 1968. Courtesy of American Medical Association Publications.)

phase. These lesions were characterized by various degrees of degeneration and accumulation of lipid-rich debris. They noticed that identifiable smooth muscle cells were responding by lipid inhibition or sequestration. The endothelial cells showed changes suggestive of disturbed metabolism which they correlated with increased permeability. These lesions were also accompanied by apparent fragmentation of the prominent internal elastic membrane. The adjacent smooth muscle cells had a thickened basement membrane which they concluded was a reaction to the fragmentation.

Studies have been recently reported[52] on miniature pigs fed high fat diets containing butter, peanut oil, sodium cholate, and cholesterol from 30-330 days. Gross and microscopic atheromatous lesions were present by 160 days in abdominal aorta. They appeared to be very similar to human lesions except that they contained more lipid. Radioautographic studies revealed that the surface cells in the proliferative lesions displayed the highest ^{3}H index. Electronmicroscopically, endothelial cell and smooth muscle cell degeneration and death became prominent when the proliferative reaction was well established. Similar, but less pronounced, findings were observed in grossly unremarkable areas of the aortas from atherogenic diet-fed swine. Since the intima was thin and there was absence of visible lipid in the same parts of aorta, they concluded that neither anoxia nor excessive lipid accumulation could be identified as the "cause" of the degenerative changes.

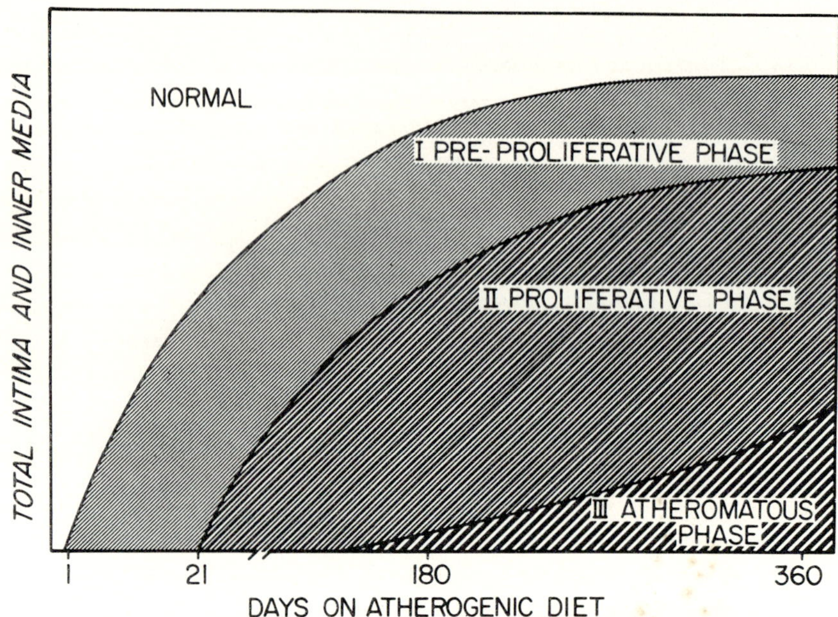

Fig. 11. Phases of cellular events in postulated pathogenesis of atherosclerosis in cholesterol-fed swine. (From Thomas, et al. *Arch. Path.*, 86:621, 1968. Courtesy of American Medical Association Publications.)

Cholesterol ester fatty acid determinations in serum, as well as in the intima-media of swine aortas, analyzed after 160 days of cholesterol feeding showed the greatest absolute increase in cholesterol oleate, linoleate, and palmitate. Triglycerides were increased four-fold in the same regions of the aortas.

In vitro incorporation of leucine ^{14}C into aortic proteins was highest in gross lesions but was also elevated in grossly unremarkable aortic regions when compared with aortic tissue of the swine fed a low fat diet containing no sodium cholate and little or no cholesterol.[52]

Scott, et al.[57] tried to identify the cell components in proliferative (non-necrotic) arterial lesions from atherosclerotic Rhesus monkeys. These lesions also closely resemble those in man. In these lesions, they identified mostly mature smooth muscle cells, as well as certain morphologic classes of cells which probably represent different maturation stages of smooth muscle cell. They also observed a few unidentified cells greatly distended with lipid. They suggested that these could either be distorted smooth muscle cells or macrophages. Foci of cellular degeneration were also frequent. It was thought that in the Rhesus monkey fed high-fat, high cholesterol diets these injured cells might stimulate intimal cell proliferation.[57]

Evaluating Pathogenetic Factors in Man

The two most critical factors in the pathogenesis of atherosclerosis in man and experimental animals appear to be the medial cell and the low density lipoprotein molecules. Therefore, recent advances in the developing practical methods of conducting large numbers of lipoprotein determinations need to be summarized.

At present, serum total lipid determinations and carefully conducted lipoprotein fractionations by paper electrophoresis, coupled with fasting triglyceride determinations and glucose tolerance tests appear to be the most desirable methods of screening large numbers of people for high-risk hyperlipemia.[58, 59, 60, 61] Lena Lewis[62] has recently published a modification of the starch-gel electrophoresis technique of Smithies,[63] which makes it possible to quantitate and to resolve the usually designated fractions of lipoproteins with little equipment other than that used for paper electrophoretic fractionation of protein. Although extensive direct comparisons have not been made, this technique appears to offer greater resolution than the usual paper electrophoretic methods. Furthermore, the results of a number of studies which are now appearing suggest that disc electrophoresis utilizing acrylamide-gel and other disc gels will result in even better high resolution results.[64, 65, 66] The only danger evident at present is that these disc methods may at times disrupt the rather unstable low density lipoprotein molecules. Each of the techniques referred to has the potential of making it possible to perform many thousands of lipoprotein determinations in a short time. These advances should make it feasible for the clinical pathologist to furnish valuable information regarding the various degree of imbalance of circulating lipoproteins which may be present in individual patients.

Lipoprotein Biochemistry

Meanwhile, the basic biochemistry of lipoproteins is also being investigated at a somewhat accelerated pace, but it is probable that the problems involved deserve much more study then they are receiving. In a recent international workshop on lipoproteins[67] held in May, 1968 the following points were recommended:

1. An attempt should be made to encourage standardization of ultracentrifugation techniques employed for the isolations and analysis of lipoproteins from normal and hyperlipemic serum. The density gradient ultracentrifugation techniques recently described deserve special consideration.

2. More knowledge is needed regarding the structural properties of the various serum lipoproteins.

3. Techniques for preparing lipid-free forms of lipoprotein must be further defined and standardized.

4. The comparative properties of lipoproteins derived from normal human and hyperlipemic sera deserve to be detailed and studied more intensively.

5. More comparative studies should be made between serum lipoproteins in man and those in experimental animals, especially those species commonly used in the production of experimental atherosclerosis.

6. Further studies are needed on the metabolism of serum lipoproteins with particular reference to defining their mode of formation, transport, and degradation, with special attention to the lipid-poor form of serum lipoproteins which appear to exist in the circulating plasma.

Evaluation of the Severity of Atherosclerosis in Man During Life

Of great importance in the study of pathogenesis and reversal of atherosclerosis in man is the perfection of in vivo coronary cinearteriography. It appears to permit premortem and postmortem study of the same coronary tree, and it provides a highly accurate means of evaluating the morphology of both normal and diseased coronary vessels.[68, 69, 70] Furthermore, it now becomes apparent that a significant proportion of patients who suffer from classic angina pectoris have normal coronary angiograms. This problem clearly requires more study and may lead to the discovery of forms of myocardial dystrophy not yet suspected. Furthermore, it appears that coronary arteriography may make it possible to follow the reversal of atherosclerosis in vivo. Methods are urgently needed for measuring quantitatively the severity of disease reflected in the arteriogram.

Quantitation of the Severity of Atherosclerosis at Autopsy

Recently, the entire question of the quantitation of atherosclerosis in human arteries has been evaluated by the Committee on Grading of Lesions of the Council on Arteriosclerosis of the American Heart Association in two separate publications in March, 1968.[70, 71] The Committee reports the reliability of the "panel method" of estimating the severity of atherosclerosis in the aorta or in the coronary artery. The panel provides a relatively simple and speedy, as well as quantitative method of comparing autopsy data on atherosclerosis among many population samples. It has the added advantage of facilitating comparisons between different geographic locations and at different times. The second paper summarizes the Committee's work on the problem of grading stenosis in the coronary artery. Postmortem arteriograms, casts and grading of surface area involved were all used on the same arteries. It appears that the use of any two of these three means of evaluating severity of coronary atherosclerosis is preferable to any other one used alone. The next stage of this study is now being undertaken, namely to correlate the degree of coronary disease as revealed by these quantitative methods and the clinical effects of the disease as expressed in damage to the myocardium.

References

1. McGill, H.C., Jr., ed. The geographic pathology of atherosclerosis. Lab. Invest., 18:465, 1968.
2. Miras, C.J., Howard, A.N., and Paoletti, R., eds. Progress in Biochemical Pharmacology: Recent Advances in Atherosclerosis. S. Karger, New York, 1968.
3. Guzman, M.A., McMahan, C.A., McGill, H.C., Jr., Strong, J.P., Tejada, C., Restrepo, C., Eggen, A.D., Robertson, W.B., and Solberg, L.A. Selected methodologic aspects of the informational atherosclerotic project. Lab. Invest., 18:19, 1968.
4. Solberg, A.L., McGarry, P.A., Moossy, J., Tejada, C., Loken, A.C., Robertson, W.B., and Donoso, S. Distribution of cerebral atherosclerosis by geographic location, race and sex. Lab. Invest., 18:604, 1968.
5. McGill, H.C., Jr., Arias-Stella, J., Carbonell, L.M., Correa, P., de Veyra, E.A., Donoso, S., Eggen, D.A., Galindo, L., Guzman, M.A., Lichtenberger, E., Loken, A.C., McGarry, P.A., McMahan, C.A., Montenegro, M.R., Moossy, J., Perez-

Tamayo, R., Restrepo, C., Robertson, W.P., Salas, Y., Solberg, L.A., Strong, J.P., Tejada, C. and Wainwright, J. General findings of the international atherosclerosis project. Lab. Invest., 18:498, 1968.

6. McGill, H.C., Jr. Fatty streaks in the coronary arteries and aorta. Lab. Invest., 18:560, 1968.

7. Robertson, W.B. and Strong, J.P. Atherosclerosis in persons with hypertension and diabetes mellitus. Lab. Invest., 18:538, 1968.

8. Restrepo, C., Montenegro, M.R., and Solberg, L.A. Atherosclerosis in persons with selected disease. Lab. Invest., 18:552, 1968.

9. Montenegro, M.R., and Solberg, L.A. Obesity, body weight, body length and atherosclerosis. Lab. Invest. 18:594, 1968.

10. Strong, J.P., Solberg, L.A., and Restrepo, C. Atherosclerotic lesions in persons with coronary heart disease. Lab. Invest., 18:537, 1968.

11. Montenegro, M.R., and Strong, J.P. Comparison in four broad causes of death groups. Lab. Invest., 18:503, 1968.

12. Geer, J.C., McGill, H.C., Jr., Robertson, W.B., and Strong, J.P. Histologic characteristics of coronary artery fatty streaks. Lab. Invest., 18:565, 1968.

13. Wissler, R.W., Vesselinovitch, D., Getz, G.A., and Hughes, R.H. Aortic lesions and blood lipids in rhesus monkeys fed three food fats. Fed. Proc., 26:2, 1967.

14. Thomas, W.A., Jones, R.M., and Lee, K.T. Electron microscopy study of preatherosclerotic aortas of cholesterol-fed swine. Fed. Proc., 27:575, 1968.

15. Groen, J.J. Recent advances in the epidemiology of atherosclerosis. *In* Progress in Biochemical Pharmacology: Recent Advances in Atherosclerosis, Miras, C.J., Howard, A.N., and Paoletti, R., eds. S. Karger, New York, 1968, Vol. 4, p. 1.

16. Groen, J.J., Dreyfuss, F., and Gutmann, L. Epidemiological, nutritional and sociological studies of atherosclerotic (coronary) heart disease among different ethnic groups in Israel. *In* Progress in Biochemical Pharmacology: Recent Advances in Atherosclerosis, Miras, C.J., Howard, A.N., and Paoletti, R., eds. S. Karger, New York, 1968, Vol. 4, p. 20.

17. Stamler, J., Berkson, D.M., Majonner, L., Lindberg, H.A., Hall, Y., Levinson, M., Burkey, F., Miller, W., Epstein, M.B., and Andelman, S.L. Epidemiological studies on atherosclerotic coronary heart disease: Causative factors and consequent prevention approaches. *In* Progress in Biochemical Pharmacology: Recent Advances in Atherosclerosis, Miras, C.J., Howard, A.N., and Paoletti, R., eds. S. Karger, New York, 1968, Vol. 4, p. 30.

18. Taylor, C.B., Mikkelson, B., Anderson, J.A., and Forman, D.T. Human serum cholesterol synthesis. *In* Progress in Biochemical Pharmacology: Recent Advances in Atherosclerosis, Miras, C.J., Howard, A.N., and Paoletti, R., eds. S. Karger, New York, 1968, Vol. 4, p. 71.

19. Ahrens, E.H., Jr. Studies of cholesterol metabolism in intact organism. *In* Progress in Biochemical Pharmacology: Recent Advances in Atherosclerosis, Miras, C.J., Howard, A.N., and Paoletti, R., eds. S. Karger, New York, 1968, Vol. 4, p. 54.

20. Krut, L.H., and Wilkens, J.H. The filtration of plasma constituents into the wall of the aorta. *In* Progress in Biochemical Pharmacology: Recent Advances in Atherosclerosis, Miras, C.J., Howard, A.N., and Paoletti, R., eds. S. Karger, New York, 1968, Vol. 4, p. 249.

21. Hollander, W., Kramsch, D.M., and Inoue, G. The metabolism of cholesterol, lipoproteins and acid mucopolysaccharides in normal and atherosclerotic vessels. *In* Progress in Biochemical Pharmacology: Recent Advances in Atherosclerosis, Miras, C.J., Howard, A.N., and Paoletti, R., eds. S. Karger, New York, 1968, Vol. 4, p. 270.

22. Robertson, L.A., Jr. Oxygen requirements of the human arterial intima in atherogenesis. *In* Progress in Biochemical Pharmacology: Recent Advances in Atherosclerosis, Miras, C.J., Howard, A.N., and Paoletti, R., eds. S. Karger, New York, 1968, Vol. 4, p. 305.

23. Bowyer, D.E., Howard, A.N., Gresham, G.A., Bates, D., and Palmer, B.V. Aortic perfusion in experimental animals. A system for the study of lipid synthesis and accumulation. *In* Progress in Biochemical Pharmacology: Recent Advances in Atherosclerosis, Miras, C.J., Howard, A.N., and Paoletti, R., eds. S. Karger, New York, 1968, Vol. 4, p. 235.

24. Christensen, S. Intimal uptake of plasma lipoprotein and atherosclerosis. *In* Progress in Biochemical Pharmacology: Recent Advances in Atherosclerosis, Miras, C.J., Howard, A.N., and Paoletti, R., eds. S. Karger, New York, 1968, Vol. 4, p. 244.

25. Billimoria, J.D., and Rothwell, T.J. Factors affecting the synthesis of individual phospholipids in the rat aorta. *In* Progress in Biochemical Pharmacology: Recent Advances in Atherosclerosis, Miras, C.J., Howard, A.N., and Paoletti, R., eds. S. Karger, New York, Vol. 4, 1968, p. 225.

26. Thomas, W.A., Lee, K.T., and Kim, D.N. Metabolic studies of protein synthesis in aortas of monkeys fed atherogenic diet. *In* Progress in Biochemical Pharmacology: Recent Advances in Atherosclerosis, Miras, C.J., Howard, A.N., and Paoletti, R., eds., S. Karger, New York, 1968, Vol. 4, p. 445.

27. McMillan, G.C., and Story, H.C. Radioautographic observations on DNA synthesis in the cells of atherosclerotic lesions of cholesterol-fed rabbits. *In* Progress in Biochemical Pharmacology: Recent Advances in Atherosclerosis, Miras, C.J., Howard, A.N., and Paoletti, R., eds. S. Karger, New York, 1968, Vol. 4, p. 280.

28. Wissler, R.W. Recent progress in studies of experimental primate atherosclerosis. *In* Progress in Biochemical Pharmacology: Recent Advances in Atherosclerosis, Miras, C.J., Howard, A.N., and Paoletti, R., eds. S. Karger, New York, 1968, Vol. 4, p. 378.

29. Hollander, W., Kramsch, D.M., and Inoue, G. The metabolism of cholesterol lipoproteins and acid mucopolysaccharides in normal and atherosclerotic vessels. *In* Progress in Biochemical Pharmacology: Recent Advances in Atherosclerosis, Miras, C.J., Howard, A.N., and Paoletti, R., eds. S. Karger, New York, 1968, Vol. 4, p. 270.

30. Hollander, W. Recent advances in experimental and molecular pathology influx synthesis and transport of arterial lipoproteins in atherosclerosis. Exp. Molec. Path., 7:248, 1967.

31. Adams, C.W.M., Abdulla, Y.H., Bayliss, O.B., Mahler, R.F., and Root, M.A. Quantitative histochemical observations on certain oxidative and lipolytic enzymes in human aortic wall. *In* Progress in Biochemical Pharmacology: Recent Advances in Atherosclerosis, Miras, C.J., Howard, A.N., and Paoletti, R., eds. S. Karger, New York, 1968, Vol. 4, p. 248.

32. Zemplenyi, T., Urhova, O., Urbonova, D., and Kohout, N. Study of factors affecting arterial enzymic activities in man and some animals. *In* Progress in Biochemical Pharmacology: Recent Advances in Atherosclerosis, Miras, C.J., Howard, A.N., and Paoletti, R., eds. S. Karger, New York, 1968, Vol. 4, p. 325.

33. Whereat, A.F. Recent advances in experimental and molecular pathology. Atherosclerosis and metabolic disorders in the arterial wall. Exp. Molec. Path., 7:233, 1967.

34. Adams, C.W.M. Vascular histochemistry. Lloyd-Lecke, London, 1967.

35. Lojda, L., and Fric, P. Lactic dehydrogenase isoenzymes in the aortic wall. J. Atheroscler. Res., 6:264, 1966.

36. Zemplenyi, T. Vascular enzymes and atherosclerosis. J. Atheroscler. Res., 7:725, 1967.

37. Beaumont, J.L. Hyperlipidemia with circulating anti-β-lipoprotein autoantibody in man. Autoimmune hyperlipidemia, its possible role in atherosclerosis. *In* Progress in Biochemical Pharmacology: Recent Advances in Atherosclerosis, Miras, C.J., Howard, A.N., and Paoletti, R., eds. S. Karger, New York, 1968, Vol. 4, p. 110.

38. Walton, K.W. The role of low density lipoproteins in the pathogenesis of human atherosclerosis. *In* Progress in Biochemical Pharmacology: Recent Advances in

Atherosclerosis, Miras, C.J., Howard, A.N., and Paoletti, R., eds. S. Karger, New York, 1968, Vol. 4, p. 159.

39. Furman, R.H., Alaupovic, P., Bradford, R.H., and Howard, R.P. Gonadal hormones, blood lipids and ischemic heart disease. *In* Progress in Biochemical Pharmacology: Recent Advances in Atherosclerosis, Miras, C.J., Howard, A.N., and Paoletti, R., eds. S. Karger, New York, 1968, Vol. 4, p. 334.

40. Carlson, L.A. Recent advances in the metabolism of plasma lipids. *In* Progress in Biochemical Pharmacology: Recent Advances in Atherosclerosis, Miras, C.J., Howard, A.N., and Paoletti, R., eds. S. Karger, New York, 1968, Vol. 4, p. 170.

41. Gould, R.G., and Swyryd, E.A. Metabolism of plasma lipids. *In* Progress in Biochemical Pharmacology: Recent Advances in Atherosclerosis, Miras, C.J., Howard, A.N., and Paoletti, R., eds. S. Karger, New York, 1968, Vol. 4, p. 191.

42. Clarkson, T.B., Bullock, B.C., and Lehner, N.D.M. Pathologic characteristics of atherosclerosis in New World monkeys. *In* Progress in Biochemical Pharmacology: Recent Advances in Atherosclerosis, Miras, C.J., Howard, A.N., and Paoletti, R., eds. S. Karger, New York, 1968, Vol. 4, p. 420.

43. Malmros, H., and Sternby, N.H. Induction of atherosclerosis in dogs by a thiouracil free semisynthetic diet, containing cholesterol and hydrogenated coconut oil. *In* Progress in Biochemical Pharmacology: Recent Advances in Atherosclerosis, Miras, C.J., Howard, A.N., and Paoletti, R., eds. S. Karger, New York, 1968, Vol. 4, p. 182.

44. Kritchevsky, D., and Tepper, S.A. Influence of special fats on experimental atherosclerosis in rabbits. *In* Progress in Biochemical Pharmacology: Recent Advances in Atherosclerosis, Miras, C.J., Howard, A.N., and Paoletti, R., eds. S. Karger, New York, 1968, Vol. 4, p. 474.

45. Mustard, J.F., Glynn, M.F., Jorgensen, L., Nishizawa, E.E., Packham, M.A., and Rowsell, H.C. Recent advances in platelets, blood coagulation factors and thrombosis. *In* Progress in Biochemical Pharmacology: Recent Advances in Atherosclerosis, Miras, C.J., Howard, A.N., and Paoletti, R., eds. S. Karger, New York, 1968, Vol. 4, p. 508.

46. Haust, M.D. Electron microscopic and immunohistochemical studies of fatty streaks in human aorta. *In* Progress in Biochemical Pharmacology: Recent Advances in Atherosclerosis, Miras, C.J., Howard, A.N., and Paoletti, R., eds. S. Karger, New York, 1968, Vol. 4, p. 429.

47. Hollander, W., and Kramsch, D.M. The distribution of intravenously administered (^{3}H) cholesterol in the arteries and other tissues. J. Atheroscler. Res., 7:491, 1967.

48. Kramsch, D.M., Gore, I., and Hollander, W. The distribution of intravenously administered (^{3}H) cholesterol in the arteries and other tissues. J. Atheroscler. Res., 7:501, 1967.

49. Knieriem, H.J., Kao, V.C.Y., and Wissler, R.W. Actomyosin and myosin in the deposition of lipids and serum lipoproteins. AMA Arch. Path., 84:118, 1967.

50. ———— Kao, V.C.Y., and Wissler, R.W. Immunohistochemical administration of smooth muscle cells in human and bovine arteriosclerosis. Amer. J. Path., 50:58, 1967.

51. Imai, H., and Thomas, W.A. Cerebral atherosclerosis in swine: Role of necrosis in progression of diet induced lesions from proliferative to atheromatous. Exp. Molec. Path., 8:330, 1968.

52. Florentin, R.A., and Nam, S.C. Dietary-induced atherosclerosis in miniature swine. I. Gross and light microscopy observations: Time of development and morphologic characteristics of lesions. Exp. Molec. Path., 8:3, 1968.
Daoud, A.S., Jones, R., and Scott, R.F. I. Electron microscopy observations: characteristics of endothelial and smooth muscle cells in the proliferative lesions and elsewhere in the aorta. Exp. Molec. Path., 8:3, 1968.
Scott, R.F., and Morrison, E.S. III. Lipid values: Cholesterol, triglyceride and phos-

pholipid and esterified fatty acid values in serum and in aortic intima-media tissue. Exp. Molec. Path., 8:3, 1968.

Kim, D.N., Lee, K.T., and Thomas, W.A. IV. Metabolic studies: *In vitro* protein synthesis by aortic strips from swine fed atherogenic diets. Exp. Molec. Path., 8:3, 1968.

Dodds, W.J., and Miller, K.D. V. Hematologic studies: Clotting factors and related hematologic values. Exp. Molec. Path., 8:3, 1968.

53. Geer, J.C., Catsults, C., McGill, H.C., Jr., Strong, J.P. Fine structure of the baboon fatty streak. Amer. J. Path., 52:265, 1968.

54. Wissler, R.W. The arterial medial cell, smooth muscle or multifunctional mesenchyme. J. Atheroscler. Res., 8:201, 1968.

55. ———— and Vesselinovitch, D. Experimental models of human atherosclerosis. *In* Atherosclerosis: Recent Advances, 1966. New York, New York Academy of Science (in press).

56. Thomas, W.A., Florentin, R.A., Nam, S.C., Kim, D.N., Jones, R.N., and Lee, K.T. "Pre-proliferative phase" of atherosclerosis in swine fed cholesterol. Arch. Path., 1968 (in press).

57. Scott, R.F., Morrison, E.S., Jarmolysch, J., Nam, S.C., Kroms, M., and Coulston, F. Experimental atherosclerosis in rhesus monkeys. I. Gross and light microscopy feature and lipid values in serum and aorta. Exp. Molec. Path., 7:11, 1967.

58. Frederickson, D.S., Levy, R.G., and Lees, R.S. Fat transport in lipoproteins—An integrated approach to mechanisms and disorders. New Eng. J. Med., 276:34, 1967.

59. ———— Levy, R.I., and Lees, R.S. Fat transport in lipoproteins—An integrated approach to mechanisms and disorders (continued). New Eng. J. Med., 276:148, 1967.

60. ———— Levy, R.I., and Lees, R.S. Fat transport in lipoproteins—An integrated approach to mechanisms and disorders (continued). New Eng. J. Med., 276:215, 1967.

61. ———— Levy, R.I., and Lees, R.S. Fat transport in lipoproteins—An integrated approach to mechanisms and disorders (concluded). New Eng. J. Med., 276:273, 1967.

62. Lewes, L.A. Broadening perspectives of electrophoresis as seen from twenty-five years of use at the Cleveland Clinic. Cleveland Clin. Quart., 34:141, 1967.

63. Smithies, O. Zone electrophoresis in starch gels; group variations in the serum proteins of normal human adults. Biochem. J., 61:629, 1955.

64. Raymond, S., Miles, J.L., and Lee, J.C.J. Lipoprotein patterns in acrylamide gel electrophoresis. Science, 151:346, 1966.

65. Margolis, S. Separation and size determination of human serum lipoproteins by agarose gel filtration. J. Lipid Res., 8:501, 1967.

66. International Workshop on Lipoproteins, Chicago. Nature, 219:10, 1968.

67. Sones, F.M. Cine coronary arteriography. Anesth. Analg., 46:499, 1967.

68. Kemp, H.G., Evans, H., Elliott, W.C., and Gorlin, R. Diagnostic accuracy of selective coronary cinearteriography. Circulation, 361:526, 1967.

69. Hermon, M.V., Elliott, W.C., and Gorlin, R. An electrocardiographic, anatomic and metabolic study of zonal myocardial ischemia in coronary heart disease. Circulation, 35:834, 1967.

70. McGill, H.C., Brown, B.W., Gore, I., McMillan, G.C., Pollak, O.J., Robbins, S., Roberts, J.C., and Wissler, R.W. Grading stenosis in the right coronary artery. Circulation, 37:460, 1968.

71. ———— Brown, B.W., Gore, I., McMillan, G., Paterson, J.C., Pollak, O.J., Roberts, J.C., and Wissler, R.W. Grading human atherosclerotic lesions using a panel of photographs. Circulation, 37:455, 1968.

SOME DIETARY ASPECTS OF ATHEROSCLEROSIS

SIGMUND L. WILENS

There is widespread interest in the question whether food plays a significant role in the development of atherosclerosis. This is understandable. If it is true, prevention of this disease process is feasible. If it is not, atherosclerosis will be much more difficult to control. The purpose of this article is to evaluate evidence and divergent opinions on this question in terms that may reflect the pathologist's viewpoint. An attempt will be made to integrate old but not necessarily invalid concepts with more recent developments. Ancel Keys [1] has published a comprehensive survey of the recent extensive literature on this subject.

The Origins of Atherosclerosis

Was it an apple or an egg that tempted the original residents of Paradise? More prosaically, was atherosclerosis a disease peculiar to humans which became manifest as civilization developed and we acquired the capacity to select and store foods according to our own tastes and in amounts that fully satisfied our appetites? Perhaps we will never be able to settle this issue, which can be attacked only indirectly by studying the incidence of atherosclerosis in the remote past or by comparing the incidence of atherosclerosis in the general population of affluent societies with that which prevails in special groups in which food intake is restricted in one fashion or another. These include primitive peoples or those who live under famine conditions, prisoners of war segregated in concentration camps, or cults in which religious practices or other scruples restrict the varieties of food consumed. As might be expected such investigations yield valuable but inconclusive results.

Atherosclerosis in the Remote Past

There is no sure way of determining whether uncivilized men prior to the days of recorded history had the same kind of arterial disease which is prevalent today. The evidence available only dates back to periods when man had already developed complicated and artificial ways of obtaining and preparing food. The systematic appropriation of mammary secretions and ova of other species must once have been considered to be bizarre dietary perversities. Data available from studying societies living under primitive conditions today or ones in which diet is restricted by ignorance, poverty, imprisonment, or voluntary eccentricity, in the main, support the view that abundant intake of foods with a high content of cholesterol or other lipids may be an important factor in the development of atherosclerosis.

The validity of this type of study can be challenged because it is seldom that only the food habits of these special groups differ from those of the general population. Primitive peoples of undeveloped countries, for example, have a high incidence of parasitic infestation, a relatively short life span, severe anemias, and relatively low blood pressures. All these might play a role in retarding or concealing the development of atherosclerosis. Dietary cultists tend to be abstemious in other ways than in food consumption. Even more pertinently, there is no accurate way to quantitate the severity of so complex and variegated a process as atherosclerosis for purposes of exact comparison in different individuals. Furthermore, the development of clinical evidence of atherosclerosis is no sure guide to the severity of the pathological process as it affects the arterial system as a whole. For example, factors other than the severity of coronary sclerosis may be concerned in the incidence of heart attacks. Pathologists are well aware that many myocardial infarcts are sufficiently asymptomatic to escape detection when they develop.

The studies of Ruffer [2] on aortic remnants recovered from the ancient Egyptian's own species of time capsule, namely securely entombed mummies, seem to establish that atherosclerosis as we know it today existed in the age of the Pharaohs (Fig. 1). This does not exclude diet as a factor in this disease, since the Egyptians had already developed intricate ways of preparing and preserving food. It does, however, eliminate many more recent developments in food processing such as canning, pasteurization, and artificial refrigeration as primary causal agents. Classical medical authorities did not recognize arterial hardening as a special or significant disease. This theory did not originate until the circulation of the blood was discovered and the consequences of disturbances in its flow were recognized. It is evident, however, from the descriptions in old medical writings that atherosclerosis has been present and widespread throughout recorded history. [3]

Spontaneous Atherosclerosis in Animals

A second approach to this problem has been through the study of spontaneous arterial disease in various animal species. A recent extensive compilation of such investigations has been edited by Roberts, Strauss, and Cooper. [4] These reports reveal that degenerative lesions of arteries are commonly found in a wide variety of

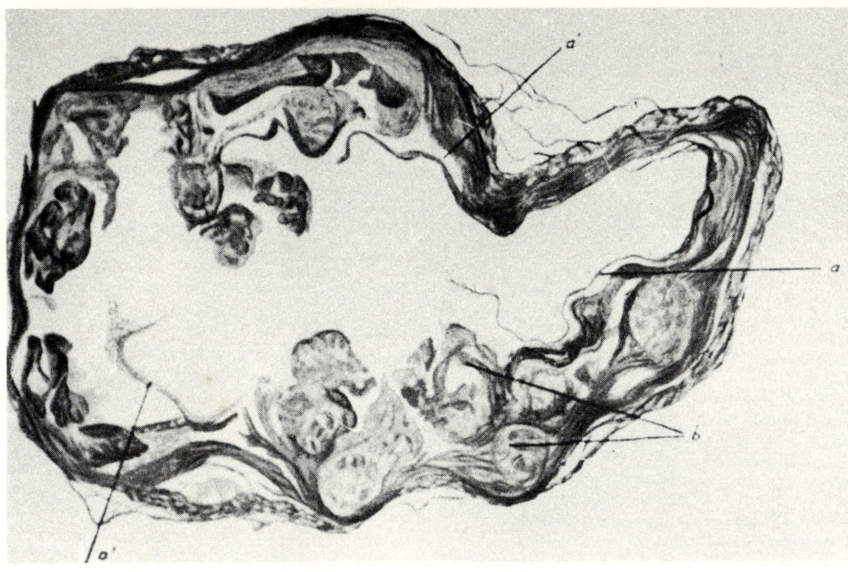

Fig. 1. Arteriosclerosis in an Egyptian mummy. Nodular, apparently calcified masses protrude into the lumen of the vessel and disrupt the continuity of its wall. (From Ruffer. J. Path. Bact., 15:453, 1911.)

animals. Whether all, some, or any of these lesions are identical or even comparable to the intimal arterial lesions of human atherosclerosis is still a debatable question. Those who consider intimal cholesterol deposition as the nidal pathogenetic factor in atherosclerosis would consider the great majority of such animal lesions to be nonatherosclerotic in nature because they are frequently associated with subintimal structural alterations in the arterial wall and usually contain a meager amount of stainable lipid.

Those who take the once predominant, broader view of the atherosclerotic process, namely that lipid deposition is only one phase of the disease, see no reason why spontaneous animal arteriosclerosis should not be equated with human atherosclerosis. In recent years, this revived viewpoint has gained increasing numbers of adherents especially among those who believe with Duguid [5] that intramural fibrin deposition plays an important role in the formation of intimal plaques. Short lived laboratory animals, such as rabbits, rats, and guinea pigs which are kept in confinement during their entire life span and are fed on usual laboratory rations, do not ordinarily exhibit lipid rich intimal plaques in their arteries at necropsy although they frequently show areas of medial fibrosis or calcification in large vessels. Absence of intimal plaques under these conditions may be related to their abbreviated survival periods rather than to the character of the food consumed.

Experimental atheromatous plaques in cholesterol fed rabbits heal very slowly even after the animals are restored to normal diets for long periods, and all evidence of excessive cholesterol deposition in other tissues has vanished. After two years the plaques have become largely fibrous, but they are still not hyalinized (Figs. 2, 3), a frequent finding in human intimal plaques. A large percentage of human in-

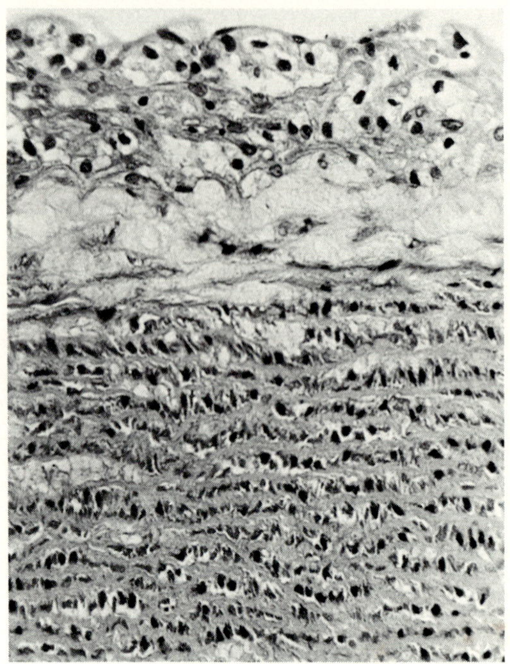

Fig. 2. Early atheromatous intimal lesion in aorta of rabbit after six weeks of cholesterol feeding.

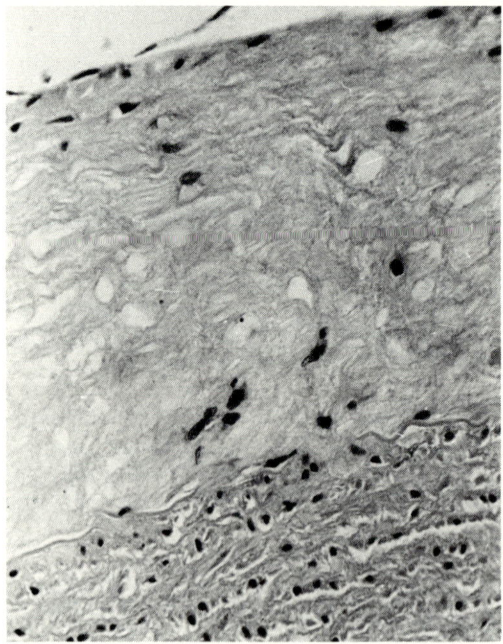

Fig. 3. Fibrous intimal lesion of aorta in rabbit maintained two years on normal rations after an eight week period of cholesterol feeding. The collagenous tissue has not become hyalinized.

timal plaques seen at necropsy may well be older than the maximum life span of most small rodents. Hyalinized scar tissue can sometimes be found in healed human surgical incisions that are less than two years old. This does not prove however that human atheromatous plaques can become hyalinized in an equally short period of time. The surprisingly slow conversion of fatty deposits in the arterial intima into fibrous tissue in experimental lesions is perhaps one of its more noteworthy peculiarities. It has been attributed to an absence of intimal capillary circulation in normal arteries.[6]

Animals in the household or in the laboratory do not consume the natural diets of wild animals even though their foods generally contain relatively little fat. Nevertheless, they enjoy some of the fringe benefits of civilized human society. Arterial lesions found in them, therefore, can not be considered to be truly spontaneous.

Role of Lipid Deposition in the Formation of Atheromatous Plaques

One of the difficulties in the assessment of the importance of lipid deposition in atherosclerotic plaques has always been that stainable lipid is frequently demonstrable as a secondary phenomenon in many degenerative lesions, eg, in old hemorrhagic cysts. Even hyaline deposits on serous surfaces sometimes contain a light film of sudanophilic material (Fig. 4). Many human atheromatous plaques contain no more than this when they are examined at necropsy. It is for this reason that the concepts of Marchand and others who stressed the importance of lipid deposition in this disease were not originally widely accepted.

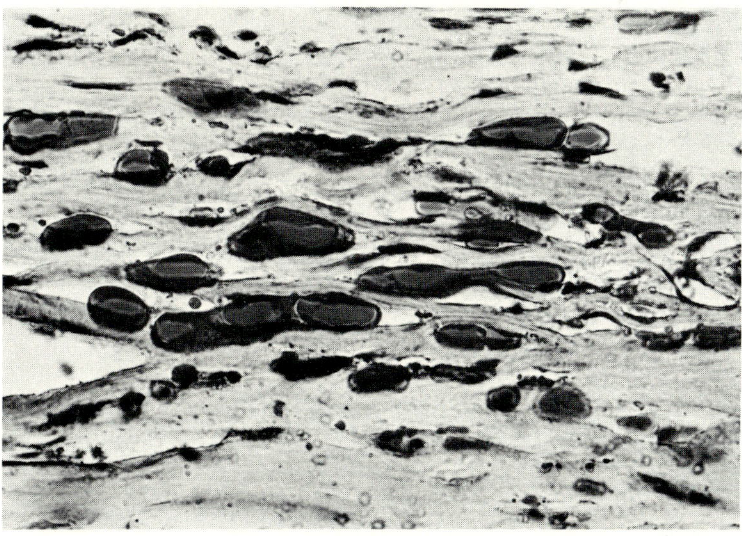

Fig. 4. Secondary lipid deposition in hyalinized splenic capsule. Lipid droplets are found in interstices of hyaline lamellae. Sudan IV stain.

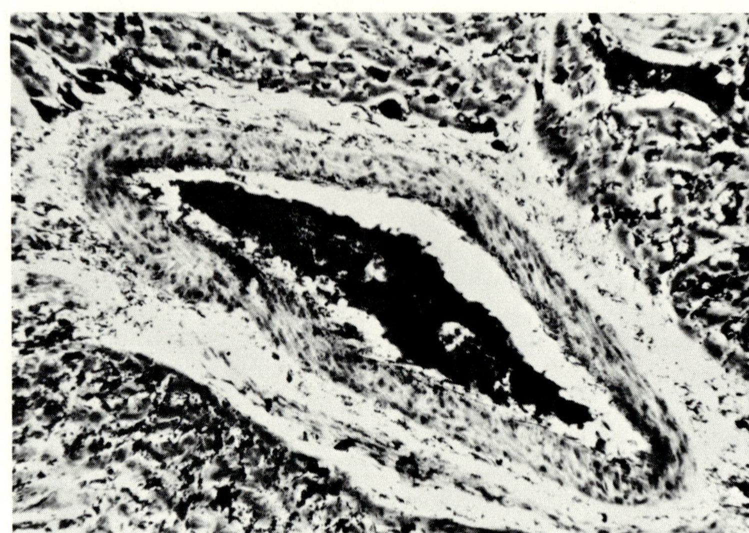

Fig. 5. Sudanophilic protein coagulum in lumen of coronary blood vessel of rabbit fed cholesterol for six weeks. When such material is found at the surface of the vessel it may be difficult to determine whether it has penetrated the intimal layer or is merely adherent to it. Oil-Red-O stain.

Those who espoused the theory of lipid deposition introduced the term atherosclerosis to distinguish this important type of arterial lesion from all others. In recent years this term has come to include a broad spectrum of arterial alterations including those in which no lesions are seen grossly and only a thin intimal film of sudanophilic material is found microscopically, and those in which lesions are grossly evident but contain only minute amounts of stainable lipid. The term atherosclerosis has thus lost most of its intended significance.

These controversial points have been intensified rather than solved by the introduction of new, more sensitive sudanophilic stains, oil Red 0 and Sudan Black. The older sudan preparations stain free fat in droplet form; the newer ones impregnate even the protein coagulum of lipemic serum (Fig. 5). Lesions once thought to contain little or no unmasked fat are now known to contain considerable amounts through the use of these newer stains. This has strengthened rather than weakened the view that lipid deposition may be only a secondary phenomenon in the atherosclerotic process.

In spite of all these considerations, certain of the spontaneous arterial lesions in animals, notably those in birds, can be composed predominantly of cholesterol rich lipid masses, and this detracts considerably from the belief that indulgences in appetite by man have led to peculiarities in diet and consequent development of arterial disease. In rebuttal it can be claimed that birds have relatively high and fluctuating blood cholesterol levels while dogs in which atherosclerosis has been found usually consumed the same foods as their masters, in addition to special rations.

Experimental Dietary Atherosclerosis

The theory that lipid deposition from the blood is largely responsible for intimal plaque formation would have undoubtedly remained a minor one had it not been demonstrated in the first decade of this century that lipid deposits can be produced experimentally in arteries of rabbits by feeding cholesterol enriched diets. This was first achieved accidentally by Ignatkowski [7] in an attempt to produce renal lesions by feeding nonvegetarian foods to rabbits. It was later found by Anitschow [8] that cholesterol in these formulas was responsible. Almost the entire concept that there is a significant dietary aspect to atherosclerosis has been fashioned subsequently from these initial discoveries. Whether they represent monstrous red herrings or the only advance of significance that has ever been made in our understanding of atherosclerosis remains yet to be proved.

That arterial lipid deposition in cholesterol fed rabbits represents the experimental reproduction of spontaneous human atherosclerosis has always aroused considerable skepticism. The ease with which blood cholesterol levels are enormously elevated on such diets, the concomitant deposition of lipid in extravascular sites, and the fact that the response was for a considerable period of time only elicited in rabbits were among the more formidable objections offered. The last of these criticisms has been effectively eliminated, since it has become possible by suitable manipulations of experimental procedures to obtain essentially the same findings in birds, dogs, monkeys, and many other species. It must now be conceded that under proper conditions the ingestion of excessive amounts of cholesterol could lead to its appearance in the walls of arteries in man as well as in other species.

Role of Diet in Human Atherosclerosis

This does not, however, solve the crucial question, namely whether or not the average amount of cholesterol usually consumed by most men is sufficient to be a significant factor in the development of atherosclerosis. It is recognized that most men with normal or even relatively low blood cholesterol levels develop appreciable degrees of atherosclerosis after the fourth decade of life and that many of these will have heart attacks or other clinical manifestations of atherosclerosis. It is difficult to prove that nutritional factors played a role in the development of arterial disease in such cases.

It is almost equally difficult to prove that overindulgence in lipid rich foods leading to obesity accelerates the atherosclerotic process in man, although insurance companies' statistics disclose a higher incidence of heart attacks in obese men than in thin ones. This has provided the chief rationale for recommending weight loss to obese persons who have clinical evidence of impaired arterial circulation, for there is no generally accepted anatomical proof that such persons tend to develop more severe atherosclerosis than thin ones, all other conditions being the same. Very obese persons, especially women, sometimes disclose surprisingly little atherosclerosis at necropsy. But this is also true of many with severe and prolonged diabetes or hypertension and even of those who have had abnormally high blood cholesterol concentrations. When all these conditions coexist it is distinctly unusual for arteries to remain unravaged by plaque formation, but even this has been observed.[9] On the other hand, pathologists are not at all surprised to find very severe atherosclerosis in elderly persons who had been thin all their lives and who always had, as far as we know, low blood pressures and low blood cholesterol levels. Such discrepancies may be the exception rather than the rule, but they cast serious doubt on the role of any of the so-called atherogenic factors as direct causal agents in this disease. It may, in fact, be seriously questioned whether any one etiological agent of over-riding importance will ever be discovered.

Role of Blood Cholesterol Levels and Nutritional Status in Human Atherosclerosis

Even morphological evidence that nutritional state and blood cholesterol concentration play subsidiary roles in the development of atherosclerosis in the average man is deficient. This is surprising in view of the fact that dietary regimes to regulate body weight and lower blood cholesterol values are so widely recommended clinically. In several statistical analyses [10] no correlation between severity of atherosclerosis observed at necropsy and state of nutrition or blood cholesterol levels could be found. There are many difficulties involved in such analyses. One of these is that there is no accurate way to assess severity of atherosclerosis as it involves the arterial system as a whole. When multiple measurements are used they soon become complex, arbitrary, and not readily adaptable to large series.

In a recent study [11] an attempt was made to obviate this latter difficulty by simply matching aortas at necropsy with ones previously selected to show the usual amounts of atherosclerosis found at different age periods throughout adult life. It was thus possible to distinguish readily the ones that had significantly greater or lesser degrees of involvement. It is perhaps not surprising that by using this technique it became obvious that a large majority of men develop roughly about the same degree of atherosclerosis of this vessel as they age. What is more surprising is that this large group with an average amount of aortic change contained many persons in whom the process should have been accelerated or retarded because they had a remarkably high or low blood cholesterol level. It also included many persons with either or both prolonged diabetes and hypertension. Under the conditions that most of us live, age is far and away the most significant factor in the development of atherosclerosis. This in turn lends substance to the ancient view that hardening of the arteries is an inevitable consequence of growing old.

The opposite side of this statistical coin is, however, considerably brighter. The same study also disclosed that about 15 to 20 percent had decidedly less aortic sclerosis than their age would warrant, and that roughly the same percentage had an even greater severity of aortic sclerosis than expected. There were rare, but far from unique, instances where men in their eighties and nineties had no more intimal plaques than men in their twenties and thirties (Fig. 6). If one assumes that what one man can do others can also achieve once they follow suit, then atherosclerosis must be listed as a potentially preventable disease even if the means of prevention still remain elusive.

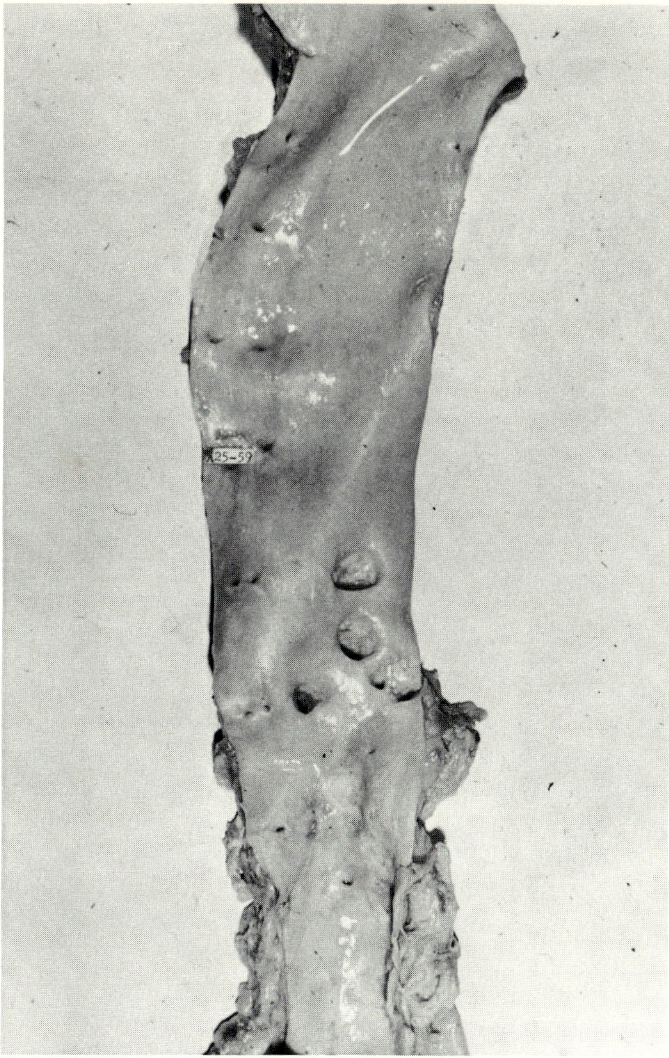

Fig. 6. Descending thoracic and abdominal aorta of a 87 year old man. Almost no intimal lesions are present.

When the minority groups with greater or lesser degrees of aortic sclerosis were scrutinized further, it was found that nutritional factors and blood cholesterol levels did play a statistically significant role (Figs. 7, 8). Within these selected categories, thin men with low blood cholesterol concentrations frequently had less and seldom more aortic sclerosis than would have been expected at their age. The opposite held true for obese men with high blood cholesterol. There was some suggestion that prolonged undernutrition was effective in retarding the development of aortic lesions, but that this could be easily negated if the blood cholesterol levels were high or at the upper limits of normal. Obese men, on the other hand, seldom had

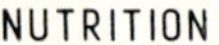

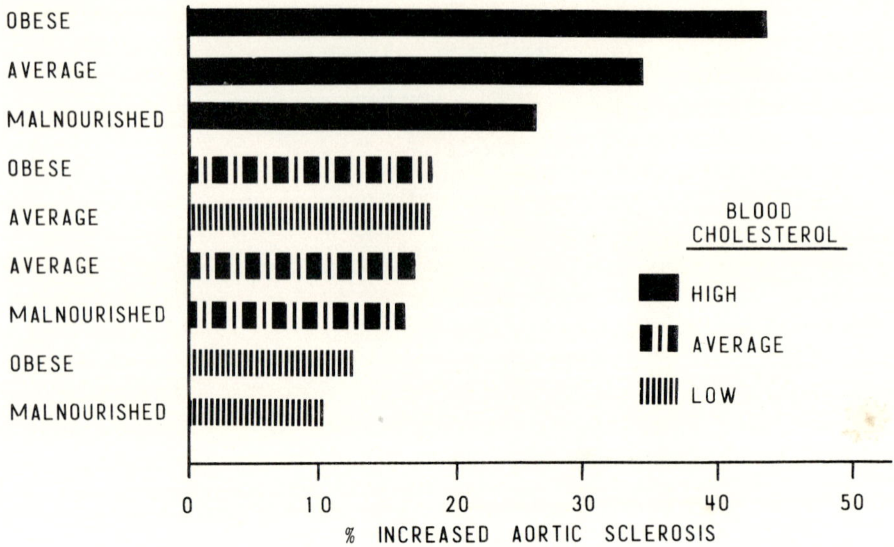

Fig. 7. Influence of blood cholesterol and nutrition on the incidence of increased aortic atherosclerosis. (From Wilens and Plair. Arch. Int. Med., 116:375, 1965.) Reproduced with permission of editors.

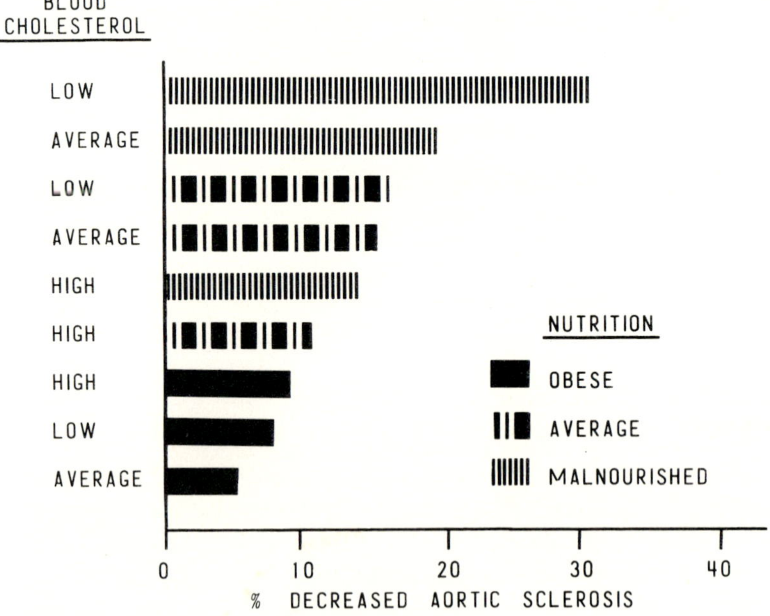

Fig. 8. Influence of nutrition and blood cholesterol on the incidence of decreased aortic atherosclerosis. (From Wilens and Plair. Arch. Int. Med., 116:376, 1965.)

less than average aortic sclerosis no matter what their levels of blood cholesterol might have been. This fragmentary evidence is limited to a small segment of the male population, but it does favor the belief that the secrets of prevention of atherosclerosis could be found in the diet.

In an organized society, sources of food supply for the majority are so channelled as to promote uniformity and conformity in diet. The shelves of one supermarket are laden with much the same assortment of items as any other. This could explain much of the uniformity with which the atherosclerotic process advances with age in most persons. If however one examines the contents of loaded food baskets as they pass through check-out counters, it is also evident that individual tastes sometimes lead to striking differences in the amounts and kinds of foods selected. It is still possible that idiosyncrasies in dietary habits which as yet have not been discovered could account for the minority groups in which nutritional factors and blood cholesterol levels do seem to affect the atherosclerotic process.

Absorption of Lipids from the Intestine

For a long time it was believed that it was necessary to dissolve cholesterol in some other fat such as olive oil or corn oil before feeding it to rabbits in order to produce arterial lipid deposits. It is ironic that many of the fat solvents used had a high content of unsaturated fatty acids in view of the widely held belief that such fats by themselves can lower blood cholesterol levels, particularly when the latter are initially relatively high, and thus possibly retard the development of atherosclerosis. It is, nevertheless, true that if crystalline cholesterol powder is simply mixed with ordinary rations or combined with unabsorbable sterols such as sito-

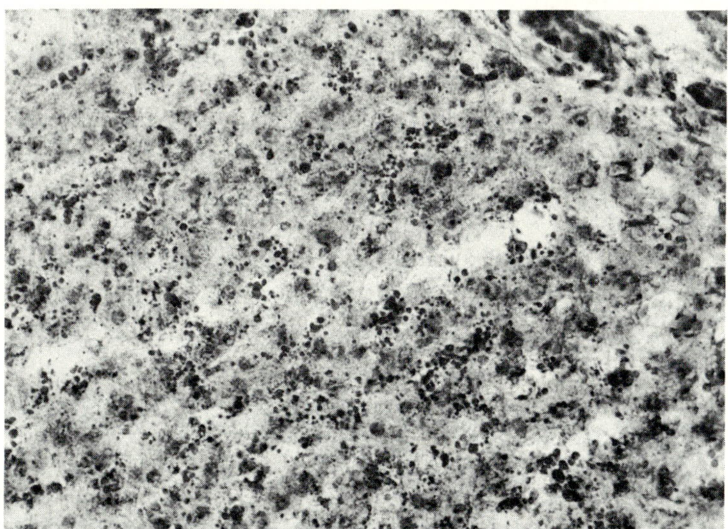

Fig. 9. Liver tissue of rabbit fed 1 g of cholesterol in 6 ml corn oil 24 hours before sacrifice. The parenchyma is studded with anisotropic fat droplets most of which are in Kupffer cells. Sudan IV stain.

sterol, it will not be absorbed in large amounts from the intestine of rabbits and the level of blood cholesterol will not be greatly increased.

If, however, cholesterol is first dissolved in a nonfatty solvent such as ether before being mixed with other food ingredients, as was done by Steiner and Kendall [12] in their classical studies on experimental atherosclerosis in dogs, it will be absorbed as readily as if it had been dissolved in fat. These observations emphasize the importance of the rate of absorption of cholesterol from the intestine in the production of experimental dietary lesions. It is perhaps equally important in the development of human ones. After a single feeding of 1 g of cholesterol in suitable form to a rabbit, sudanophilic deposits can be demonstrated in the Kupffer cells 24 hours later, indicating the speed with which it can be absorbed and so deposited (Fig. 9). This experiment has apparently not been performed in man although it might disclose marked individual variability with which such ingested material enters the blood stream under different circumstances. In any case the total amount of cholesterol consumed is obviously not an exact measure of the amount absorbed, and if there is a dietary aspect to atherosclerosis, the latter consideration is of far greater importance.

Atherosclerosis in Chronic Alcoholism

Theoretically, the rate of absorption of cholesterol and other lipids from the intestinal tract may be of significance in one special group of dietary eccentrics, chronic alcoholics. Since this group obtains a good portion of caloric requirements from alcohol, it may be presumed that in many the intake of fat and cholesterol must be relatively low. It might be expected, therefore, that if the consumption of fatty substances is important in the development of atherosclerosis, chronic alcoholics should enjoy relative immunity.

Every pathologist of experience has seen instances at necropsy in which the arteries of elderly alcoholics have been singularly free from atheromatous change. Such isolated observations fortify the belief that dietary factors can play an important role in this disease. Unfortunately, similar freedom from atherosclerosis is occasionally seen in elderly nonalcoholics whose diet, as far as is known, was not peculiar in any way. Furthermore, many heavily alcoholic men have an average or even greater than average degree of atherosclerosis at necropsy. In at least one statistical analysis [13] no significant difference in severity of this process was noted in large groups of alcoholics and nonalcoholics. Recent unpublished data from a series of necropsies in which the matching plan of comparing aortas was used amply confirmed this initial finding.

Effect of Estrogenic Hormones on Atherosclerosis

Such observations may be disturbing to those who believe that unrestricted ingestion of cholesterol is primarily responsible for human atherosclerosis. This is especially true, since there is at least one other theoretical reason why heavy alcohol consumption might protect against the formation of intimal arterial plaques. Such indulgence should lead to periodic liver injury and thus impede estrogen degradation. This is supported by the well-known fact that chronic alcoholics are prone to develop cirrhosis and that they sometimes lose body hair, develop gynecomastia, and that prostatic enlargement is often absent or develops at a later age than usual.[14]

The relative freedom from atherosclerosis of premenopausal women who are neither diabetic nor hypertensive is widely attributed to the influence of circulating estrogenic hormones on the character of blood lipoproteins. There is also substantial, if controversial, evidence that prolonged administration of steroids to men with prostatic carcinoma can retard the progression of atherosclerotic lesions.[15] Unpublished data from the series of necropsies by Wilens and Plair support this observation although it is obvious that retardation does not occur in all men so treated.

Since the regression of prostatic cancer under estrogenic therapy is also capricious and unpredictable, it is likely that in at least some men the hormones administered are ineffective. Alcoholic addiction generally begins at a relatively early period in adult life before substantial degrees of atherosclerosis have developed. If increase in circulating estrogens is a factor in preventing arterial lipid deposition, its effects should be more obvious in a series of alcoholics than in a group of elderly men with prostatic cancer. On the other hand, estrogen blood levels in the latter group are much higher than in chronic alcoholics. This is evidenced by differences in histological patterns in the type of gynecomastia observed in the two groups.[16]

In any case, if dietary influences and circulating lipoproteins play significant roles in atherosclerosis, the bulk of chronic alcoholics should be relatively protected. The evidence cited here does not support this. Since there are marked individual differences in the drinking and eating habits of chronic alcoholics, they can hardly be considered to represent a homogeneous group; eg, some consume alcohol during or just prior to eating while in others alcohol has no consistent relationship to food intake. It is possible that absorption of cholesterol and other lipids from the intestines may be influenced by such practices.

Local Factors in the Development of Atherosclerotic Plaques

Atherosclerosis of the aorta is of particular interest to those concerned with the pathogenesis of this disease and to vascular surgeons who sometimes remove aneurysms that have developed in the vessel. It is not of equal importance to clinicians since it is well known that, in itself, aortic atherosclerosis may not lead to symptoms. Aortic disease may be misleading if it is used as a measure for the severity of atherosclerosis in smaller arteries such as the coronaries and cerebrals. At necropsy extreme degrees of aortic sclerosis are frequently found in men with normal brains and hearts, and even in those who had no difficulties with circulation in the legs. On the other hand a man may die of myocardial or cerebral infarction and have less severe sclerotic change in his aorta than is usually seen in his own age group.

It is obvious, therefore, that local factors at the site of plaque formation play an important and perhaps sometimes decisive role in the development of intimal lesions, even if the materials in them are derived in part from the blood and indirectly from food. This has always been a vexing feature of atherosclerosis to those who classify this disease as purely one of disturbed lipid metabolism. Aschoff[17] first propounded the basic tenets of the lipid infiltration theory in his well-known preface to Cowdry's book on arteriosclerosis. He suggested that it was the aging changes which become manifest in the arterial system during middle age, such as loss of elasticity and also enlargement and changes in composition of interstitial fluid, which make arteries vulnerable to increased lipid deposition or retention, thus implying that the composition of the blood need not change at all to initiate this process.

This concept is appealing because it fits in so well with actual observations. No striking pertinent changes have been detected during middle age in the composition of blood other than changes in lipoprotein molecules, particularly in postmenopausal women. There is still insufficient evidence that such changes play a decisive role in the penetration of lipid into arteries. Furthermore, lipid deposits found in adolescents and young adults tend to remain in superficial streaks or films without forming many discrete plaques. It is, therefore, reasonable to assume that something has happened to arteries of aging persons which make them attract or hold lipid within their intimas.

There is considerable evidence that a variety of injuries to the arterial media can accelerate the formation of intimal plaques in the same region. It was well recognized that in syphilitic mesaortitis, intimal atheromatous changes were frequently accentuated. In fact, the latter could so overshadow the medial lesion as to obscure its presence. Striking plaque formation has been described in endothelialized false passages of dissecting aortic aneurysms even though these have been present for only a few months (Fig. 10). The luminal surface of homologous arterial transplants is often covered by extensive plaque formations. It is true that fibrosis is often much more in evidence than lipid deposition in such secondary intimal thickenings. But in most examples of this type, capillary circulation has penetrated to the inner surface so that the process of organization is facilitated.

There is also considerable experimental evidence that damage to an arterial wall can promote intimal lipid deposition in the same area provided the cholesterol content of the blood is high. Schmidtmann,[18] and more recently Hass et al[19] found unusually severe aortic intimal lesions when medial calcification was produced with irradiated ergosterol in cholesterol fed rabbits. Application of silver bands to the external surface of arteries also leads to local intimal lipid deposition in cholesterol fed rabbits.[20] Analogous findings have been obtained by Taylor[21] and others who traumatized segments of aortic wall in a variety of ways during the period of cholesterol feeding. Waters[22] produced lipid deposition in the coronary arteries of dogs, previously injured by treatment with adrenalin or allylamine, by intravenous injection of lipid rich emulsions.

Such experiments however do not necessarily prove that medial injury is necessary for the formation of significant intimal plaques.

A recent unpublished study suggests that in hyperlipemic, cholesterol fed rabbits, lipid does not deposit in the intima of segments of mesenteric and renal arteries with acute, adrenalin-produced, medial necrosis provided that the internal elastic membrane remains intact (Fig. 11). The internal elastic lamella probably serves as an important barrier to the penetration of lipid into the media. This is indicated by the fact that if excised,

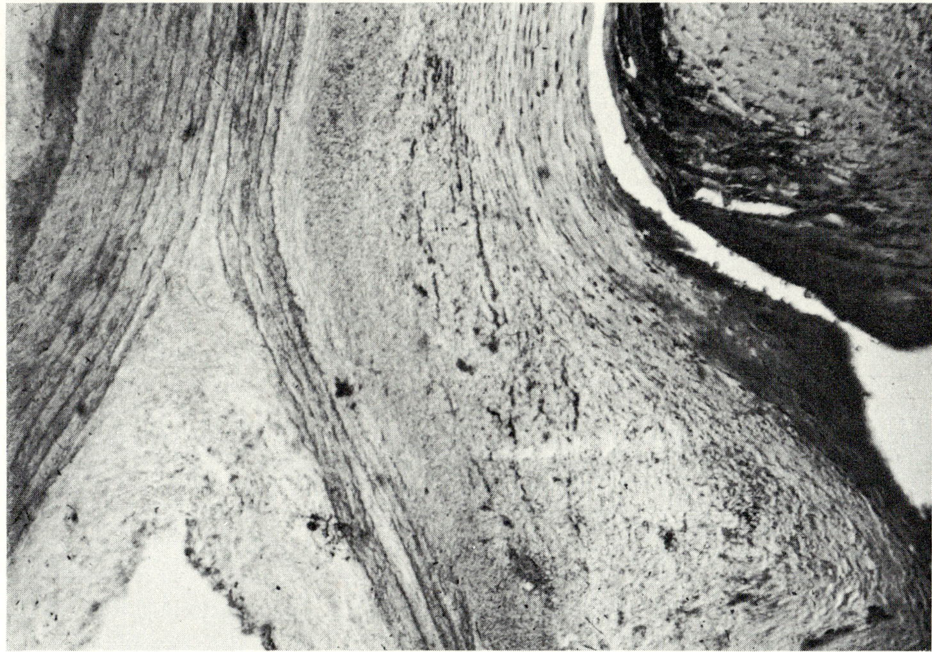

Fig. 10. False passages in dissecting aneurysm of aorta present for seven months. The space at lower left is lined by fibrous tissue. The walls of the passage at upper right are impregnated with sudanophilic material. Sudan IV stain of frozen section.

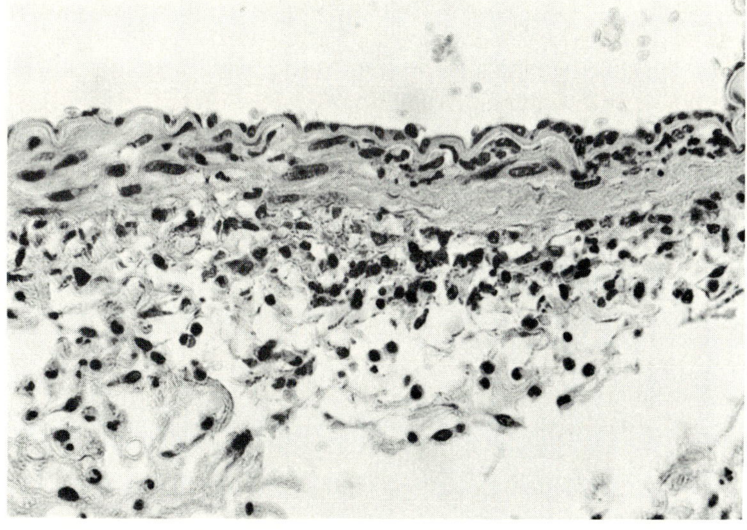

Fig. 11. Main renal artery of cholesterol-fed, hypercholesterolemic rabbit sacrificed four days after multiple small intravenous injections of adrenalin. There is cellular infiltration of the adventitia and partial necrosis of the media. The internal elastic lamella, however, is intact and no lipid deposits have formed.

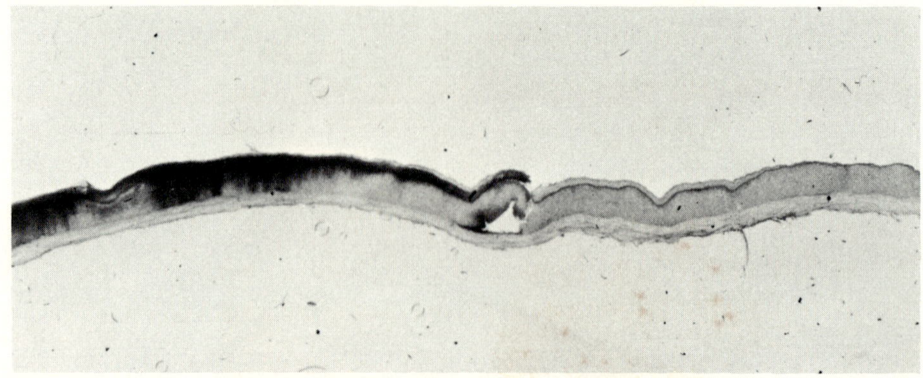

Fig. 12. Frozen section of human femoral artery through which normal human blood serum was filtered for 48 hours at pressure of 200mm Hg. Defect at center represents point of ligature. The arterial wall to the left was subjected to filtration. Sudanophilic material has impregnated the intima primarily but has streamed through the media at places. No lipid is seen in segment at right of defect not subjected to filtration. Sudan IV stain.

unfixed segments of arteries are used as filtration membranes against normal blood serum under pressure, serum lipid will deposit against this membrane as fluid passes through the wall [23] (Fig. 12).

If such experiments are carried out in rabbits when the blood cholesterol is normal, very little or no intimal proliferation may occur. It is usually impossible to demonstrate significant structural alterations in the subintimal region underlying most intimal lipid plaques in cholesterol fed rabbits and in human atherosclerosis. Moreover, severe medial calcification and syphilitic mesaortitis do not always lead to acceleration of intimal plaque formation. These diverse findings can be readily reconciled by applying Aschoff's theory of a dual mechanism. If the lipid patterns of blood serum are sufficiently abnormal, it is assumed according to this theory that lipid can be deposited in the inner layer of arteries even if these are structurally intact. If blood cholesterol levels rise well above 1,000 mg%, cholesterol may be deposited in extraarterial sites as in cutaneous eruptions. It is noteworthy that even in such extreme conditions it is not ordinarily deposited in the walls of veins.

One curious exception is the occasional finding of lipid deposits in large pulmonary veins in diabetics with mitral stenosis (Fig. 13). It should be noted that the pulmonary veins transport oxygenated blood and may derive their nutrition by intimal permeation in the same fashion as arteries. It should be noted that in mitral stenosis the pressure in these veins is considerably augmented. Lipid deposits are seldom found in sclerotic varicose veins [24] unless they contain organized and recanalized thrombi (Fig. 14).
The lesions of arteriolar sclerosis are thought to be quite different in pathogenesis than atheromatous plaques of large arteries, chiefly because they can be quite severe in relatively young hypertensives in whom the large arteries show very little atherosclerosis. Lipid when present in hyalinized arterioles is thought to represent a secondary phenomenon (Fig. 15). However, Versé [25] pointed out that the follicular arterioles of the spleen, unlike most other arterioles, are regularly impregnated with lipid in cholesterol fed rabbits (Fig. 16). These arterioles frequently become hyalinized in man even in the absence of hypertension.

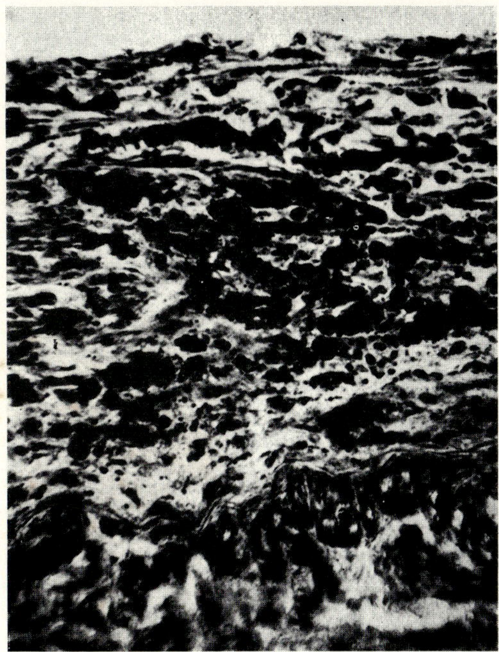

Fig. 13. Pulmonary vein of 28 year old woman with mitral stenosis and diabetes. A large amount of sudanophilic material is deposited in thickened intima. Sudan IV stain. (From McCluskey and Wilens. Amer. J. Path., 29:83, 1953.)

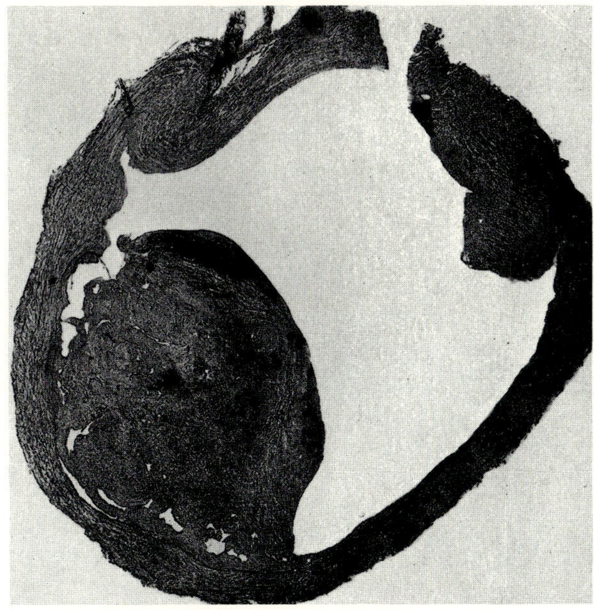

Fig. 14. Frozen section through varicose leg vein containing an organized fibrous parietal thrombus. The surface of the fibrous mass contains a large deposit of sudanophilic material, but none is seen in the vein wall. (From McCluskey and Wilens. Amer. J. Path., 29:83, 1953.)

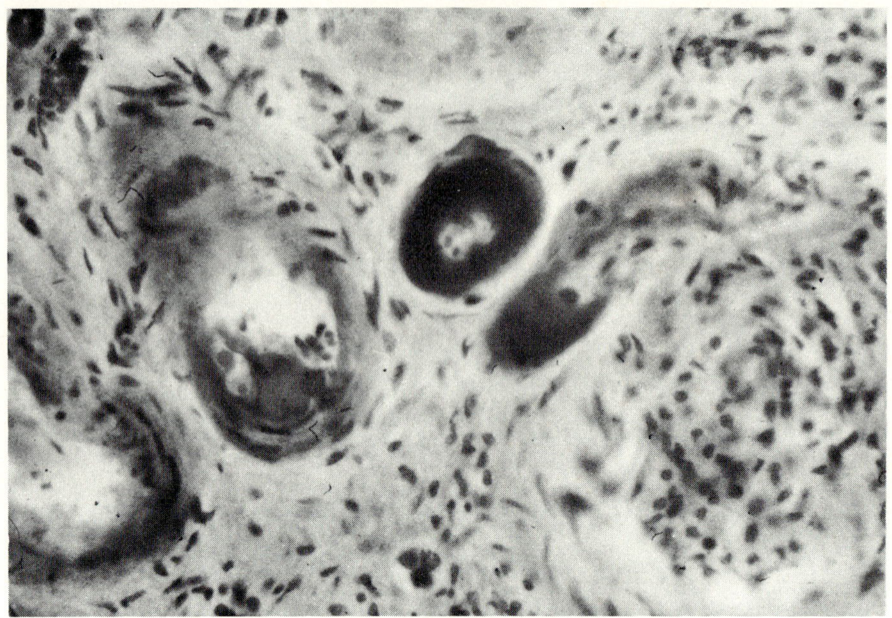

Fig. 15. Sudanophilic material in hyalinized sclerotic renal arterioles in arteriolar nephrosclerosis. Sudan IV stain on frozen section.

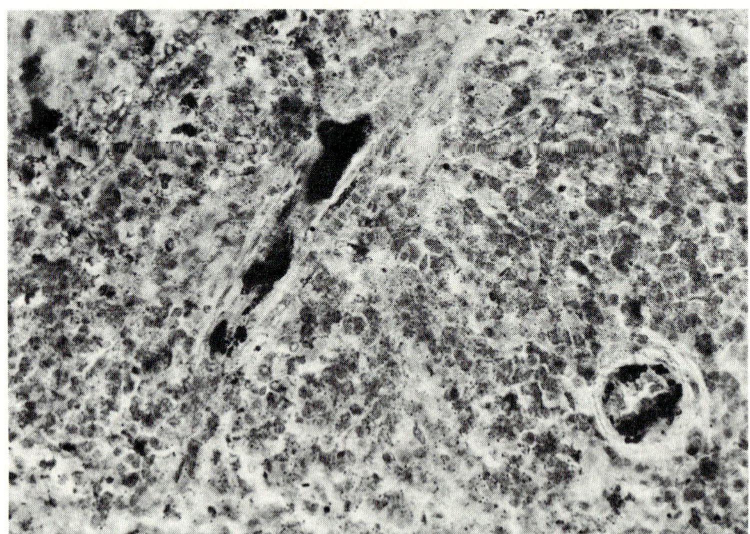

Fig. 16. Sudanophilic deposit in follicular arterioles of spleen in a rabbit with blood cholesterol of 1225 mg/% after four weeks of cholesterol feeding. There were no grossly visible lipid deposits in any large artery in this rabbit. Sudan IV stain.

If areas of arterial wall are altered, lipid presumably can also be deposited even if serum lipid composition is not abnormal. It is likely that in most individuals morphological aging changes in arterial structure play the most conspicuous role in initiating the changes that appear in middle age and increase progressively with advancing years. This is suggested not only by the fact that the majority of men develop atherosclerosis to approximately the same extent as they age, but also because a fairly predictable pattern of distribution of lesions is usually found.

However, when atherosclerosis develops precociously in the arteries of one organ and is obviously more pronounced in this location than in other arteries, it may be presumed that these vessels have been altered functionally if not structurally in such a way as to favor intimal lipid deposition. This latter situation probably obtains in most men who have heart attacks before the age of 50 and in a high percentage of even older ones.

Initial Size of Major Coronary Arteries in Relation to Vulnerability to Myocardial Infarction

Relatively little attention has been paid to individual variations in size of the major coronary arteries as a factor in the pathogenesis of myocardial infarction due to coronary atherosclerosis. Our own observations[26] indicate that infarcts seldom occur in human hearts in which the original surface area of the epicardial branches of the coronary arteries is greater than 7 sq cm/100 g of heart weight but are common in hearts in which they measure less than 6 sq cm/100 g of heart weight. These observations indicate that there may be a threshold value in the size of the vessels which is of considerable importance in determining whether the heart will be vulnerable to infarction when the arteries become sclerotic. If this reasoning is correct, the likelihood of sharply reducing the incidence of such attacks by regulation of the diet alone would seem to be bleak. It would probably require a regimen that would reduce blood cholesterol levels found in most animals which do not ordinarily develop lipid-rich plaques, ie, less than 150 mg%. This is a goal that would be difficult to achieve by dietary control alone.

Summary

Although the evidence supporting the view that dietary factors are significant in the development of atherosclerosis is formidable, it is far from conclusive. Frequently but not invariably the persistence of high concentrations of cholesterol in the blood leads to acceleration of the atherosclerotic process. Nevertheless, atherosclerosis develops in most men even though their blood cholesterol and blood pressure levels remain within average limits. In the majority of men the arterial lesions as a whole progress to approximately the same extent with advancing age. This is true very frequently even if such atherogenic factors as diabetes and hypertension are present. In sizable minorities the atherosclerotic process appears to be either accelerated or retarded in development. In these minority groups nutritional factors and blood cholesterol levels appear to play a significant role. It is questionable, however, that atherosclerosis in the general population will ever be controlled by voluntary regulation of diet alone.

The focus of attention of many investigators appears to have shifted from the study of the regulation of blood lipids to a closer scrutiny of the factors involved in the entrance and retention of lipid within the arterial wall. Development of therapeutic procedures designed to promote the elimination of lipid from the arterial intima, if feasible, would seem to offer the best prospects of controlling this disease.

References

1. Keys, A. The role of the diet in human atherosclerosis and its complications. *In* Atherosclerosis and Its Origin. Sandler, M., and Bourne, G. H., eds., New York, Academic Press, Inc., 1963, Ch. 8, pp. 263–299.
2. Ruffer, M. A. On arterial lesions found in Egyptian mummies (1580 B.C.–525 A.D.). J. Path. Bact., 15:453, 1911.
3. Long, E. R. The development of our knowledge of arteriosclerosis. *In* Arteriosclerosis. Cowdry, E. V., ed., New York, Macmillan Company, 1933, pp. 19–52.
4. Roberts, J. C., Strauss, R., and Cooper, M. S., eds. Comparative Atherosclerosis: The Morphology of Spontaneous and Induced Atherosclerotic Lesions in Animals and Its Relation to Human Disease. New York, Paul B. Hoeber, Inc., 1965.
5. Duguid, J. B. Pathogenesis of atherosclerosis. Lancet, 2:207, 1952.
6. Wilens, S. L. The comparative vascularity of cutaneous xanthomas and atheromatous plaques of arteries. Amer. J. Med. Sci., 223:4, 1957.
7. Ignatowski, A. Über die Wirkung des Tierischen Eiweisses auf Aorta. Virchow Arch. Path. Anat., 198:248, 1909.
8. Anitschow, N. Über Veränderungen der Kaninchen-Aorta bei Experimenteller Cholesterinsteatose. Beitr. Path. Anat., 56:379, 1913.
9. Wilens, S. L. Bearing of the nutritional state on atherosclerosis. Arch. Intern. Med., 79:129, 1947.
10. Moses, C. Atherosclerosis: Mechanisms as a Guide to Prevention. Philadelphia, Lea & Febiger, 1963, p. 157.
11. Wilens, S. L., and Plair, C. M. Blood cholesterol, nutrition and atherosclerosis. Arch. Intern. Med. (Chicago), 116:373, 1965.
12. Steiner, A., and Kendall, F. E. Atherosclerosis and arteriosclerosis in dogs following ingestion of cholesterol and thiouracil. Arch. Path. (Chicago), 42:433, 1946.
13. Wilens, S. L. The relationship of chronic alcoholism to atherosclerosis. J.A.M.A., 135:1136, 1947.
14. Stumpf, H. H., and Wilens, S. L. Inhibitory effects of portal cirrhosis of liver on prostatic enlargement. Arch. Intern. Med. (Chicago), 91:304, 1953.
15. Rivin, A. U., and Dimitroff, S. P. The incidence and severity of atherosclerosis in estrogen treated males, and in females with a hypoestrogenic or hyperestrogenic state. Circulation, 9:533, 1954.
16. Schwartz, I., and Wilens, S. L. The formation of acinar tissue in gynecomastia. Amer. J. Path., 43:797, 1963.
17. Aschoff, L. Arteriosclerosis. Cowdry, E. V., ed., New York, Macmillan Company, 1933, pp. 1–18.
18. Schmidtmann, M. Vigantolversuche. Verh. Deutsch. Gesellsch., 24:75, 1929.
19. Hass, G. M., Trueheart, R. E., and Hemmens, A. Experimental athero-arteriosclerosis due to calcific medial degeneration and hypercholesterolemia. Amer. J. Path., 38:289, 1961.
20. Wilens, S. L. The distribution of intimal atheromatous lesions in the arteries of rabbits on high cholesterol diets. Amer. J. Path., 18:63, 1942.
21. Taylor, C. B. The reaction of arteries to injury by physical agents. With discussion

of arterial repair and its relationship to arteriosclerosis. Symposium on Atherosclerosis, National Acad. Sciences, National Research Council Pub. 338, Washington, D.C., 1954, p. 74.

22. Waters, L. L. Studies on the pathogenesis of vascular disease. The effect of intravenous egg yolk emulsions on inflammatory lesions of the aorta and coronary arteries of dogs. Yale J. Biol. Med., 29:9, 1956.

23. Wilens, S. L. The experimental production of lipid deposition in excised arteries. Science, 114:389, 1951.

24. McCluskey, R. T., and Wilens, S. L. The infrequency of lipid deposition in sclerotic veins. Amer. J. Path., 29:71, 1953.

25. Versé, M. Zur Frage der Experimentelle Atherosklerose. Zbl. Allg. Path., 34:614, 1924.

26. Wilens, S. L., Plair, C. M., and Henderson, D. The size of the major epicardial coronary arteries: Its relation to age, heart weight, and myocardial infarction. J.A.M.A. 198:1325, 1966.

Addendum

Cassius M. Plair

When invited to substitute for the late Sigmund L. Wilens, former associate, colleague and respected mentor, I experienced mixed feelings about accepting the assignment. On the one hand I felt honored, privileged, and, perhaps, duty-bound in view of my prior close association with the author of the original article; however when consideration is given to Wilens' expertise in the field of atherosclerosis and to the excellence of his literary style, I am somewhat awed by the undertaking. Ideally, one should like to append a note which captures the mood and style of the original author, such that the reader feels that the addendum is a continuum of the original writing, interrupted only by time and events, and is scarcely aware that a change in penman had occurred. The ideal might not be realized but satisfaction will be achieved if I should be convinced that the expanded treatment of the subject would elicit the approbation and concurrence of Sigmund L. Wilens were he in a position to appraise it.

The general tenor of the treatise on certain dietary aspects of atherosclerosis as espoused by Wilens in 1967 was one of deliberate skepticism regarding the role of dietary factors in the development of the atherosclerotic lesion in the arterial system of humans. Closely entwined with this attitude was a subtle appeal that more attention be directed to local factors which influence the entrance and retention of lipid within the arterial wall in our search for means of eliminating or arresting the progress of this widespread disease process which, from all indications at the present time at least, is inextricably associated with the aging process.

In the intervening eight years, many opinions regarding the relation of diet to atherosclerosis have been expressed. These have been based upon theoretical, experimental, statistical, and epidemiologic studies with varying degrees of emphasis applied to various influences according to the interest and experiences of the various investigators.[1-13] Almost universally there is the attitude that the genesis and progression of atherosclerotic lesions are multifactorial and that dietary factors are only one of many categories of influences converging into a common final pathway leading to atherosclerosis. Opinions as to the relative significance of dietary factors in atherogenesis vary from those who hold that they are of major importance to those at the opposite end of the spectrum who feel that they are of little or of unproven effect. In this latter regard certain observations of Altschule are worthy of cognizance.[8, 9, 16] This writer gets the impression that the written expressions of most authorities on the subject embody a strong element of caution in their attempts to relate causally dietary components to atherogenesis, be they cholesterol, triglycerides, lipoproteins, or even carbohydrates. In spite of numerous studies showing the relationship of diet to atherosclerosis, the cautious approach to the assessment of dietary lipid composition as a factor in atherogenesis is perhaps a natural consequence of certain observations such as the following:

1. Critical analyses of statistical studies have shown that methods of observation and experimentation often lead to conclusions which are not justified.[8, 22, 23] Many studies purporting to relate diet to atherosclerosis, though otherwise inculpable. may lack statistical integrity.
2. There are increasing reports of the significant effects of a variety of local factors (ie. within the arterial wall) in the genesis and progression of the atherosclerotic lesion.[6, 11, 16, 20, 27] Among these factors the relevance of vascular enzymes as revealed by Zemplényi may be cited specifically [24]
3. Evidence that certain nonlipid, nondietary, or not necessarily dietary blood factors such as trace elements, circulating catecholamines, and carbon monoxide play a role in atherogenesis.[21, 25, 26]
4. Evidence that neurogenic and nondietary environmental factors, including the psychosocial, play a significant role in atherogenesis.[6, 20, 21, 25, 27]

Many early studies in which experimental animals were fed inordinately high concentrations of lipid, often with some other manipulations such as thyroidectomy or use of an adjuvant, to produce atherosclerotic lesions have been used to establish a classic cause and effect relationship. These methods, so blatantly artificial, can scarcely provide a parallel to the true pathogenesis of the atherosclerotic lesions in humans. Therefore, it is perhaps fitting to direct attention to the work of Stout and Bohorquez in which over 400 autopsies of mammals and birds representing 162 species revealed, in a significant number, spontaneous atherosclerotic lesions.[20] These were especially common in avian species and, in the birds, could not be correlated with the type of diet consumed in captivity or in nature — whether the diet were fish, meat, grain, or insects. In sea lions and seals fibrous intimal plaques contained no stainable lipid, suggesting some method other than lipid insudation as a cause of smooth muscle cell proliferation in the intima. It is of interest that in the atherosclerotic plaques of giant anteaters and aardvarks, central plaque necrosis appeared to precede lipid accumulation.

These findings lend some support to those who feel that lipid deposition may not be a primary event in the formation of the atherosclerotic plaque.[27-29] Interesting observations of Lindsay and Chaikoff on spontaneous atherosclerosis in animals also tend to deemphasize diet and to enhance the importance of other factors.[27] It may be stated that events which take place in the lower animal milieu are not necessarily indicative of the course of events in humans. True. However, if animal experiments purporting to show the effects of diet on atherosclerosis are constantly presented to us, it is only proper that those which show other facets of the problem also be given a fair share of the limelight.

The importance of local factors is again emphasized while simultaneously acknowledging a role of serum lipids (presumed to be dietary-dependent to some extent) in the hypothesis of atherogenesis mentioned by Robertson and referred to in part here.[12] Studies based on short-term culture techniques applied to the isolation of human arterial intimacytes have revealed two types of atherophils, one genetically susceptible and the other genetically resistant—susceptibility being based on the cells' response to incorporation of homologous serum lipids in vitro. Thus susceptible atherophils, in the presence of other influences—increased perfusion of lipoprotein secondary to hypertension, elevated serum lipids, and increased endothelial permeability (from fibrin deposition, platelet aggregation, or trauma)—become lipid-laden atherocytes. Genetically resistant atherophils, on the other hand, either do not respond or respond to a limited extent only. With great and/or prolonged elevation of serum lipoproteins, the resistance of the resistant atherophils may be overcome and fatty streaks produced.

Since the hypothesis recognizes a combination of consequential influences, it may answer many, if not all, of the objections which may be raised. The vital role accorded genetic factors may very well explain certain vagaries observed in individuals who differ little if at all from other members of a group with respect to dietary habits, age, physical activity ambient influences, and the like but show serious differences in the onset, distribution, severity, and progression of atherosclerotic lesions.

Eight years later the questions raised by Wilens have not been answered satisfactorily. We still do not know "whether it was an apple or an egg that tempted the original residents of Paradise"; but there seems to have been established among workers in the field a definite trend in thinking and doing which fosters an openmindedness, a receptivity to new concepts, a constant critical reevaluation of established principles, and a willingness to conduct searching expeditions for truths which will perhaps provide the answers to the many questions raised about the effect of diet on atherosclerosis. Such a trend is certainly consonant with the general theme of the original article on this subject.

References

1. Robbins SL: Pathologic Basis of Disease. Philadelphia, Saunders, 1974, pp 586–601
2. Keyes A, Aravanis C, Blackburn H, et al: Probability of middle aged men developing coronary heart disease in 5 years. Circulation 45:815, 1972
3. Turpeinen O: Diet and coronary events. J Am Diet Assoc 52:209, 1968

4. Kannel WB: The role of cholesterol in coronary atherogenesis. Med Clin North Am 58:363, 1974

5. Kuo PT: Hyperlipidemia and coronary artery disease Principles of diet and drug treatment. Med Clin North Am 58:351, 1974

6 Lee KT, Nam SC, Florentin RA, Thomas WA: Genesis of atherosclerosis in swine fed high fat-cholesterol diets. Med Clin North Am 58:281, 1974

7 Kahn HA: Change in serum cholesterol associated with changes in the United States civilian diet, 1909–1965. Am J Clin Nutr 23:879, 1970

8. Altschule MD: Foreword. Med Clin North Am 58:243, 1974

9. Altschule MD: The etiology of atherosclerosis. Med Clin North Am 58:397, 1974

10. Kannel WB: Serum lipid precursors of coronary heart disease. Hum Pathol 2:109, 1971

11. Robertson AL: Hypothesis on pathogenesis of human atherosclerosis. In Netter F (ed): The Ciba Collection of Medical Illustrations. New York, Colorpress, 1971, p 213

12. Robertson AL: Factors in etiology of atherosclerosis. In Netter F (ed): The Ciba Collection of Medical Illustrations. New York, Colorpress, 1971, p 213

13. Master AM, Jaffe HL: Coronary (ischemic) heart disease. In Conn HL, Kuo P (eds): Practice of Medicine. New York, Harper & Row, 1970

14. Stamler J: Nutrition, metabolism, and atherosclerosis — A review of data and theories, and a discussion of controversial questions. In Ingelfinger FJ, Relman AS, Finland M (eds): Controversy in Internal Medicine Philadelphia, Saunders, 1966, p 27

15. Albrink MJ: The dietary prophylaxis of atherosclerosis requires the control of triglycerides, not of cholesterol, in the plasma. In Ingelfinger FJ, Relman AS Finland M (eds): Controversy in Internal Medicine. Philadelphia, Saunders, 1966, p 60

16. Altschule MD: The uselessness of diet in the treatment of atherosclerosis. In Ingelfinger FJ, Relman AS Finland M (eds): Controversy in Internal Medicine. Philadelphia, Saunders, 1966, p 69

17. Koumerell B: The significance of blood coagulation in atherosclerosis. J Atheroscl Res 2:233, 1962

18. Michaels L: Etiology of coronary artery disease: an historical approach. Br Heart J 28:258, 1966

19. Keys A: The role of the diet in human atherosclerosis and its complications. In Sandler M, Bourne GH (eds): Atherosclerosis and Its Origin. New York, Academic Press, 1963, ch. 8, p 263

20 Stout LC, Bohorquez F: Intimal arterial changes in nonhuman vertebrates. Med Clin North Am 58:245, 1974

21. Rosenman RH, Friedman M: Neurogenic factors in pathogenesis of coronary heart disease Med Clin North Am 58:245, 1974

22. Yerushalmy J: On inferring causality from observed associations. Med Clin North Am 58:659, 1974

23. Wynder EL: The identification of causal factors in noncommunicable diseases by statistical means. Med Clin North Am 58:649, 1974

24. Zemplényi T: Vascular enzymes and the relevance of their study to problems of atherogenesis. Med Clin North Am 58:293, 1974

25. Astrup P, Kjeldsen K· Carbon monoxide, smoking, and atherosclerosis. Med Clin North Am 58:323, 1974

26 Schroeder HA: The role of trace elements in cardiovascular diseases. Med Clin North Am 58:381, 1974

27. Lindsay S, Chaikoff I: In Sandler M, Bourne GH (eds): Atherosclerosis and Its Origin, New York, Academic Press, ch. 10, pp 349–437

28. Moon HD, Rinehart JF: Histogenesis of coronary arteriosclerosis. Circulation 8:481, 1952

29. Taylor HE: Role of mucopolysaccharides in pathogenesis of intimal fibrosis and atherosclerosis of human aorta. Am J Pathol 29:871, 1953

MESENTERIC VASCULAR OCCLUSION STUDIED BY POSTMORTEM INJECTION OF THE MESENTERIC ARTERIAL CIRCULATION*†

LEOPOLD REINER

Unlike some other circulatory units, the vasculature of the abdominal viscera has been a rather neglected field of systematic pathologic investigation. This may be related to a lack of clinical urgency, on the one hand, and to the tediousness of anatomic dissection necessitated by the vastness of the vascular bed, on the other. There has been an upsurge of interest in the general field in recent years, the result of tremendous advances in vascular surgery that have changed situations of hopelessness into therapeutic triumphs.[1]

We set ourselves the task to study systematically the vasculature of the abdominal viscera by means of a postmortem injection technic.[2] In particular, the emphasis was, first, on the extent and topography of stenosing and occlusive disease in an autopsy population predominantly unselected with respect to the status of the abdominal viscera; second, on clinical manifestations and anatomic sequelae of vascular disease; and, third, on the vascular substrate of intestinal infarction versus that of lesser degrees of mesenteric arterial decompensation.

* The article appeared first in *Medical Science*, 12:229–242, 1962. It is here being republished in a revised and illustrated form with the kind permission of J. B. Lippincott Company.

† The work here described was supported by a Research Grant of the National Heart Institute, National Institutes of Health, Public Health Service.

In the subsequent text the celiac, superior mesenteric, and inferior mesenteric arborizations are viewed as the constituents of a single circulatory unit which may be called the celiacomesenteric circulation. For reasons of brevity it will be referred to simply as the mesenteric circulation. Beyond the anatomic and hemodynamic justification for this unitarian interpretation, it is also true that from the clinical viewpoint vascular disease of the celiac branches is relatively unimportant.

Technic

Following en bloc removal of the abdominal viscera, glass cannulae are inserted into the aortic ostia of the celiac, superior mesenteric, and inferior mesenteric ar-

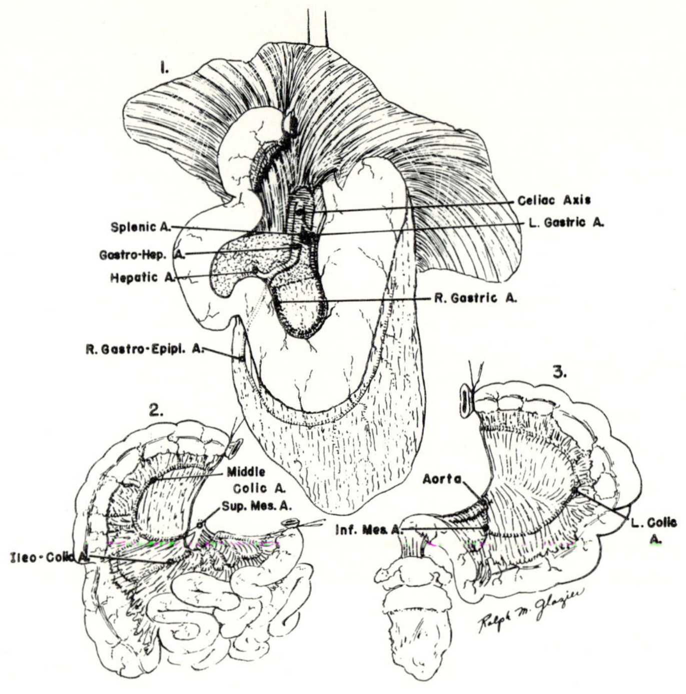

Fig. 1. Partitioned abdominal viscera. 1. Celiac artery specimen. Note the rotation and consequent upward sweep of the duodenum. The root of the superior mesenteric artery remains with the celiac artery but is here hidden behind the pancreas. 2. Superior mesenteric artery specimen comprising the intestine from the middle of the first jejunal loop to the midtransverse colon. 3. Inferior mesenteric artery specimen extending from the midtransverse colon to the anus. The pelvic viscera (uterus and bladder) are attached.

teries. In order to retard postmortem autolysis and bacterial action, generous quantities of sublimate ($HgCl_2$) in saline are instilled into the lumen of the gastrointestinal tract by needle and syringe and by numerous transmural portals. Injection is carried out at a final pressure of 200 mm of mercury attained by stepwise increments of 50 mm and employing a highly viscous radiopaque mass of barium sulfate in gelatin. By adding a measured amount and concentration of formalin just prior to use, the mass

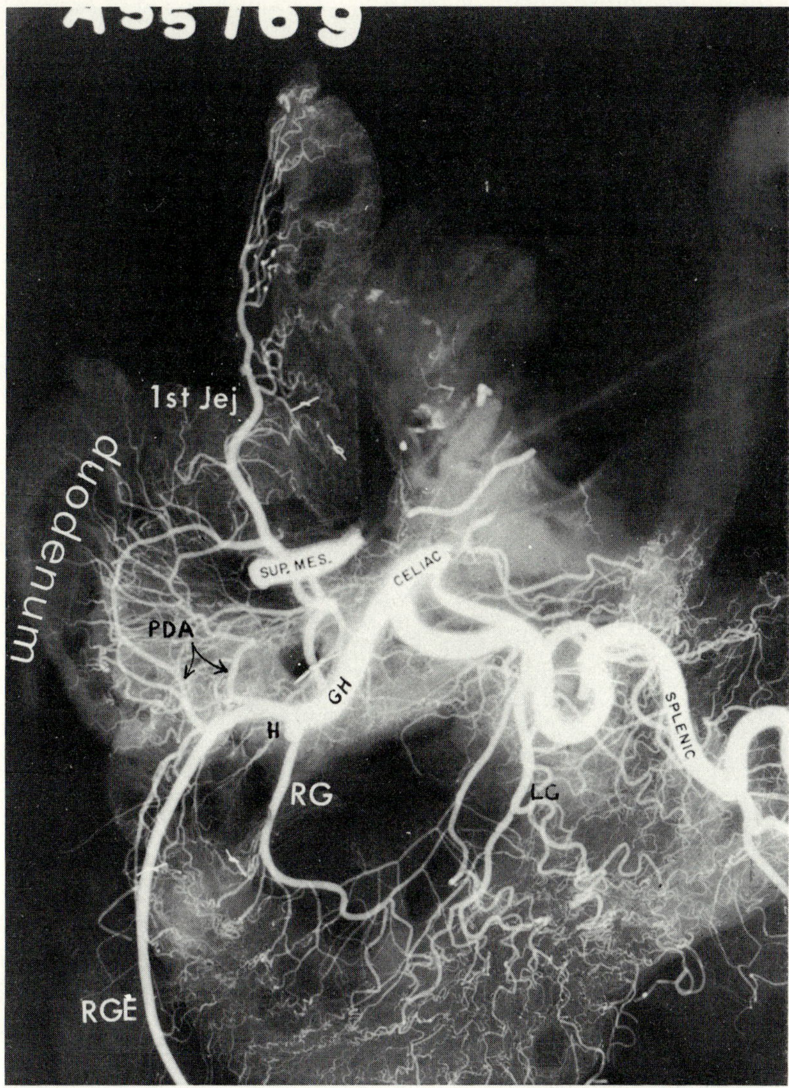

Fig. 2. Celiac arteriogram with duodenum rotated upward. Even though postmortem injection was carried out only via the superior mesenteric artery there is complete vessel filling of the celiac arborization via collaterals including the pancreaticoduodenal arcades (PDA). These two arcades fuse to become the inferior pancreaticoduodenal artery which in turn opens into the first jejunal rather than the superior mesenteric artery. Contrary to most texts this is the usual finding. GH, gastrohepatic; H, hepatic; LG, left gastric; RG, right gastric; RGE, right gastroepiploic.

is made to solidify intravascularly within a predetermined period of time. Although the mass penetrates into vessels of arteriolar dimensions quite regularly, it does not ordinarily cross the capillary bed. For technical details the reader is referred to previous publications.[2,3]

The injection procedure is complemented by triple partitioning of the abdominal viscera in accordance with the distribution of the three "constituent" (celiac, superior mesenteric, and inferior mesenteric) arborizations (Fig. 1). In order to retain the vascular interrelations, the root of the superior mesenteric artery down to and including the first jejunal artery is left attached to the celiac artery specimen,

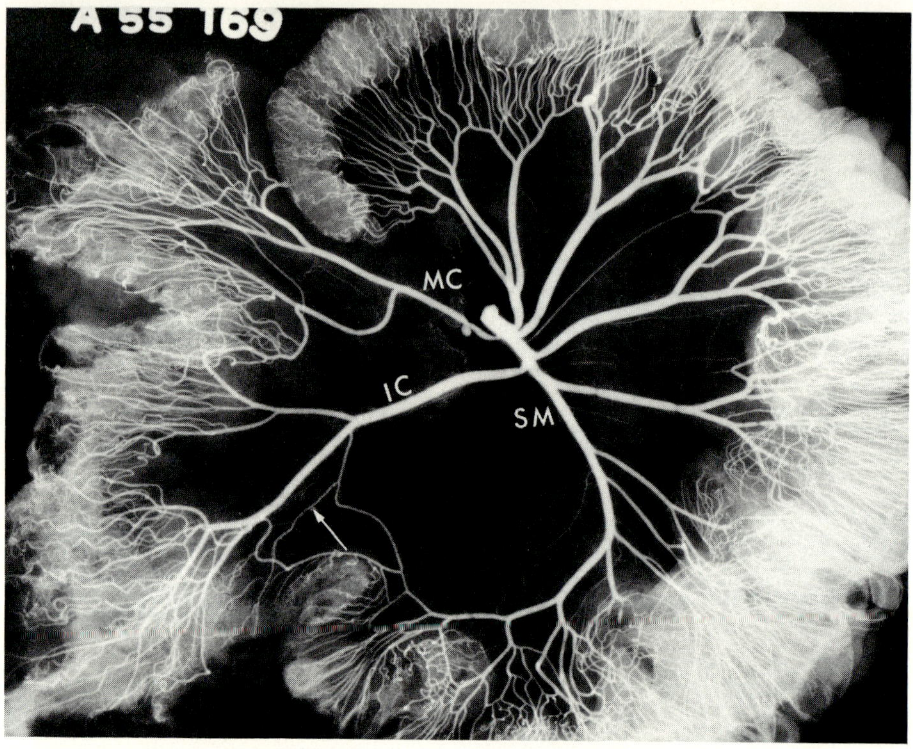

Fig. 3. Superior mesenteric arteriogram. Same case as Figure 2. Note the separateness and the considerable length of the appendiceal artery (arrow). IC, ileocolic; MC, middle colic; SM, superior mesenteric.

thereby preserving the anastomoses between the two arborizations, including the pancreaticoduodenal arcades (Fig. 2). Radiographic arteriograms of the arborizations so isolated yield pictures such as illustrated in Figures 2 to 4. They are useful both for anatomic study and for ready identification of vascular stenoses and occlusions. Moreover, if taken stereoscopically and viewed with stereobinoculars, superb three-dimensional arteriograms are obtained, as lucid and instructive as any anatomic dissection and vastly less time-consuming, especially with respect to the celiac arborization (Fig. 5). In searching for a way to facilitate still further the interpretation of the complex vasculature about the duodenum and the head of the pancreas,

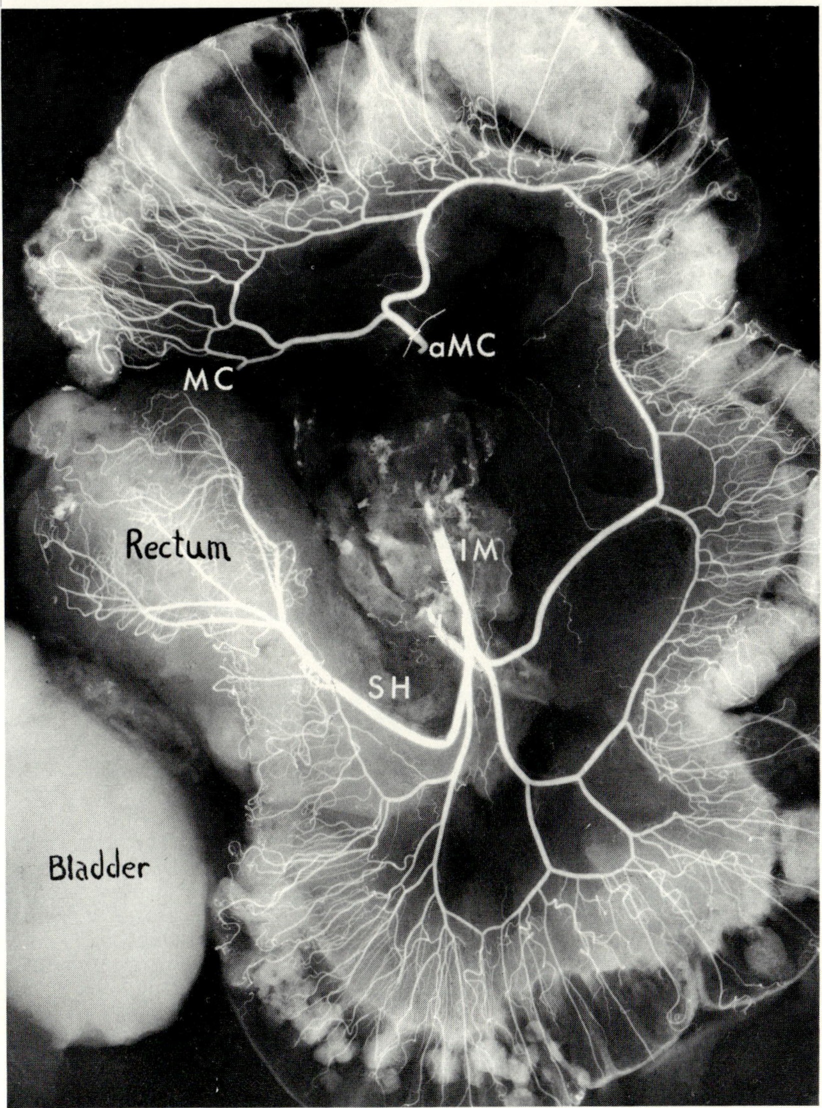

Fig. 4. Inferior mesenteric arborization. Same case as Figures 2 and 3. Excellent anastomotic filling via the middle colic (MC) and accessory middle colic (aMC) arteries. The latter vessel was divided between two wire markers, one of which is readily seen in this photograph; the other can be seen in Figure 2, just to the left of the gastrohepatic artery. This technique of marking vessels with flexible copper wire during the partitioning procedure is often useful for later radiographic identification. Notice the dichotomous vessel pattern in the rectum as against the arcading arrangement in the remainder of the gastrointestinal tract. Delicate adipose tissue arteries may be seen coming off the visceral arteries, e.g., the marginal ("Drummond's") artery. With arteriography being carried out in eviscerated specimens the vessels of the extraintestinal pelvic viscera (e.g., bladder) do not become filled because the anastomoses between the (inferior) mesenteric and extramesenteric vessels are destroyed upon evisceration. IM, inferior mesenteric; SH, superior hemorrhoidal.

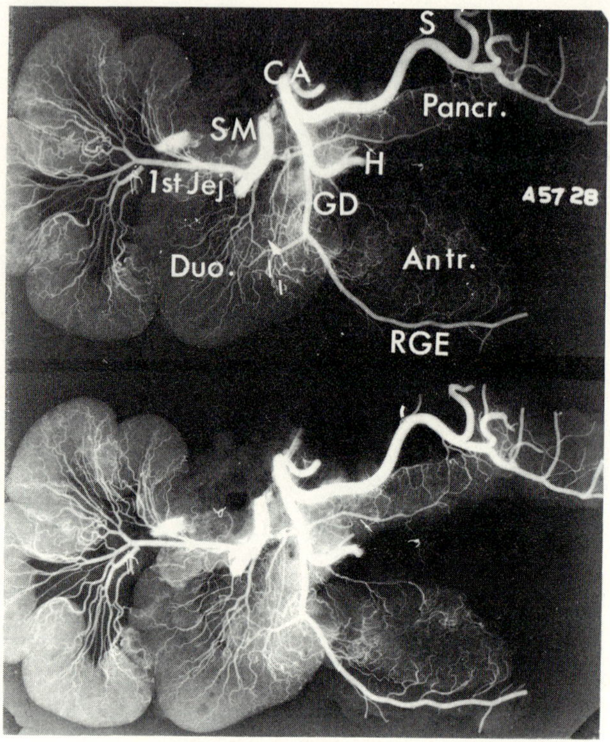

Fig. 5. Stereoscopic angiogram of the celiac arborization. The corpus has been ablated retaining only the antrum (Antr.) of the stomach. The duodenum (Duo.) has been rotated in order
to unfold the pancreaticoduodenal arcades seen to arise from the gastroduodenal artery (GD)
and running along the lesser curvature of the duodenum. For stereoscopic examination the
illustration has to be turned 90 degrees. CA, celiac artery; H, hepatic; RGE, right gastroepiploic; S, splenic; SM, superior mesenteric.

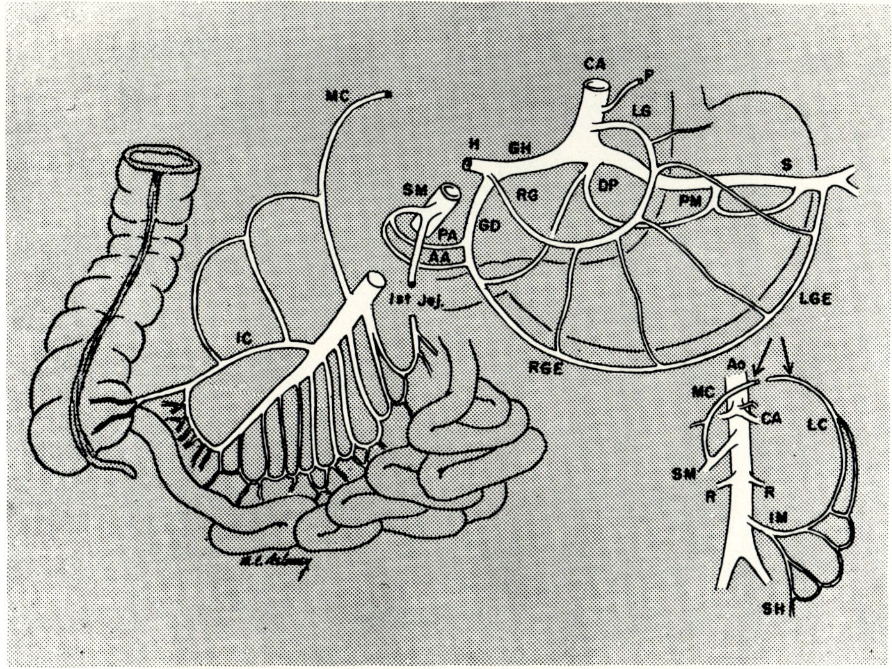

Fig. 6. Diagram of mesenteric arterial circulation based on the roentgenographic appearance of the three constituent arborizations, following partitioning of the abdominal viscera. Note that the root of the superior mesenteric artery (together with the first jejunal and pancreaticoduodenal arcades) is left with the celiac arborization. The superior and inferior mesenteric arborizations anastomose with each other via the middle and left colic arteries (Riolan's arch, arrows) as shown in the diagram of the aorta (right lower inset). AA, anterior pancreaticoduodenal arcade; Ao, aorta; CA, celiac artery; DP, dorsal pancreatic; GD, gastroduodenal; GH, gastrohepatic; H, hepatic; IC, ileocolic; IM, inferior mesenteric; 1st Jej, first jejunal; LC, left colic; LG, left gastric; LGE, left gastroepiploic; MC, middle colic; P, phrenic; PA, posterior pancreaticoduodenal arcade; PM, pancreatica magna; R, renal; RG, right gastric; RGE, right gastroepiploic; S, splenic; SH, superior hemorrhoidal; SM, superior mesenteric.

a rotational procedure of these two structures was discovered which greatly reduces the vessel overlap in the celiac arteriograms (Figs. 1, 2, and 5). A diagrammatic representation of the triple-partitioned mesenteric vasculature is shown in Figure 6.

Collateral Circulation

The collateral potential of the mesenteric circulation was studied in vitro—first, by isolated injection of each of its constituent arborizations and, second, by ligation experiments. It could be shown that isolated injection of any one of the three constituent arteries (celiac, superior mesenteric, inferior mesenteric) was capable of filling the other two. In general, the quality of collateral filling was best upon injection of the superior mesenteric (Figs. 2 to 4) and least upon injection of the inferior mesenteric artery. Injection of the celiac axis yielded intermediate results. These in vitro differences are paralleled in vivo. The likelihood that damage will occur in the target organs is vastly greater upon occlusion of the superior mesenteric main

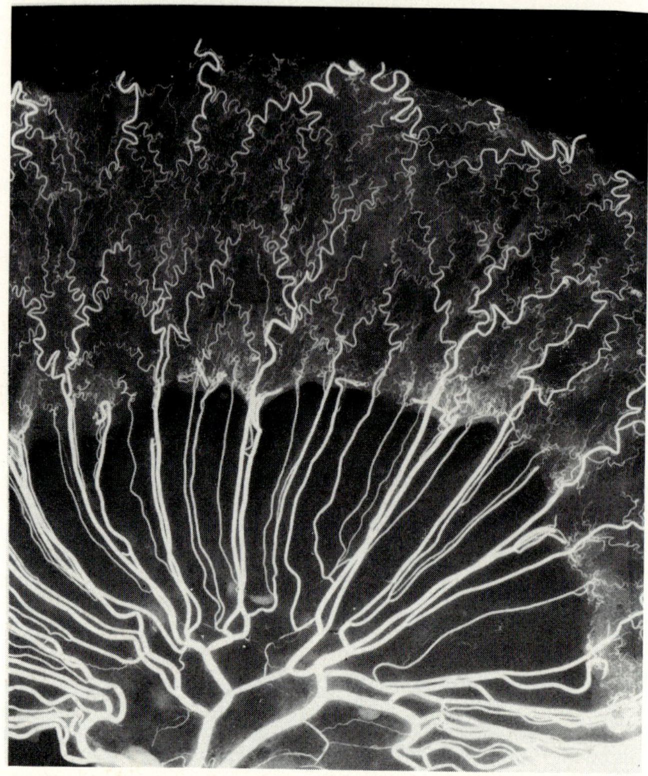

Fig. 7. Vascular pattern of small intestine. The jejunum has been opened close to the mesentery, thereby transecting approximately one half of the number of mural vessels. The mural vessels are tortuous and anastomose with each other both laterally and circumferentially. The vasa recta are of variable diameter depending on their destination: the most delicate ones supply the intestine about the mesenteric insertion; the thickest go to the antimesenteric circumference. Notice the fine adipose tissue arteries within the arcades at the bottom of this photograph.

stem than upon occlusion of the main stem of either of the other two constituents of the mesenteric circulation.

Collateral flow between the celiac and the superior mesenteric arborizations, and between the superior and the inferior mesenteric circuits, is facilitated by preformed anastomoses (Fig. 6). These are located respectively in and about the pancreas (e.g., the pancreaticoduodenal arcades) and along the transverse colon (via an arch made up of the middle and the left colic arteries and occasionally referred to as Riolan's arch). Depending on anatomic variations in number and size of these and other anastomoses, the results of a single-artery injection disclose individual differences of appreciable magnitude. It is inferred that such individual differences may influence the clinical and pathologic sequelae of naturally occurring vascular occlusions.

The vascular arcade so characteristic of the extraintestinal course of the superior and inferior mesenteric arborizations is found in modified fashion also in

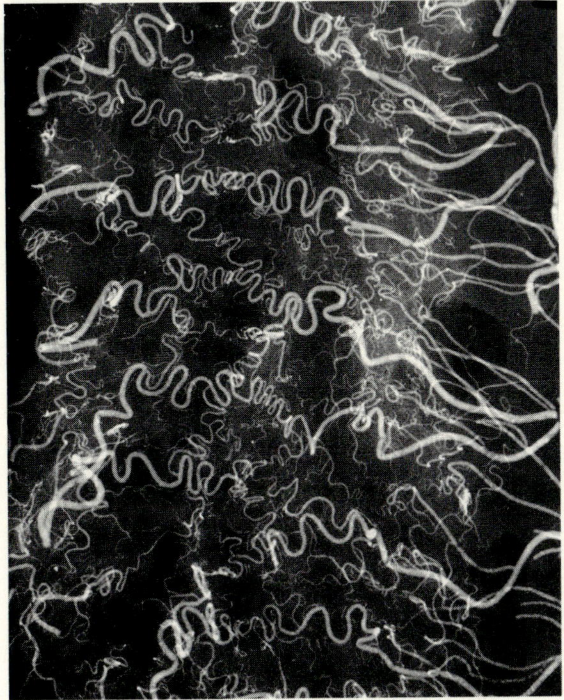

Fig. 8. Ascending colon. The intestine is rather contracted, and the arteries are highly tortuous. Note the prominence of the circumferential anastomoses.

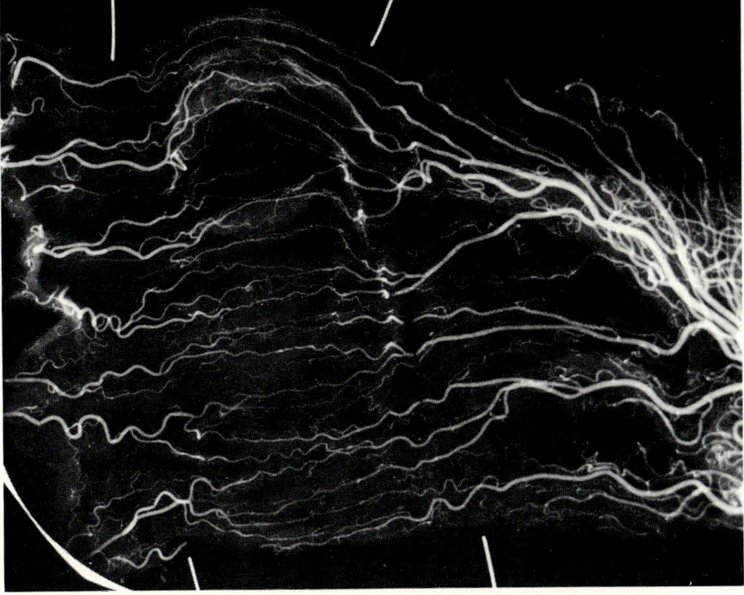

Fig. 9. Ascending colon in a distended state. Compare with Figure 8. The wires mark the position of the tenias.

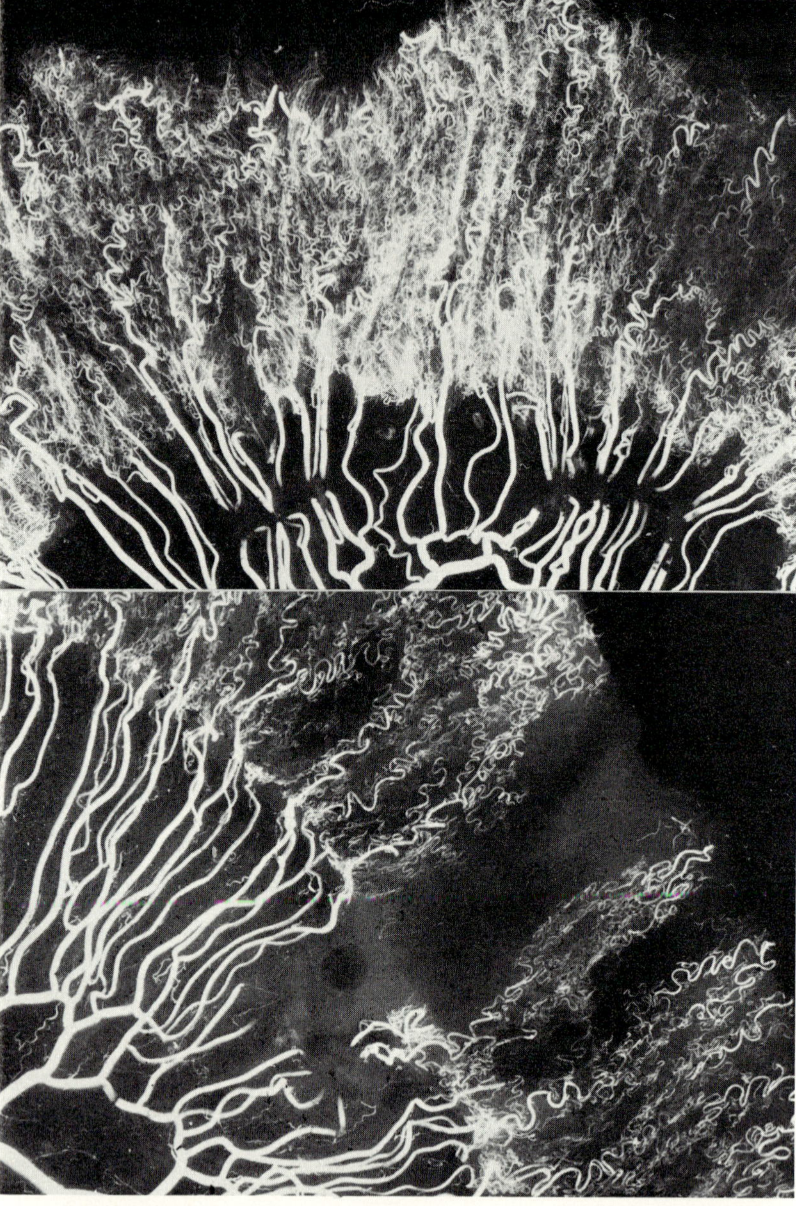

Fig. 10. Experimental ligation of the vasa recta in series, twice in the top photograph and once in the bottom photograph. The two loops of small intestine illustrated are from two different cases which were injected under similar conditions. The pictures illustrate the variability in collateral potential of the mural vasculature between different cases and between different segments even of the same case.

relation to the stomach (the two gastric and the two gastroepiploic arteries) and along the duodenum (the pancreaticoduodenal arcades). The arcading principle is also encountered in the wall of the small (Fig. 7) and large (Fig. 8) intestine. Here the anterior and posterior branches of the vasa recta anastomose with each other both circumferentially and laterally. The sinusoidal tortuosity characteristic of these anastomoses is admirably adapted to allow for changes in diameter and length of the intestine during peristalsis (Fig. 9). This mural vasculature has only a limited capacity to compensate for obstruction of the vasa recta. Ligation of the latter leads to variable injection defects in the target area of the intestinal wall (Fig. 10). In no case were the mural anastomoses capable of compensating for ligation of contiguous vasa recta in excess of 4 cm of intestinal wall (as measured in the small intestine attached to its mesentery). In striking contrast complete filling of the mural vasculature was obtained after ligation of the arborization placed at any level proximal to the vasa recta (Fig. 11).

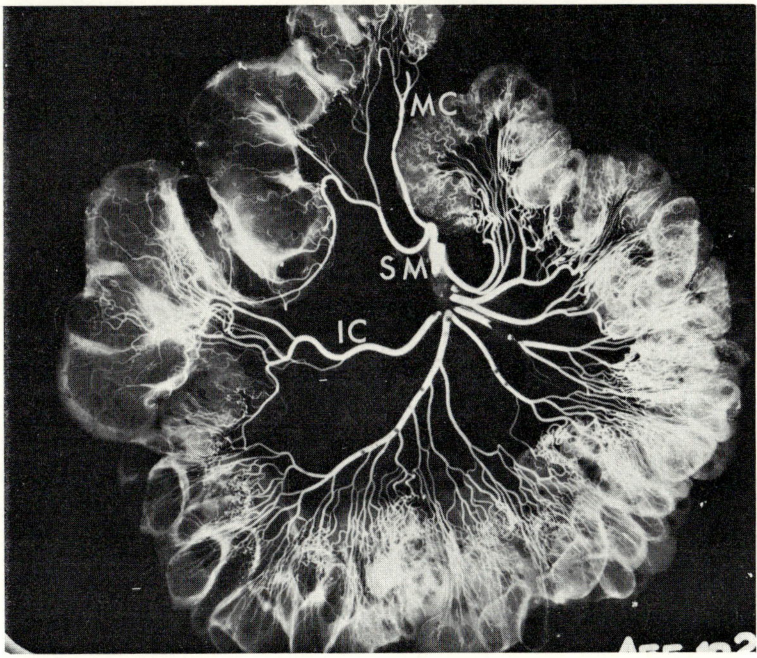

Fig. 11. Superior mesenteric arborization. Pre-injection ligation of the superior mesenteric main stem including two jejunal and the ileocolic (IC) arteries. There are no circumscribed injection defects, but the overall injection quality of the ileum is less than that of the jejunum. MC, middle colic; SM, superior mesenteric. (From Reiner et al. Surgery, 45:820, 1955.)

Subsidiary to the visceral branches of the mesenteric circulation, there exists a little-known system of delicate vessels that supply the adipose tissues of the mesentery and mesocolon (Figs. 4 and 7). These vessels originate from the main stems as well as from their visceral branches and communicate with each other in a seem-

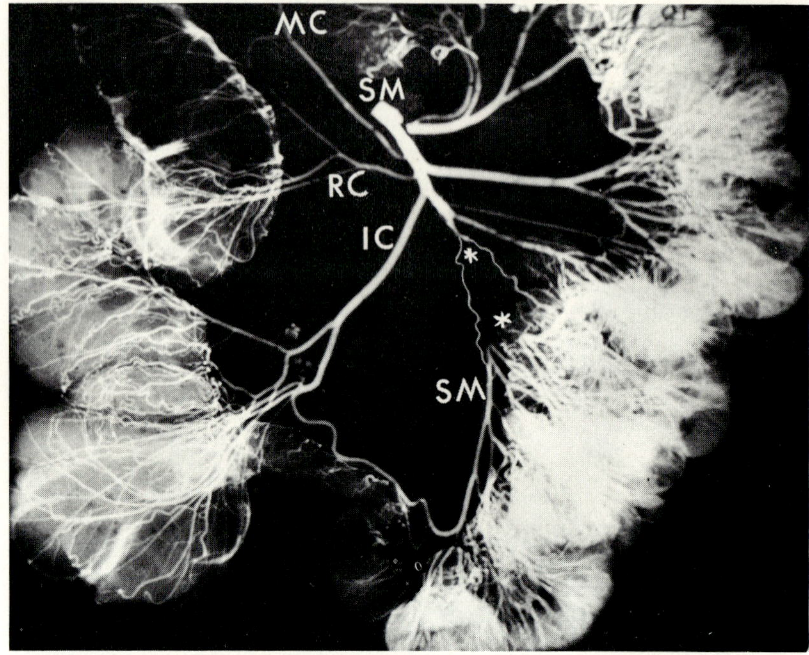

Fig. 12. Silent embolic occlusion of superior mesenteric (SM) main stem (and sixth enteric artery) distal to the ileocolic (IC) artery in a patient with mitral stenosis and left auricular thrombosis. The occlusion is old and blocks the segment, as indicated by the two asterisks. Note the prominently enlarged tortuous adipose tissue arteries which flank the whole length of the occlusion. Obviously, this enlargement took place after the occlusive episode and cannot be held responsible for the absence of either clinical or anatomic disease referable to the intestine. MC, middle colic; RC, right colic.

ingly haphazard fashion, widely transgressing the anatomic boundaries of their parent arcades. They may communicate directly with the aorta, especially in relation to the inferior mesenteric arborization. Injection studies have shown that these delicate vessels may appreciably enlarge and thus act as collaterals about sites of stenosis and occlusion of visceral branches (Fig. 12). It is not improbable that these vessels contribute to the hemorrhagic component in intestinal infarction by carrying arterial blood around sites of arterial occlusion.

Apart from the adipose-tissue arteries of aortic origin, the mesenteric circula-

---

Fig. 13. Superior (A) and inferior (B) mesenteric arteriograms in a case of aortoiliac thrombosis. There were occlusions of the ostia of the superior (SM) and inferior (IM) mesenteric arteries which were effectively bypassed on account of enormous enlargement of Riolan's arch comprising the middle (MC) and left (LC) colic arteries. The enlargement is continued into the superior hemorrhoidal artery (SH), which for technical reasons had to be clamped proximal to its destination, accounting for the lack of vascular injection in the rectum. Injection was via the celiac artery, imitating the situation as it existed prior to the supervention of a terminal embolus that occluded the ostium of the celiac axis and thereby caused infarction of the entire small intestine and proximal colon. The stomach did not become infarcted. In this case, the superior mesenteric vein became injected, the only example ever observed by us and considered an artefact. Note in B the great enlargement of adipose tissue arteries (arrows) several of which extend from the aorta (Ao) to the colon. IC, ileocolic.

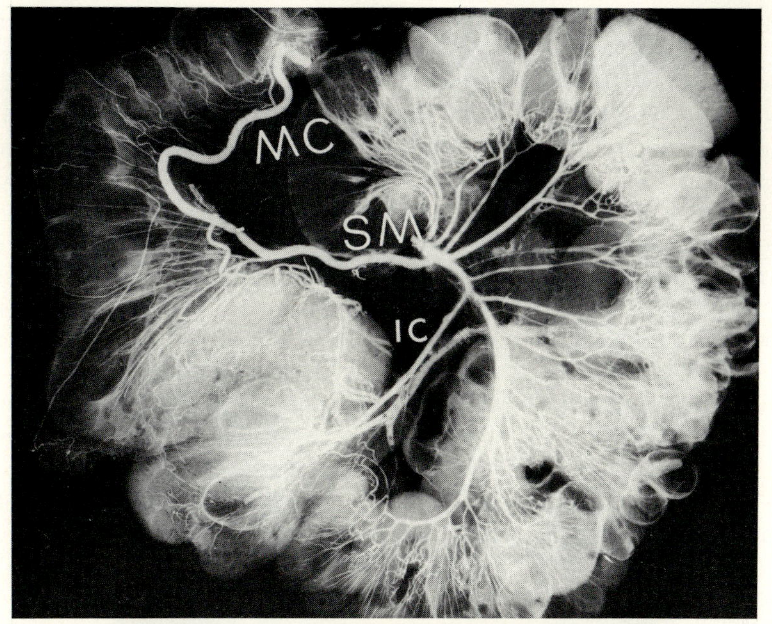

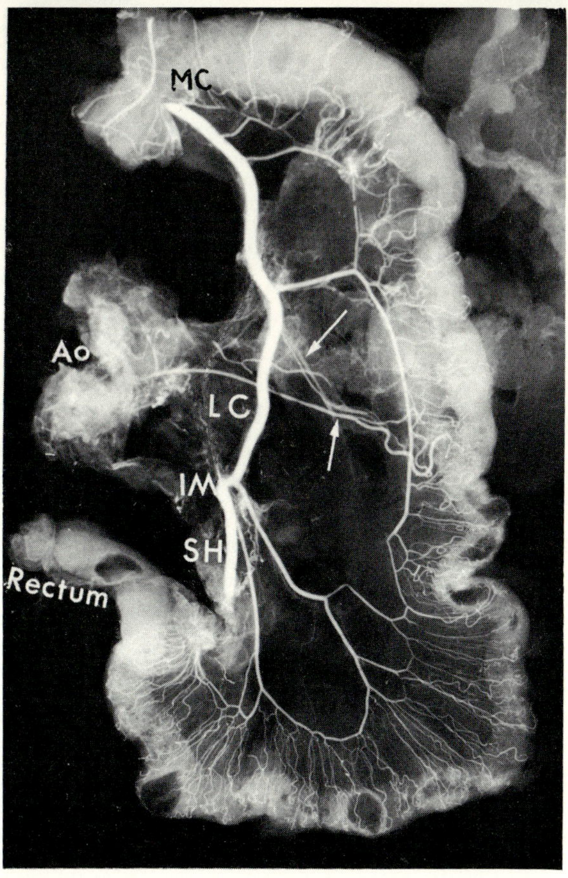

Fig. 13. See legend on facing page.

tion is to be viewed as a largely self-contained unit. Indeed the visceral branches have few or no communications with extramesenteric arteries except about the cardia above (and thus indirectly with the adrenal and renal arteries) and the rectum below. The communications at the former site with the phrenic and paraesophageal arteries no doubt account for the rarity of gastric infarction in occlusions of the celiac artery. At the latter site the superior hemorrhoidal artery, derived from the inferior mesenteric artery, communicates with the middle and inferior hemorrhoidal arteries, derived from the iliac arteries. These communications are believed capable of compensating for each other in resective bowel surgery of the rectum and distal sigmoid colon.[4] In addition, we have observed cases of occlusive aortoiliac thrombosis in which the hemorrhoidal vessels—together with strategically located branches of the superior and inferior mesenteric arteries—became enormously enlarged. Thereby not only was intestinal damage prevented but also the mesenteric circulation was enabled to bypass such an aortoiliac occlusion and to furnish an important source of blood supply to the pelvic viscera and lower extremities (Fig. 13).

Mesenteric Arterial Occlusions

We have studied two series of cases by postmortem mesenteric arteriography. Series I comprised 8 patients specifically selected for arteriography because of intestinal infarction. Series II comprised 84 patients subjected to arteriography for the sole purpose of investigating in an unbiased and systematic fashion the status of the mesenteric arterial circulation in the adult autopsy population of the "acute" general hospital. In this second series there were 11 patients with occlusive disease in the mesenteric arterial circulation but without intestinal infarction, an incidence of 13 per cent.* In Table 1 the two series are listed by sex and age, and in Table 2 by pertinent associated conditions. The 84 unselected patients of Series II were further divided into three groups: Group A comprised the 11 patients with mesenteric arterial occlusion; Group B comprised 53 patients with (nonocclusive) mesenteric arteriosclerosis with or without luminal stenoses; Group C (20 patients) showed neither occlusions nor mesenteric arteriosclerosis. These groups are expressive of nosologic profiles and consequently useful in clinical diagnosis. Attention is drawn, first, to the high incidences of hypertensive and arteriosclerotic heart disease, congestive failure, peripheral vascular disease of legs, and diabetes mellitus in all patients with mesenteric arterial occlusion, i.e., in Series I and in Group A of Series II. Second, there is an exceptionally high incidence of embolic manifestations in the systemic circulation in the patients with intestinal infarction. In view of the difficult histopathologic distinction between local thrombosis and thromboembolism, this last item supports the contention of those authors who, like the writer, find intestinal infarction to be more commonly due to mesenteric embolization than to local thrombosis. Assuming that mesenteric (and other systemic) thromboemboli usually arise in the heart, one may also infer from the figures in Table 2 that the embolic event occurs with about equal frequency on the basis of valvular and of ischemic heart disease. Moreover, the absence of a mural thrombus in the left side

---

* This is more than 400 times greater than the incidence of intestinal infarction which has been reported as 0.03 per cent in an unselected hospital population.[5]

Table 1. Distribution of Cases by Sex and Age

	SERIES I INTESTINAL INFARCTION		SERIES II NO INTESTINAL INFARCTION					
			Group A Mesenteric Occlusions		*Group B* Mesenteric Arteriosclerosis; No Occlusions		*Group C* No Mesenteric Arteriosclerosis; No Occlusions	
	(8 patients)		(11 patients)		(53 patients)		(20 patients)	
Age	M	F	M	F	M	F	M	F
20-29			1		1			
30-39					1		1	1
40-49			1		2	1	2	3
50-59	1		2	1	7	7	1	5
60-69	3	1	1	3	8	9		3
70-79	2	1		1	9	7	2	
80-89				1	1		1	1
Range	50-75		28-88		28-83		28-86	
Mean	66		60.4		62.3		57.4	
Median	67		62		56		57	

Table 2. Incidence (Percentage) of Associated Conditions

| | SERIES I
INTESTINAL INFARCTION | SERIES II
NO INTESTINAL INFARCTION | | |
| | | *Group A*
Mesenteric
Occlusions | *Group B*
Mesenteric
Arteriosclerosis;
No Occlusions | *Group C*
No Mesenteric
Arteriosclerosis;
No Occlusions |
	(8 patients)	(11 patients)	(53 patients)	(20 patients)
Cardiac hypertrophy*	87%	82%	77%	50%
Congestive heart failure	75	82	53	5
Coronary arteriosclerosis†	63	82	72	30
Myocardial infarction	63	82	57	20
Auricular fibrillation	50	45	12	10
Valvular disease	50	27	11	20
Mural thrombi, left side of heart	50	36	8	5
Embolic manifestations, systemic	87	18	32	20
Peripheral vascular disease (legs)**	87	64	31	0
Diabetes mellitus	50	64	14	5

* Heart weight above 400 g in men and above 300 g in women.

† Occlusions or severe stenosis.

** Including cases of thromboembolism.

of the heart at autopsy does not necessarily militate against the cardiac origin of a peripheral embolus.

Table 2 is interesting also because it shows that nonocclusive mesenteric arteriosclerosis (Group B, Series II) is also commonly associated with severe coronary arteriosclerosis, ischemic heart disease, congestive failure and cardiac hypertrophy. Finally, the data are in keeping with observations reported elsewhere [6] that the chance of severe mesenteric atherosclerosis being associated with severe coronary arteriosclerosis is two to two and one half times greater than the reverse, a one-sided correlation also observed with respect to aortic arteriosclerosis.

Occlusive disease in the mesenteric arborization is associated with a broad spectrum of clinical and anatomic manifestations. At one extreme are the patients with intestinal infarction. At the other are those in whom the occlusions are altogether silent. The spectrum is completed by an intermediate group of cases with relative, incomplete, or chronic mesenteric arterial insufficiency characterized by purely functional derangement (e.g., angina abdominalis), segmental anatomic injury of a lesser extent than intestinal infarction, or both. Of the 11 cases in Group A of Series II, 4 were intermediate and 7 were silent.

These variants of mesenteric arterial occlusion show little relation to the number of arborizations or the number of individual vessels affected.[7] They do, however, bear a relation to such qualitative factors of occlusion as arborization affected, site (main stem versus branches), mechanism (thromboembolism versus local thrombosis), extent and speed of secondary clot propagation, individual variations of vessel size and anatomy, and possibly the enlargement of collaterals by preceding stenosing mesenteric arteriosclerosis. For example, in every one of our infarct cases there was occlusion of the main stem of the superior mesenteric artery. In the majority, at a ratio of about 6 or 7 to 1, this was due to thromboembolism rather than to local thrombosis.

At the same time there were several patients with embolic or thrombotic occlusion of the superior mesenteric main stem without intestinal infarction and, indeed, with few or no clinical manifestations. An analysis of this unexpected contrast led to the postulate [8] of a critical segment of the superior mesenteric main stem, extending anywhere from the origin of the second jejunal and middle colic arteries down to, and to a variable extent beyond, the origin of the ileocolic artery (Fig. 14). It was occlusion of this segment that was associated with intestinal infarction. Occlusions located either proximal or distal (Fig. 12) to this critical segment, regardless of their nature, were not necessarily so related. These observations may be explained by anatomic and hemodynamic factors related to the anatomic pathways of collateral flow, on the one hand, and to the transmission of pressure head, on the other. In our experience occlusion of vasa recta by embolic shattering or by stagnant thrombosis was neither a necessary prerequisite nor a frequent concomitant of infarction, as has been claimed.[9] The good clinical results of superior mesenteric embolectomy also minimize the importance of vasa recta occlusion.

The foregoing considerations are not meant to imply that infarction does not take place in the distribution area of the inferior mesenteric artery, i.e., in the distal colon. Indeed, among the 8 patients with infarction of the small intestine, thromboemboli to the inferior mesenteric arborization were noted in 3, with necrosis in the

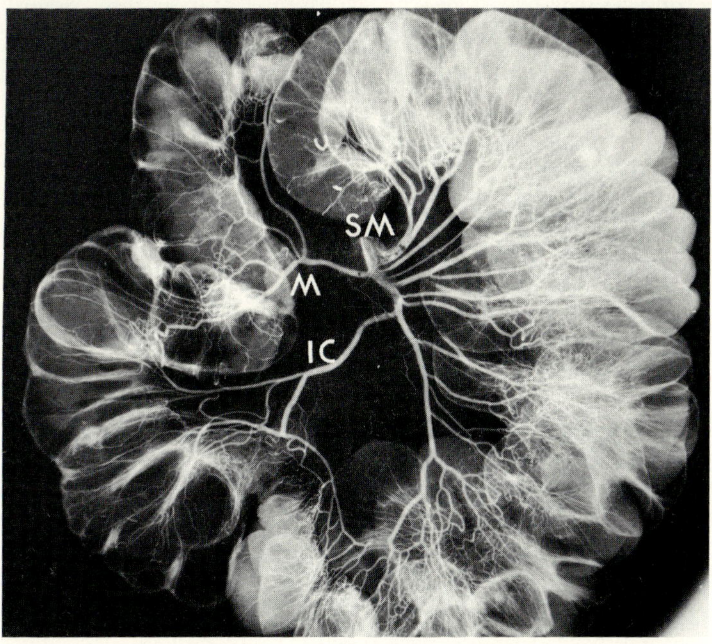

Fig. 14. Superior mesenteric arteriogram in a case of infarction involving the small intestine and proximal colon in a 70 year old man with mitral stenosis, auricular thrombosis, and fibrillation. There is occlusion by a thromboembolus which extends from the second jejunal (appearing in the arteriogram as the first small-intestinal branch) past the middle colic (M) and down to but not including the ileocolic (IC) artery. In this case, the occlusion involved also the more proximal portions (not shown) of the superior mesenteric (SM) main stem. The injection quality of the intestine is quite good and thereby recapitulates the picture obtained after experimental ligation of the superior mesenteric artery illustrated in Figure 11. This resembles the experience in postmortem coronary artery injection: depending on pre-existent interarterial anastomoses the territory of a myocardial infarct may be—and more often than not, actually is—well injected.

distal colon in 2. However, as a naturally occurring phenomenon isolated infarction of the distal colon seems to be a rare occurrence. In a single observation of mitral valve disease with atrial fibrillation, an isolated thromboembolic occlusion at the aortic ostium of the inferior mesenteric artery occurred without any clinical or pathologic manifestations. It thereby differed from 2 of the above 3 infarct cases in which the emboli had lodged in the terminal arcades. This asymptomatic embolic occlusion of the main stem ostium of the inferior mesenteric artery is in accord with other evidence, obtained by postmortem injection and by surgical experience: 1) the *proximal* components of this arborization are dispensable, 2) the distal colon can be supplied very efficiently by collaterals from above, i.e., from the superior mesenteric artery (via Riolan's arch), and from below, i.e., from the internal iliac arteries (via the inferior and middle hemorrhoidal arteries).

Nonetheless, we have observed 2 patients presenting with *isolated* ischemic disease of the distal colon (p. 339). Even though the changes were qualitatively those of intestinal infarction, they were of limited dimensions and, at least in 1 of them, self-healing. Neither patient died from his intestinal disease. In both instances

the colonic disease was occasioned by widespread and severely stenosing arteriosclerosis with superimposed occlusive thrombosis.

Intestinal Infarction

VASCULAR SUBSTRATE.   As stated previously, all 8 patients with intestinal infarction exhibited occlusions of the superior mesenteric main stem with or without
extension into its branches. This was due to thromboembolism in 6 and to local
thrombosis on the basis of arteriosclerosis in 1. In the eighth case (Fig. 13) thrombosis of remote vintage occluded the aortic ostia of both the superior and inferior
mesenteric arteries, and circulatory compensation was afforded via collateral channels with the celiac arborization. Not until these collateral sources became blocked
by a thromboembolus at the aortic ostium of the celiac axis did the target area of
the superior mesenteric artery become infarcted. Neither the stomach nor the distal
colon were involved, obviously because of effective communications with extramesenteric vessels about the cardia and rectum, respectively.

Occlusive disease in our infarct cases was not necessarily confined to the
superior mesenteric arborization. Indeed, in 6 of the 8 patients the main stems
and/or branches of the celiac and inferior mesenteric arborizations were involved
as well. As in the superior mesenteric main stem, these occlusions were thromboembolic and fresh in the majority of instances. Ischemic necrosis in the distal large
intestine, spleen, and pancreas ensued in several of these patients.

In this connection a word may be said about the extreme rarity of infarction of
the stomach. The subject has been discussed by Cohen [10] and Dassel,[11] who reported on a total of 5 patients. In 4 of them, the infarction involved the entire
stomach and was associated with infarction of all or part of the small and large
intestines. The superior mesenteric artery was patent in 2 cases and probably also
in a third one. The celiac axis was patent in 2 and freshly occluded in the remaining
2 patients. Among the latter, infarctive phenomena were observed also in the spleen,
liver, and pancreas.

We have studied a relevant case (not included in the series) by postmortem
arterial injection and dissection.[12] No occlusions or stenosis were demonstrated in
any of the three constituent arborizations of the mesenteric circulation, even though
the entire stomach, the small intestine, and part of the large intestine were involved.
In this elderly man with cardiomegaly and rheumatoid arthritis, mesenteric arterial
insufficiency was probably brought about by suppression of endogenous adrenal
secretion secondary to abrupt and self-imposed withdrawal of cortisone medication,
which the patient had taken continuously for several years. Adrenal unresponsive-
ness in the face of bodily stress is known to cause a breakdown of circulatory competence by a decrease in plasma volume and vascular tone.[13]

The foregoing data and more cited below suggest that gastric infarction, if it
occurs at all, is usually associated with intestinal infarction and that this combination speaks to a considerable extent against organic occlusions in the superior
mesenteric and celiac arteries.

PATHOLOGY.   The gross anatomic findings of intestinal infarction do not require description. However, some comments are presented for conceptual reasons

and also to draw attention to certain facets of the anatomy of intestinal infarction.

It is my belief that intestinal infarction is not necessarily and probably not even commonly due to a complete and sustained cessation of blood flow. Rather its critical reduction is responsible, i.e., an uncompensated disproportion between blood supply and metabolic requirements of the target tissues.* This belief is based on the result of animal experimentation in vivo, on observations made on postmortem mesenteric arteriography, and, finally, on histopathologic interpretation of intestinal infarction itself.

Khanna [14] has shown that experimental ligation of the main stem of the superior mesenteric artery in the living rat causes early cessation of circulation in the intestinal wall. Following this there is rapid though incomplete resumption of blood flow in both arteries and veins. Yet, the mucosa fails to survive (or recover), which is an expression of its particular vulnerability on the one hand and of the inadequacy of the reestablished circulation on the other. The same work has also shown—at least with respect to the experimental rat—that the bleeding into and from the mucosa takes place from its sinuses upon receipt of blood from the reestablished circulation and then ceases. In other words, the bleeding is not a continuous phenomenon but occurs as a single episode.

Secondly, one may reasonably infer that with all the reduction of pressure head and the changes in vascular tonus distal to an occlusion a measure of arterial blood may still be brought in from neighboring fields with an intact circulation. This inference is made plausible by postmortem angiography in man, which has disclosed a rich collateral potential residing in the arterial arcades.[2] Finally, the survival of partial thickness of the intestinal wall and the demarcation of the inner necrotic layers by an inflammatory zone—a common finding in intestinal infarction and, in my opinion, its diagnostic hallmark—are difficult to conceive without the assumption of at least some measure of arterial inflow.

Total or near-total cessation of blood flow may occur with occlusions that involve a very large proportion of the total vascular bed (Fig. 15). However, in such cases, which are observed only rarely, infarction will be preponderantly anemic. Yet even here small amounts of arterial blood may trickle slowly and focally into the infarct territory by the route of the delicate adipose-tissue arteries described previously. It follows that anemic infarction will be essentially transmural. Conversely, transmural infarction need not be anemic. The reasons are inherent in the preceding discourse and are related to such factors as duration, extent of occlusion, and involvement of vasa recta.[15]

In several cases we have noted gas bubbles in the wall of the infarcted intestine. This probably resulted from the invasion of gas-forming bacteria into the devitalized tissue. It was not a postmortem phenomenon, since it had already been observed during surgery and in antemortem roentgenographic films of the abdomen.

In the usual case of hemorrhagic infarction, intestinal necrosis will be transmural only segmentally (mainly in the central portions of the infarcted segment)

---

* The alternate or complementary possibilities that the effects upon the target tissues caused by thrombotic and especially by thromboembolic occlusions are reinforced by vasculospastic phenomena and aided by smooth muscle spasm of the target intestine itself (followed by muscular atony of vessels and intestine) do not alter the validity of the tenets here expressed.

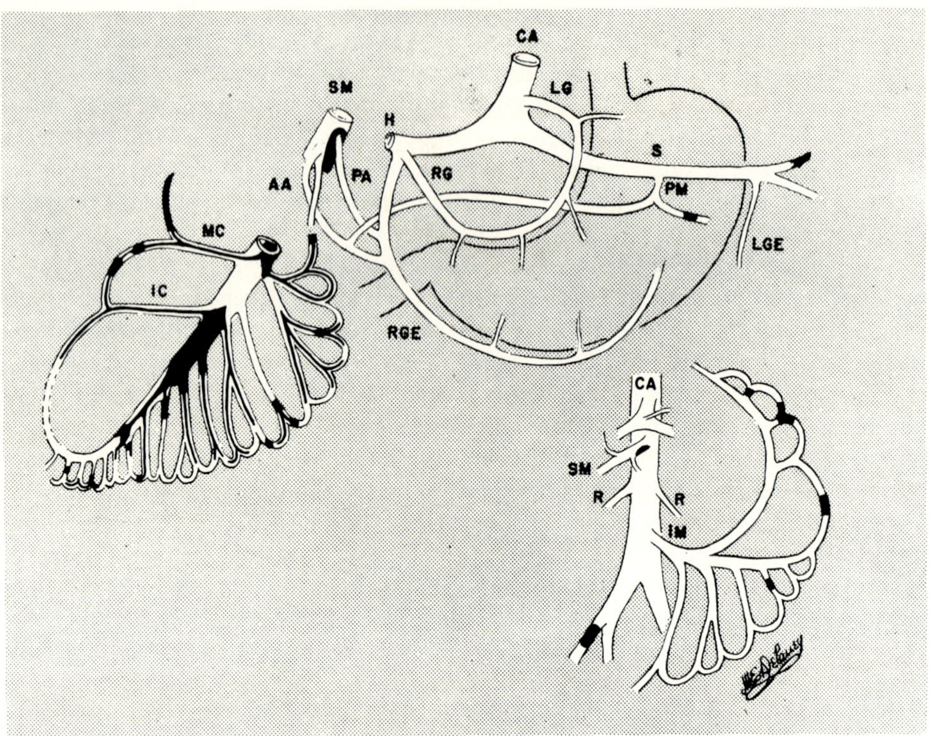

Fig. 15. Mesenteric arteriogram showing widespread thromboembolic occlusions of the three constituent arborizations and including the marginal (Drummond's) arcade of the inferior mesenteric artery. There were also occlusions of the vasa recta in the superior mesenteric arborization (not shown). The small and proximal large intestine showed transmural infarction, much of it anemic. In the descending colon infarction was patchy and confined to the antimesocolic circumference. AA, anterior pancreaticoduodenal arcade; CA, celiac artery; H, hepatic; IC, ileocolic; IM, inferior mesenteric; LG, left gastric; LGE, left gastroepiploic; MC, middle colic; PA, posterior pancreaticoduodenal arcade; PM, pancreatica magna; R, renal; RG, right gastric; RGE, right gastroepiploic; S, splenic; SM, superior mesenteric. (Case made available for study through the courtesy of Drs. J. C. Ehrlich and R. Platt.) (From Reiner et al. Gastroenterology, 39:747, 1960.)

and becomes more or less superficial as one approaches the viable intestine. In fact, the ischemic constellation may be of such low magnitude as to cause no more than diphtheritic or pseudomembranous inflammations (Fig. 16). Such anatomically superficial injuries of the mucosa are nonetheless serious, since they cause a loss of fluids and electrolytes as endangering as the more deeply extending forms of wall necrosis.

Since pseudomembranous and diphtheritic inflammations of the intestine are known to occur with a diversity of agents [16] other than mesenteric arterial occlusions (e.g., antibiotics, uremia, bacterial action, radiation), one may postulate that the particular agents operate via a common, i.e., nonspecific, final pathway. Such a common pathway, for example, might be provided by local impairment of circulatory competence due to organic or vasculospastic phenomena by involving the vascular arborization at any level from main stem to mucosal capillaries and back to the venous circulation. It may be provided by the intestinal flora acting on the mucosa in either a primary or a secondary capacity. Or, alternately,[14] the injured mucosa may become vulnerable to the action of intestinal digestive enzymes. At any rate, the phenomenon of identical lesions from dissimilar causes may be interpreted as the expression of a strictly limited reactivity to injury on the part of the tissues.

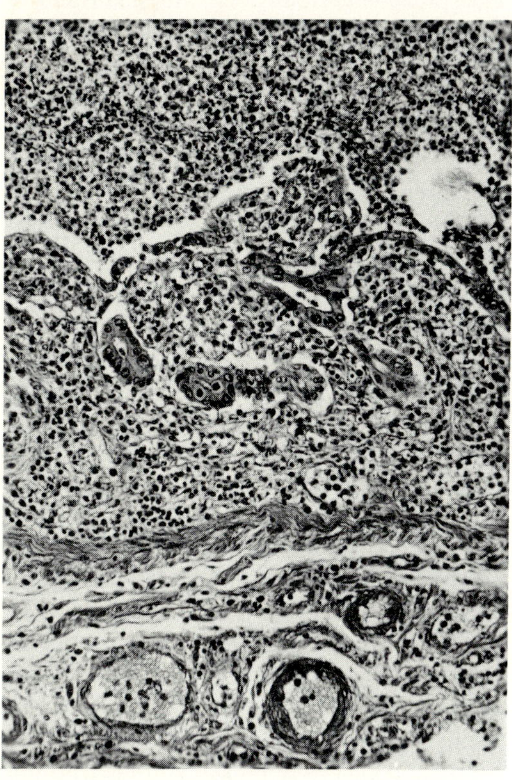

Fig. 16. Pseudomembranous inflammation of the ileum secondary to thromboembolic occlusion of the superior mesenteric main stem. The photograph represents not an isolated field but, together with diphtheritic phenomena,[16] the predominant gross and microscopic pathology.

Remote as they may seem to the subject under discussion, the foregoing considerations do serve as a convenient means to point out that the morphologic manifestations of ischemia in the target tissues overlap with inflammatory reactions initiated by other pathogenetic agencies. It follows that the ischemic etiology of a given intestinal lesion cannot be deduced with certainty from its histomorphology unless there is (arterial) infarction as currently understood, i.e., necrosis demarcated by a zone of inflammatory reaction. Even this statement may be questioned on the grounds that diphtheritic inflammation meets these criteria of infarction and yet may be due to causes other than ischemia. It is thus a truism to state that infarction refers not only to tissue phenomena but also to etiology.

In this connection, reference must be made to quite a number of papers which have appeared especially in the recent literature dealing with cases of intestinal "infarction" in which meticulous dissection (no postmortem injection) failed to disclose any significant disease in the mesenteric circulation. By and large, these patients were elderly subjects suffering from chronic heart disease, congestive heart failure, and other debilitating conditions. Various pathogenetic mechanisms have been proposed including intestinal capillary breakdown, immunologic processes, and vasculospastic phenomena.

In a pertinent series by Ming and Levitan [17] designated by the authors as "acute hemorrhagic necrosis of the gastrointestinal tract" emphasis was placed, first, on the widespread involvement in the small and large intestine. Unlike the classical intestinal infarct necrosis was segmental and thus did not conform to any vascular pattern. Second, the predominant confinement was to the mucosa; and third, there was constant involvement of the stomach. The last feature has special relevance to what has been said elsewhere with respect to infarction of the stomach.

In two important contributions, Corday et al.[18,19] have shown that the mesenteric circulation plays an important role, by means of marked vasoconstriction in the intestinal wall, in maintaining circulatory homeostasis of the body in states of reduced cardiac output, such as during congestive heart failure, after coronary arterial occlusion, and during acute hypotension. While this compensatory vasoconstriction allows for a shunting of blood to more vital tissues, enough blood may be diverted from the gastrointestinal tract to lead to ischemic manifestations especially of the mucosa. By topography, by metabolic requirements, and by its immediate proximity to the intestinal contents the mucosa is the most vulnerable of the gut's coats, as indicated above. This shunting phenomenon is, of course, analogous to the pathogenetic mechanism of acute tubular necrosis of the kidney or "lower nephron nephrosis."

Mesenteric Occlusions of Intermediate Type

The intermediate cases, as mentioned, exhibit functional and/or anatomic manifestations. Although qualitatively similar, they are quantitatively of a lesser degree than intestinal infarction. In other words, the intermediate type of mesenteric arterial disease bears a relation to intestinal infarction similar to that which exists between angina pectoris and coronary insufficiency on the one hand and myocardial infarction on the other. The relationship between vascular disease and its effects upon the target organs may be schematized as in Table 3.

Table 3. Spectrum of Mesenteric Arterial Occlusions

	MANIFESTATIONS	
Type of Case	Anatomic	Clinical
Intestinal Infarction	+	+
Intermediate		
A	+	+
B	+	+
C	0	+
Silent	0	0

FUNCTIONAL MANIFESTATIONS.   Abdominal pain of an intermittent and usually postprandial nature has long been accepted as the functional criterion and indeed the only manifestation of impaired efficiency in the mesenteric arterial circulation, as shown by some of the terminology applied: intermittent anemic dysperistalsis,[20] abdominal intermittent claudication,[21] chronic midgut ischemia,[22] intestinal angina,[23], visceral angina,[24] and, most commonly, abdominal angina. Some authors believe—and our retrospective perusal of the clinical records tends to be in accord —that incomplete, relative, or chronic arterial insufficiency may also give rise to other symptoms. They include changes in intestinal dynamics and bowel habits, malabsorption phenomena, transient ileus, and blood in the stools. These manifestations may occur either alone or in association with abdominal angina (for literature, see reference 7).

Our observations [7] and those of others [1,24] suggest that abdominal angina is usually associated with a characteristic vascular constellation. It comprises occlusion at the aortic ostia of two of the three main stem arteries, notably including the superior mesenteric artery. Though characteristic, the correlation is not obligatory, since a like vascular substrate may long remain silent (personal observations not included in the present series). Conversely, intermittent abdominal pain of otherwise unexplained etiology may be encountered in patients without the usual number or sites of ostial occlusions.[24] In one such case, postprandial abdominal pain mistakenly ascribed to a duodenal ulcer—not confirmed at autopsy—was associated with stenosing rather than occlusive disease at the aortic ostia of all three main stems. There were no symptoms of mesenteric arterial decompensation until intercurrent myocardial infarction led to a deterioration of the total cardiovascular status, including a sustained drop of blood pressure from hypertensive to normotensive levels. This sequence of events is in keeping with the concepts of Lapiccirella.[25] At no time was the pain excruciating or incapacitating.

This case illustrated, as did others *with* ostial occlusions, certain points: 1) the intensity of ischemic intestinal pain may vary from case to case, as indeed it may from episode to episode in the same patient; 2) the symptoms are prone to be misdiagnosed clinically and ascribed to peptic ulcer, pancreatic disease, and others; and 3) apart from the classical and fullblown case of abdominal angina with excruciating episodic, i.e., postprandial pain, fear of eating, and weight loss, there exist milder cases of ischemic abdominal pain that may neither request nor receive particular medical attention. Whether such milder forms deserve to be designated as abdominal angina or not will depend on one's viewpoint.

It is the writer's opinion that a disease entity is not determined by its severity or clinical purity but by the total complex of clinical and anatomic findings and their plausible correlation. When found in association with the characteristic vascular substrate of abdominal angina, episodic abdominal pain, even if not strictly postprandial and not excruciating, may reasonably be considered ischemic if other causes can be excluded. Such atypical pictures may perhaps be more credible if it can be accepted that, as in the case of angina pectoris, attacks of abdominal angina too may be mediated by neurogenic and emotional stresses rather than by mechanical (digestive) effort. This broadening of concept does complicate still further an already difficult problem of clinical diagnosis.

ANATOMIC MANIFESTATIONS. Anatomic lesions in the intermediate group of cases [8] manifest themselves as single or multiple ulcers of variable depth. In the large intestine they may resemble stercoraceous ulcers (Fig. 17). This is of interest,

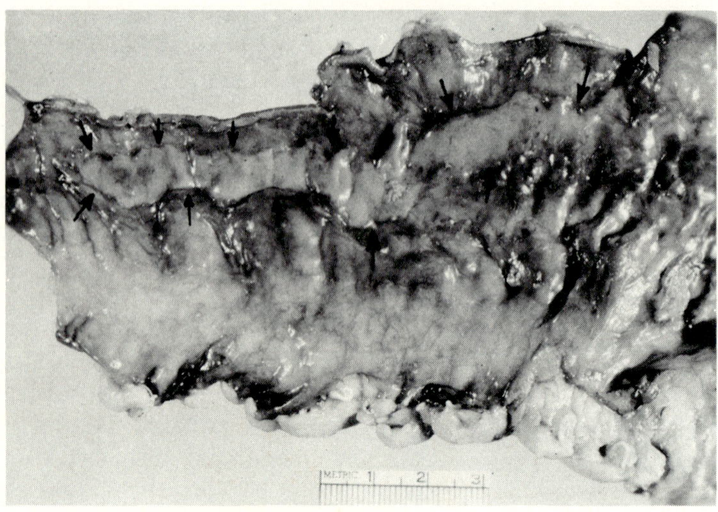

Fig. 17. Large slough ("stercoraceous" ulcer) on the antimesenteric circumference in the large intestine, ascribed to advanced stenosing and occlusive arteriosclerosis involving, among others, the colonic branches of the superior and inferior mesenteric arteries. The lesion was an active one and associated with localized serositis. Patient was admitted to the hospital for a myocardial infarct from which he died.

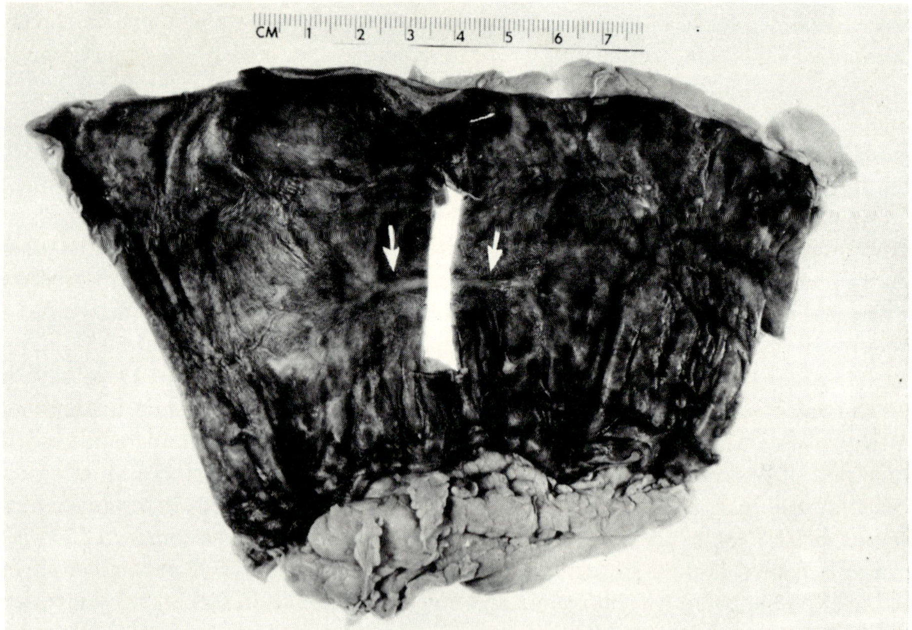

Fig. 18. A linear scar in the descending colon located about the antimesocolic circumference and associated with severely stenosing and occlusive arteriosclerosis of the branches of the inferior mesenteric artery including the marginal arcade of Drummond. The lesion is arranged in the long axis of the intestine and is thought to be the healed stage of a lesion such as illustrated in Figure 17.

since some authors [26] believe that all stercoraceous ulcers of the colon have an ischemic background with the inspissated feces acting in decubitus fashion as a subsidiary or precipitating cause. Fecal inspissation, one may argue with good reasons, is altogether the result rather than a cause of stercoraceous ulceration and is brought about by local dysperistalsis, increased water absorption or both.

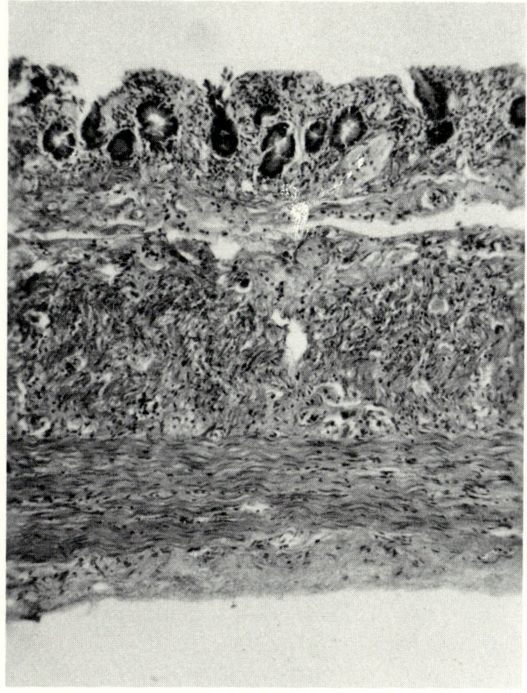

Fig. 19. Mucosal atrophy and loss of villi in the small intestine in a case of abdominal angina. There were also recurrent ulcers in both the small and large intestines.

Be that as it may, more severe ischemic lesions appear as necrotic sloughs and ulcers that involve the intestine in a segmental fashion. The necrosis is associated with a zonal and demarcating inflammatory reaction which, when deep, may be associated with active serositis. In principle, these colonic sloughs are intestinal infarcts. However, they are of limited dimensions (formes frustes) and are thus less prone to cause fetal losses of fluids and electrolytes. One such case was associated with repeated episodes of severe but painless melena. Lesions of this type may heal by scarring (Fig. 18). Here also belong cases of segmental infarction in the small intestine described in the literature [27,28] which upon healing cicatrize and thereby imitate segmental enteritis.

As to the vascular correlate, we have observed such ulcerative disease in the large intestine against the background of widespread stenosing and occlusive mesenteric arteriosclerosis but with the occlusions confined to colonic branches of the mesenteric circulation. In one case not included in the present series but briefly reported elsewhere [7] ulcerative disease involved both the large and small intestines. Again, the occlusions were in branch arteries but involved those of both the large and small intestine. There were additional occlusions at the aortic ostia of the superior and inferior main stems. In retrospect the patient displayed a characteristic case of abdominal angina. With intestinal ischemia for well over a year this patient also developed widespread atrophy in the small intestine characterized notably by loss of villi (Fig. 19). Although not searched for in this particular case, such villous atrophy may lead to a malabsorption syndrome, as mentioned earlier.

Epicrisis

A measured parallelism will have been recognized by the reader between the terms and concepts here expressed and those evolved and widely accepted in the field of ischemic heart disease. This applies particularly to the spectrum of clinical and anatomic manifestations and perhaps also to the somewhat unpredictable correlation between the anatomy of vascular disease and its effects upon target tissues. Both these features are greatly influenced by the topical availability of a collateral circulation which in the case of the mesenteric circulation is innate but which in the coronary circulation is usually acquired through local or systemic disease.

Allowing for some degree of variability within each group as well as for overlap between the groups, the preferential vascular substrate of intestinal infarction is fresh and usually embolic occlusion of the main stem of the superior mesenteric artery at some distance from the aortic ostium, with varying involvement of the branches of the same and neighboring arborizations. A good topographic correlation exists between site of occlusion and length and identity of intestine infarcted. The more proximal the occlusion the more of the intestine will be involved. Consequently, occlusions at or proximal to the origin of the middle colic artery will involve most of the small intestine as well as the ascending and proximal half of the transverse colon.

Relative mesenteric arterial insufficiency other than abdominal angina is usually associated with multiple branch occlusions on an arteriosclerotic basis, notably in relation to the colon. They are associated with anatomic injury of segmental distribution. Abdominal angina, by contrast, has its usual correlate in main stem occlusions located at the aortic ostia and involving two of the three constituent arborizations. They have either an embolic or, more frequently, an arteriosclerotic basis. The principal difference between the topography of occlusion in abdominal angina and the majority of intestinal infarcts lends support to our experience that abdominal angina has no outstanding propensity to terminate in infarction.

Cases to the contrary reported in the literature are difficult to evaluate on account of generally inadequate anatomic descriptions. Nonetheless, one may anticipate this sequence of progressive vascular decompensation as well as other less catastrophic events: 1) if additional occlusions or stenoses develop affecting critical pathways of the collateral circulation, or 2) if there is a deterioration of the total cardiovascular status as from congestive heart failure, myocardial infarction, or shock states without any new changes in the mesenteric arterial tree. This is different from cases in which the anginal syndrome actually represents the prodrome of intestinal infarction that develops on the basis of slowly evolving *thrombosis* of the midsuperior mesenteric artery, as contrasted to the more usual sudden blockage by thromboembolism.

References

1. Morris, G.C., and DeBakey, M.E. Abdominal angina: Diagnosis and surgical treatment. J.A.M.A., 176:89, 1961.
2. Reiner, L., Rodriguez, F.L., Platt, R., and Schlesinger, M.J. Injection studies on the mesenteric arterial circulation. I. Technique and observations on collaterals. Surgery, 45:820, 1959.
3. Schlesinger, M.J. New radiopaque mass for vascular injection. Lab. Invest., 6:1, 1957.
4. Lockhart-Mummery, H.E. The colon. *In* Textbook of British Surgery, Souttar, Sir Henry, ed. London, Wm. Heinemann Medical Books, Ltd., 1956, Vol. 1, p. 449.
5. Egeblad, K. Occlusion of mesenteric vessels. Ugeskr. Laeg., 123:1589, 1961.
6. Reiner, L., Jimenez, F.A., and Rodriguez, F.L. Atherosclerosis in the mesenteric circulation. Observations and correlations with aortic and coronary atherosclerosis. Amer. Heart J., 66:200, 1963.
7. ——— Mesenteric arterial insufficiency and abdominal angina. Arch. Intern. Med., 114:765, 1964.
8. ——— Rodriguez, F.L., Jimenez, F.A., and Platt, R. Injection studies on mesenteric arterial circulation. III. Occlusions without intestinal infarction. Arch. Path., 73:461, 1962.
9. Cokkinis, A.J. Mesenteric Vascular Occlusion. New York, William Wood & Company, 1926.
10. Cohen, E.B. Infarction of the stomach. Report of three cases of total gastric infarction and one case of partial infarction. Amer. J. Med., 11:645, 1951.
11. Dassel, P.M. Roentgen demonstration of gangrene of the stomach and intestine. A late finding in infarction of the gastrointestinal tract. Amer. J. Roentgen., 91:819, 1964.
12. Klickstein, G.D., and Reiner, L. Diarrhea, shock and paralytic ileus, Clinicopathologic Conference. New York J. Med., 61:3478, 1961.
13. Greenberg, A.D., and Morgan, H.R. Cortisone and infection. New York J. Med., 61:455, 1961.
14. Khanna, S.D. An experimental study of mesenteric occlusion. J. Path. Bact., 77:575, 1959.
15. Reiner, L., Platt, R., Rodriguez, F.L., and Jimenez, F.A. Injection studies on the mesenteric arterial circulation. II. Intestinal infarction. Gastroenterology, 39:747, 1960.
16. ——— Schlesinger, M.J., and Miller, G.M. Pseudomembranous colitis following aureomycin and chloramphenicol. Arch. Path., 54:39, 1952.
17. Ming, S.C., and Levitan, R. Acute hemorrhagic necrosis of the gastrointestinal tract. New Eng. J. Med., 263:59, 1960.
18. Corday, E., and Williams, J.H. Effect of shock and of vasopressor drugs on the regional circulation of the brain, heart, kidney and liver. Amer. J. Med., 29:228, 1960.
19. Corday, E., Irving, D.W., Gold, H., Bernstein, H., and Skelton, R.B.T. Mesenteric vascular insufficiency. Intestinal ischemia induced by remote circulatory disturbances. Amer. J. Med., 33:365, 1962.
20. Schnitzler, J. Zur Symptomatologie des Darmarterienverschlusses. Wien. Klin. Wschr, 51:505, 568, 1901.
21. Seymour, W.B., and Liebow, A.A. "Abdominal intermittent claudication" and narrowing of the celiac and mesenteric arteries. Ann. Intern. Med., 10:1033, 1937.
22. Mavor, G.E., and Michie, W. Chronic midgut ischemia. Brit. Med. J., 2:534, 1958.
23. Mikkelsen, W.P., and Berne, C.J. Intestinal angina. Surg. Clin. N. Amer., 42:1321, 1962.

24. Fry, W.J., and Kraft, R.O. Visceral angina. Surg., Gynec. Obstet., 117:417, 1963.
25. Lapiccirella, V., and Weber, G. La claudicaziona mesenterica sindrome di alarme della malattia coronarica. Arch. De Vecchi Anat. Pat., 19:112, 1953.
26. Siegmund, H. Einfache Entzündungen des Darmrohres, *In* Handbuch der speziellen pathologischen Anatomie und Histologie, Henke, F., and Lubarsch, O., eds. Springer Verlag, 1920, Vol. 4, part 3, p. 304.
27. Wolf, B.S., and Marshak, R.H. Segmental infarction of the small bowel. Radiology, 66:701, 1956.
28. Hawkins, C. F. Jejunal stenosis following mesenteric-artery occlusion. Lancet, 2:121 1957.

THE INTENSIVE CARE UNIT
AND THE PATHOLOGY OF PROGRESS *

G. A. FATTAL
JOHN P. WYATT

The time has been, that when the brains were out, the man would die, and there an end. But now they rise again. . . .

MacBeth, Act III, Scene IV, line 68.

Pathology and Intensive Care

One contemporary viewpoint expressed about pathology as a discipline in the investigation of disease has been that it is bankrupt; it can offer nothing further through the autopsy room. Such a viewpoint, nihilistic at its worst and erosive at its best, clearly neglects the knowledge that the evolution of disease processes is constantly being altered by developments in medical care. It is our viewpoint that the Theatre for Information in analyzing the changing faces and masks of disease is the pathologist's atelier. This is particularly so in the consideration of the functions of a modern intensive care unit. This unit is a new center of hospital activity in which an investigative autopsy can play a most important role in the recognition, analysis, and communication of changing trends in our medical care environment.

What is an intensive care unit? It has been said that one should not speak of a ward as being allocated to intensive care unless there is continuing mortality of at least 25 percent. This trenchant comment reflects the desperate nature of the condition of the patients admitted, and, like Polyphemus, the unit exacts a daily toll. Historically, the intensive care units have developed from the head injury wards of the

* This contribution would not have been possible without the cooperation and interest of Dr. Brian Kirk, Physician-in-Charge, Intensive Care Unit (I.C.U.), Winnipeg General Hospital.

late 1930's. The significant reduction in the tragic complications of decerebrate rigidity and "lame brains"[1, 2, 3] has been a major impetus in extending the use of these specialized facilities to other conditions associated with a high incidence of grave complications.

The intensive care unit (I.C.U.) is the resuscitative care area in a hospital in which there is the maximum concentration of the most sophisticated therapeutic procedures and the minimum time for the evaluation of their effect. This unit is constantly concerned with decisions involving Homeric salvation procedures and the meticulous supervision of bioelectronic channels monitoring the critically ill. But it is not our intention to leave the impression that intensive care is a recent development. Toulouse-Lautrec has depicted a common emergency procedure of the late nineteenth century in his painting *The Tracheotomy* (Fig. 1).[4] (Unfortunately, either the title is incorrect or the physician is committing an error in anatomical judgement!)

The careful clinical study during life of deranged organs requires a matched

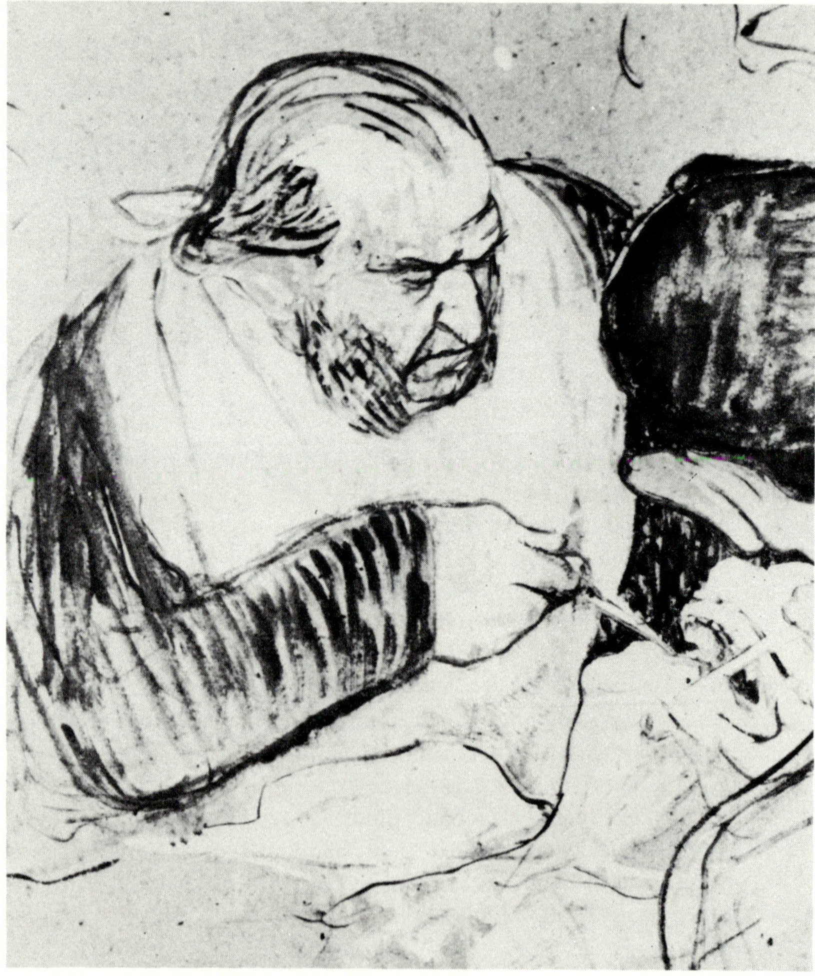

Fig. 1.   Toulouse-Lautrec: *The Tracheotomy*. (Courtesy of Sterling and Francine Clark. Institute of Art, Williamstown, Mass.)

performance from the autopsy teaching unit. The clinicians expect a comparable and ongoing analysis from the investigative autopsy unit to complement the precise physiologic studies of cardiorespiratory function, cerebral state, and hepatic and renal behavior measured during the life of the critically ill patient. Coupled with artificially supported respiration, precise electrolyte balance, and instant monitoring of vital organ systems, the rewards of the I.C.U. are now more readily perceived clinically.[5] To validate these clinical impressions, it is imperative that an investigative aura dominate the autopsy performance. To do this, a distinction should be made between the investigative autopsy and the "routine" autopsy, which contributes solely to hospital statistics.

The orientation of intensive care units varies. Where cardiologists dominate, the emphasis is on the cardiac pump; if the unit leadership is from the respiratory division, the diffusion of gases into the tissues is of paramount concern. One contribution that the pathologist can make is the prevention of polarization of therapeutic efforts into a single avenue of endeavor; he is the ballast against subdiscipline bias.

Although this essay is primarily concerned with a delineation of patterns of pathology that are characteristically related to intensive care areas, the emotional charge of therapeutic "pyrrhic victories" is not being levelled.[6] Some of the patterns of pathology are often unavoidable complications which follow Aesculapian inter-

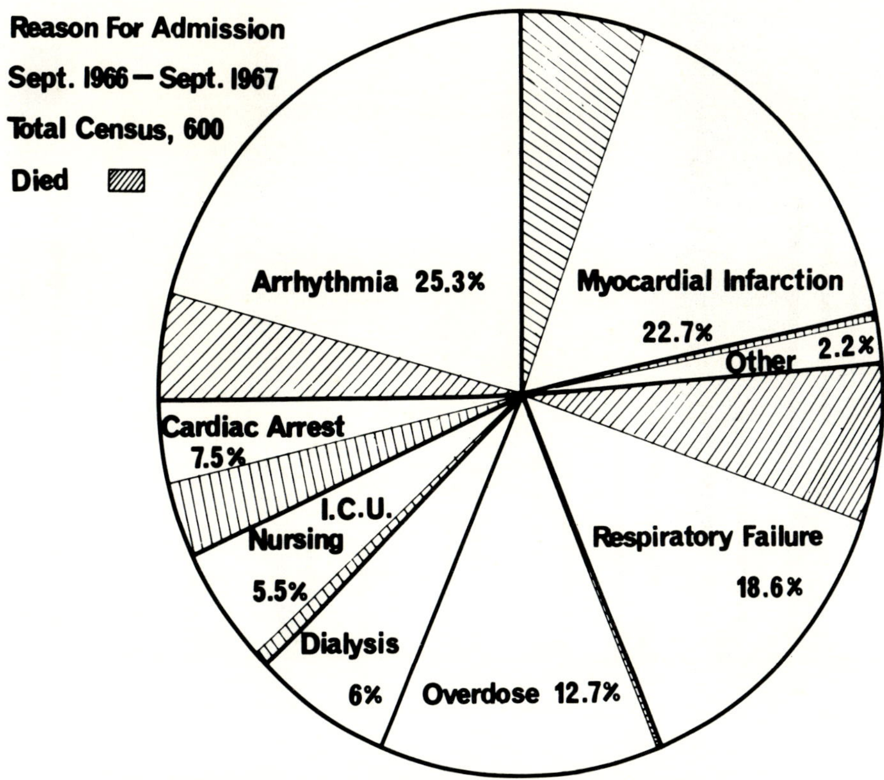

Fig. 2.   Case Distribution in the I.C.U.

ventions, obligatory in any operation concerned with intensive care. The physician may walk the I.C.U. with the "two-edged sword—Iatrogenesis" in his hand,[7] but all its ills are not necessarily of his making.

Case Distribution and a Prototype

The nature of the cases admitted to our unit reflected a broad variety of primary pathologic disorders (Fig. 2), but the admission diagnosis was of necessity a physiologic one. As a practical point, for example, preliminary information from earlier biopsy studies may restrain expensive therapeutic undertakings. One of our cases, showing diffuse radiographic infiltration of the lung fields, was unsuccessfully but intensively treated for acute respiratory failure. If the pathologic diagnosis of disseminated malignant reticulosis based on the lung biopsy performed a few days before final admission had been forwarded earlier, three days of intensive care might have been avoided.

In the two years of the I.C.U. operation (1966-1968), approximately 1,200 cases of critically ill patients have been admitted. Of these, 200 were directly from casualty. Sixty were transferred from hospital wards in their first 24 hours. An equal number were transferred from the general hospital beds as long as two weeks after their initial entry into hospital. Eight percent of the total number of patients were

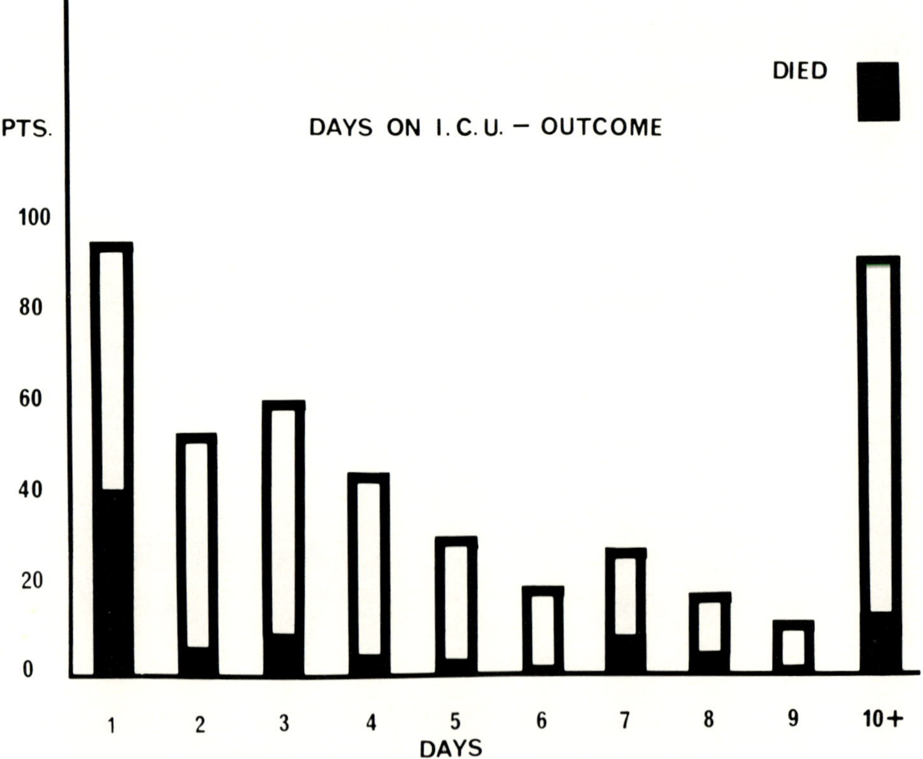

Fig. 3.   Length of stay and mortality distribution of patients in the I.C.U.

from the recovery room. The majority of patients were males, except for the third and fourth decade, where the male:female ratio was approximately one (Fig. 3).

In the year 1967, for example, 134 patients with respiratory failure were admitted; 70 percent of these were diagnosed as having acute pulmonary insufficiency uncomplicated by a previous lung disorder. In the same interval, 80 patients with myocardial infarction were seen; the three commonest physiopathologic diagnoses applied to their mode of death were shock, cardiac arrhythmia, and severe cardiac failure. One-half of the deaths in these coronary catastrophes were due to a refractory rhythm disturbance. Of the patients with myocardial infarction coming to the intensive care area, a large proportion died in the first 24 hours from irreversible cardiogenic shock (Fig. 2).

The following case represents a prototype of the patients admitted to the I.C.U. and illustrates the interwoven complexities of disease processes and therapy. The unravelling of the multiple factors involved in these case makes the unitary concept of understanding the physiopathologic derangements often difficult, always frustrating, and certainly subject to challenge.

CASE 1. This 20-year-old, white female, a known diabetic who had been on 60 U of NPH Insulin daily, was brought to the casualty ward cyanosed and in a comatose state. A blood glucose determination of 50 mg/100 ml led to the admitting diagnosis of hypoglycemic shock. A spinal tap was done on admission without any significant findings being noted in the fluid. Support of the circulation, administration of antibiotics, correction of metabolic state, hypothermia, tracheostomy, curare relaxation, and mechanical ventilation were instituted. X-ray film of the chest showed diffuse bilateral pulmonary infiltration. Acidosis persisted and signs of renal failure were noted. From the third day on, 100 percent oxygen was used continuously. The patient was never hypercarbic. Marked bronchial breathing was heard over both lungs. The patient remained comatose and died on the fourth day. Three consecutive EEGs showed diffuse slow activity of very low amplitude. The postmortem showed multiple organ involvement, particularly cerebral, respiratory, cardiovascular, and renal.

These pathologic alterations have been seen separately or combined in many of our I.C.U. patients. This essay deals, at some length, with three of the structural changes as delineated in Case 1. They are dealt with under the following headings: respiratory, cardiovascular, and central nervous system derangements.

Respiratory Derangements

Ventilator Cuff Necrosis

The endotracheal passage of any artificial ventilatory tube almost invariably creates some degree of tracheitis,[8] with loss of epithelium and progressive degrees of metaplasia probably related to the length of time the tube is retained.[9]

The use of endotracheal intubation, particularly with cuffed tubes, has aroused clinical discussion because of its frequent association with a circumscribed, indolent form of erosion ulcer. At the level of the cuff, probably due to continuous or intermittent pressure (Figs. 4 A, B) there is an ischemic loss of mucous membrane. The cuff or the end of the plastic tracheotomy tube excoriates the trachea and produces

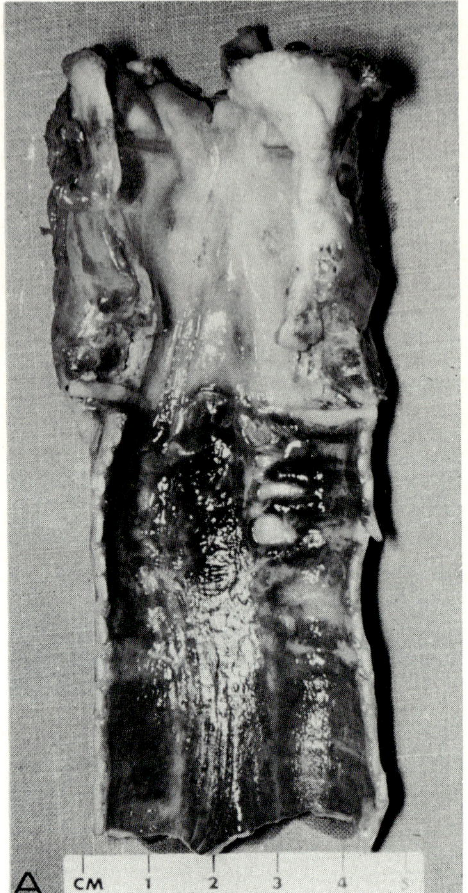
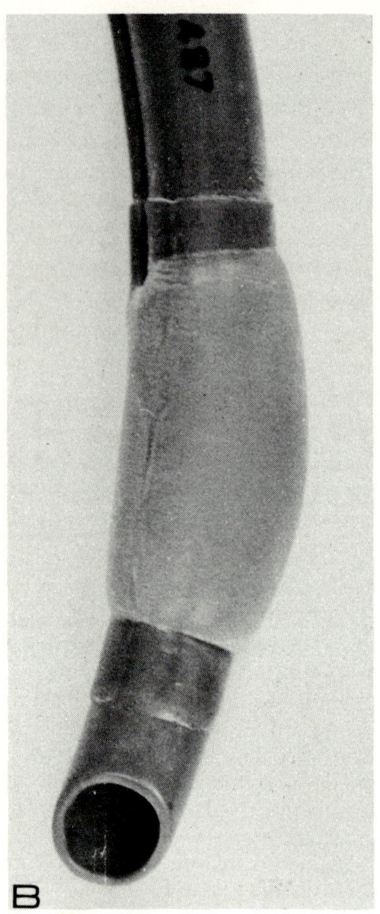

Fig. 4.   A. Trachea showing circumscribed ulceration, ecchymoses, and edema. B. Ventilator tube with pressure cuff.

a large, deep ulcer. This circumscribed lesion is often on the anterolateral surface of the trachea. The piston-like motion of the tracheotomy tube induced by IPP respirators may be an additive factor, producing shearing forces between the inflated cuff and the partially fixed trachea. The semirigidity of the tracheal cartilaginous plate obviously offers a resistance to the inflated pressure cuff. This lesion is much more frequently observed in elderly patients with circulatory difficulties. In some ways, this tracheal erosion is a symbol of unrelieved tissue compression, like buttock bed sores were for so many years.

Serious and chronic complications, such as tracheoeosophageal strictures, arising from the plastic tube have been documented in the literature.[10]

The "Respirator Lung"

Prior to a more specific discussion of the "respirator lung," comments on the deranged physiopathology and the multiple influences which can operate within a single pair of lungs are essential. Virtually 20 percent (Fig. 2) of the admission problems in the resuscitative area are of a respiratory nature. Therefore, the analysis of these lung disturbances will remain a continuing and preceptive task.

The lung, owing to its simple air-blood membrane and the relative ease of cell migration into air spaces, most effectively reflects the influence of therapeutic agents. The suppressive action of antibiotics, protracted perfusion through maintenance of cardiac action, and the countervailing effect of assisted respiration facilitating gas diffusion are influences long maintained by intensive care measures. The lung is, therefore, an excellent field to study the impress of prolonged care upon reparative responses to injury and the natural history of respiratory diseases.

The variety of pathologic problems, both of pulmonic and extrapulmonic nature, which present themselves to the unit are often well advanced down a final common pathway. The term "respiratory insufficiency," used by the I.C.U., may actually have a morphologic reflection. The concept is gaining credence that a common lung reaction may be observed in autopsy material, and yet the causative factors are widely divergent. In patients who have suffered from shock, severe trauma, sepsis, extensive burns, and prolonged extracorporeal circulation, or who have absorbed large amounts of degenerating tissue products, the lung often showed the common pathologic picture of "congestive atelectasis," capillaries packed with erythrocytes, and a heavy mononuclear and histiocytic infiltrate.

A second montage of linked factors within the lung are the often neglected physiologic considerations which are operative in the critically ill. Chronic airway obstruction, for example, is a common clinical entrance diagnosis, but its pathologic causative mechanisms may be many. A most important factor in airway obstruction is the underlying physiologic change. From the rare tracheal stricture[10] to the common bronchitis-emphysema complex, it is the "physiologic" derangements which are of importance to the gravely ill. Patients with peritonitis or upper abdominal surgery develop diaphragmatic or thoracic limitations of motion impeding ventilation. Small dosages of narcotics, curare (frequently used in the I.C.U.), and barbiturates, as well as cerebral infarction, will precipitate respiratory center depression, particularly in the patient with antecedent chronic airway obstruction. Equally profound ventilatory/perfusion ($\dot{V}/\dot{Q}$) inequalities (Fig. 5 B) may follow lung collapse or induced hyperventilation, due to the adaptive physiologic shunting which ensues. These physiopathologic deviations may gravely alter the normal cascade relationships that exist from the apex to the base of the lung.[11] Pathologists should be concerned with these $\dot{V}/\dot{Q}$ derangements rather than the putative I.Q. value of static morphology.

Disturbances in cardiac force and rhythm will seriously compromise the pulmonary circulation and produce physiologic diversions of blood and dramatic changes in the ventilation:perfusion ratio. Such physiologic alterations may precipitate hypoxia and acidosis and thus induce further compromise of the vascular bed. Significant changes in the rheologic behavior of the blood follow and lead to an abrupt increase in the blood viscosity and erythrocyte packing in the pulmonary capillaries. The "congestive atelectasis" seen at the autopsy table may be an expression of altered blood viscosity as well as cardiac perfusion.

These background comments lead us now to consider a contemporary lung derangement that plagues all intensive care units. In the last 18 months we have observed 14 patients who were treated in the I.C.U. for severe respiratory difficulties and at autopsy had distinctive, noncompliant, heavy, indigo-blue lungs. We have labelled these "respirator lungs"; the I.C.U. physicians favor the term "solid lung syndrome." The principal reason for our colloquial label was that, regardless of the

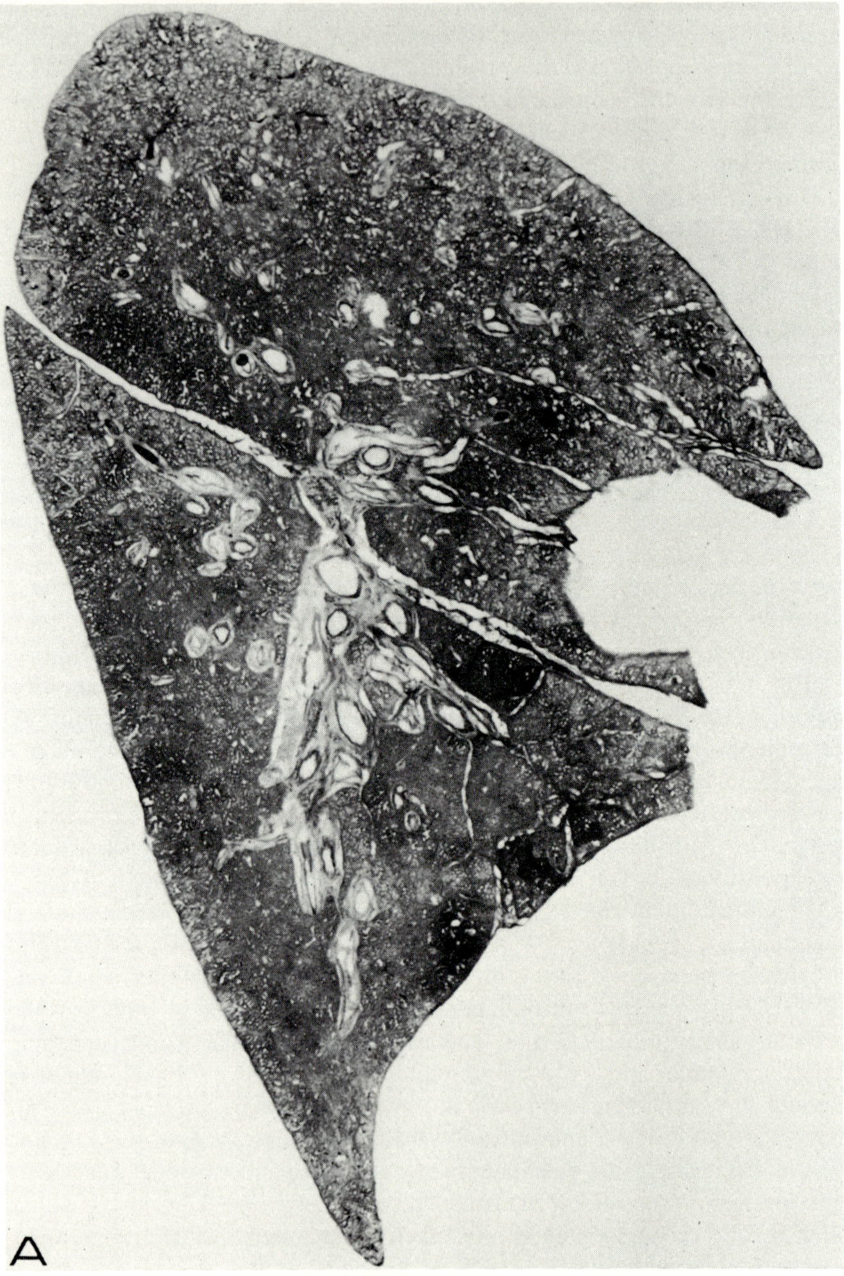

Fig. 5. A. Whole lung (left) paper section. Case 1 illustrates an example of "respirator lung." The changes are homogeneously distributed throughout the lung. One-fourth actual size.

nature of the disease leading to admission, its complications, or the therapy received during the intensive care period, all of these patients had assisted ventilation for varying periods of time.

The recognition of the "solid lung syndrome" has been equally distinctive for the I.C.U. physician. The progressive solidification of the lung was clinically recorded by the progressive development of diffuse bronchial breathing, matched by generalized "frothy" radiographs. Although most of these patients survived seven to ten days, they eventually succumbed to hypoxia but the pCO_2 was consistently normal. Except for the last 24 hours, the arterial oxygen saturation had been maintained close to 100 percent, but mounting increments in the inspired alveolar oxygen levels were required. To achieve this delivery of oxygen and to overcome the in-

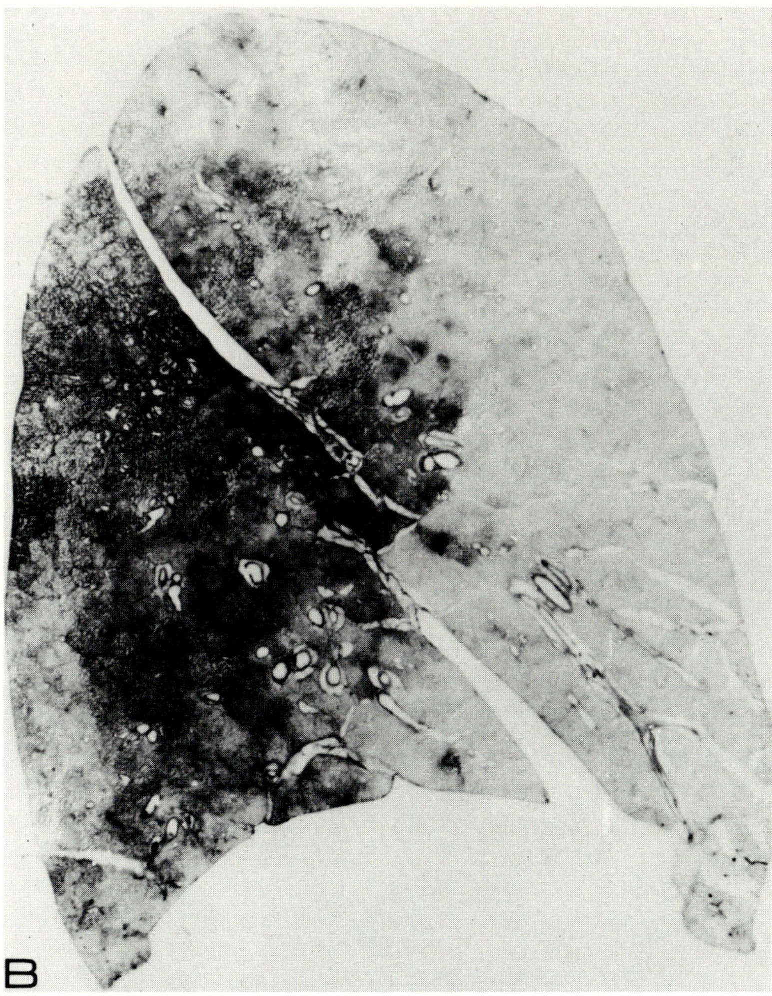

Fig. 5. (cont.)   B. Whole lung paper section of another "respirator lung" (left). Severe congestion and hemorrhage in posterolateral location suggest the likelihood of redistribution of pulmonary blood flow and hyperventilation in the upper and anterior parts of the lung. One-fourth actual size.

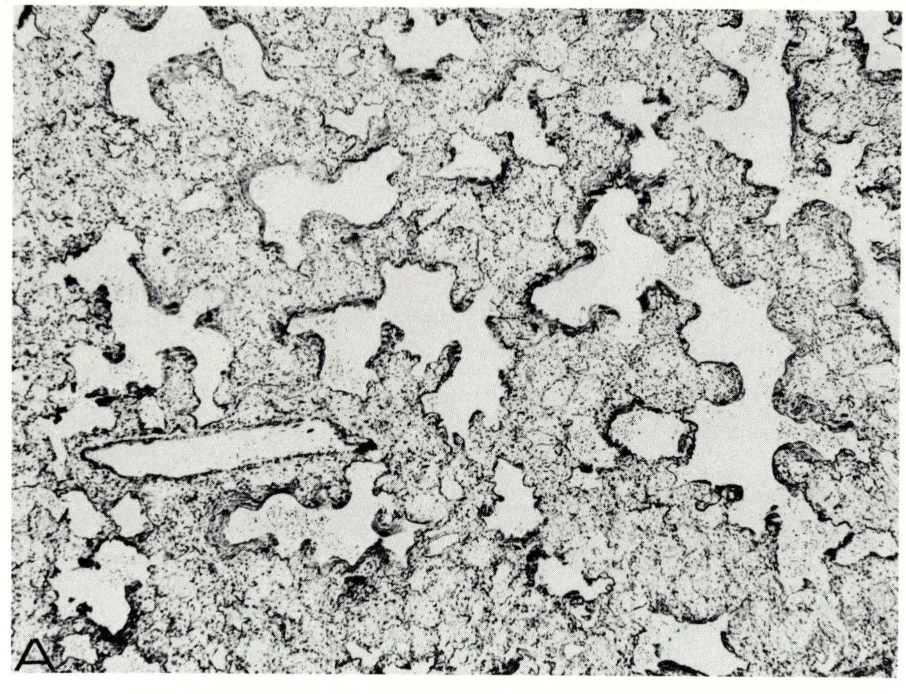

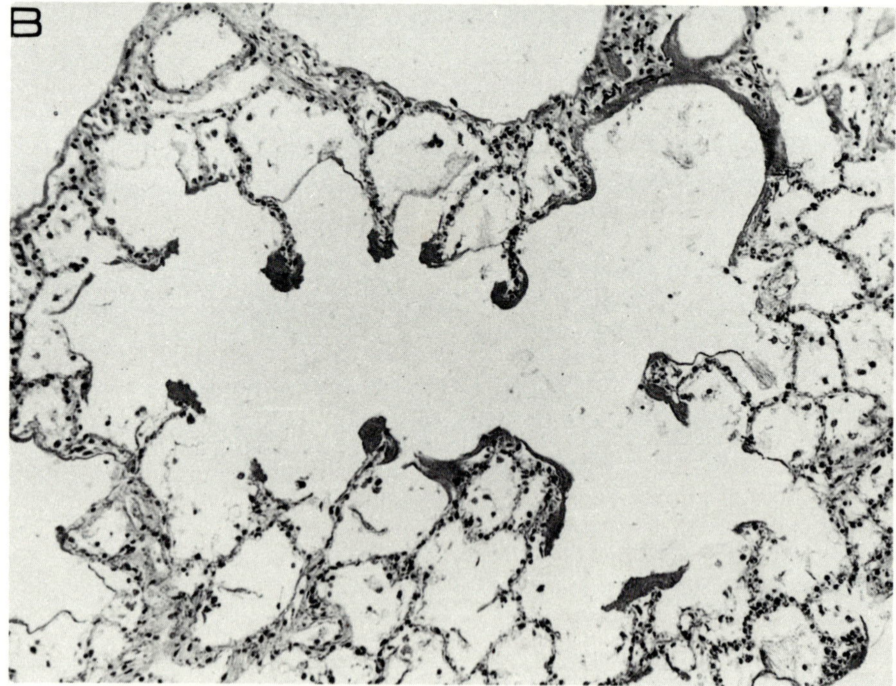

Fig. 6. Photomicrograph of "respirator lung" demonstrating the presence of hyaline membranes in terminal respiratory bronchioles. H & E. A, X25; B, X65.

creasing elasticity of the lung (noncompliance), continuing adjustments in the machine ventilatory force were needed.

Grossly, these lungs were bulky; their combined weight ranged from 1,600 to 2,200 g. The cut surfaces had a homogeneous solid appearance which was quite different from the gross impression in pneumonias and remarkably similar to the lung in hyaline membrane disease of infants (Figs. 5 A, B). Both intra-alveolar and interstitial edema was frequently observed. The most striking feature was the presence of hyaline membrane-like structures which lined the terminal respiratory bronchioles (Figs. 6 A, B), and in protracted cases there were the beginnings of organization and collagen deposition. The alveoli were, in general, fairly heavily sprinkled with macrophages (Fig. 7). Within the broadened alveolar septa, a similarly increased cell population was encountered with the occasional aggregate of polymorphonuclear leucocytes. These cells were not the major component of the infiltrate. Giemsa stains demonstrated clearly the heterogeneity of the migratory cell population (Fig. 8). The eosinophilic hyaline membrane was PAS-positive and sudanophilic. Barter, et al.[21] have emphasized the spatial relationships between these membranes and bundles of elastic fibers. Similar observations were made in our series (Fig. 6).

The location of the hyaline membranes characteristically on the elastic spurs of the air ducts infers a highly selective functional or biochemical derangement. In

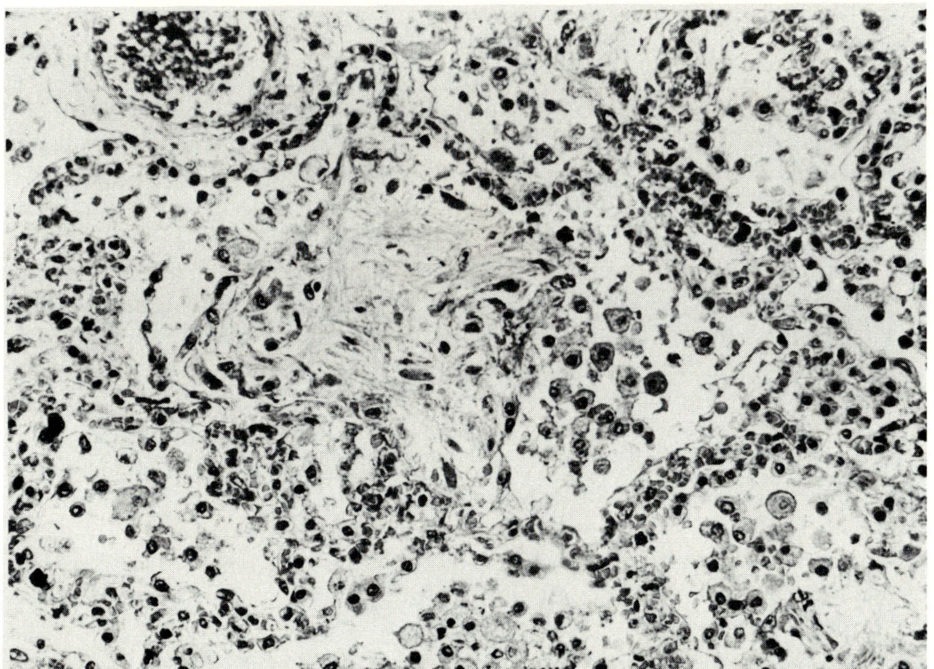

Fig. 7. Alveoli containing many histiocytes and early deposition of collagen, in the absence of significant acute inflammatory response. X160.

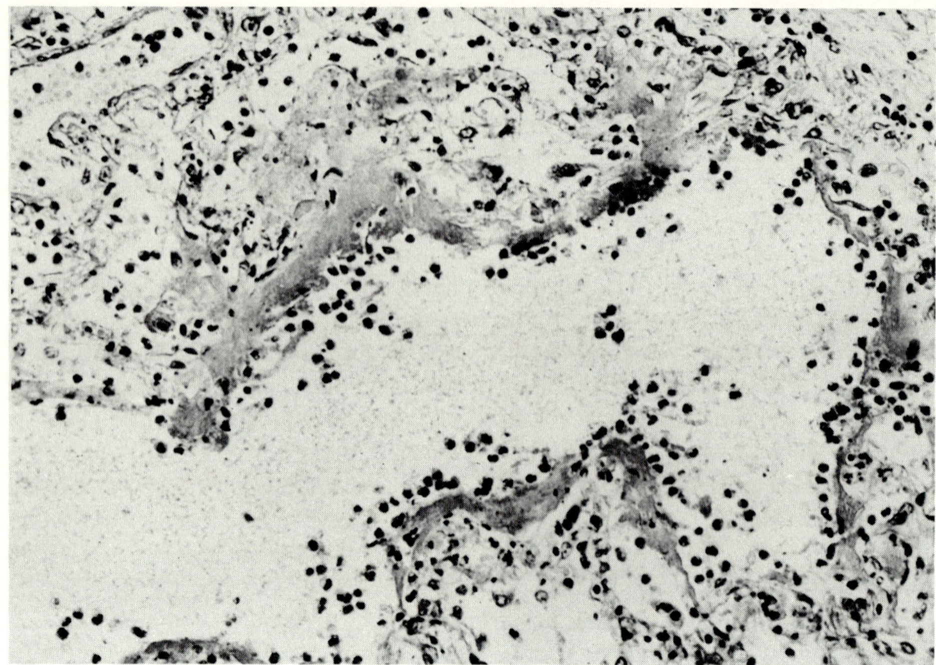

Fig. 8.   Air duct lined by hyaline membrane showing its relationship to a mixed migratory cell population. X160.

terms of clinicopathologic interpretation the concentration of the hyaline membranes at the respiratory bronchiole and air ducts probably interferes with lobular air flow. The respiratory bronchiole site and the close apposition to the lobular artery is a strategic physiologic control area, and, as in certain special pathologic conditions, derangements at this centrilobular level may influence perfusion.[19] The progressive thickening of the septa with fluid and cell infiltrates, as well as air sac filling, means impaired oxygen diffusion.

Case 1 in this essay is an example of the "respirator lung," but it also emphasizes the variety of factors (hypotension, shock, and other conditioning mechanisms) which complicate the understanding of the causation of this distinctive lung disorder.

One of the commonest therapeutic agents utilized in the intensive care ward is oxygen.[12] In 1899, Lorrain Smith[13] experimented with oxygen at several atmospheres of pressure, indicating that the lung may undergo an imperceptible transition from the physiologic to the pathologic, but this early warning was unheeded. Lung tissular effects have been searched for only since the recent therapeutic enthusiasm for hyperbaric oxygen and the appreciation of the vasospastic effects of oxygen on the developing retrolental tissues of the neonate. From the early report of capillary proliferation[14] to the more recent and widely bruited effects of oxygen upon the premature lung,[15, 16] investigative studies have now been redirected to the air-blood membranes of the adult lung and, more specifically, to the characteristic endothelial capillary damage.[17, 18, 19] Several groups of investigators[20, 21, 22] have clearly implicated high concentrations of oxygen as being the primary noxious agent producing distinctive morphologic alterations both in the newborn and the adult lung requiring oxygen assistance.

The use of oxygen, at present an irreplaceable therapeutic agent in the I.C.U., usually means that perfusional or ventilatory difficulties existed in the critically ill patient. It is our contention that to single out oxygen as the sole toxic agent responsible for new respiratory distress syndromes neglects the existence of pre-conditioning factors in the lung.

In the neonate requiring mechanically assisted ventilation, immaturity of the lung and altered vascular permeability are the two main abnormalities present which antedate the use of oxygen. Shanklin and Wolfson[15] refer to hemorrhage as being another manifestation of damaged vasculature in premature infants. The eclectic premise of Northway, et al.[16] is that the "respirator lung" in infants receiving oxygen therapy is a prolongation of the healing phase of hyaline membrane disease (respiratory distress syndrome: R.D.S.) combined with generalized oxygen toxicity.

In the adult, the conditioning factors existent in the lung before oxygen therapy are legion in number and polyvalent in character. The adult respiratory distress syndrome of Ashbaugh,[22] Barter's[21] adult cases of "oxygen poisoning" developing in the Bird respirator, and Nash's[20] large series of a similar pulmonary disability, emphasize the frequency, divergence, and overlapping nature of antecedent pathodynamic factors operating in I.C.U. patients. Direct chest trauma, hypotension, impaired cardiac function, multiple bone fractures with pulmonary fat embolism, metabolic and biochemical imbalance, uremia, hypoxia, and tracheobronchial infections are all conditioning factors[23] of major significance in the development of adult hyaline membrane disease.

The premature lung is vulnerable due to its tissue immaturity and ventilatory-perfusional difficulties induced by the pathologic alterations of R.D.S. prior to oxygen therapy. Similarly, disparate conditioning factors have an equally prominent preparative and synergistic role in the so-called "respirator lung" of the adult.

Cardiovascular Derangements

Vascular Manipulations

The introduction of various inert materials into vascular channels for a variety of diagnostic and therapeutic purposes is a well-established procedure.[24] This practice is particularly common in the intensive care unit. The desperate nature of the illness being treated usually means a large variety of intravascular manipulations.

In a large proportion of the patients, the central venous pressure (C.V.P.) is monitored through a catheter introduced into the superior vena cava usually via the basilic vein. Following catheter introduction, thrombosis in this vein is fairly common; however, extension of this thrombosing process into the great veins of the neck and superior vena cava is extremely rare. We have encountered three such cases. In all three, the catheters had been left in place for unusually long periods of time. One such example of massive intravascular thrombosis is illustrated in Figure 9.

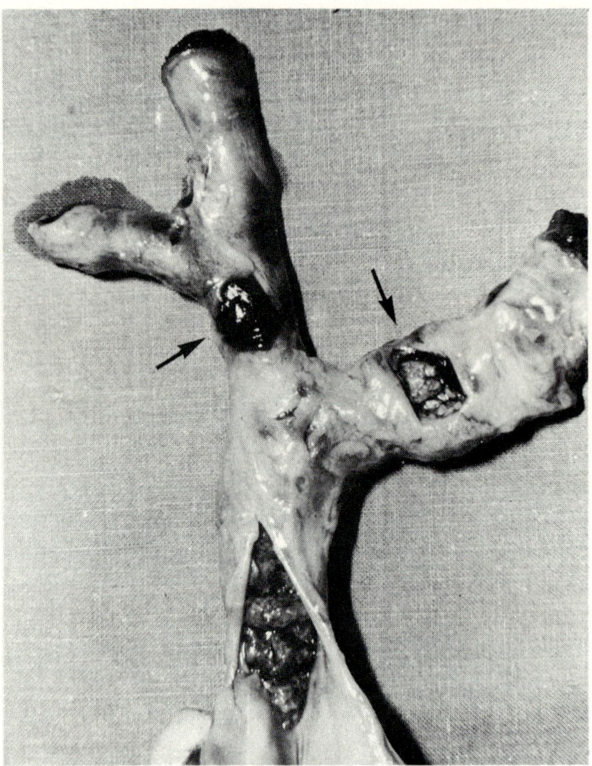

Fig. 9. Thrombosis of superior vena cava and tributaries (arrows point to windows made in right subclavian and innominate veins).

CASE 2. A 31-year-old woman was admitted to the hospital for multiple and severe injuries sustained in a car accident. The traumatic lesions were corrected surgically, but she remained seriously ill and was transferred to the I.C.U. because of cardio-respiratory complications. A C.V.P. catheter was inserted into the left basilic vein, and a thrombus developed. This catheter was removed and another one was introduced into the right basilic vein. A progressive and eventually massive edema appeared in the upper extremities, neck, and face. The prothrombin time was 16 sec (control 12 sec), and circulating macromolecular fibrinogen breakdown products were demonstrated.

Despite heparin and antibiotic therapy, she died 10 days after admission. At autopsy there was a massive thrombosis of the superior vena cava and its immediate tributaries (Fig. 9). Multiple small and peripheral pulmonary thromboemboli were also found, presumably a direct result of the thrombotic phenomenon described. The thrombi around the catheters were bland. No inflammatory reaction was found in the vein walls. There appeared to have been in this patient an increased propensity for intravascular clotting; the cause of this hypercoagulability is outside the scope of this essay.

Polyvinyl tubing is the material most commonly used in the manufacture of C.V.P. and intravenous infusional catheters. In severely ill patients who require frequent analyses of arterial blood or the direct monitoring of arterial blood pressure, a teflon tube is introduced into a medium-sized artery. Transvenous cardiac pacing electrodes are sheathed in silicon rubber tubing, which is alleged to be more inert than other synthetic materials used in medicine.

Teflon tubing was associated with arterial thrombosis in only one case. Nine patients with cardiac pacemakers came to autopsy; seven had permanent subcutaneous pacemakers, while in the other two the electrodes had been introduced for temporary pacing in severe acute myocardial infarction. In the seven, the pacemaker catheter was enveloped in a synovia-like sheath in the subcutaneous and deeper connective tissues of the body, and throughout its intravascular and intracardiac course it was invariably accompanied by some degree of thrombosis. The thrombotic material was the conventional layered red thrombus (Figs. 10 A, B). All seven cases of permanent pacemakers exhibited small "red sleeve thrombi" loosely investing the intracardiac portions of the catheters. The tips of four out of seven catheters were deeply embedded in the apical muscle of the right ventricle, passing obliquely through secondary trabeculae carnae and enclosed in an endothelial lined fibrous canal. The superior vena cava was extensively thrombosed and occluded in three patients with permanent pacemakers. Out of nine patients, three showed multiple small pulmonary thromboemboli. An example of massive intravascular thrombosis associated with a permanent pacemaker in a 70-year-old man with Stokes-Adams syndrome is illustrated in Figure 10A.

In spite of the possibility of triggering a thrombotic event, vascular manipulations unquestionably remain a mandatory component of the I.C.U. operation. Notwithstanding the development of more and more allegedly inert synthetic materials and the ultrarefinement of the intravascular techniques, thrombosis will remain an occasional annoyance to the I.C.U. physician.

There appears to be a great deal of individual variability in catheter-related thrombogenicity. I.C.U. physicians have noted many times that some patients develop venous thrombi almost immediately following the insertion of a polyvinyl C.V.P. catheter, while others tolerate this intravascular tubing for many days or weeks. The association of distal peripheral thrombi with intravascular catheters is common; the development of deep major vessel thromboses is uncommon. In the latter instance the centripetal spread of the thrombotic phenomenon does not appear to be directly related, either to phlebitis or embolism. This is borne out by the absence of thrombophlebitis in the juxtapositional deep veins and by freedom of the distal vein segments from propagated thrombus. This suggests that the thrombosing phenomenon is an in situ process throughout the intravenous or intracardiac course of the catheter. Further evidence for this postulate was the development of thrombi in two patients who had temporary pacing devices and were on anticoagulant therapy.

Our concern with iatrogenesis has been, up to this point, with catheter-related thromboses, but on rare occasions other vascular complications are encountered. Case 3 demonstrates a rare arterial catastrophe associated with angiography.

Case 3.   During a parade, a 43-year-old soldier suddenly experienced dizziness and blurring of vision. Twenty-four hours later his speech became slurred and he had a questionable right-sided hemiparesis. These symptoms persisted, and unequal pupils were noted. In an effort to localize the cerebral lesion, a carotid angiography was attempted, but some difficulty was encountered and repeat punctures proved necessary. The films eventually showed some filling of the cerebral arteries. The patient suddenly became comatose, and an emergency tracheostomy was performed. After transfer to the I.C.U. the following day, another angiography was attempted. This time good filling was obtained in the external carotid system but none in the internal carotid artery. The patient remained in a deep coma and succumbed 36 hours after the second angiography.

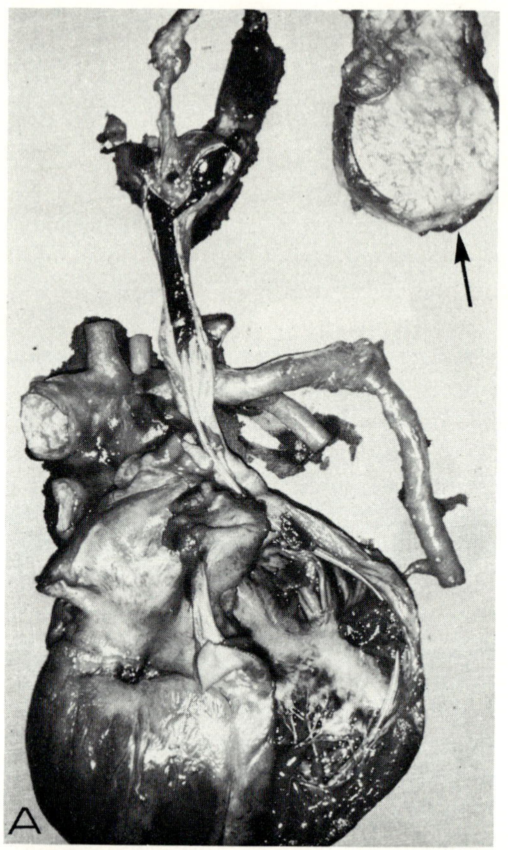

Fig. 10. A. Pacemaker (indicated by arrow) and catheter. The latter is encased in a thrombus within the superior vena cava. B. Same case. A view of the intracardiac portion of the catheter. Sleeve thrombi are clearly visible (arrow A). The tip of the catheter (arrow B) is embedded in the right ventricular myocardium and is surrounded by thin endothelialized fibrous sheath.

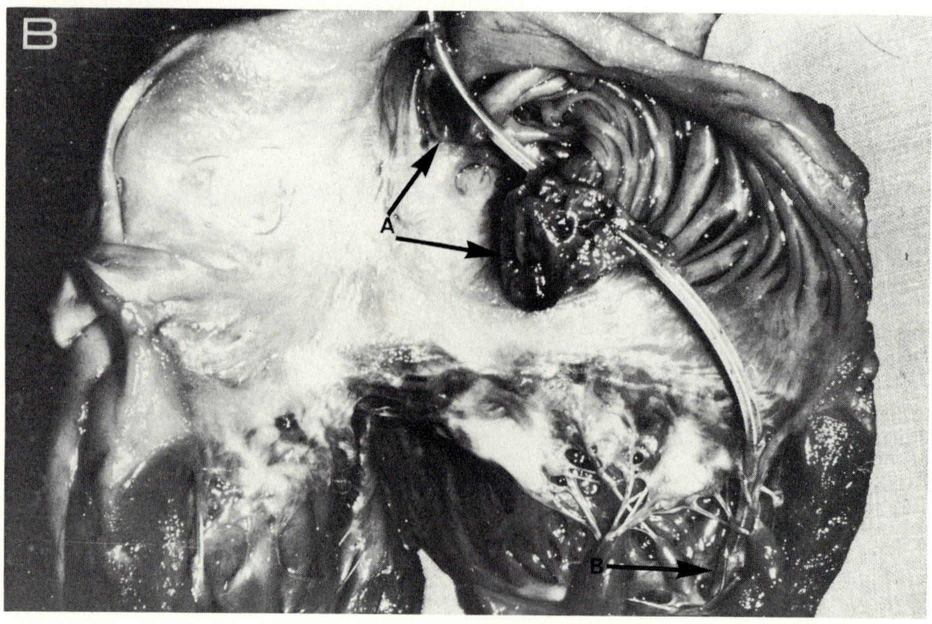

At autopsy several needle puncture marks were noted in the wall of the carotid artery at the point of bifurcation. Microscopic examination revealed an intimal tear which communicated with an intramural hematoma. The dissection of the media of the internal carotid artery had progressed upwards into the region of the carotid siphon, and the corresponding cerebral hemisphere had been recently infarcted. A postmortem radiograph of the excised arterial specimen revealed the presence of contrast medium within the intramural hematoma. The findings indicated that the initial angiographic attempt was responsible for the introduction of contrast medium in the wall of the vessel and its subsequent dissection.

Of much greater import than rare vascular catastrophies are the existence of intravascular thromboses associated with indwelling catheters, the influence of catheter materials on blood coagulability, and the clinical impact of these adventitious thrombi.

Cardiac Massage

The technique of external cardiac massage (E.C.M.) has been widely adopted as an emergency resuscitative measure. In the I.C.U. a significant proportion of cases with circulatory arrest received compressive cardiac stimulation. A smaller proportion (12 percent) received E.C.M. on the general hospital wards or the casualty department before admission to the I.C.U.

Our primary objective with those cases who had had cardiac massage was the morphologic reflections of this act as observed in tissues. The major complications (fractures of the ribs, marrow embolism, myocardial contusions, pneumothorax, pneumomediastinum, ruptures of the liver and diaphragm) are well known hazards.[25] In this essay we have confined our analysis to marrow and fat embolism.

In a retrospective review of patients who had received E.C.M., we reexamined the autopsy protocol and microscopic slides (Table 1). For contrast purposes, we

Table 1. Incidence of Marrow Emboli in "Routine" Autopsy

	Cases
E.C.M.	24
Rib fractures	12
Emboli	1

analyzed in greater detail a prospective study group of 12 cases. The technique was as follows: multiple histologic sections with appropriate fat stains from each lobe of the lung; radiography of the excised fourth, fifth, and sixth ribs; and thick histologic sections of the latter. All of these patients had been subjected to closed-chest massage by a physician (Table 2).

Table 2. Incidence of Marrow Emboli in a Prospective Study

	Cases
E.C.M.	12
Fracture or cartilage dislocation	3
Emboli	6

In the retrospective series of cases, a cursory examination of one histologic section from each lung, the incidence of marrow embolism was approximately 4 percent, even lower than the early survey of Baringer.[26] In the prospective group of 12 consecutive (E.C.M.) autopsies, six cases of marrow embolism were encountered, three without evidence of gross fracture. These findings are comparable to those of Yanoff.[27]

In analyzing the mechanism of closed-chest massage and the pathologic finding of pulmonary fat embolism, the fourth, fifth, and sixth grossly nonfractured ribs of each patient were examined in greater detail. Radiographic examination of the ribs was not helpful in the search for fractures in the diploe. Multiple sections of these ribs revealed trabecular fractures associated with intramedullary ecchymoses. Jagged irregular margins of these broken fragments and longitudinal splits of the trabeculae were found in situ in the areas of hemorrhage. Small fragments of recognizable bone marrow were found in blood vessels at the sites of the microtrabecular fractures. These changes were not present in a control group. Our observations suggest a cause-effect relationship between these microtrabecular fractures and pulmonary marrow and fat embolism.

The vigor of the external cardiac massage and the reestablishment of blood circulation probably are the two most important components of this "marrow pumping mechanism" (Fig. 11). Although it is apparent that a high proportion of patients undergoing closed-chest cardiac massage develop pulmonary fat and marrow embolism, the functional effects in surviving patients are difficult to appraise.

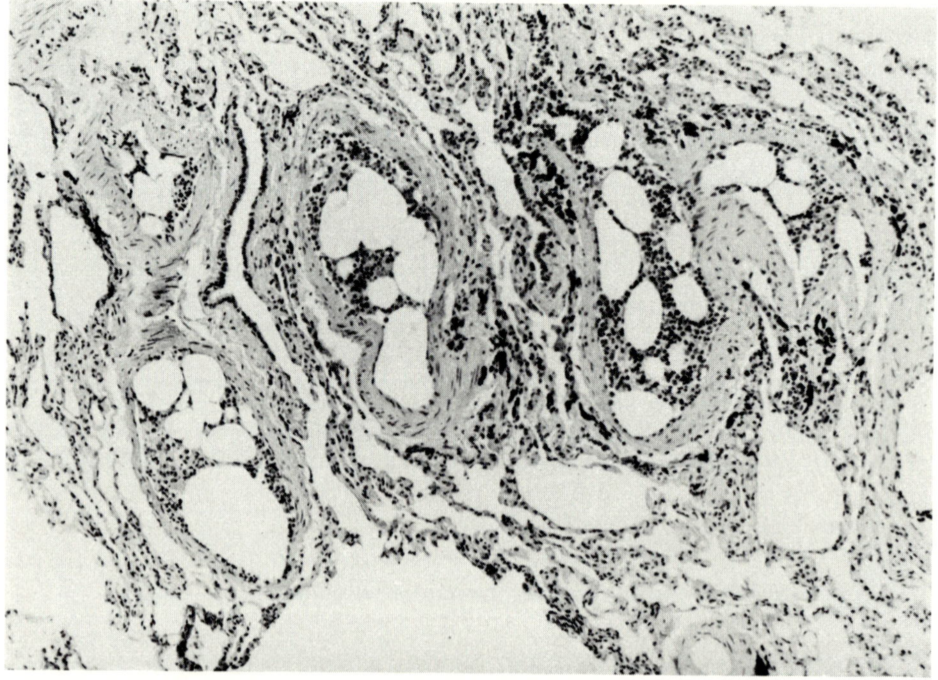

Fig. 11.   Multiple pulmonary blood vessels plugged with bone marrow emboli. X60.

Central Nervous System Derangements

One of the major system disturbances of cardinal concern to the I.C.U. physician is the functional assessment of the central nervous system in the comatose patient. Meaningful interpretations of electroencephalographic evidence of cortical function and the current inability to analyze deep ganglionic centers electronically have contributed to the physician's hesitancy in pronouncing somatic death. The final diagnosis—death—has thus become more difficult to establish, due largely to the new worship given to sophisticated instrumentation. The I.C.U. physician is still in as great a dilemma as was William Congreve, who in 1697 wrote, "Is he then dead? What dead at last, quite, quite forever dead."[28]

This fresh uncertainty in the recognition of somatic death has created a new problem for the pathologist. At autopsy certain organs show surprising degrees of advanced autolysis even though autopsy is performed soon after the final diagnosis. The pathologist's most dramatic evidence of this "premortem" autolysis is in the central nervous system—the "melted brain syndrome." Because of this observation we have introduced in the morgue the practice of infusing fixing solutions into the carotid arteries of dead I.C.U. patients. This procedure is routine if scrutiny of the hospital chart reveals extremely low amplitude in electrical activity of the brain or bursts of equipotentiality.

Twenty-four examples of EEG cases with prolonged irregular or absent electrical activity were studied. The pattern of most of these corresponded to the C and D profiles reported by Pampiglione and Harden.[29] Our current effort is directed at a search for a temporal relationship between severity of morphologic changes in the brain and the monitored parameters of patient care. In Table 3 the data from 10 randomly selected cases out of the 24 are reported. As prototypes, Case 5 and Case 8 in Table 3 are presented in greater detail.

CASE 4. (No. 5 in Table 3).   A 53-year-old man was admitted unconscious from carbon monoxide poisoning. Despite hyperbaric oxygen, he remained flaccid and areflexic. Throughout the seven day period in the resuscitative area, the electrolytes and the blood urea nitrogen were always within normal range. At autopsy an unsuspected recent large myocardial infarction of the left ventricle was discovered, as well as bilateral extensive laminar necrosis of the cerebral hemispheres.

CASE 5. (No. 8 in Table 3).   A 50-year-old man, a known psychotic, had been on barbiturates (long- and short-acting) and tofranil for at least three years. Two previous hospitalizations had been due to overdose of barbiturates. He was found unconscious and readmitted. Respiration was shallow and rapid (40 to 50 per min), and the patient was cyanosed (blood gas measurements showed moderate hypoxia but no hypercarbia). Assisted ventilation was started and continued until his death two weeks later. X-ray examination of the chest showed progressive infiltration of both lungs. One of the major problems in this patient was maintaining sufficient oxygen tension. Neither carbon dioxide retention nor abnormalities in electrolyte balance were recorded throughout his course. Temperature remained high (102 to 105° F), and the patient gradually deteriorated and died in shock.

At autopsy, apart from the extensive cortical liquefaction of the brain, both lungs were extremely heavy, noncompliant, and solid. There was a generalized stuffing

**Table 3.   Correlative Study Between C.N.S. Lesions and Electroencephalogram:
March 1967-1968**

	CLINICAL DATA				LESIONS*			
No.	Diagnosis	Age	Days In I.C.U.	E.E.G.	Cerebral Cortex	Globus Pallidus	Hippocampus	Cerebellar Cortex
1	Diabetic, delayed death from hanging	58	6	0/2 days	Focal laminar	–	+	0
2	Multiple bone and visceral injuries	32	3	0/1 day	0	0	++	0
3	Congestive heart failure	62	6	0/4 days	+	+	+	0
4	Myocardial infarction	70	10	0/4 days	+	++	+	0
5	CO poisoning; Myocardial infarction	53.	5	Arythmic, irregular for 4 days; 0 for 1 day	Generalized multilaminar ++++	++	++	+++
6	Nicotine sulphate poisoning	19	4	0/1 day	++	++	+	++
7	Gouty nephritis, congestive failure	68	4	0/2 days	+	0	+	+
8	Barbiturate overdose and coma; 2 episodes 3 days apart	50	7	0/4 days	++	+	+	+
9	Diabetic; hypoglycemic shock	20	4	Low amplitude 2 days; 0/1 day	+++	0	++	++
10	Chronic bronchitis-emphysema with hypoxia; renal failure	57	10	0/3 days	+	+	++	+

* 0 represents lack of phasic activity or absence of morphologic lesion.

of the air sacs with hyaline membranes interwoven with fibroblasts, histiocytes, and collagenous matrix. This lung alteration, already discussed in an earlier section, clearly contributed to generalized cellular hypoxia, with extremely vulnerable tissues (brain) showing greater degrees of structural damage.

An extensive and severe postmortem dissolution of the brain, particularly the cerebral cortex, is not infrequent in individuals who have been deeply unconscious for a week or more (Figs. 12 A, B). The persistence of cardiac action would suggest that stimuli to the sinoatrial conducting bundle continue to arise from the deep ganglionic brain centres which are spared ischemic and autolytic changes for a

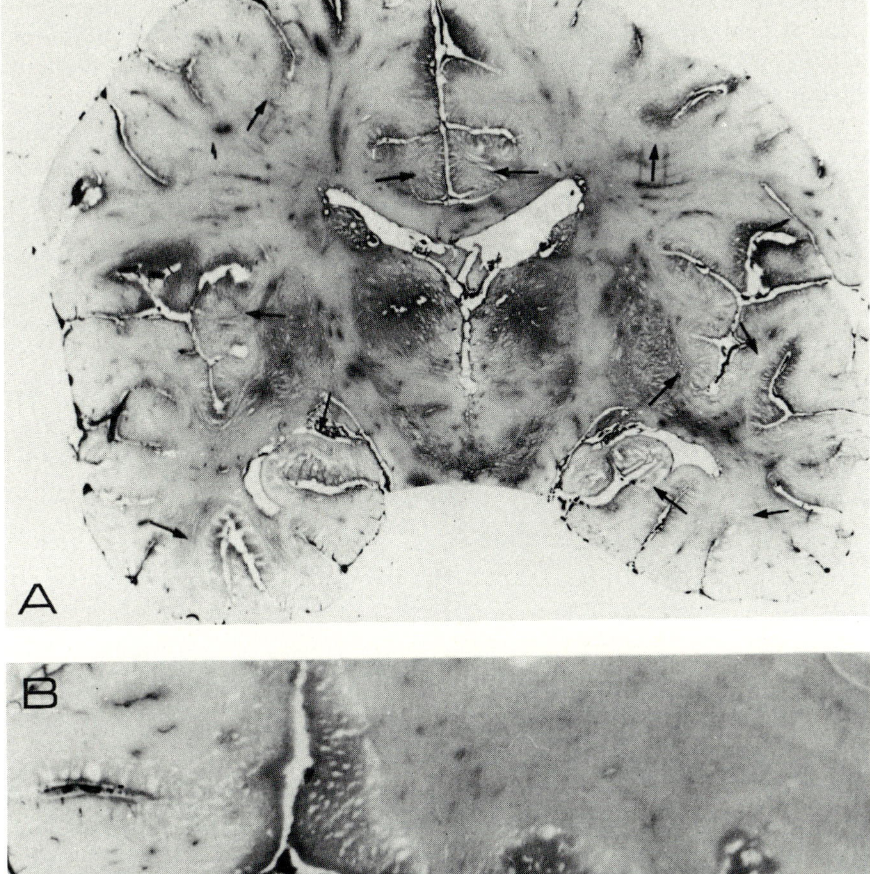

Fig. 12.   A. Whole brain paper section, 300 μ in thickness, demonstrates patchy laminar necrosis of cortex and patchy tinctorial irregularities of white matter. One-half actual size. B. Same section as shown in A. X 3.

greater period of time. These brains, particularly their cortices, often have a "toothpaste" appearance, and give off a rather distinctive odor, probably related to anerobic tissue breakdown. The greater the degree of breakdown of cerebral lipoproteins (Fig. 13), the less successful the fixation with formalin.

Edema and liquefactive necrosis of the brain may be quite pronounced, although the interval of time between the clinician's decision to withdraw all forms of mechanical assistance and the performance of the autopsy may only have been one or two hours. The greatest concentration of dissolution is usually cortical, with punctate mottling at the base of the convolutions the most prominent feature. With progression of the liquefactive necrosis, the extent of laminar necrosis is more noticeable (Fig. 12B). The selective erasure of the middle neuronal strata in the sesquilaminated cortex is observed in the hypoxic as well as hypoglycemic brain. Extreme degrees of pericellular edema and perivascular dissolution without the histologic companion of granulocytic infiltration are morphologic hallmarks of this form of brain death.

Budd,[30] as early as 1852, indicated that organ changes appear to become aggravated after death. Loss of cytoplasmic structure and nuclear karyorrhexis are now well recognized as tissue effects often associated with postmortem change.

The degree of dissolution in I.C.U. cases suggests that there has been a premortem liberation of lysosomal enzymes which brings about colliquation while the pumping action of the heart is still effective. Investigations into autolysis have indicated that factors other than the release of hydrolytic enzymes influence cell dis-

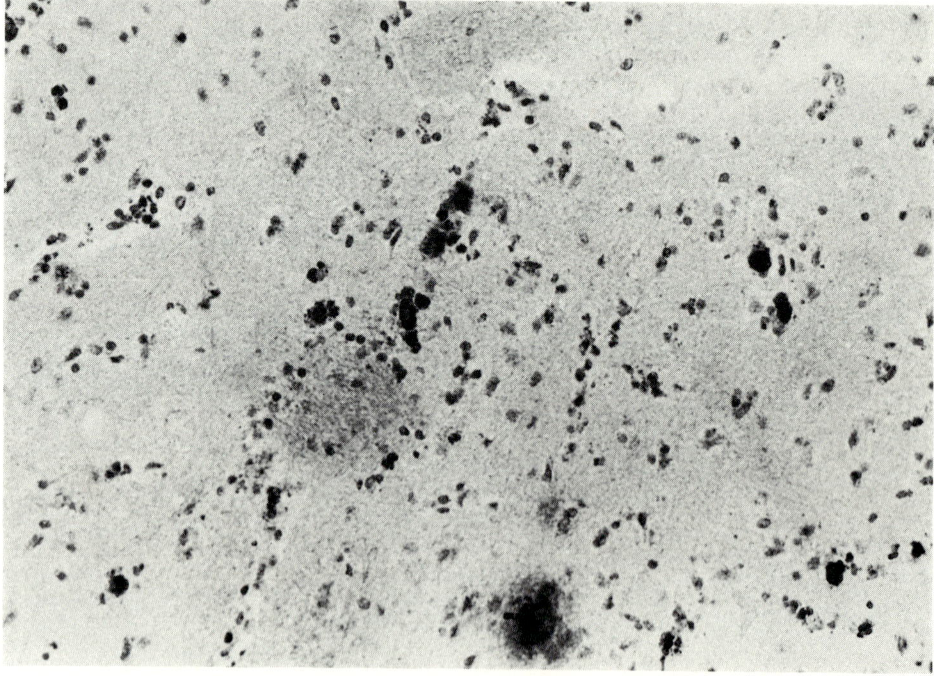

Fig. 13.   Brain showing multiple lipid droplets, mostly perivascular in location, free and intracellular. Oil red O. X160.

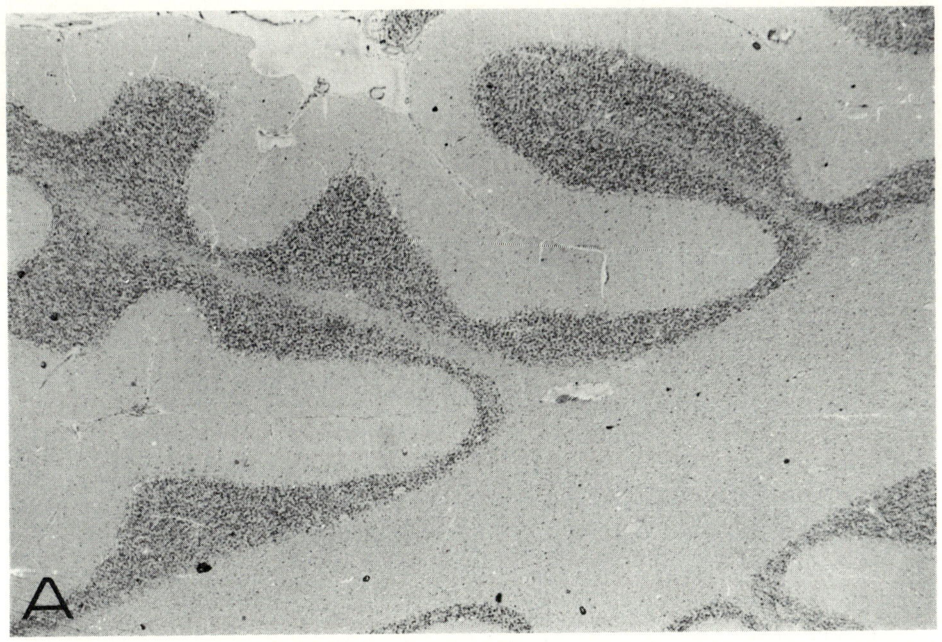

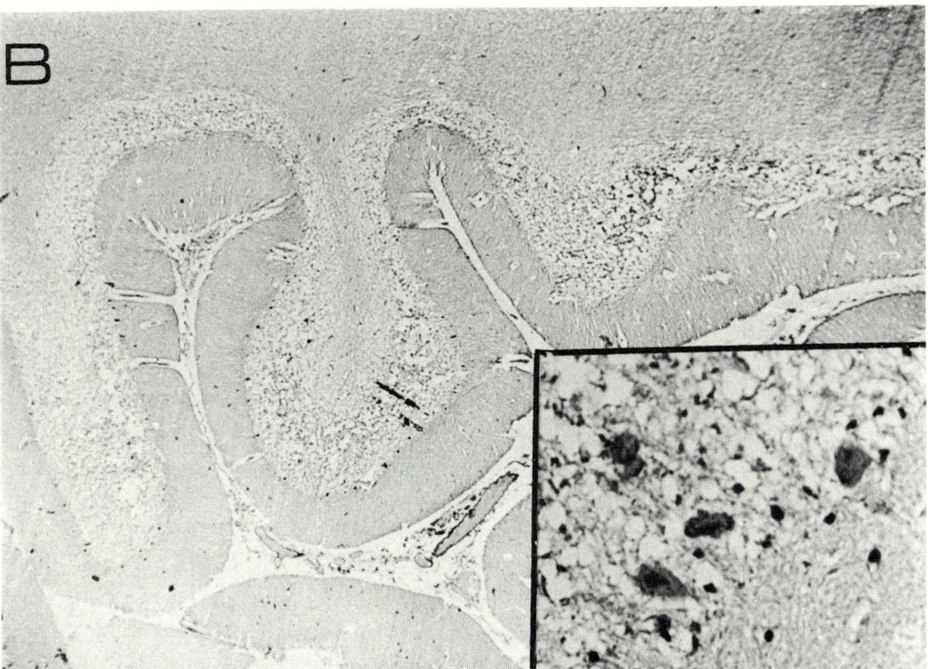

Fig. 14.   A. Normal cerebellar folia. H & E. X10. B. Massive conglutination of cerebellar folia. H & E. X10. Inset demonstrates neuronal degeneration. X125.

solution. For example, the dependence of autolysis on oxygen tension is well recognized.

In the patient on IPP and without activity in the electroencephalogram for several days, a consideration of the factors concerned in brain necrobiosis, although speculative, is of current interest. Since subnormal oxygen tensions would be present in the hypoxic brain fields, carbon dioxide, due to its rapid diffusability, might not influence the acidity of the tissues which favors autolysis. The total effect may be a form of controlled autolysis. Diffusion of oxygen and amino acids would be impaired in the hypoxic fields. The integrative action of these factors would further control autolysis by inhibiting the production of —SH groups. Inhibition of —SH groups favors the liberation of the intracellular proteolytic enzymes and accordingly enhances tissue liquefaction.[31]

Selective vulnerability of cell fields to disintegration is a distinguishing feature of tissue hypoxia. Older theories contended that this tissue susceptibility to hypoxic injury was related to the distance of the circulatory pathway, or certain cell fields with specialized intracellular metabolic cycles were more readily influenced by lack of oxygen. In rare events, the substrates of the cell involved in oxygen usage might be lacking (oxyachrestic hypoxia). A recent postulate[32] is that the neurones of the cortex, due to their large surface area (cell + axon + dendrites) are readily susceptible to minor degrees of hypoxia. This built-in susceptibility would foster, after the cell membrane has been injured, an early liberation of proteases and cathepsins, thus advancing tissue necrosis. The cerebellum seems to be peculiarly prone to conglutinative changes probably due to altered metabolism induced either by ischemia or electrolyte derangements (Figs. 14 A, B).[33, 34]

Experimental work on the blood flow to a rabbit brain has revealed that certain areas remain ischemic, even after restoration of circulation. In as short a period as five minutes obstruction, no reflow develops in these areas. A spastic narrowing of the vascular lumen, not microcirculatory thrombosis, appears to be the pathogenetic mechanism. The prompt development of glial swelling, a central nervous injury of polyvalent etiology, may impinge upon capillaries and produce the irreversible phenomenon of no reflow.[35, 36] Failure of electrolyte transfer and accumulation of extravascular water increase blood viscosity and compound the microcirculatory cerebral problem.

Certain of our cases had greater destruction of the central nervous system than others. A comatose state, provoked by selective hypnotics or cellular poisons such as nicotine, seems to be associated with a limited neuronal damage. Case 5, a combination of cardiac failure (circulatory hypoxia) and carboxyhemoglobin poisoning (anemic hypoxia), showed the greatest degree of cerebral damage (Figs. 12 A, B). An interesting feature of this case was that the EEGs, although arythmic and irregular, always revealed some evidence of electrical activity. This case illustrates the synergistic action of two forms of hypoxia. To some extent, this is an anatomic recapitulation of earlier experimental studies by Scholz and Schmidt.[35]

Selective vulnerability of brain matter was not clearly demonstrated in our 10 cases (Table 3). This morphologic disparity may well represent a blurring of the traditional patterns of hypoxia—the result of sustained care.

Summary

In dealing with problems arising from the I.C.U., the hospital pathologist quickly becomes aware that there is no retreat into the sanctuary of factual morphology. He cannot ignore the pathobiologic derangements which developed during the period of sustained life. The morphologic alterations observed by the pathologist in the morgue are the culmination of complex, interwoven but often disparate, functional, biochemical, and physical phenomena. The nature of these changes is further compounded by the multiple, active, and continuous lines of medication, along with other iatrogenic efforts by the I.C.U. staff.

To decipher the maze of available information and constantly to devise ways and means of increasing the interpretative values of pathology at the autopsy table are the tasks of the hospital pathologist. "The alveoli are filled with granulocytes." Is this enough evidence to state that pneumonia was the cause of death if the patient was afebrile, receiving appropriate antibiotics, on a balanced fluid intake, with normal blood gases and satisfactory cardiac action? Are other pathways of death being overlooked?

The pathologist must ask fundamental questions about the mechanisms of death, time of visceral and somatic death, criteria for viability of tissues, and other changing parameters of life and death. As the intensive care unit is an ever changing one, the hermeneutics of morphology must be reflective of that change.

Due to the glamorous nature of intensive care units, numerous efforts to compare mortality rates, salvable ratios, and resuscitative procedures have produced a deluge of reports.[37, 38, 39] Beginning with the admission policy of the unit to the codification of pathology findings on the fatal cases, there is a clear need for the establishment of common methods of reporting. Both from the clinical and morphologic viewpoints, conscientious quantitation of the disease process, the procedures, and the pathology should be the dominant theme of the hospital record.

To those of us convinced of the necessity of a new educational approach to the postmortem examination, it is apparent that the traditional routine autopsy is all but inadequate for the purpose at hand. To achieve this aim, we suggest a prospective collaboration between the I.C.U. physician and the autopsy teaching unit staff on a few fatal cases selected each week. In the intensive care unit clinical and morphologic translations can be analyzed to provide an understanding not only of the progress of disease but also the diseases of progress.

References

1. MacIver, I.N., Lassman, L.P., Thompson, C.W., and McLeod, I. Decerebrate rigidity reduced from 80 percent to 40 percent. Lancet, 2:544, 1958.
2. Editorial. Severe head injuries. Lancet, 1:514, 1968.
3. Lewin, W. Mortality of head injuries fall from 9 percent to 3.5 percent over eight years. Proc. Roy. Soc. Med., 60:1208, 1967.
4. Henri de Toulouse-Lautrec: The Tracheotomy. (Courtesy of Sterling and Francine Clark, Institute of Art, Williamstown, Mass.)
5. Lown, B., Fabhro, A.M., Hood, W.B., and Thorn, G.W. Coronary care unit: New perspective and directions. J.A.M.A., 199:188, 1967.

7. Hildreth, E.A. The significance of iatrogenesis. J.A.M.A., 193:386, 1965.

8. Yarington, C.T., and Frazer, J.P. Complications of tracheotomy. Arch. Surg., 91:652, 1965.

9. Friedberg, S.A., Griffith, T.E., and Hass, G.M. Histologic changes in the trachea following tracheostomy. Ann. Otol., 74:785, 1965.

10. Gibson, P. Aetiology and repair of tracheal stenosis following tracheostomy and intermittent positive pressure respiration. Thorax, 22:1, 1967.

11. West, J.B., Glazies, J.B., Hughes, J.M.B., and Maloney, J.E. Recent work on the distribution of pulmonary blood flow and topographical differences in alveolar size. *In* Form and Function in the Human Lung. London, E. & S. Livingston, 1968, Sec. 3, pp. 111-124.

12. Schiff, M.M., and Massaro, D. Effect of O_2 administration by a Ventura apparatus on arterial blood gas values in patients with respiratory failure. New Eng. J. Med., 277:950, 1967.

13. J. Lorrain Smith. The pathological effects due to increase of oxygen tension in the air breathed. J. Physiol., 24:19, 1899.

14. Pratt, P.C. The reaction of the human lung to enriched oxygen atmosphere. Ann. N.Y. Acad. Sci., 121:809, 1965.

15. Shanklin, D.R., and Wolfson, S.L. Therapeutics O_2 as a possible cause of pulmonary hemorrhage in premature infants. New Eng. J. Med., 277:883, 1967.

16. Northway, W.H., Jr., Rosahn, R.C., and Porter, D.Y. Pulmonary disease following respirator therapy of hyaline-membrane disease: Bronchopulmonary dysplasia, New Eng. J. Med., 276:357, 1967.

17. Kistler, G.S., Caldwell, P.R.B., and Weibel, E.R. Development of fine structural damage to alveolar and capillary lining cells in oxygen-poisoned rat lungs. J. Cell Biol., 32:605, 1967.

18. Buckingham, S., and Sommers, S.C. Pulmonary hyaline membranes. Amer. J. Dis. Child., 99:216, 1960.

19. Bowden, D.H., Wyatt, J.P., and Adamson, I.Y.R. The reaction of the lung cells to a high concentration of oxygen. Arch. Path., 86:671, 1968.

20. Nash, G., Blennerhassett, J.B., and Pontoppidan, H. Pulmonary lesions with oxygen therapy and artificial ventilation. New Eng. J. Med., 276:368, 1967.

21. Barter, R.A., Finlay-Jones, L.R., and Walters, M.N.I. Pulmonary hyaline membrane: Sites of formation in adult lung after assisted respiration and inhalation of oxygen. J. Path. Bact., 95:481, 1968.

22. Ashbaugh, D.G., Bigelow, D.B., Petty, T.L., and Levine, B.E. Acute respiratory distress in adults. Lancet, 2:319, 1967.

23. Clowes, G.H.A., Zuschneid, W., Turner, M., Blackburn, G., Rubin, J., Toala, P., and Green, G. The pathogenesis of pneumonitis associated with severe infections in other parts of the body. Ann. Surg., 167:630, 1968.

24. Comparative Study on Cardiac Catheterization. Braunwald, E., and Swan, H.J.C., eds. Circulation, Vol. 37, Suppl. 3, 1968.

25. Saphir, R. External cardiac massage. Medicine (Balt.), 47:73, 1968.

26. Baringer, J.R., Salsman, E.W., Jones, W.A., and Friedlich, A.L. External cardiac massage. New Eng. J. Med., 265:62, 1961.

27. Yanoff, M. Incidence of bone marrow embolism due to closed chest cardiac massage. New Eng. J. Med., 269:837, 1963.

28. William Congreve. The Mourning Bride. 1697.

29. Pampiglione, G., and Harden, A. Resuscitation after cardiocirculatory arrest. Lancet, 1:1261, 1968.

30. Budd, G. Diseases of the Liver, 2nd ed. Philadelphia and London, J. Churchill, 1852.

31. Bradley, H.C. Autolysis and atrophy. Physiol. Rev., 18:173, 1938.

32. Dixon, K.C. Cerebral vulnerability to ischemia: An hypothesis. Lancet, 2:289, 1967.
33. Olsen, S. Acute selective necrosis of the granular layer of the cerebellar cortex. J. Neuropath. Exp. Neurol., 18:609, 1959.
34. Ikuta, F., Hirano, A., and Zimmerman, H.M. An experimental study of postmortem alterations in the granular layer of the cerebellar cortex. J. Neuropath. Exp. Neurol., 22:581, 1963.
35. Scholz, W., and Schmidt, H. Durchblutungsstorungen bei Hypoxamie (Asphyxia). Arch. Psychiat. Nervenkr., 189:231, 1952.
36. Chiang, J., Kowada, M., Ames, A., Wright, R.L., and Majno, G. Cerebral ischemia: III. Vascular changes. Amer. J. Path., 52:455, 1968.
37. Lawrie, D.M., Greenwood, T.W., Goddard, M., Harvey, A.C., Donald, K.W., Julian, D.G., and Oliver, M.F. A coronary-care unit in the routine management of acute myocardial infarction. Lancet, 2:109, 1967.
38. Yu, P.N., Imboden, C.A., Fox, S.M., and Killip, T. Coronary care unit: I. A specialized intensive care unit for acute myocardial infarction. Mod. Conc. Cardiovasc. Dis., 34:23, 1965.
39. Partridge, J.F., and Gedees, J.S. A mobile intensive-care unit in the management of myocardial infarction. Lancet, 2:271, 1967.

INDEX